The Child Protection Handbook

The Child Protection Handbook

Edition 4

RACHAEL CLAWSON

Associate Professor of Social Work
University of Nottingham
UK

LISA WARWICK

Associate Professor of Social Work
University of Nottingham
UK

RACHEL FYSON

Professor of Social Work
University of Nottingham
UK

ELSEVIER

First edition 1995
Second edition 2001
Third edition 2007
The rights of Rachael Clawson, Lisa Warwick and Rachel Fyson to be identified as author(s) of this work has been asserted by them in accordance with the Copyright, Designs and Patents Act 1988.

Notices

Practitioners and researchers must always rely on their own experience and knowledge in evaluating and using any information, methods, compounds or experiments described herein. Because of rapid advances in the medical sciences, in particular, independent verification of diagnoses and drug dosages should be made. To the fullest extent of the law, no responsibility is assumed by Elsevier, authors, editors or contributors for any injury and/or damage to persons or property as a matter of products liability, negligence or otherwise, or from any use or operation of any methods, products, instructions, or ideas contained in the material herein.

ISBN: 978-0-7020-7977-1

Content Strategist: Robert Edwards
Content Project Manager: Kritika Kaushik/Suthichana Tharmapalan
Design: Miles Hitchen
Marketing Manager: Deborah Watkins

Printed in India

Last digit is the print number: 9   8   7   6   5   4   3   2   1

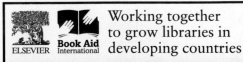

CONTENTS

EDITORS' PREFACE TO THE FOURTH EDITION

In the 15 years that have passed since the third edition of *The Child Protection Handbook* (edited by Kate Wilson and Adrian James) was published, much has changed. Setting aside for a moment the immense social, political and technological changes unleashed by the COVID-19 pandemic, the past decade and a half has seen various attempts to improve child protection services and outcomes for the children, families and young people who need those services. New models of child protection practice such as Signs of Safety and Family Group Conferences have been popularised with largely good effect. New legislation has reshaped some areas of child protection work, and the Children Act 1989 has been amended to reflect 16 as the legal age at which capacity must be assumed. Innumerable legislative changes have shaped and re-shaped youth justice processes. The law – in theory at least – offers greater recognition and support for young carers. New concepts such as coercive control have entered the lexicon and helped us to rethink our understandings of domestic abuse and intimate partner violence, including where teenagers are either victims or perpetrators. New forms of abuse – including technology-facilitated abuse, child sexual exploitation, criminal exploitation, forced marriage, female genital mutilation and faith-based abuse – are increasingly recognised and understood. We have finally begun to recognise that sexually abused and exploited children are not making 'life choices'. The pain of women and families whose children are removed, particularly those experiencing repeat removals, is beginning to be acknowledged. The need for safeguarding to be 'everybody's business', including organisations whose primary purpose lies in other areas such as education, health or sport and leisure, is now accepted. These things feel like progress.

At the same time, little has changed. The Children Act 1989 continues to be the bedrock of child protection legislation in England and Wales (with the Children (Scotland) Act 1995 and the Children (Northern Ireland) Order 1995 fulfilling the same functions in Scotland and Northern Ireland, respectively). Both children's rights and family rights are often undermined or overlooked in our criminal justice and social care systems. Children and young people continue to suffer abuse, neglect and exploitation at the hands of those who should be nurturing and supporting their journey to adulthood. Child death inquiries continue to highlight failures in interprofessional practice. Children from Black, Asian and minority ethnic families are still disproportionately likely to experience children protection interventions. Disabled children are still disproportionately likely to experience abuse or neglect. Certain groups of parents – including parents with learning disabilities, parents experiencing mental distress and young parents – continue to face increased risk of having their children removed. Children cared for by the local authority are still, on average, less likely than other children to do well at school and progress on to university or an apprenticeship. Children continue to live in poverty, with families dependent on charitable donation to foodbanks, in one of the wealthiest nations on earth. Many of these things feel like retrograde steps.

Looking beyond the immediate horizon of child protection services, the social changes of the past 15 years have impacted hugely on how these services are funded and provided. The economics of austerity which followed the 2008 financial crash have cast a long shadow. Local authority budgets have been drastically reduced, resulting in fewer 'children in need' and preventative services – thresholds for access to support have risen, resulting in a 'revolving door' system, with families repeatedly falling between the cracks of referrals, case closures and re-referrals. Funding for non-statutory work with children and families has been badly affected, with both preschool and youth services suffering, while the number of children removed from the care of their families has also risen. At the same time, the advances in technology – internet, mobile phones, tablets and laptops – have irrevocably altered the norms of communication, particularly for children and young people who are now growing up as 'digital natives'. Social media and online gaming, which have risen on the back of these technologies, has brought both significant benefits and additional risk into the lives of children and young people. Importantly, in many families it has exacerbated the usual generational divide – with children growing up as 'digital natives' while many parents (and many professionals whose role is to protect children from harms) unable to keep up with the fast changes of the online world.

Beyond the digital, but driven in part by social media, Black Lives Matters protests have reminded us of the ongoing impact of the UK's legacies of colonialism and the urgent need for culturally sensitive child protection practice. Our withdrawal from the EU and political challenges to the role of the European Court of Human Rights threaten the legal protections currently afforded by the Human Rights Act 1998, not least Article 8 the (qualified) right to a private and family life. And, overlaying and re-shaping all of these experiences, has been the global COVID-19 pandemic whose full societal impacts are still unravelling. What we do know is that children were hit hard by the pandemic. All children experienced losses of different kinds during and beyond the pandemic. Many experienced bereavement. The social development of babies and young children, and the normal trajectory towards independence for older children, was interrupted by extended lockdowns. Nurseries, schools and colleges closed or delivered education online, to the detriment of the poorest children who lacked the technology to stay connected. The impacts of housing inequality were laid bare: families in overcrowded conditions or without gardens suffered disproportionately from 'stay at home' rules; working parents who were not on furlough struggled to balance employment with home education; and there was a sharp rise in domestic violence and abuse. We will discuss the impacts of the pandemic on child protection practice further in the conclusion (Chapter 23).

And yet, despite the social upheavals of the past decade and a half, the child protection challenges identified by Professor Olive Stevenson in her concluding chapter of the third edition of this handbook remain prescient. Her verdict was that the child protection system needed to focus its energies on:

- *Dealing with the widening and changing understanding of child maltreatment and the circumstances in which it occurs*
- *Coming to terms with the cultural issues raised for child protection practice in multi-cultural Britain*
- *The widening of professional and community involvement in protecting children from maltreatment*
- *Working together – inter-agency and inter-professional activity*
- *Managing tensions between political and professional worlds*
- *Critical issues for practice, education and professional development*

Stevenson (2007, p. 532)

We believe that these matters are as relevant today as they were then. We hope that this restructured, revised and extended fourth edition of *The Child Protection Handbook* gives readers a broad understanding of the complexities involved in addressing these persistent issues. This edition revisits the challenges highlighted in previous editions but also reflects the social changes which have created new contexts in which children and young people are experiencing harm and abuse.

The handbook is organised into three parts. Part one addresses *the context for safeguarding* and the contexts in which child protection work takes place; it also seeks to establish the underpinning ethos of all that follows, namely the need for a child protection system which recognises the inherent worth of people and values them as human beings. Ray Jones' introductory chapter reflects on 50 years of child protection policy and practice and provides an overview of how we got to where we are and an analysis of the current climate of child protection practice. This is followed by Carolyne Willow contribution, focusing on the rights of the child, which reminds practitioners of the imperative to not only recognise power imbalances between adults and children but also to use this in considering how children's position in society impacts upon child protection definitions, processes and effectiveness. Willow emphasises that children are not 'people-in-the-making'; they are people now, with thoughts and feelings and a right to a child protection system which affirms their dignity and helps them recover from harm. Jagwida Leigh and Clare Webster then provide an example of how one project sought to deliver humane child protection practices, identifying both the challenges and rewards of this approach. Moving the focus to the impacts of poverty, Brid Featherstone and Anna Gupta's chapter notes the clear correlation between social deprivation and a child's chances of being subject to child protection plans and being removed into public care. They call for poverty-aware practice which recognises the material and affective impacts of poverty. More than ever, there is a need for practitioners to move away from a focus on individual blame and to instead recognise the impacts of systemic and multiple deprivations on child welfare. Subsequent chapters from Ann Potter and Sarah Dennis, Sarah Goff and Angie Bartoli set out (respectively) the legal and policy framework, consider the ongoing importance of effective interagency working and explore the crucial role supervision plays in ensuring that frontline practitioners remain supported in their role.

Part two explores *key issues in child safeguarding.* It opens with a contribution from Sarah-Jo Lee and Helen Woods who explore the cumulative risks of harm which children may experience in families where mental distress, substance misuse and domestic abuse intersect with poverty and social disadvantage to create an environment in which children may suffer multiple harms. It continues with a chapter from Diana Bentley, who outlines what we have termed 'enduring forms of abuse' – neglect, physical, emotional and future harm – issues which remain at the centre of child protection work. The following chapter we have called '*new forms of abuse*' and addresses areas of child protection practice which are emerging in response to societal change and where we are only beginning to develop an understanding of the impacts on children and families. This chapter starts with Amanda Taylor-Beswick's exploration of how the rapidly shifting socio-technical context can exacerbate risks of abuse, with a particular focus on technology-assisted child sexual abuse. Donna Peach and Grace Ellen Robinson then consider the related fields of child sexual exploitation

and child criminal exploitation. Next, Lisa Curtis and Nigel Bromage address radicalisation – including the targeting of vulnerable young people to promote extremist political views and engage in violent political acts – as an area of growing concern within the child protection arena. The final three sections of the chapter share a focus on the cultural contexts within which some forms of abuse occur, highlighting the need for culturally competent practice. Rachael Clawson sets out the risk of forced marriage for both boys and girls, including those with learning disabilities; Leethen Bartholomew provides guidance for practitioners working to protect girls from female genital mutilation (FGM); and Mor Dioum and Stephanie Yorath identify the origins of child abuse linked to faith abuse or belief and make recommendations for improved practice.

The penultimate chapter in part two considers *characteristics that may accentuate vulnerability to abuse.* Whilst there are many individual factors that may serve to either increase a child's vulnerability or protect them from abuse, there are some groups of children where there is strong evidence to show a broad-based increased risk compared to children without that characteristic. With this frame in mind, Anita Franklin provides an overview of child protection practice with disabled children; Robin Sen sets out the additional difficulties faced by looked-after children; Kelly Devenney considers the needs of child refugees and asylum-seekers; and Jo Aldridge gives a critical account of the (lack of) support and protection for young carers. The last chapter in this part of the book considers the particular needs of children *From 10s to teen: working with young people.* The inclusion of these contributions is intended as a reminder to students and practitioners that child protection is not only about babies and young children: older children and teenagers are also vulnerable to harm and in need of protection. These needs are clearly established in the anchor section by Leslie Hicks and Mike Stein who consider the specific needs of teenagers within the child protection system. This is followed by contributions from Jo Dixon, addressing the needs of care leavers; by Joe Yates and Stephanie Yates, who explore the child protection needs of young people in conflict with the law; by Stuart Allardyce and Peter Yates, who take a closer look at children and young people who display harmful sexual behaviours; and by Helen Bonnick, who discusses teenagers who are violent or abusive towards their parents or carers.

The third and final part of the Handbook moves away from the consideration of particular forms of harm or vulnerability to take a wider perspective on *Child Protection Practices*. It begins by establishing, through the contribution of Cath Williams, the need for culturally sensitive child protection practice. Siobhan McLean then goes on to explore different models of child protection practice and Martin Charles Calder unpicks the challenges for practitioners assessing children at risk of harm. This is followed by two chapters that examine the legal frameworks that impact on child protection, with Kim Holt providing an overview of child protection legislation in emergency situations and John Williams exploring the interactions between our child protection and criminal justice systems. Next, we turn to the interpersonal interactions which lie at the heart of all child protection practice, and Michelle Lefevre explains the importance of direct work with children and suggests principles which should guide such work. The extended chapter which follows focusses on working with parents and explores capacity and resilience in parenting as well as identifying the potential for discriminatory practice when working with certain groups of parents. It contains contributions from multiple authors and considers the particular needs of parents with learning disabilities (Danielle Turney & Beth Tarleton), parents experiencing mental distress (Kirsten Morley & Andrew Murphy), young parents (Caroline Lynch) and parents at risk of repeat removal of their children through care proceedings (Karen Broadhurst, Claire Mason, Lisa Morriss and Bachar Alrouh). Part three of the book concludes with a trio of chapters which look at specific contexts for safeguarding – which we would define as preventative child protection work. Mike Cullen and Mary Baginsky explore safeguarding in educational settings, Maria Clark and Louise Isham look at safeguarding in health settings, and Nick Slinn and Michelle North consider the often-overlooked need for effective safeguarding of children who participate in sport and leisure activities.

Child protection is a huge field of practice. It does – or should – extend into all homes, organisations and areas of society where children are present, or where decisions are made which will impact on children. As editors, we are aware that new areas of child protection practice emerge continually in response to wider social changes. We have attempted to address some of these areas whilst also recognising that new areas of practice will continue to emerge that we have been unable to address. With that in mind, we remind our readers that, at its core, child protection is about protecting those with less power from those who have more power. All those who seek to protect children from harm must therefore also reflect on their own power and seek ways to ensure that they use those powers responsibly, minimally, and always with the aim of empowering children, young people and parents.

RACHAEL CLAWSON, RACHEL FYSON, LISA WARWICK

LIST OF CONTRIBUTORS

RACHAEL CLAWSON
Associate Professor of Social Work, University of Nottingham

Rachael Clawson is Associate Professor of Social Work and Director of the Centre for Social Work at the University of Nottingham. She is a qualified social worker, registered with Social Work England. Rachael has a wealth of child protection experience having worked in a variety of frontline social work and management roles within local authorities. She has been teaching on social work qualifying programmes for over 20 years, firstly as a visiting practitioner and for the past 11 years as a social work academic. Rachael's research interests are mostly focused on improving safeguarding policy and practice for children and adults with learning disabilities. She has written extensively on the topic of forced marriage of people with learning disabilities and has undertaken a number of research projects on this issue. Rachael has worked closely with HM Government Forced Marriage Unit and wrote the first UK Government guidelines on forced marriage and people with learning disabilities.

PROFESSOR RACHEL FYSON
Professor of Social Work, University of Nottingham

Rachel Fyson is Professor of Social Work and Head of School of Sociology & Social Policy at the University of Nottingham, where she has taught on social work qualifying programmes for over twenty years. Prior to becoming an academic, Rachel worked with children and adults with physical, sensory and learning disabilities in both the statutory and voluntary sectors. Since enter-ing academia her research interests have centred largely on learning disabilities and safeguarding, concerning children as well as adults. Her work on children's issues has included a study of foster fathers (undertaken with Professor Kate Wilson, co-editor of the third edition of *The Child Protection Handbook*); a study of young people with learning disabilities who sexually harm others (undertaken in collaboration with the Ann Craft Trust); and work on forced marriage of people with learning disabilities (work led by Rachael Clawson, co-editor of this edition of *The Child Protection Handbook*).

DR. LISA WARWICK
Associate Professor of Social Work, University of Nottingham

Lisa Warwick is an Associate Professor of Social Work at the University of Nottingham. Lisa's research is largely focused on child and family social work, specifically relational interactions between professionals, children and families. Lisa has been involved in a range of research projects relating to child and family social work; most recently in her work Lisa has focused on supervision practices, organisational cultures and how mothers are conceptualised in child protection work. Lisa has also been involved with a musical production of the care system with LUNG theatre group. Lisa has worked in a variety of areas within child and family social work, mostly with children in residential and foster care. Outside of her academic work, Lisa is Chair of the Board of Trustees for New Beginnings Greater Manchester, a trauma informed service that works with parents whose children are on the edge of care.

PROFESSOR RAY JONES

Emeritus Professor of Social Work, Kingston University

Ray Jones is Emeritus Professor of Social Work at Kingston University and St. George's, University of London, and a registered social worker. From 1992 to 2006 he was director of social services in Wiltshire, was the first chief executive of the Social Care Institute for Excellence and has been chair of the British Association of Social Workers. From 2008 to 2016 he was professor of social work at Kingston University and St George's, University of London. He led inquiries following the deaths of children and adults, chaired Bristol's Safeguarding Children Board and was appointed to oversee children's services improvement in five areas across England. His eight books include *The Story of Baby P: Setting the Record Straight,* and he is a regular media commentator. In 2017 he received the Social Worker of the Year Award for 'Outstanding Contribution to Social Work', in 2021 was awarded an honorary doctorate in civil law by the University of East Anglia, and in 2022 was appointed to undertake the independent review of Northern Ireland's Children's Social Care Services.

CAROLYNE WILLOW

Director of Article 39

Carolyne Willow is a Social Worker and the Founder Director of Article 39, a charity that fights for the rights of children in institutional settings. She started her career in child protection in the 1980s, then moved into children's rights specialist roles amid widespread revelations of abuse in the children's care system. Between 2000 and 2012, she was head of the Children's Rights Alliance for England, during which time she led the charity's fight for transparency in restraint techniques in child prisons and successfully pressed for new legislation and statutory guidance around listening to children.

Carolyne has worked closely with children's rights bodies at the United Nations and the Council of Europe and written extensively on children's rights. Poet and musician Benjamin Zephaniah, who was incarcerated as a child, said of her publication *Children Behind Bars: Why the Abuse of Child Imprisonment Must End,* 'this book tells our truth'. Carolyne won the Social Worker of the Year (Championing Social Work Values) Gold Award in 2017 and the Sheila McKechnie Foundation Outstanding Leadership Award in 2020.

DR JADWIGA LEIGH

CEO of New Beginnings Greater Manchester and Senior Lecturer in Social Work, Lancaster University

Jadwiga Leigh is a part time Senior Lecturer in Social Work in the School of Sociology. Prior to becoming an academic, Jadwiga worked with children and families in both the statutory and voluntary sectors. Since entering academia her research interests have centred largely on organisational culture, blame and safeguarding in the child protection arena. Jadwiga now spends most of her time on New Beginnings, a charity which she founded in 2018 in collaboration with Stockport Local Authority. New Beginnings is a community project that works with primarily in the child protection process using a trauma-attachment informed approach. Its aim is to support parents who have experienced significant harm at some point in their lives.

CLARE WESTERN

Post Programme Support Worker, New Beginnings

Clare Western is the Post Programme Support Worker for New Beginnings. As a former New Beginnings graduate and peer mentor Clare uses her lived experience of the child protection system, mental health advocacy and SEND needs in children and adults to help support parents and families at New Beginnings. Clare works with parents with the aim of helping families proactively take further steps in their journeys after completing New Beginnings to meet their ongoing support needs. Clare is also currently studying towards a level 3 diploma in Counselling and uses her academic studies to help support a family's well-being.

Professor Anna Gupta

Professor of Social Work, University of London

Anna Gupta is Professor of Social Work at Royal Holloway, University of London. Anna is a qualified and registered social worker. Prior to joining academia over twenty years ago, she worked with children and families as a social worker, team manager and Children's Guardian in London. At Royal Holloway she has taught on social work qualifying, post-qualifying and PhD programmes for over twenty years. Her research interests include child protection and poverty, social work with racially minoritised children, families and communities, children in care and adoption. She has also undertaken participatory projects with parents who have experienced child protection interventions. Her publications include a co-authored a book with Professors Featherstone, White and Morris on a Social Model for protecting children and supporting families and a co-edited a book on unaccompanied asylum-seeking young people. She has recently been part of a study exploring the impact of the pandemic and racial inequalities on Black, Asian and minority ethnic young people and their families.

Professor Brid Featherstone

Professor of Social Work, University of Huddersfield

Brid Featherstone is Professor of Social Work at the University of Huddersfield. She has a long standing interest in researching families' experiences of child protection and family support services with a particular focus on gender relations and the experiences of fathers. She was a member of the Child Welfare Inequalities Project, a research project led by Professor Paul Bywaters. This project has been highly influential in highlighting the links between deprivation and child's chances of being looked after or subject to child protection interventions. She is co-investigator currently on a Nuffield funded project exploring intersecting inequalities in domestic abuse and child protection: https://www.nuffieldfoundation.org/project/rethinking-domestic-abuse-in-child-protection-responding-differently

Dr Ann Potter

Independent Academic and Registered Social Worker

Ann Potter spent just under twenty years as a practising social worker. She worked in local authorities, as an independent social worker and expert witness in the Family Court, and as a Children's Guardian within Cafcass. On moving into academia, Ann taught on pre-qualifying and post-qualifying social work programmes over thirteen years, developing a specialism in teaching, training and research relating to social work law (children and families) and court skills. Ann's doctoral research focused on legal evaluations of social work evidence in care proceedings, and the social processes involved in inter-disciplinary communication as a professional witness. She has also undertaken DfE evaluation research with carers and young people involved in the Shared Lives programme. Ann now works as an associate for NHS Research and Development North West, within a project to build research capacity and develop 'practitioner researchers' within the social work and social care workforce. In a voluntary capacity, Ann chairs the board of trustees of the charity New Beginnings Foundation.

Sarah Dennis

Lecturer in Social Work and PhD Candidate, Manchester Metropolitan University

Sarah Dennis is a part-time Lecturer in Social Work at Manchester Metropolitan University, a role which started in September 2022. Previously, Sarah had been a social worker for 16 years, working in child protection, as a Children's Guardian for Cafcass, and as an independent social worker. Alongside her lecturing role, Sarah is undertaking a part-time PhD at Manchester Metropolitan University, which is funded by the Economic and Social Research Council. Sarah's PhD research is exploring the well-being of families involved in care proceedings and how their experiences of court could be improved. This will include creative groupwork with families, a courtroom ethnography and analysis of family justice data. Sarah is interested in how families' experiences of court could become less alienating and traumatic, and the ways in which therapeutic approaches (such as those used in the Family Drug and Alcohol (FDAC) court) could be used more widely in 'mainstream' court settings.

SARAH GOFF
Young people's Development Manager, Ann Craft Trust

Sarah Goff is Young People's Development Manager at the Ann Craft Trust based at the University of Nottingham. A children's social worker, she has worked for nearly thirty years in practice in a variety of roles from residential, community and hospital based social work posts, at Child-Line, then chairing child protection conferences. The voice and experience of the child and a whole family approach have been a key focus. Sarah currently co-chairs the National Working Group on Safeguarding Disabled Children and is studying for a professional doctorate at Bedfordshire University looking at sexual abuse of learning disabled and neurodiverse children. Her research focus has included work on sexual exploitation and learning disabled children, on needs of parents in preventing sexual abuse with Professor Anita Franklin and Dr Alex Toft published by NSPCC, on the voice and right to complain of Looked After and placed away children, and a study about disabled young people's experiences of domestic abuse led by Sarah with Anita Franklin published by Ann Craft Trust.

DR ANGIE BARTOLI
Principle Lecturer in Social Work, Nottingham Trent University

Dr Angie Bartoli is a qualified and registered social worker and currently a Principal Lecturer in Social Work and Student Experience Manager at Nottingham Trent University. Prior to becoming an academic Angie worked with children and families as a practitioner and social work manager in the statutory and voluntary sectors. Angie has a keen interest in equality and diversity which is reflected in her publications. Her research focuses on the transition from the role of social work practitioner to manager and professional supervision. Angie has facilitated and contributed to the national Practice Supervisors Development Programme funded by the Department of Education and coordinated by Research in Practice. As the Vice Chair for the British Association of Social work, Angie has developed an interest in the often-overlooked role of social work in disasters and as co-edited a book on this area of practice.

DR SARAH-JO LEE
Senior Lecturer in Social Work at De Montfort University

Sarah-Jo has worked with domestic abuse issues for over thirty years. Her PhD research examined group programmes for male perpetrators of domestic abuse when these were new to the UK. Her research highlighted risks as well as potential benefits of such work and contributed to the wider landscape of activity that sought to shape its development. Sarah-Jo went on to develop and facilitate group perpetrator programmes for a voluntary organisation, before taking up the position of Domestic Abuse Policy Officer with Nottinghamshire Council. Here, she was responsible for leading the local authority's policy and practice responses to domestic abuse and for supporting inter-agency partnership work to address domestic abuse. Sarah-Jo later trained and qualified as a social worker; she worked in child protection where domestic abuse often featured in the lives of the children and families she worked with. Sarah-Jo joined DMU in 2017 where she teaches on social work qualification programmes and is an active member of the Domestic and Sexual Violence Research Network.

DR HELEN WOODS
Senior Lecturer, Nottingham Trent University

Helen Woods is a Senior Lecturer in social work where she teaches on a range of qualifying social work programmes. Helen worked as a social worker for 18 years before completing her doctorate and working in academia. Helen commenced her social work career in the probation service, moving on to work in youth offending, child protection and the voluntary sector with families affected by substance misuse. Helen retains a connection to criminal justice social work via her work with BASW. Helen's research interests concern the experience of children in residential care and the care system more widely. Helen is also keen to raise the profile of different types of social and care work, such as that which takes place in substance misuse, criminal justice and domestic abuse settings.

DIANA BENTLEY
Principle Child and Family Social Worker, Nottinghamshire County Council

Diana Bentley is the Principal Child and Family Social Worker for Nottinghamshire County Council and chair of the East Midland's regional principal social work network with more than 25 years' experience as a practising social worker and practice supervisor in children and family social work services. In their current role they have a lead role for developing a culture where excellent children and families social work practice can thrive. Particular areas of interest include compassionate care and relational practice in a child protection context and ensuring children and young people are seen, heard and have genuine opportunities for participation.

DR AMANDA TAYLOR-BESWICK
Director of Digital Transformation, University of Cumbria

Dr Amanda Taylor-Beswick is currently the Director of Digital Transformation at the University of Cumbria, but prior to this was a Social Work Academic at the University of Central Lancashire and Queens University Belfast. Amanda's research interests focus on socio-technical intersections and the preparation of social work students for life and work in a digitally complex world. Amanda's current Directorship involves delivering on whole organisation digital transformation – including leading on the development of an academic portfolio that has real-world relevance, to people, places and partnerships. Amanda is a registered social worker and continues to provide digital knowledge exchange to the social work and social care fields.

DR DONNA PEACH
Senior Lecturer in Social Work, University of Salford

Donna Peach is a Senior Lecturer in Social Work at the University of Salford. Donna has enjoyed a rewarding career in social work since 1985 with roles that included being an expert witness in the family courts. Donna remains a registered social worker and undertakes child practice reviews. Donna's doctoral research explored the experiences of prospective adoptive parents. Her research interests are situated within a critical social psychology paradigm, and she supervises doctoral candidates who use a qualitative, mixed-method or pluralistic methodology in topics with a focus on health, education and communities. Donna has acted as the Principal Investigator for several projects including the Rotherham CSE Needs Analysis study. Donna has published on topics including social work skills and child sexual abuse and exploitation. She currently sits on the expert panel advising the HMICFRS national review of the police response to group-based child sexual exploitation. Donna remains optimistic about the future of social work providing we hear the voices of children, families and those who work with them.

DR GRACE ROBINSON
Founder and CEO of Black Box Research and Consultancy

Grace is the Founder and CEO of Black Box Research and Consultancy, a nationwide criminal justice consultancy specialising in forced labour, criminal exploitation and County Lines drug supply. Having completed her PhD on Urban Street Gangs, Child Criminal Exploitation and County Lines, Grace is able to offer contemporary insights into an area with little existing literature. She has worked on over 250 modern slavery cases as an expert witness - providing her expertise to the criminal courts and assisting in asylum tribunals - comprising drugs and weapon offences, fraud, burglary and robbery. Grace previously worked within the 'Rights Lab' at the University of Nottingham's 'Rights Lab', where she led on projects (1) exploring the impact of COVID-19 on County Lines, and (2) examining the intersection between cognitive impairment and exploitation.

She was also involved in research investigating the prevalence of trafficking and online sexual exploitation of children in the Philippines. Grace continues to spread awareness of criminal exploitation by delivering training and participating in podcasts, radio interviews and documentaries.

Lisa Curtis
Deputy CEO, Ann Craft Trust

Lisa Curtis is a Learning Disability Nurse, Head of Safeguarding Adults and Young People and Deputy CEO at the Ann Craft Trust. Lisa had a long career in health and social care working in operational roles and compliance before joining the Ann Craft Trust 6 years ago. Prior to joining the Ann Craft Trust, Lisa led on projects to support people with a learning disability and autism to leave long stay hospitals and successfully connect with communities. Lisa maintains a close interest in this subject now. Lisa has supported various research projects whilst at the Ann Craft Trust, such as the forced marriage of people with learning disabilities work led by Rachael Clawson, and is currently involved in a research project regarding the exploitation of people with a cognitive disability. Always keen to develop resources that support practitioners, Lisa's interest in the area of radicalisation developed after meeting Nigel Brommage, co-author of the chapter 'Radicalisation', as well as hearing from practitioners about practical challenges they face in recognising and addressing radicalisation.

Nigel Bromage
CEO & Founder of Small Steps Consultants & Exit Hate UK

Nigel Bromage is a previous far-right activist with nearly 20 years of involvement. Using his unique inside insight, Nigel now seeks to create a positive out of a negative.

He established Small Steps Consultants in 2015, which provides training on far-right extremism nationwide, and in 2017 he set up Exit, which today operates as Exit Hate, a charity which offers free, non-judgmental support to people involved in extremism, with the aim of getting them to reject extremism and families who have a loved one involved. An advisor to Sadiq Khan on extremism Nigel has assisted in developing far-right storylines for mainstream soaps like Hollyoaks and Eastenders, with the aim of raising awareness of the dangers of extremism and showing people with support can change. For more information, please visit: www.exithate.org

Leethen Bartholomew
PhD Candidate, University of Sussex

Leethen has worked in frontline social work and is a safeguarding expert specialising in female genital mutilation and other harmful practices. He previously worked as the Head of the National Female Genital Mutilation Centre in the UK. Leethen is currently a Trustee of Oxford Against Cutting, a UK charity providing top-quality education and community support to help tackle female genital mutilation, honour-based abuse, and harmful body alterations of girls and women. He works internationally as a trainer and consultant on safeguarding children and harmful practices. Leethen is a student at the University of Sussex, where he is reading for a PhD in Social Work and Social Care. His thesis focuses on the experiences and outcomes for accused children and non-accused siblings of witchcraft and spirit possession and the effectiveness of professional responses.

Dr Mor Dioum
Co-Founder and Director, Victoria Climbié Foundation UK

Mor Dioum is the co-Founder and Director at The Victoria Climbié Foundation UK. The VCF continues to monitor and campaign for improvements in child protection policies and practices following the Victoria Climbié inquiry led by Lord Herbert Laming. Mor played a pivotal role in guiding Victoria's parents, and thereafter to establish the organisation that he now leads, advocating for family inclusion and involvement in child protection processes and child death reviews. His longstanding advocacy work has been vital to securing justice for families in racially motivated cases (including Stephen Lawrence) whilst working at The Monitoring Group. Mor has lobbied extensively for the rights of Black and minority ethnic (BME) children to be upheld alongside the dominant community. He took on leadership of the National Working Group on Child Abuse Linked to Faith (2014-2017) and a remit for national research to explore practitioner knowledge. Mor has an honorary doctorate from the University of East London and is an Executive member of the BME-Migrant Advisory Group (B-MAG); Safeguarding Children and Young People.

DR STEPHANIE YORATH
Programme Director, Victoria Climbié Foundation UK

Stephanie Yorath is VCF's programme director and was instrumental in developing a support structure for children, young people and families from primarily, though not limited to, Black and minority ethnic (BME) communities. Stephanie is co-author of a joint research paper supporting social workers to deliver quality services to children, in addition to her role as a practice educator for social work students to develop their practice skills within an advocacy-based environment. Stephanie oversees advocacy casework support for family's subject to Section 17 or 47 assessments and participates in research, case reviews and court-directed work seeking specialist advice on culture or faith. Stephanie delivered family support during the criminal investigation into the tragic death of Kristy Bamu, amid further efforts to address faith-based abuse and beliefs in witchcraft or spirit possession. Stephanie has an honorary doctorate from the University of East London (UEL) and is an Executive member of the BME-Migrant Advisory Group (B-MAG); Safeguarding Children and Young People.

PROFESSOR ANITA FRANKLIN
Professor of Childhood, University of Portsmouth

Anita Franklin is Professor of Childhood Studies at the University of Portsmouth, UK. Prior to becoming an academic, Anita worked within the voluntary sector developing policy, and undertaking research, within major children's organisations. Her background is in children's social care and policy, and her research has mainly focused on disabled children and young people's voice, rights, participation and protection. Specifically, Anita has contributed unique insight into the abuses and protection of disabled children and young people ensuring that their voices and experiences inform the development of policy and practice in this area. Her work has highlighted specific risks to exploitation and abuse of children and young people with learning disabilities, and neuro-divergent young people, and sought to explore appropriate multi-agency responses. Anita has also developed a methodology for co-leadership with disabled young people within research studies. For over a decade she has worked in partnership with groups of disabled young people to support evidence generation to facilitate policy and practice change, and activism, which is led by disabled young people.

DR ROBIN SEN
Lecturer in Social Work, University of Edinburgh

Robin Sen is a lecturer in social work at the university of Edinburgh where he teaches on qualifying social work programmes and an Honorary Research Fellow at the University of Sheffield. He practiced as a social worker in Glasgow, principally in the area of statutory child and family work. His research and writing has focused on different aspects of child and family social work including aspects of support for children and young people in state care, child protection practice and family support. Over recent years he has developed an interest in the political governance of social work and the policy-making processes related to child and family social work. He is the co-editor of *Practice: Social Work in Action* and is also co-editor of a forthcoming edited collection *The Future of Children's Care, Critical Perspectives on Children's Services Reform* which will be published by Policy in 2023.

Dr Kelly Devenney

Senior Lecturer in Social Work and Social Policy, University of York.

Kelly Devenney is a Senior Lecturer in Social Work and Social Policy in the School for Business and Society, University of York. Kelly is a qualified social worker who worked with young people and young offenders before pursuing an academic career. She has been teaching Social Work, Social Policy and Children & Young People's Studies for seven years. Kelly's research has focused largely on migrant, refugee and asylum-seeking children and young people. Her work includes studies of refugee and asylum seeking children leaving care, explorations of the family relationships of refugee children and work on the role of social work professionals with unaccompanied asylum seeking children. Kelly continues her research on migrant and refugee children whilst also pursuing interests in promoting anti-racist practice in UK Social Work and researching refugee camps in the Global South.

Professor Jo Aldridge

Emeritus Professor of Social Policy, Loughborough University

Jo Aldridge is Emeritus Professor of Social Policy in the School of Social Sciences and Humanities at Loughborough University. She started research on young carers and their families and co-founded the Young Carers Research Group in the early 1990s. Her research in this field has focused on the rights and needs of children with caring responsibilities and has influenced the development of national and international policy and practice on young carers. Jo has worked with a wide range of health and social care agencies, government departments and charitable organisations in promoting a whole family approach to working with and supporting young carers. Her most recent book, *Can I Tell You About Being A Young Carer?* (2018, Jessica Kingsley Publishers), is aimed at children, families and professionals who support young carers and their families. Jo's wider research on vulnerable and marginalised groups has led to advances in participatory research methods and research ethics.

Dr Leslie Hicks

Associate Professor in the School of Health and Social Care, University of Lincoln

Dr Leslie Hicks is an Associate Professor in the School of Health and Social Care at the University of Lincoln. She came to academic life after working in the field of residential child care. Leslie has long-standing research interests in services for children, young people and families; safeguarding and child protection; and well-being and social inclusion. She teaches at undergraduate, postgraduate and post-qualifying levels, mainly in the areas of research methods and research-informed practice, child and adolescent well-being, and international social work. She has held university responsibility for research ethics. Leslie served a three-year term as Associate Editor for Child and Family Social Work and acts as a reviewer for several journals and research councils. She has worked with many organisations to enable staff to conduct their own research about practice, and to make appropriate use of research findings to support the development of their work. Leslie's specialist area lies in research related to adolescent welfare and the experiences of and care for looked after children and young people.

Professor Mike Stein

Professor of Social Work, University of York

Mike is an Emeritus Professor in the Department of Social Policy and Social Work at the University of York. A qualified social worker, he has worked in probation and children's services. At Leeds and York Universities, he has led pioneering research studies on young people moving on from care, the neglect and maltreatment of teenagers and those who go missing from home and care.

Mike was a founder member of the International Research Network on Transitions to Adulthood from Care (INTRAC) and an adviser to the rights movement for young people in care in England. He also acted as the academic adviser to the Quality Protects research initiative and was a member of the Laming Review on 'Keeping Children in Care out of Trouble'.

Mike has also been involved in the preparation of guidance and training materials for Leaving Care legislation in the UK. He has published extensively on leaving care, neglected and maltreated teenagers (with Dr Leslie Hicks), the children's rights movement and child welfare history and policy.

Dr Jo Dixon

Senior Lecturer in Social Work, University of York

Jo Dixon is a Social Work Lecturer and Research Fellow in Social Policy and Social Work, within the School for Business and Society at the University of York. Since coming to York in 2000, Jo has carried out research focused on policy, practice and experiences of children and young people in foster and residential care and those leaving care. She has carried out research across England, Scotland and Ireland. Over the past decade, Jo has led a number of evaluations of innovative interventions to improve outcomes for care-experienced young people. Most recently this has included research on accommodation options for care leavers and exploring factors associated with the education and employment outcomes for children in care and care-experienced young adults. Jo's work also includes practice development via her teaching and involvement in research, working groups and programmes aimed at improving and supporting children's social care practitioners. Jo is a mixed-methods researcher with an interest in using participatory approaches that directly involve care-experienced young people in research as respondents, advisors and as peer researchers.

Professor Joe Yates

Professor of Criminology and Social Policy and Pro-Vice-Chancellor, Liverpool John Moores University

Professor Joe Yates is a Professor of Criminology and Social Policy and Pro-Vice-Chancellor, Faculty of Arts Professional and Social Studies at Liverpool John Moores University. He has held positions as Director of the School of Humanities and Social Science, Head of Criminology and Director of the Centre for the Study of Crime, Criminalisation and Social Exclusion (which he co-founded). He also led the development of the Liverpool Centre for Advanced Policing Studies. He has researched and published in the field of youth justice with a particular focus on policy responses to marginalised children involved in crime and antisocial behaviour. He has conducted research for the Home Office and the Youth Justice Board of England and Wales as well as for a range of community groups, non-governmental organisations and charities. Prior to working in Higher Education, Professor Yates worked in the Criminal Justice Sector, working with young people as a youth worker, social worker, youth justice officer and policy and performance manager. He is a trained a probation officer and a qualified social worker.

Steph Yates

Lecturer, King George V College, Merseyside

Steph Yates lectures post 16 Criminology at King George V College in Southport, Merseyside. She is a qualified social worker and confirmed probation officer with extensive experience of working in the statutory and voluntary sector. She has worked as a probation officer, residential social worker in probation bail hostels and worked with vulnerable people in complex multi-agency settings. She has professional experience of working with, and advocating for, young people and adults with physical, sensory and learning disabilities in a variety of settings and has managed NHS partnership residential settings for learning disabled adults. She has taught social work at HE level at degree and masters level, leading the preparation for practice placement modules, coordinating placement education and undertaking the role of practice educator in addition to participating in service user/carer forums.

STUART ALLARDYCE
Director, Lucy Faithfull Foundation

Stuart Allardyce is a social worker who has specialised in tackling child sexual abuse for more than 20 years, with a particular emphasis on work in relation to children and young people who have displayed harmful sexual behaviour. He is a director of the UK child protection charity The Lucy Faithfull Foundation with responsibilities for Stop It Now! services in Scotland as well research across the wider charity. He is vice chair of the National Organisation for the Treatment of Abuse (NOTA) and a visiting honorary researcher at Strathclyde University. He was a member of the Scottish Government's Expert Working Group on preventing sexual offending amongst adolescents. Alongside Peter Yates he is co- author of *Working with Children and Young People who Have Displayed Harmful Sexual Behaviour* (Dunedin Press, 2018) as well as 'Sibling sexual abuse: A Knowledge and Practice Overview' (Centre of Expertise in Child Sexual Abuse, 2021) along with a range of journal articles and book chapters on preventing child sexual abuse.

PETER YATES
Lecturer in Social Work, University of Edinburgh

Peter Yates is a Lecturer in Social Work at the University of Edinburgh. He is a qualified social worker with over ten years' experience of complex child protection including particular experience of working within a specialist service supporting children and young people who have displayed harmful sexual behaviour. He has a national and international profile and reputation for research and scholarship on harmful sexual behaviour and sibling sexual abuse and is co-chair (with Anna Glinski) of the Association of Child Protection Professionals' special interest group on child sexual abuse. He has published a number of papers on the subject of harmful sexual behaviour and sibling sexual abuse and is co-author of *Sibling Sexual Abuse: A Knowledge and Practice Overview* (Centre of Expertise on Child Sexual Abuse, 2021) and Working with Children and Young People Who Have Displayed Harmful Sexual Behaviour (Dunedin Academic Press, 2018).

HELEN BONNICK
Independent Social Worker

Helen Bonnick is a social worker who has built an expertise over the last fifteen years in the issue of child to parent violence and abuse (CPVA). Qualifying in 1983, she spent the next twenty years working in a local authority patch social services team, and then in schools, before becoming a practice educator for a number of universities. Studying for a Masters in Child Studies in 2004, Helen made access to support for families experiencing CPVA the subject of her research and eventually went on to work for the development of better understanding in this area, and more effective and timely support for those impacted. She runs the website Holes in the Wall, which acts as an international resource and knowledge hub; has written a practitioners' guide and a set of briefing papers; and is regularly called on to act as a consultant in research, in publications and in the media. She is passionate about the need for a joined up response to the issue, recognising the needs of the whole family.

CATH WILLIAMS
Assistant Professor of Social Work, University of Nottingham

Cath Williams is Assistant Professor in Social Work in the Centre for Social Work at the University of Nottingham where she teaches modules on social work theory and practice. Cath has taught on social work qualifying programmes for nearly twenty years. As a former social worker she has worked in the area of safeguarding disabled children as well as with vulnerable adults in different local authorities. Cath also has extensive work experience in working within black communities, and this is one of her major areas of interest. She recently worked with Siobhan Laird on a project exploring Cultural Competence in Social Work with child-in-need and child protection social workers to safeguard children and support families from Black and minority ethnic backgrounds. Cath is also completing a PhD research project exploring the impact of migration on Black family relationships.

Siobhan Maclean
Independent Social Work Educator

Siobhan is an independent social work educator; she works with a number of Universities and is a Visiting Professor at the University of Chester. Siobhan delivers training for many local authorities, largely around the topics of theory and critical reflection. Siobhan has written widely about social work theory and is committed to making the knowledge base accessible for busy practitioners. Siobhan's practice background is varied, but she has worked with children and their families in a range of social work settings. Siobhan worked for the International Federation of Social Workers for a number of years and maintains strong international links in her work. Siobhan is an editorial board member of the International Journal of Practice Teaching and Learning. Siobhan has been working to support social workers experiencing moral injury and ethical distress over the last few years, and as a result of her work in this area she has recently set up a reflective retreat for social workers in Northern Ireland.

Martin Charles Calder
Director of Calder Training and Consultancy Limited

Prior to establishing his own company Martin worked as a social worker in the field of child protection before going on to manage the child protection and domestic abuse services in Salford. He is also affiliated with Queens University in Belfast as a Senior Honorary Research Fellow. Martin's enduring interest has been about harvesting the best of the available evidence and developing accessible assessment frameworks to guide busy frontline workers. He has also challenged the problematic guidance issued by government across a range of areas that distract from good and safe practice. Martin has published extensively on the assessment materials he has developed and was the lead author in the development of the Scottish risk assessment framework as well as recently working to introduce a risk assessment framework in Abu Dhabi. He disseminates these materials across the UK by commission and licenses some for use by agencies.

Professor Kim Holt
Professor of Childhood Studies, University of Northumbria

Kim Holt is Professor of Family Law at Northumbria University. Kim practises as a Barrister exclusively in the field of family law proceedings. Within this area she has developed a high-profile practice specialising in both public law and private law proceedings. Kim practised as a social worker and children's guardian for over 20 years in the northwest of England. Kim was called to the bar in 2005 and continues a career in child protection and family law that spans over 30 years. Kim has been involved in serious case reviews as a chair, author and committee member for 32 years.

Professor John Williams
Emeritus Professor of Law, Aberystwyth University

John Williams is Emeritus Professor of Law at Aberystwyth University. His research centres on law and social care with reference to children and to older people. Safeguarding is a key feature of his work. He has published widely in academic and practitioner journals and before retirement was one of the principal investigators in a research project on access to justice for older victims of abuse. John has presented at many national and international conferences. He is a regular presenter at Harvard Medical School's Program in Psychiatry and the Law. Throughout his career he has given evidence to government and parliamentary committees on aspects of the law and social care. John is involved in several third sector organisations including CAB, MIND, and West Wales Domestic Abuse Service. He is currently chair of Age Cymru. He is a member of the All-Wales Specialist Fertility Group and the Welsh Health Specialised Services Committee. In 2012 he was appointed to the Expert Group Meeting of the United Nations Open-Ended Working Group on the Human Rights of Older Persons.

PROFESSOR MICHELLE LEFEVRE
Professor of Social Work, University of Sussex

Michelle Lefevre is Professor of Social Work at the University of Sussex, where she is Director of the Centre for Innovation and Research in Childhood and Youth (https://www.sussex.ac.uk/esw/circy/). Her research interests centre around practice improvement in children's services, and direct work with children, young people and parents in the context of safeguarding. Currently, Michelle leads the Innovate Project (www.theinnovateproject. co.uk), a four year study funded by the Economic and Social Research Council, which is exploring how local authorities and social care organisations transform practice methods and systems to address extra-familial risks and harms encountered and experienced by young people beyond the home, such as child exploitation. Prior to her academic career, Michelle practised as a social worker and psychotherapist with children and families in the context of child protection concerns. Michelle was awarded a National Teaching Fellowship in 2015 for her work on developing social workers' skills in engaging and communicating with children.

PROFESSOR DANIELLE TURNEY
Emeritus Professor of Social Work, Queen's University Belfast

Danielle Turney is Emeritus Professor of Social Work in the School of Social Sciences, Education and Social Work at Queen's University Belfast. She worked with children and families in the statutory sector before moving into academic life where she was involved in social work education at qualifying and post-qualifying levels for 20+ years. Her work is underpinned by an interest in using theory to inform, support and develop social work practice, addressing three broad areas: critical thinking and professional judgement in assessment and decision making; relationship-based practice; and child protection and family support. She has published widely in these areas. Recent research activity has included an ESRC-funded Knowledge Exchange project, with Professor Gillian Ruch, developing an innovative framework for reflective supervision, and

working with Beth Tarleton exploring 'successful practice' with parents with learning difficulties where there are child protection concerns. Danielle continues to focus on issues of family support with reference to parents with learning difficulties and to explore the place of care/relational ethics in social work.

BETH TARLETON
Senior Lecturer, University of Bristol

Beth Tarleton is a Senior Lecturer at the University of Bristol. Beth has undertaken applied research with/for people with learning difficulties/disabilities for over twenty years and always seeks to ensure that the research findings are accessible through outputs such as easy read briefings and videos. For over 17 years, Beth's research has focused on positive support for parents with learning difficulties/learning disabilities. She had mapped the issues and services available, evaluated specialist services for parents and investigated how services regarded as 'successful' in supporting parents are organised. She is currently investigating how Adult Services work with parents. Beth co-ordinates the Working Together with Parents Network (www.bristol.ac.uk/sps/wtpn/) which provides free support to professionals working with parents with learning difficulties/disabilities and has written many articles, chapters and resources on this topic. Beth is also programme director for the Masters in Policy Research and Masters in Social work research and lectures on ethics, disability and qualitative/inclusive research.

KIRSTEN MORLEY
Assistant Professor of Social Work, University of Nottingham and AMPH, Nottingham City Council

Kirsten Morley is a practising social worker and Approved Mental Health Professional (AMHP) who teaches in the role of Assistant Professor in Social Work at the University of Nottingham. Having worked in adult social care for over 26 years, Kirsten's experience encompasses a range of service user groups in various settings with a focus on mental health and learning disability. Kirsten also works as a volunteer with the organisation Social Workers Without Borders supporting asylum seekers, refugees and those impacted by borders. Kirsten has a keen interest in values-based and trauma-informed practice in social work as well as social approaches to mental distress and radical social work. Tensions between human rights, self-advocacy and the use of compulsion under the Mental Health Act 1983 are also areas of research interest as is the relationship between the state, social work and social justice.

ANDREW MURPHY
Associate Professor of Social Work, University of Nottingham

Andrew Murphy is an Associate Professor in social work at the University of Nottingham. He has taught social work for six years. He is Programme Director for the MA in Social Work and teaches modules on mental distress and social work with adults and families. His research includes work on the retention and support of managers in Children's Social Care and gender equality in universities. Andrew has worked in secondary schools, homeless charities and with adults with learning disabilities. Andrew qualified as a social worker in 2001 and worked in local authorities for 15 years, predominantly in services for adults with mental health problems. He has worked as a senior practitioner and team manager. He was also an Approved Mental Health Professional, working within the Mental Health Act 1983.

CAROLINE LYNCH
Principle Legal Advisor, Family Rights Group.

Caroline Lynch is Principal Legal Adviser at Family Rights Group where she takes a leading role in the charity's work in influencing child welfare law, policy and the family justice system. She leads strategic litigation activity and oversees the development of tailored online advice resources. Called to the bar in 2003, Caroline has specialised in children's public law for nearly 20 years. Prior to joining Family Rights Group, she practiced at the independent bar and within a local authority legal team. She has represented families, children and local authorities in a range of complex public law matters under the Children Act 1989 and Adoption and Children Act 2002. Caroline has led action research examining the experiences and needs of young parents involved with child welfare processes. She designed and led a knowledge inquiry into the use of section 20 voluntary arrangements, the precursor to the charity's intervention in the Supreme Court matter of Williams-and-LB Hackney. Caroline was part of the team facilitating the 2018 Care Crisis Review and sits on the Public Law Working Group.

PROFESSOR KAREN BROADHURST
Professor of Social Work, Lancaster University

Karen Broadhurst is Professor of Social Work in the Department of Sociology at Lancaster University, Co-Director of the University's Data Science Institute, elected Fellow of the Academy of Social Sciences and ESRC ADR UK Ambassador. Karen's interests are in child and family justice, and she is recognised nationally and internationally for high quality, high impact research that has catalysed measurable change in policy and practice. With colleagues at Lancaster University, Karen led a programme of research to quantify rates of women's repeat appearances in care proceedings. Karen and colleagues also initiated the high profile Born into Care series, funded by the Nuffield Family Justice Observatory, which is transforming preventative services for the very youngest children in family court proceedings, and their parents. Karen collaborates with colleagues in Australia, Europe, the US and in China, through joint programmes of research on family justice and children in care. Karen remains very close to social work practice through enduring partnerships of reciprocal benefit, with local authorities, charities, advocacy groups and parent collectives.

CLAIRE MASON
Research Fellow, Lancaster University

Claire Mason is a Research Fellow at The Centre for Family Justice at Lancaster University. Claire's work focuses particularly on the lived experience of families within the child protection and family justice systems. Claire has worked on a range of research projects at local, regional and national levels including a national project investigating the issue of women in recurrent care proceedings and most recently the Born into Care series examining newborns in care proceedings. Claire is currently co-leading a Nuffield Family Justice Observatory-supported project to develop new national guidelines to improve practice when a baby is separated from their parents at birth.

DR LISA MORRISS
Lecturer in Social Work, Lancaster University

Lisa Morriss is a Lecturer in Social Work at Lancaster University. Prior to entering academia, she worked as a social worker in Community Mental Health teams in London and in Greater Manchester for over ten years. Lisa completed her ESRC funded 1+3 PhD in 2014. Since entering academia, Lisa's research interests have focused on mental health, visual and creative research methods. More recently, Lisa has written about mothers who have had their children removed through the Family Court, particularly in relation to stigma, shame, and hauntology. She completed a project on the tattoos of mothers living apart from their children funded by the Sociological Review. Most recently, funded by the ESRC Impact Acceleration Account, Lisa co-created a resource on Letter Exchange for birth families and adoptive families with the Common Threads Collective. Based at WomenCentre in Kirklees, the Collective are mothers living apart from their children and Siobhan Beckwith who facilitates their work. Lisa is the European Editor of the Sage journal *Qualitative Social Work*.

DR BACHAR ALROUH
Research Fellow, University of Lancaster

Bachar is a research fellow in the Department of Sociology at Lancaster University. He is on the leadership team of the Centre for Child & Family Justice Research at Lancaster University, which works in partnership with Cafcass, Cafcass Cymru and the Nuffield Family Justice Observatory (NFJO), and is a member of the Family Justice Data Partnership team at the NFJO. Bachar is a data scientist with over 20 years of experience in academia. His background is in Information Systems and Computing, and he has an extensive knowledge of the family justice system gained through lengthy engagements with multiple family justice research projects as the lead data analyst. His work on family justice has included the evaluation of the Family Drugs and Alcohol Court (FDAC); the contribution of supervision orders and special guardianship to children's lives and family justice; the Born into Care series; and mothers in recurrent care proceedings in England and Wales.

MIKE CULLERN
Safeguarding Advisor to Education and Local Authority Designated Officer, Barking and Dagenham

Mike Cullern has worked in front line child protection services for over 19 years. He worked for a number of those years as a social worker on the front line of child protection, supporting children and families under Child in Need, Child Protection and looked after children frameworks. He formed part of the team to create and implement the local Multi-Agency Safeguarding Hub (MASH) and managed the service for several years. He is currently the Safeguarding Advisor to education settings and the Local Authority Designated Officer (LADO). He contributes to the implementation of local policy and procedures, participates in the quality assurance of social work practice, and provides training to schools and multi-agency partners on safeguarding with the aim to improve practice, multi-agency working arrangements and to drive improvements for the safety and best outcomes of children.

Dr Mary Baginsky
Senior Research Fellow, Kings College London

Dr Mary Baginsky is Senior Research Fellow in the Health and Social Care Workforce Research Unit in the Policy Institute, King's College London. She has considerable experience in social research and evaluation across academic, public, voluntary and private sectors. While working at NSPCC she developed a programme of research that provided accurate data on the responses of local authorities, teacher training institutions and schools to their responsibilities within safeguarding and child protection. Before joining King's College she was Assistant Director of the Children's Workforce Development Council and then Professional Advisor in the Department for Education. She has recently led an ESRC funded project that examined the role of schools in a multi-agency approach to child protection and safeguarding. She has published very widely on this subject and others, and was lead author on *Protecting and Safeguarding Children in Schools: A Multi-agency Approach* (Policy Press, 2022).

Dr Maria Clark
Associate Professor of Associate Professor of Graduate Entry Nursing, University of Nottingham

Maria Clark is an Associate Professor of Graduate Entry Nursing (GEN) at the School of Health Sciences, University of Nottingham. A registered nurse and specialist community public health nurse (health visitor) by background, she has held extensive teaching and research roles focused on pre and post qualifying programmes for health and social care professionals. Her combined interests involve safeguarding women and children's health, integrated care and sustainability and well-being.

Dr Louise Isham
Lecturer in Social Work, University of Birmingham

Louise Isham is a Lecturer in Social Work at the University of Birmingham. Louise teaches on the undergraduate and postgraduate social work qualifying programmes and supervises postdoctoral research students. Before moving into research and teaching-focused work, Louise worked in range of roles in the voluntary and statutory sector in the field of children and families' social work and support for victim-survivors of sexual violence. Louise's research has focused on the lived experience of violence, abuse and care relationships - issues that disproportionality impact women and girls – across the life course. Her research is also interested in people's experiences accessing social work, health and voluntary sector services. Louise's work draws on qualitative and mixed-methods approaches, and she is committed to ensuring people with lived experience play a central role driving and creating research through co-produced and participatory methods.

Nick Slinn
Independent Safeguarding Consultant

Nick Slinn is a former social worker and manager with more than forty years safeguarding practice experience. Initially Nick worked in a Local Authority, in generic duty and long-term children's teams. After working as a guardian ad litem, he moved to the NSPCC to provide therapeutic services for abused children and risk assessment services. In 2002 he joined the newly-formed NSPCC Child Protection in Sport Unit (CPSU) - established to support sports organisations across the UK. Its services included overseeing the application of sports safeguarding standards; developing sector-specific safeguarding policies, procedures and support materials; providing case advice; developing and delivering a wide range of safeguarding training; and representing and advocating for the sector with government departments and other bodies (including the DBS). Following a brief spell managing the CPSU Nick retired from the NSPCC in 2019, but has continued to work on specific projects as an independent consultant. Recently he authored a modular Lead Safeguarding Officer diploma course for FIFA, and he chairs the Welsh Rugby Union's independent safeguarding advisory group.

MICHELLE NORTH
Service Head, NSPCC's Child Protection in Sport
Unit

Michelle North is the Service Head of the
NSPCC's Child Protection in Sport Unit. Michelle
joined the CPSU in 2013 and become Service
Head in 2020. This role includes working with
sports organisations and funders across the
country to advocate for the safety of young people
in sport. Prior to this she worked for the NSPCC
Safeguarding in Education Service. Both of these
units work with professionals to improve the
safeguarding arrangements in those sectors.
Before joining the NSPCC, Michelle was an education welfare officer with over 10 years' frontline
experience for Nottingham City Council, which
involved working with families and young people
to address poor schools attendance. Later she was a
senior manager with responsibility for prosecutions
and case management across the service.
Currently she is responsible for managing the
unit's staff across England, Northern Ireland
and Wales. She also manages relationships with
the respective Sports Councils and with our key
partners in sport and physical activity.

ACKNOWLEDGEMENTS

We would like to thank Emeritus Professor Kate Wilson and Emeritus Professor Adrian James, editors of previous editions of *The Child Protection Handbook,* for entrusting the editing of this fourth edition to us. Their work provided a sound basis from which this edition has developed; we hope we have done justice to their legacy.

We would also like to thank the team at Elsevier, particularly Suthi Tharmapalan and Kritika Kaushik, for their support and encouragement (and gentle nagging) without which we would not have made it to the finishing line.

Finally, we would like to thank the authors. Writing was made all the more complicated by the outbreak of the COVID-19 pandemic. Thank you for sticking with it in the most difficult of times.

This book is dedicated to child protection practitioners. They do an important and complex job, often in the most difficult of circumstances.

PART 1 The Context for Child Safeguarding

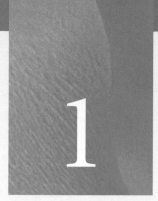

1

FROM RELATIONSHIPS AND COMMUNITY TO RISK AND COMPLIANCE: REFLECTIONS ON FIFTY YEARS OF PROTECTING CHILDREN

RAY JONES

KEY POINTS

- How the range of child protection concerns has expanded.
- The increasing proceduralisation of child protection.
- The generation and impact of blame and compliance cultures.
- From help and assistance to monitoring and surveillance.
- The impact of deprivation.
- Lessons learnt and better practice.

INTRODUCTION

It was the 1970 Local Authority Social Services Act, following the recommendations within the 1968 Seebohm Report (Seebohm Committee, 1968), which sought to tackle the complexity and fragmentation of social work services in England and Wales and to create family and community personal social services (Jones, 2020a). The 1970 Act legislated for the creation of local authority social services departments where generically educated and qualified social workers would be employed to work with individuals and families across the lifespan and would be based in teams embedded within communities. They were to help those in difficulty but also to take action to prevent crises from arising, promote well-being, and to harness and develop resources within the communities of which they were to be a part.

At the same time a unified profession of social work was created across the United Kingdom, with one social work qualification (the Certificate of Qualification in Social Work), one professional association (the British Association of Social Workers), and with the organisational base for most social workers to be within the new large local authority social services departments led by directors of social services who were almost invariably social workers and where social work was to be the lead profession.

But it was not without conflict. The move away from, for example, medical social workers and childcare officers, was not seen as positive by some who particularly valued specialist experience and workers (Butrym, 1977; Holman, 1998, 2001). And some social workers saw the big social services departments as threateningly bureaucratic and hierarchical 'Seebohm factories' (Simpkin, 1979).

THE PLOT TURNS

It was, however, the killing of 7-year-old Maria Colwell in 1973 which was to have an early impact on how social services departments and the focus of social workers was to develop. Maria was killed by her stepfather, and following campaigning by the local newspaper and Member of Parliament the government ordered a public inquiry. This was novel and exceptional at the time. For example, the 1945 inquiry into the killing of Dennis O'Neil while in foster care was not held in public and was completed in 5 days (Monkton, 1945). The Colwell Inquiry was to last much longer and took evidence in public over 41 days. At the public hearings, the social worker was described by the chair of the Inquiry as 'the defendant' and she required police protection when arriving at and leaving the public hearings because of threats and abuse (Butler and Drakeford, 2011). It was a herald of how future and frequent inquiries would focus on and target social workers.

The Inquiry report (Committee of Inquiry into the Care and Supervision Provided in Relation to Maria Colwell, 1974) was published with extensive media coverage in 1974 and included concerns about communication and information sharing between the local authority social worker, her supervisor, a National Society for the Prevention of Cruelty to Children (NSPCC) inspector, a health visitor, and housing officer. It had two quick consequences. First, social workers and managers in the still new local authority social services departments recognised that they too could potentially be the focus of the media and public if a child died as a consequence of abuse or neglect. Child protection was now to be their first and primary concern. Second, the government issued statutory guidance putting in place local child protection structures and processes. These were to include a multi-agency area review committee of senior managers to oversee policies and practices to tackle child abuse, multi-professional case conferences to determine whether a child should be the subject of what were

introduced as child protection plans, a local 'at risk' register of children with child protection plans, and guidance on information sharing (Parton, 1979). In essence, the structures, procedures and processes which were put in place in 1974 are still the foundations of child protection today.

The focus, however, was on the physical abuse of children. This in itself was an expansion of the late 1960s concerns about 'battered babies' and the 'shaken baby syndrome', which were imports from medical studies in the United States. Indeed, it was doctors who had been seen to be the lead profession in identifying and responding to the physical abuse of (young) children (Renvoise, 1974). The Colwell inquiry and the government's response broaden the attention beyond babies and young children and also led to a greater investigative role for the police in identifying and responding to child abuse (Rogowski, 2013).

THE NEW PLAYERS ON THE STAGE

The Colwell Inquiry had crossed a threshold and set a trend. Having agreed to one lengthy independent and semi-judicial public inquiry following media and public demands, any government would then find it difficult to resist demands for similar inquiries when the deaths of other children caught the media's attention and which then caused public outrage.

And so it was that the in the 1980s increasingly frequent inquiries were held leading the period to be called 'the age of inquiry' (Stanley and Manthorpe, 2004) and with lawyers chairing inquiries as the new players within child protection (see, e.g. London Borough of Brent, 1985; London Borough of Lambeth, 1987; London Borough of Greenwich, 1987).

When a child died, then as now, it was never known whether it would attract attention beyond the immediate area and limited short-term coverage in the local newspapers. It would, for example, depend on how full news agendas were at the time, whether there was a national reporter located nearby or a local reporter selling the story on to national newspapers, or a local Member of Parliament (MP) or councillor seeking wider coverage.

Inquiries became not only more frequent, but their reports became lengthier, each adding layers of recommendations to add to policy and practice guidance (Reader and Duncan, 2004). The inquiries also continued – with help from the press – the targeting and condemnation of social workers who were now very firmly the lead professionals being held accountable for not foreseeing and preventing a child's death (Munro, 2004). The increasing blame culture meant that child protection became an even greater workload priority for generic social workers in social services area teams, but one strength of the community team model was that social workers, community and hospital health professionals, police officers, school leaders and others working in the same neighbourhoods and areas did know each other which helped working together, communication and building local knowledge.

REFLECTIVE QUESTION

Is there an awareness of the threat of blame if a child dies or is seriously injured, and is it impacting on workers and decision-making?

THE SCOPE BROADENS

The scope of child protection was enlarged during the 1980s and 1990s with the recognition of sexual abuse within families and by those who had access to children, including the increasing knowledge about sexual as well as physical abuse within residential schools and children's homes (see, e.g. Levy and Kahan, 1991; Kirkwood, 1993; Waterhouse et al., 2000).

As a social worker and social services team manager in the 1970s and early 1980s responding to the physical abuse of children was a significant part of my workload, but on only one occasion was there concern about the sexual abuse of a child, and she was living in a small private children's home. By the end of the 1980s, however, sexual abuse was a significant, albeit heavily contested, concern, and when I was a deputy director of social services, we were undertaking major investigations with the police into long-standing sexual abuse in, for example, boarding schools. It was at this time that the sexual abuse of children became a national story.

THE 1987 CLEVELAND INQUIRY

The inquiry (Report of the Inquiry into Child Abuse in Cleveland, 1987), chaired by Lady Butler-Sloss, followed concerns that children were possibly being erroneously assessed as having been sexually abused within their families. The assessment was largely based on a diagnosis by two paediatricians who used a test of anal dilation to identify abuse. Within 5 months 121 children were diagnosed as having been anally abused. Social workers and their managers largely acted on the diagnosis of the paediatricians, as did magistrates in authorising the place of safety orders. The conclusions of the Inquiry were that 'the problems of child sexual abuse have been recognised to an increasing extent over the past few years by professionals in different disciplines. This presents new and particularly difficult problems for the agencies concerned with child protection'. The Inquiry panel criticised the paediatricians 'for the certainty and over-confidence with which they pursued the detection of sexual abuse in children referred to them', but there was also a conclusion and concern that 'we hope that professionals will not as a result of the Cleveland experience stand back and hesitate to act to protect the children'.

So what messages and lessons to take from the Cleveland Inquiry? First, sexual abuse was now being acknowledged and tackled. Second, assessing sexual abuse was not simple or straightforward. Third, the importance of remaining reflective and not dogmatic but also not being afraid to act. Fourth, medical diagnosis is an important finding and opinion, but it should form part of a wider assessment which should include listening to children. Fifth, multi-agency working gets stressed under pressure and needs to be given greater attention at those times. And, finally, the events and conclusions about Cleveland have been heavily contested (Campbell, 1988; Richardson and Bacon, 1991; Stevenson, 1999; Daily Mail, 2008) indicating that child protection is often inevitably immersed in uncertainty based on incomplete knowledge and information and challengeable judgements.

It has been assumed and stated that the Cleveland Inquiry led to the 1989 Children Act but as with other inquiries, such as the Dennis O'Neil inquiry in 1945 and the 1948 Children Act (Parker, 1983) and the Victoria Climbie Inquiry and the 2004 Children Act (Purcell, 2020), the inquiries became a symbol and badge for legislative change which was already in train (Jones, 2020b).

A DRAMA IN TWO ACTS

The 1989 Children Act was based on the principle that it was the welfare of the child which was to be the paramount consideration in both private and public law proceedings concerning children. It stressed that local authorities should assist and promote the upbringing of 'children in need' by their families by consulting and working in partnership with parents whilst taking into account the views of children (Tunstill and Thoburn, 2020). In essence, the Act sought to rebalance the focus to help children and families alongside what had become the predominant activity of child protection. It followed research during the 1980s on families' disempowering experience of their contact with social workers and local authority social services (Department of Health and Social Security, 1985a) and a review of childcare law (Department of Health and Social Security, 1985b).

Section 47 of the 1989 Act reinforced the duty of local authorities to undertake investigations if children were suspected of suffering or likely to suffer significant harm and new orders, such as child assessment orders, were made available to assist in protecting children and promoting their welfare but based on the 'no order' principle so that statutory and coercive powers should only be used when necessary to get cooperation and compliance from parents and carers. However, as noted by Thoburn (2019), funding restrictions and a continuing flurry of inquiries and reviews set the scene for heavily rationed help for families and a concentration on child protection.

The 1989 Children Act was implemented at the same time as the 1990 National Health Service (NHS) and Community Care Act. The latter Act had the implication that local authorities should separate the purchasing and arranging of services, what became known as commissioning and care management, from the provision of social care services for older and younger disabled adults. The 1989 Act, by contrast, emphasised partnership working rather than competition between providers within a commercial market of care. There were now different philosophies, organisational arrangements and practice requirements for children's and adults' social work and social services. The consequence was a separation within social services departments in England (there was not the same tensions and requirement within the other UK nations) into separate divisions for children's services and adults' services and with social workers based in either children's teams or adults' teams.

But separation and specialisation went much further than the creation of divisions for children's and adults' services. The determination of central government and civil servants to see the 1989 Act implemented led to ten volumes of regulations and guidance being issued totalling almost 1000 pages. The detail of the separate guidance on, for example, family support, children with disabilities, foster placements, and adoption also led to more specialisation within children's social services. There was the creation of separate teams, among others, for referral and assessment, disabled children, children in need, child protection, court proceedings, children looked after, permanency, and children and young people leaving care.

Increasingly specialisation also led to a withdrawal from communities with task-focussed separate teams located more centrally rather than being embedded within the communities where children and families lived. This also led to fragmenting the knowledge and relationships with workers within other agencies as there was less coterminosity in areas covered and less commonality in the children and families being assisted.

REFLECTIVE QUESTION

Are local organisational arrangements helping or hindering multi-professional and inter-agency working?

'WORKING TOGETHER' AND SERIOUS CASE REVIEWS

One further significant change pre-dated the 1989 Act by a year. Prompted by the concern about events in Cleveland there was a debate in Parliament with demands that the government issue a child protection 'code of practice' (Meacher, 1987). The government's response in 1988 (Department of Health and Social Security and the Welsh Office, 1988) was to publish 'Working Together'. In 1988 it had 72 pages, in 1991 it was increased to 124 pages (Home Office et al., 1991), and by 2010 it had been enlarged to 390 pages.

What drove the increasing expanding guidance was, in part, another development at the end of the 1980s. It was to be a requirement that when a child was significantly harmed or died as a consequence of abuse or neglect a serious case review (SCR) had to be commissioned by what were now called area child protection committees, which replaced area review committees. The executive summaries of the SCRs were to be published.

About 150 to 200 SCRs have been undertaken each year, and reviews were reported, on average, to have 47 recommendations (Brandon et al., 2011). The total number of recommendations over the past 30 years, therefore, is about 150 reviews × 47 recommendations × 30 years = 211,500 recommendations! These then get incorporated in policies and practice guidance which helps explain how 'Working Together' came to dramatically increase its pages. It also explains why and how organisations have become constipated and clogged up with the bureaucracy of more policies and procedures which then generate compliance and audit cultures within agencies.

SCRs, however, have not only produced more bureaucratic cultures. They have also contributed to intensifying blame cultures. Local, and sometimes national, media scan the reports to identify what are described as 'failings' by workers across and within all agencies which had contact with a family. Almost invariably there are comments that more should have been communicated and shared between workers. All is now judged with the benefit of hindsight and with little attention paid to the context of workload pressures, the organisational change and disruption in which the workers are often immersed, and that at the time assessments are being made and actions taken information will inevitably be incomplete and not everything will be known, unlike what will become known by the SCR process of drilling down in depth over months of dedicated attention to one case.

Even the best-performing workers and agencies, and despite developing technology, do not have fully functioning crystal balls to be able in advance to see that something terrible will happen to, for example, one of the 400,000 children in need known to local authorities in England at any one time. Indeed some tragedies and terrible killings of children are so unpredictable that the child may not have been seen as a child in need let alone one needing protection.

INSPECTIONS

Along with public inquiries and SCRs, a further contribution to the blame culture encapsulating and engulfing those involved in working with children and families has been the advent since the early 2000s of external inspections of children's services as part of what was termed the 'modernisation' of the personal social services (Secretary of State for Health, 1998). It has led to the publication of reports with overall ratings of services and front-loaded with recommendations about what needs to be improved. The impact was heightened when the Office for Standards in Education, Children's Services and Skills (OFSTED) in 2007 became the inspectorate of children's social services in England with inspection methodologies which were experienced as harassing and judgements which were undermining (Puffett, 2013).

It is not that reviews, inquiries and inspections are necessarily and inherently destructive and damaging. It is sensible and wise to reflect when there is a terrible tragedy and to review and revise when necessary and appropriate. As noted by Munro (1996), the difficulty occurs when there is no concern for context and no attention to uncertainty with inevitably incomplete information which is the reality of child protection practice. The history and legacy of reviews, inquiries and inspections are that they have generated actions and activities to show procedures are followed and data sets are acceptable rather than recognising, developing and promoting professional practice and, necessarily tentative and tenuous, professional judgements and assessments.

VICTORIA CLIMBIE, EVERY CHILD MATTERS AND THE 2004 CHILDREN ACT

One inquiry which has had a significant impact on social work and social services for children followed the killing in 2000 by her aunt and the aunt's boyfriend of 8-year-old Victoria Climbie. The inquiry (Laming, 2003) was chaired by Lord Laming, a former probation officer, director of social services and chief inspector of social services in the Department of Health.

It found a catalogue of concerns about leadership, management and practice across all the agencies which had, or should have had, contact with Victoria. It is erroneously assumed that it was the Laming Inquiry which directly led to the 2004 Children Act, but the move to bring education and schools and children's social services together into a local authority children's service led by a director of children's services was already underway. It was based on the New Labour government's commitment to tackle social exclusion through integrating public services, including local authority responsibilities for children. It was based on the learning from Sure Start with cross-cutting services for young families based in local areas (Eisenstadt, 2011) and with the 2003 Every Child Matters green paper (HM Treasury, 2003) setting a framework to promote the well-being of all children.

There were three particular consequences from the 2004 legislative reforms in England for child protection. First, there was a further separation of children's and adults' social workers within local authorities, and yet they each still worked with, for example, parents with mental health difficulties, learning disabilities, or who were drug and alcohol misusing and where there were also concerns about children. Secondly, local authority children's services came to be led, at least in the mid and late 2000s, by senior managers with experience in teaching and education administration rather than social work and the social services. Thirdly, the broader focus on children and their welfare and safety led to a widening of safeguarding concerns rather than more targeted attention to child protection, and this was reflected in the replacement of area child protection committees (ACPCs) by local safeguarding children boards (LSCBs). As Eileen Munro stated in a British Broadcasting Corporation (BBC) Panorama television programme following the death of Peter Connelly (see below), 'If you're looking for a needle [serious abuse] in a haystack then you are going to make things much harder by making the haystack even bigger' (BBC, 2008; Fox, 2009).

The 2004 Act changes might all have settled down, bedded in, and found a balance over time, but the new arrangements were disturbed and disrupted by the death of another little child which attracted considerable media attention.

THE STORY OF 'BABY P'

Peter Connelly, known in media reporting as 'Baby P', was 17 months old when he was killed in Haringey in London in August 2007. In November 2008 his mother, her boyfriend and the boyfriend's brother were each found guilty of 'causing or allowing' Peter's death.

Following the findings of guilt, the media launched their coverage of Peter's death, coverage which had been in preparation for months. The Sun newspaper in particular, and led by its editor Rebekah Brooks, day after day through mid and late November carried front and full pages targeting and demanding the sacking of the social worker, her managers and Sharon Shoesmith, Haringey's director of children's services. The Sun published a front-page headline of 'BLOOD ON THEIR HANDS' above the faces of the social worker and managers. David Cameron, the leader of the Conservative opposition, along with the local Liberal Democrat MP, joined The Sun's campaign targeting the social worker and her managers and Labour-controlled Haringey council.

Under the media pressure, Ofsted senior managers changed their rating of Haringey's children's services from 'good' to 'inadequate', and Ed Balls – the secretary of state for children, schools and families – was told that if he did not remove Sharon Shoesmith from her post, he would become the media's target (Balls, 2016). Not only did he do what was demanded by The Sun and others, but he also rejected the comprehensive serious case review and commissioned a second SCR which ignored concerns about the police, Haringey's legal services and the paediatric service provided in Haringey by Great Ormond Street Hospital but was damning of Haringey's children's services. The council subsequently dismissed its director of children's services, head of children's social care, child protection lead and the team manager and social worker, all of whom with their families were threatened and made unsafe. It was later concluded by the Court of Appeal that Sharon Shoesmith had been scapegoated and Patrick Butler commented "for the British political class it was a shameful episode" (Butler, 2014).

What reflections on the media and political behaviours are recounted above? First, the impact was immediate and widespread. Not only were those named and vilified left threatened and in danger from media-incited vigilantes, but it quickly became difficult to recruit social workers and paediatricians to work with vulnerable children. Second, although the social workers and their managers lost their employment and their careers working with children, Rebekah Brooks, David Cameron, the Liberal Democrat MP (Lynn Featherstone, now Baroness Featherstone) and Ed Balls all went on to thrive in different ways. Third, and most concerning, the impact on and skewing of services working with children and families continues. And, fourth, there has been no indication that the press or politicians have reflected and changed their behaviour with vengeance and vilification still targeted at, in particular, social workers when a child is killed (Jones, 2014).

As commented in the box above, the impact of the media's shaping and telling of the 'Baby P' story was immediate. Within weeks there was an escalation in the number of care proceedings being initiated by local authorities. They jumped from 482 in September 2008 and 496 in October to 716 in December, the month immediately after the launch of the media story targeting social workers and the Haringey council. What is also noticeable is that, just like the continuing referencing in the media of 'Baby P' when there are reports of another child being killed, there has also been a continuation of the increase in child protection workloads. In 2009 to 2010 there were 89,300 1989 Children Act Section 47 investigations in England, and in 2018 to 2019 this had increased by a massive 125 per cent to 201,170 investigations. On 31 March 2008 there were 29,200 children in England with child protection plans, and by 31 March 2019 this had increased significantly by 86 per cent to 52,600 children.

Not only is this having a major impact on the workload of children's services statutory and voluntary sector social workers but is also taking the time of early years workers, teachers, police officers, doctors and other health professionals, along with social workers working in adult social services. Contributing to and preparing reports for Section 47 investigations, initial and subsequent child protection case conferences, core groups, managing and implementing child protection plans, and preparing and presenting care proceedings are all time-consuming activities. And they now have to be undertaken amid politically chosen austerity targeting poor children and families and public sector services and workers. Not only are poor families being made much poorer as a consequence of continuing and deepening cuts in welfare payments, and with life expectancy reducing for people in the most economically deprived areas (Marmot et al., 2020), but the assistance that might have been available from, for example, Sure Start family centres and youth services has also been decimated (Action for Children, 2019; Bulman, 2019).

DEPRIVATION AND CHILD PROTECTION

This helps to explain the strong correlation between deprivation, child protection activity and the increasing numbers of children looked after by local authorities, which has increased in England from 60,000 in 2009 to 80,850 in 2021 (Bilson et al., 2016; Bywaters et al., 2016; Hood et al., 2016), and 79% of children are now looked after by local authorities as a consequence

of a care order made in the courts compared to 59% in 2010, and the proportion of children in care through voluntary agreements with parents has reduced from 33% to 15%. So there has been a 36% increase between 2009 and 2021 in the number of children in care, and for a greater proportion, this is through court care proceedings leading to compulsory, coercive order rather than through an agreement with parents.

Parenting well when stressed and exhausted gets more and more difficult. The concern should be that more and more children and parents are getting caught in the child protection net with the threat and fear of child protection investigations and procedures not only because of defensive practice resulting from the blame culture which has percolated into and permeated children's services but also because more families are struggling amid more intense deprivation, and for some destitution, with less help available.

This conclusion is supported by the reasons children are being made the subject of child plans. Unlike what is probably understood by the public, it is not physical abuse or sexual abuse and sexual exploitation (despite the horrific networked abuse exposed in Rochdale, Rotherham and elsewhere) which accounts for the majority of child protection activity. On 31 March 2021, it was neglect (48%) followed by emotional abuse (38%) which were the primary concerns leading to child protection plans (and different local child protection systems seem to differentially favour one of these categories compared to the other).

So in March 2021, 86% of child protection plans in England were the consequence of concerns about chronic neglect and emotional abuse and only seven per cent were the result of physical abuse and four per cent because of sexual abuse. Neglect and emotional abuse reflect on a lack of parenting competence and capacity. They are the type of concerns that may have been responded to before from the now largely lost family support and 'early help' services for children in need rather than being responded to through the surveillance and monitoring which characterises much child protection activity and fuels the increase in looked after children.

REFLECTIVE QUESTION

Are concerns about the neglect of children significant within your workload and the overall work of your agency?

Research on the controversial 'Troubled Families' programme supports the concern expressed above. A study of families involved in one programme found that the parents – primarily mothers on their own with no more than two or three children – were exhausted, depressed and physically unwell as a consequence of enduring and draining poverty and poor insecure housing. Many had also experienced previous violence from partners and were isolated from extended families and neighbours. They had little energy or routine to give to their children, it was a struggle to get through the week with more bills and court summonses arriving, and they were feeling guilty about what was happening for their children (some pre-school as well as school age). Children might be poorly fed and clothed, not getting to school, and might themselves be anxious and angry at having to care for mothers who were overwhelmed and withdrawn. May be surprising because of the assertiveness of the workers, the mothers appreciated the more intensive attention and time they were getting from the 'Troubled Families' multi-disciplinary team. They felt that someone was beside them as an ally, giving structure and practical help, providing them with personal attention and care, and negotiating on their behalf across agencies. In contrast, they experienced the short monitoring visits from the local authority children's social workers as harassing rather than helpful (Jones et al., 2015).

It seems awful, however, that it was the shaming and stigmatising 'Troubled Families' programme which was well funded by the government and provided intensive interventions rather than the Sure Start, family centres and other services which have had their funding reduced or ended. These were services which were non-stigmatising, area-based and integrated into communities, and which had developed to be both a universal resource but also with more targeted intensive and pervasive help for those families in most difficulty.

NEGLECT

With over 24,000 of the 50,000 children in England in March 2021 with child protection plans because of concerns about neglect, it might be particularly important to be reflecting upon the nature of neglect and how best to seek to tackle it.

A TYPOLOGY OF NEGLECT

PASSIVE NEGLECT

Parent(s) are overwhelmed and exhausted by poverty, are isolated and withdrawn, and have little energy to care for themselves or their children who are also immersed in poverty and deprivation and without structure or the resources available to give to their children. Respond by being beside the parent(s) providing practical help and emotional care and with positive compensatory experiences for the children and look to link the parent(s) with neighbourhood networks of friendships and activities. The family of Hamza Khan (Bradford Safeguarding Children Board, 2013) might be an example of passive neglect which led to Hamza's death.

CHAOTIC NEGLECT

Parent(s) have had poor childhood experiences themselves, have limited parenting and home-making skills, have little understanding of the needs of their children and may be quite focussed on their own needs for love and affection. They are not lacking energy, but their own and their children's lives are chaotic. Dangers in the home might not be recognised, children might be left unsupervised and

hygiene may be an issue along with, for example, irregular meals. Poverty may be a compounding factor. Respond by challenging the parent(s)' behaviours, provide parenting programmes to promote awareness of children's needs, give practical help and coaching on home-making skills and also seek to build the self-esteem of the parents whilst not losing a focus on the children. The family of Peter Connelly (Haringey Local Safeguarding Children Board, 2008) might be an example until Peter's mother's boyfriend and his brother moved into the family home.

ACTIVE NEGLECT

This is deliberate targeted neglect to impose threat and fear and to assert power. It is particularly dangerous as it may quickly escalate to serious physical abuse. It may be linked with domestic violence by a controlling partner. The child who is targeted by a jealous and controlling partner may be a reminder of, in particular, the mother's previous relationship(s). This may require a response from the police to secure the safety of children by constraining and removing the perpetrator. Daniel Pelka's (Coventry Safeguarding Children Board) family might be an example (Jones, 2016).

LOOKING FORWARD

The media coverage and professional crisis which followed the death of Peter Connelly led to the Munro Review of Child Protection (Munro, 2011) and the Social Work Task Force (2009) and the Social Work Reform Board (2012). Each brought forward proposals which would potentially strengthen social work and its practice. If implemented and sustained, there would be a reduction in targets and tick boxes and a focus on professional practice and judgements within a social worker's career development shaped by the Professional Capabilities Framework.

Some of the constructive changes which were proposed in England, such as the College of Social work and *one* chief social worker to champion social work and to be an advisor across government, have already been undermined by the government. So has the recommendation that initial social work qualifying education and training should remain generic but followed by specialist post-qualifying education and training. Indeed the government's funding and favouring foreshortened, specialised initial qualifying training outside of universities undervalues the time required to build the knowledge, competencies and confidence to practice social work and to sustain a career which might include moving across client groups and work settings. The imposition of government-shaped and controlled accreditation for children's social workers in local authorities also has every danger of destabilising further a fragile workforce which is already heavily dependent on short-term agency social workers and newly qualifying social workers. Retention is now more of an issue than recruitment but is unrecognised by government.

But the greatest threat is the potential privatisation and commercialisation of statutory children's social work and social services since changes in statutory regulation opened up to the marketplace of outsourcing companies the provision of social work services and decision-making for children in need, child protection and looked after children (Jones, 2019). It will lead to increasing competition, churn and change when what is needed is more stability, continuity and a focus on partnership working within communities.

The challenge to inter-agency partnership working is also likely to be a consequence of the abolition of local safeguarding children's boards which spanned all agencies and workers involved with children and families in a local authority area. A structure to coordinate and promote inter-agency and multi-professional working is even more needed as academy and free schools assert their independence and inward-looking isolationism and health services in England are separated and parcelled up between commercial providers.

On the ground there are, however, developments, many recounted in this book, which demonstrate learning from the past and also constructive developments for the future. For example, stronger models and methods of practice (Oliver, 2017), more openness and explicitness in work and relationships with families, the strengthening of the voice of children, and the re-building of teams within communities which include children's and families' social workers alongside mental health, drug and alcohol workers, and domestic violence workers, are all developments which may help to rebuild what has been described as humane relationship-based practice (Featherstone et al., 2014, 2018).

The UK has had a lower incidence of known child deaths from abuse and neglect compared to anywhere else in the world where there are comparative statistics (Pritchard and Williams, 2010). This will in no small part be due to the commitment, care and diligence of social workers and others working with children and families. Their work has been informed by 50 years of learning about protecting children and helping parents and families. Increasing deprivation, cuts to services and the time workers can give to children and families, and the continuing occasional flaring up of media-generated blame, all make the task harder. However, as demonstrated throughout this book, social workers and others know how to protect children and do it every day, despite the inevitable uncertainty which means that not all child deaths can be anticipated and prevented.

REFLECTIVE QUESTIONS

- Are child protection procedures being applied to too many children and families?
- How best to respond to the neglect of children?
- Will the new models of social work practice make children safer?
- Is privatisation a danger for child protection?

FURTHER READING

Featherstone, B., Gupta, A., Morris, K., White, S., 2018. Protecting Children: A Social Model. Policy Press, Bristol.

Jones, R., 2019. In: Whose Interest? The Privatisation of Child Protection and Social Work. Policy Press, Bristol.

Purcell, C., 2020. The Politics of Children's Services Reform: Re-Examining Two Decades of Policy Change (1997–2020). Policy Press, Bristol.

REFERENCES

Action for Children, 2019. The Result of Cuts and Children's Centre Closures. https://www.actionforchildren.org.uk/news-and-blogs/policy-updates/2019/june/the-result-of-cuts-and-children-s-centre-closures/.

Balls, E., 2016. Speaking Out: Lessons in Life and Politics. Hutchinson, London, pp. 284–291.

Bilson, A., Martin, K., 2016. Referrals and child protection in England: one in five children referred to children's services and one in nineteen investigated before the age of five. Br. J. Soc. Work 47 (3), 793–811. https://doi.org/10.1093/bjsw/bcw054.

Bradford Safeguarding Children Board, 2013. A Serious Case Review: Hamzah Khan: The Overview Report. Bradford Safeguarding Children Board, Bradford.

Brandon, M., Sidebotham, P., Bailey, S., Belderson, P., 2011. A Study of Recommendations Arising From Serious Case Reviews 2009–2010. Department for Education, London.

British Broadcasting Corporation (BBC), 2008. Panorama: What Happened to Baby P? BBC One. 17 November.

Bulman, M., 2019. Youth Services 'Decimated By 69 Percent' in Less Than a Decade Amid Surge in Knife Crime, Figures Show. https://www.independent.co.uk/news/uk/home-news/knife-crime-youth-services-cuts-councils-austerity-ymca-a9118671.html.

Butler, I., Drakeford, M., 2011. Social Work on Trial: The Colwell Inquiry and the State of Welfare. Policy Press, Bristol.

Butler, P., 2014. Foreword. In: Jones, R. (Ed.), The Story of Baby P: Setting the Record Straight. Policy Press, Bristol.

Butrym, Z., 1977. Book Review of 'Reforming the Welfare' (op cit). Community Care.

Bywaters, P., Bunting, L., Davidson, G., Hanratty, J., Mason, W., McCartan, C., et al., 2016. The Relationship Between Poverty, Child Abuse and Neglect: An Evidence Review. Joseph Rowntree Foundation. https://www.jrf.org.uk/report/relationship-between-poverty-child-abuse-and-neglect-evidence-review.

Campbell, B., 1988. Unofficial Secrets: Child Sexual Abuse and the Cleveland Case. Virago Press, London.

Committee of Inquiry into the Care and Supervision Provided in Relation to Maria Colwell, 1974. Report of the Committee of Inquiry Into the Care and Supervision Provided by Local Authorities and Other Agencies in Relation to Maria Colwell and the Co-Ordination Between Them. Her Majesty's Stationery Office, London.

Coventry Safeguarding Children Board, 2013. Serious Case Review re Daniel Pelka: Overview Report. Coventry Safeguarding Children Board, Coventry.

Daily Mail, 2008. The Women Who Went Through an Ordeal Beyond Belief. https://www.dailymail.co.uk/femail/article-438208/The-women-went-ordeal-belief.html.

Department of Health and Social Security, 1985a. Social Work Decisions in Child Care: Recent Research Findings and their Implications. HMSO, London.

Department of Health and Social Security, 1985b. Review of Child Care Law: Report to Ministers of an Interdepartmental Working Party. HMSO, London.

Department of Health and Social Security and the Welsh Office, 1988. Working Together: A Guide to Arrangements for Inter-Agency Co-Operation for the Protection of Children From Abuse. HMSO, London.

Eisenstadt, N., 2011. Providing a Sure Start: How Government Discovered Early Childhood. Policy Press, Bristol.

Featherstone, B., White, S., Morris, K., 2014. Re-Imagining Child Protection. Policy Press, Bristol.

Featherstone, B., Gupta, A., Morris, K., White, S., 2018. Protecting Children: A Social Model. Policy Press, Bristol.

Fox, C., 2009. A Needle in a Haystack. LocalGov. https://www.localgov.co.uk/A-needle-in-a-haystack/23796.

Haringey Local Safeguarding Children Board, 2008. Serious Case Review of 'Child A'. Department for Education, London.

HM Treasury, 2003. Every Child Matters, Cm 5860. Stationary Office, London.

Holman, B., 1998. Child Care Revisited: The Children's Departments 1948–1971. Institute of Childcare and Social Education UK, London.

Holman, B., 2001. Champions for Children: The Lives of Modern Child Care Pioneers. Policy Press, Bristol.

Home Office, Department of Health, Department of Education and Science, and Welsh office, 1991. Working Together Under the Children Act 1989. HMSO, London.

Hood, R., Goldacre, A., Grant, R., Jones, R., 2016. Exploring demand and provision in English child protection services. Br. J. Soc. Work 46 (4), 923–941. https://doi.org/10.1093/bjsw/bcw044.

Jones, R., 2014. The Story of Baby P: Setting the Record Straight. Policy Press, Bristol.

Jones, R., 2016. The Conundrum of Neglect. Professional Social Work, pp. 22–23.

Jones, R., 2019. In: Whose Interest? The Privatisation of Child Protection and Social Work. Policy Press, Bristol.

Jones, R., 2020a. A History of the Personal Social Services in England. Palgrave Macmillan, London.

Jones, R., 2020b. The impact of scandal and inquiries on social work and the personal social services. In: Bamford, T., Bilton, K. (Eds.), Social Work – Past, Present and Future. Policy Press, Bristol, pp. 191–213.

Jones, R., Matczak, A., Davis, K., Byford, I., 2015. 'Troubled Families': a team around the family. In: Davis, K. (Ed.), Social Work With Troubled Families: A Critical Introduction. Jessica Kingsley, London, pp. 124–158.

Kirkwood, A., 1993. The Leicestershire Inquiry 1992. Leicestershire County Council.

Laming, L., 2003. The Victoria Climbie Inquiry, Cm 5730. The Stationary Office, Norwich.

Levy, A., Kahan, B., 1991. The Pindown Experience and the Protection of Children: The Report of the Staffordshire Child Care Inquiry 1990. Staffordshire County Council.

London Borough of Brent, 1985. A Child in Trust: The Report of the Panel of Inquiry into the Circumstances Surrounding the Death of Jasmine Beckford. London Borough of Brent.

London Borough of Greenwich, 1987. A Child in Mind: Protection of Children in a Responsible Society: The Report of the Commission of Inquiry into the Circumstances Surrounding the Death of Kimberly Carlile. London Borough of Greenwich.

London Borough of Lambeth, 1987. Whose Child? The Report of the Public Inquiry Into the Death of Tyra Henry. London Borough of Lambeth.

Marmot, M., Allen, J., Goldblatt, P., Boyce, T., McNeish, D., Grady, M., et al., 2020. Fair Society, Healthy Lives: The Marmot Review. www.ucl.ac.uk/marmotreview.

Meacher, M., 1987. Child abuse Cleveland, house of commons debate. Hansard. 119, 528–538. https://api.parliament.uk/historic-hansard/commons/1987/jul/09/child-abuse-cleveland.

Monckton, S.W., 1945. Report on the Circumstances Which Led to the Boarding-Out of Dennis and Terence O'Neill at Bank Farm, Minsterly, and the Steps Taken to Supervise Their Welfare, Cmnd 6636. HMSO, London.

Munro, E., 1996. Avoidable and unavoidable mistakes in child protection work. Br. J. Soc. Work 26 (6), 793–808.

Munro, E., 2004. The impact of child abuse inquiries since 1990. In: Stanley, N., Manthorpe, J. (Eds.), op cit, pp. 75–91.

Munro, E., 2011. The Munro Review of Child Protection: Final Report: A child-centred system. The Stationary Office, London.

Oliver, C., 2017. Strengths-Based Child Protection: Firm, Fair and Friendly. University of Toronto Press, Toronto and London.

Paley, J., Thorpe, D., 1974. Children: Handle with Care. National Youth Bureau, Leicester.

Parker, R., 1983. The gestation of reform: the Children Act 1948. In: Bean, P., MacPherson, S. (Eds.), Approaches to Welfare. Routledge and Kegan Paul, London, pp. 196–217.

Parton, N., 1979. The natural history of child abuse: a study in social problem definition. Br. J. Soc. Work 9 (4), 431–451.

Pritchard, C., Williams, R., 2010. Comparing possible 'Child-Abuse-Related-Deaths' in England and Wales with the major developed countries 1974–2006: signs of progress? Br. J. Soc. Work 40 (6), 1700–1718.

Puffett, N., 2013. NCAS Conference: Tough OFSTED Inspections Having Detrimental Effect of Child Services Standards. https://www.cypnow.co.uk/news/article/ncas-conference-tough-ofsted-inspections-having-detrimental-effect-on-child-services-standards.

Purcell, C., 2020. The Politics of Children's Services Reform: Re-Examining Two Decades of Policy Change (1997–2020). Policy Press, Bristol.

Reader, P., Duncan, S., 2004. From Colwell to Climbie: inquiring into fatal child abuse. In: Stanley, N., Manthorpe, J. (Eds.), op cit, pp. 92–115.

Renvoise, J., 1974. Children in Danger. Harmondsworth, Penguin.

Report of the Inquiry into Child Abuse in Cleveland, 1987. Cm 412. HMSO, London.

Richardson, S., Bacon, H. (Eds.), 1991. Child Sexual Abuse: Whose Problem? Reflections From Cleveland. Venture Press, Birmingham (revised edition 2018, Policy Press, Bristol).

Rogowski, S., 2013. Critical Social Work With Children and Families: Theory, Context and Practice. Policy Press, Bristol.

Seebohm Committee, 1968. Report of the Committee on Local Authority and Allied Personal Social Services. Cmnd 3703HMSO, London.

Secretary of State for Health, 1998. Modernising Social Services: Promoting independence, Improving Protection, Raising Standards, Cm 4169. The Stationary Office, London.

Simpkin, M., 1979. Trapped Within Welfare Surviving Social Work. Macmillan Press, London.

Social Work Reform Board, 2012. Building a Safe and Confident Future: Maintaining Momentum. Department for Education, London.

Social Work Task Force, 2009. Building a Safe, Confident Future. Department for Education, London.

Stanley, N., Manthorpe, J., 2004. The Age of the Inquiry: Leaning and Blaming in Health and Social Care. Routledge, London.

Stevenson, O., 1999. Children in need and abused. In: Stevenson, O. (Ed.), Child Welfare in the UK. Blackwell Science, Oxford, pp. 107–108.

Thoburn, J., 2019. Policy and Funding shifts 'subverted' Act, 29 October, Children and Young People Now. https://www.cypnow.co.uk/features/article/the-children-act-1989-30-ds-on.

Tunstill, J., Thoburn, J., 2020. The 1989 England and Wales Children Act: the high-water mark of progressive reform. In: Bamford, T., Bilton, K. (Eds.), Social Work Past, Present and Future. Policy Press, Bristol, pp. 157–172.

Waterhouse, R., Clough, M., le Fleming, M., 2000. Lost in Care: Report of the Tribunal of Inquiry Into the Abuse of Children in Acre in the Former County Council Areas of Gwynedd and Clwyd Since 1974. HMSO, London.

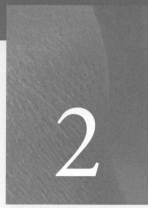

2 THE RIGHTS OF THE CHILD

CAROLYNE WILLOW

KEY POINTS

- What a children's rights approach to child protection means.
- The development and importance of the United Nations Convention on the Rights of the Child.
- That children are human beings today, not people-in-the-making. All children, including babies, have thoughts and feelings and are able to communicate.
- Recognising power imbalances between adults and children.
- Considering how children's position in society impacts upon child protection definitions, processes and effectiveness.
- Whether children in contact with the child protection system are experiencing this as affirming their dignity and rights, and helping them to recover from harm.

INTRODUCTION

Children's rights to protection and recovery from harm confirm their moral status as human beings with inherent dignity, and the growing legitimacy of state interference in the privacy of the home and family relationships from the 19th century to date (Freeman, 1989; Hendrick, 2003; Cunningham, 2005; Flegel, 2009). This is not to suggest that deeply entrenched beliefs about parental ownership and authority over children have completely transformed from previous centuries. In England, parents retain a special legal defence which can be invoked if we are charged with assaulting our children (see below). But we are a very long way off from 1889, when Parliament passed the first law to protect children from cruelty nearly seven decades after similar legislation for animals. As one of the leading parliamentary champions for the legislation explained at the time:

> *Children have very few rights in England, and by this Bill I am really only anxious that we should give them almost the same protection that we give under the Cruelty to Animals Act and the Contagious Diseases Act for domestic animals.*
> *Mundella (cited in House of Commons Hansard, 1889)*

A children's rights approach to child protection operates on many levels – from positive support to parents and families, to public education, to fighting socio-economic inequality, to sensitive, age-appropriate communication and respectful help for children who have endured violence and other forms of harm. It is concerned with children feeling and being safe wherever they are – within their families, at school, in their communities and within institutional settings. But it also challenges power imbalances between children and adults (Cloke and Davies, 1995; Willow, 2010; Davies and Duckett, 2016), at both the interpersonal and societal, structural levels. Families can be the smallest democracies on earth; they can also be tyrannies where children are terrorised and degraded. The same applies to group-based living and institutional settings – children's homes, mental health units, prisons and immigration detention, for example. Children rights' advocates strive to make children – their

15

interests, concerns and feelings – truly visible, within families, communities and wider society (Schofield and Thoburn, 1996; Willow, 2009; Ferguson, 2017).

WHAT ARE CHILDREN'S RIGHTS?

Children's rights are the obligations and duties which states and public authorities have towards children, who are defined in both domestic and international law as human beings up to the age of 18 years (Children Act 1989, United Nations Convention on the Rights of the Child).

Like all other rights, the rights of children entitle them to particular treatment, freedoms and help. This includes the entitlement to be treated with dignity, respect and equal worth; to enjoy personal and social protections (such as the right to physical and psychological integrity, the right to a fair hearing and effective participation, and the right to social security and an adequate standard of living); and to have remedies when there have been rights violations.

Rights allow individual children and groups of children, or those acting on their behalf – independent advocates for example – to make claims on public authorities when they have not fulfilled their legal obligations. So, for example, in England and Wales section 47 of the Children Act 1989 requires local authorities to investigate when a child in their area is suffering, or is likely to be suffering, significant harm in order to decide whether to take action to safeguard or promote that child's welfare. Section 47(5A) of the Children Act 1989 requires that the child's wishes and feelings about the actions to be taken by the local authority are ascertained and given due consideration. These rights of the child to be protected, and for their wishes and feelings to be taken into account as an integral part of this protection, are supported by international law. Article 19 of the United Nations Convention on the Rights of the Child (UNCRC) grants children the right to protection from all forms of violence and mistreatment, and Article 12 gives every child the right to express their views and to have these given due weight in all matters affecting them, in accordance with their age and maturity. Article 39 grants children who have been abused the right to recover in environments where their health, self-respect and dignity are nurtured – this 'right to recovery' in the UNCRC reflects the local authority duty in section 47 to take action to safeguard or promote the child's welfare.

Alongside adults, children in the United Kingdom are also protected by the Human Rights Act 1998. Section 6 of the Human Rights Act 1998 requires public authorities – which includes schools, hospitals, the police, prisons and local authorities – to act compatibly with the rights in the European Convention on Human Rights (ECHR). Article 8 of the ECHR protects the right to private and family life and entitles children (and adults) to psychological and physical integrity; Article 3 provides protection from inhuman or degrading treatment or punishment; and Article 2 is the right to life. The age and vulnerability of children are highly relevant when courts determine whether they have suffered violations of their rights and assess the severity of any breaches.

CASE STUDY 2.1: THE RIGHT TO PROTECTION FROM INHUMAN AND DEGRADING TREATMENT

In 2012, the High Court found that two teenage brothers had suffered 'irreparable harm' while in a series of foster placements supposedly awaiting adoption. The boys had entered care as infants and orders were made for their adoption. The local authority had not returned to court after abandoning this course of action for the boys. All contact with their birth family had ended, and the boys were sexually and physically abused while in foster care. Human Rights Act proceedings were brought by the eldest boy (aged 16 at the time of the judgment) and the Official Solicitor[a] acting on behalf of the youngest (aged 14). A declaration was made against the local authority and the boys' independent reviewing officer for a catalogue of rights breaches, including failure to protect the boys' 'physical and sexual safety and their psychological health' (A and S (Children) v Lancashire County Council). The boys were subsequently awarded £9.6 million in damages which included amounts for loss of future earnings and care and Court of Protection fees (Farleys, undated).

---

[a]The Official Solicitor is empowered to act as a 'litigation friend' for children and for adults who lack capacity.

Dignity is at the centre of a children's rights approach to child protection. Recognising each child's human dignity is to understand that they have their own, distinct place and value in the world. A child rights approach is clear that children are people with their own thoughts, feelings and perspectives (Munro, 2011, p. 16) whose rights and interests must always be separately and carefully considered from parents and other caregivers.

Paternalism and rescue exemplify the welfare approach to child protection – where adults believe they know best and *do unto* children. Conversely, children's rights accentuate the child's integrity, their self-respect and empowerment. The manner in which 121 children were treated by professionals and removed from their families in the northeast of England in 1987 illustrates the damage that can be done when procedures take priority over the people they are intended to help. The Cleveland child abuse inquiry led by Lady Elizabeth Butler-Sloss (a High Court judge when appointed to the role) is wrongly associated with false findings of child sexual abuse. Research by the writer Beatrix Campbell reveals confidential government papers from the period recorded that "an independent medical assessment [concluded] that the diagnoses of sexual abuse were correct in at least 80% of the 121 cases" (Campbell, 2023, p. 17). For children's rights advocates, two sentences from the inquiry report endure as a guard against losing the child in child protection:

> *There is a danger that in looking to the welfare of the children believed to be the victims of sexual abuse the children themselves may be overlooked. The child is a person and not an object of concern.*
> **Butler-Sloss (1988, p. 12)**

The UNCRC provides a shared value base and a philosophy of respect towards children, as well as a comprehensive set of economic, social and cultural and civil and political rights. Arguably every single provision in the treaty is concerned with child protection – whether this is the right to protection from all forms of violence (Article 19), the right to social security and an adequate standard of living (Articles 26 and 27), the right to be heard and taken seriously (Article 12), the right to be diverted from criminal proceedings and sanctions (Article 40), the right of child refugees to humanitarian assistance (Article 22) and the right to protection from hazardous work and economic exploitation (Article 32). Anyone working with children, including in roles specifically defined as child protection, will require an understanding of what children need to enjoy happy, safe and fulfilled childhoods. The UNCRC is the international standard for this, and when the UK ratified the treaty in 1991, it undertook to implement its provisions for all children, without any form of discrimination.

The treaty confirms children as rights holders and as equal members of the human family. No longer can children be disregarded as 'not-yet' people (Willow, 2021), as empty vessels, unformed and unready. The Convention demands that they be respected as full persons in the here-and-now; they are human *beings* not human *becomings* (Qvortrup, 1985). The adult tendency of treating childhood as simply a stepping stone to adulthood, with no intrinsic value or worth of its own, was strikingly encapsulated by a child who took part in a consultation some years ago:

> *One group felt angered that children are often not listened to in their own right [because] children are treated as less important than adults. One child summed this up powerfully – 'they think we're there to become adults – you're only a child because you can't be born as an adult'.*
> **Morgan (2003, p. 16)**

COMMITTEE ON THE RIGHTS OF THE CHILD

Nominated by UN member states, the Committee on the Rights of the Child's (CRC) 18 independent experts are drawn from a wide range of professions concerned with children's rights and well-being. They meet in Geneva in Switzerland four times a year to review the compliance of individual countries with the Convention, and they produce detailed guidance ('general comments') on different aspects of the treaty to help governments and others interpret and implement the treaty's requirements.

When the CRC examined the UK in 2016, it made nearly 40 recommendations concerning children's right to protection. These included improving information-sharing and developing comprehensive support for sexually exploited and abused children. Prohibition of corporal punishment within the home was once again recommended, and the Committee pressed for government action to 'promote positive and non-violent forms of discipline and respect for children's equal right to human dignity and physical integrity' (CRC, 2016, para. 41(c)). It also urged legal protection from cruelty for 16- and 17-year-olds. Currently the law states that only children aged 15 and under can be a victim of a child cruelty offence. Other recommendations such as the abolition of pain-inducing restraint in child prisons, the prohibition of the use of Tasers by police and an increase in the minimum age of recruitment to the armed forces from 16 to 18 (CRC, 2016) are not typically viewed as child protection matters, even though they concern children's fundamental safety. In 2023, the CRC's recommendations for the UK included an end to the 'hostile environment' in immigration policy and practice; the legal prohibition of strip-searching; and ensuring that children who have suffered abuse or neglect can access community-based trauma care.

From April 2014, the Committee has been able to consider complaints from children (or others acting on their behalf) about breaches of their rights under the CRC, once all remedies have been exhausted in the children's own country. The UK Government has not accepted this procedure, so it is unavailable here.

GENERAL PRINCIPLES

Four articles – 2, 3, 6 and 12 – were selected as general principles by the first CRC. Together, they establish an overarching framework for the full enjoyment of the Convention's rights. Two of the general principles, the right to be heard and taken seriously (Article 12) and the requirement to treat the child's best interests as a primary consideration (Article 3), are mirrored in domestic legislation (see box below).

The right to life had been part of the Universal Declaration of Human Rights (1948) and the International Covenant on Civil and Political Rights (1966), but in Article 6 UNCRC the standard was heightened for children to *maximum survival and development*. The other general principle, non-discrimination in the enjoyment of rights (Article 2), is a stock feature of all international human rights instruments.

CHILD'S BEST INTERESTS AND THE RIGHT TO BE HEARD – PROTECTED IN DOMESTIC AND INTERNATIONAL LAW

ARTICLE 3, UNCRC – IN ALL ACTIONS CONCERNING A CHILD OR GROUP OF CHILDREN, THE CHILD'S BEST INTERESTS MUST BE A PRIMARY CONSIDERATION

Some illustrative examples from UK law:

- Section 1(1) Children Act 1989 and section 1(2) Adoption and Children Act 2002 both require the family court to treat the child's welfare as their paramount consideration
- Section 11 Children Act 2004 requires local authorities and a wide range of other agencies to discharge their functions having regard to the need to safeguard and promote the welfare of children
- Section 1(1)(a) Children and Social Work Act 2017 lists acting in the best interests of looked after children among the 'corporate parenting' principles which local authorities must have regard to when carrying out their functions

ARTICLE 12, UNCRC – CHILD'S RIGHT TO EXPRESS THEIR VIEWS FREELY AND TO HAVE THESE VIEWS GIVEN DUE WEIGHT

- Section 1(3)(a) Children Act 1989 and section 1(4)(a) Adoption and Children Act 2002 lists the child's ascertainable wishes and feelings among the factors that the family court must have regard to
- Section 17(4A) Children Act 1989 requires local authorities to ascertain and give due consideration to the child's wishes and feeling before deciding what (if any) services to provide to a child in need. This duty is to be carried out so far as is reasonably practicable and consistent with the child's welfare, and the due consideration element must have regard to the child's age and understanding
- Section 20(6) Children Act 1989, as above relating to the provision of accommodation
- Section 22(4) Children Act 1989, as above relating to looked after children
- Section 47(5A) Children Act 1989, as above relating to child protection enquiries
- Section 46(3)(d) Children Act 1989, in respect of emergency police protection, requires the police to take such steps as are reasonably practicable to discover the wishes and feelings of the child;
- Section 1(4) Adoption and Children Act 2002 requires family courts and adoption agencies to have regard to the ascertainable child's wishes and feelings (considered in the light of the child's age and understanding)
- Section 1(1)(b)-(c) Children and Social Work Act 2017 lists encouraging children to express their views, wishes and feelings, and then taking these into account, among the 'corporate parenting' principles which local authorities must have regard to when carrying out their functions

BEST INTERESTS OF THE CHILD

Children's best interests being *a* primary consideration in the UNCRC, rather than *the* primary consideration, creates legitimate space for other matters, including the interests of adults. However, when it comes to decision-making about individual children, the CRC effectively encourages paramountcy of children's best interests:

> *Viewing the best interests of the child as 'primary' requires a consciousness about the place that children's interests must occupy in all actions and a willingness to give priority to those interests in all circumstances, but especially when an action has an undeniable impact on the children concerned.*
> *CRC (2013, p. 6)*

Children's best interests can be a slippery, nebulous concept in practice, and practitioners should be able to show their 'working out'. The CRC states 'the ultimate purpose of the child's best interests should be to ensure the full and effective enjoyment of the [Convention's] rights' (CRC, 2013, p. 7). This means that all of the rights which are germane in a given situation, including a child's right to know and be cared for by their parents, must be considered together. Children's views, their wishes and feelings, are integral to determining their best interests: the notion that children can either have their welfare secured *or* their perspective and feelings attended to is a false binary (Marshall, 1997; Willow, 2021). A child who feels unheard and invisible is not a protected child.

PROTECTION FROM ALL FORMS OF VIOLENCE

Article 19 of the UNCRC grants all children the right to protection from all forms of violence, abuse, neglect and exploitation no matter where they are living. The CRC emphasises the responsibility of states to prevent violence:

> *Securing and promoting children's fundamental rights to respect for their human dignity and physical and psychological integrity, through the prevention*

CLOSER LOOK: ACTING IN ACCORDANCE WITH THE CHILD'S BEST INTERESTS

In 2011, the UK's Supreme Court held that the best interests of children overrode the state's decision to deport their mother who had 'an appalling immigration history'. The two children, aged 9 and 12 years at the time of the judgment, were born in the UK and are British citizens. Deportation of their mother would have resulted in the children having to leave their home, being deprived of their education and losing their friends and their community. They would 'lose the advantages of growing up and being educated in their own country, their own language and own culture'. The court held the children should not be blamed or held responsible for the actions of their parents (*ZH Tanzania*).

Why is it vital that those making decisions about parents – in the context of immigration, social security or criminal justice for example – always separately and carefully consider the potential impact of decisions on the child's best interests?

How does the principle of not holding children responsible for the conduct of their parents apply in your work with children and families?

Does respect for children's best interests help you to have a more humane approach in your work with families?

> *of all forms of violence, is essential for promoting the full set of child rights in the Convention.*
> *CRC (2011, para. 13)*

When Poland first proposed an international human rights treaty for children, there wasn't a single country where children were fully protected in law from parental violence. Sweden was the first to outlaw corporal punishment in the family home, in 1979. A Swedish Government publication charting the development of the law, and its impact, explains:

> *At the beginning of the 20th century it was still implicitly assumed that the child should obey its parents and authorities without murmur. Children were ascribed no independent standing and as a rule were not allowed to voice their opinions. Corporal punishment followed in the wake of this insistence on unconditional obedience. Gradually society has changed. Independent thinking and*

the sense of responsibility, both for oneself and for others, have come to be seen as increasingly important prerequisites of the democratic social order. The concept of the child as an independent individual with rights of its own has become more prominent. This calls for a form of child education based on interaction, care and mutual respect.

Hindberg (2001, pp. 11–12)

Today, children enjoy the same protection from assault as adults in around a third of the world's countries – though not in England (or Northern Ireland). Although corporal punishment has been prohibited in schools, childminding and nurseries, foster care and children's homes across the UK, it continues to be permitted within the family in England. Children are the only people in our society who can be legally hit. This makes our system of child protection fundamentally flawed. The UK Parliament last voted on whether to provide children with the same protection from assault as adults in 2004. Baroness Uddin, a former social worker, supported an outright ban on smacking, explaining:

As a mother of five children, I accept the ambivalence that we have all faced from time to time. But I also speak as one who has worked as a professional social worker and a child protection officer for many years ... Anyone who has witnessed the pain of children would not argue for anything less than the fact that violence is totally unacceptable.

Whereas adults frequently refer to 'light taps' and 'smacks', when young children were first ever consulted, they overwhelmingly described smacking as hitting. One of the questions put to them through the medium of a storybook was why adults smack children, but children don't smack adults. A 7-year-old boy exclaimed:

That's simple! Because it's very rude to smack your parents because they're bigger and older and they might hurt you back and they might be silly when they're drunk and they might hit you.

Willow and Hyder (1998, p. 60)

A 7-year-old girl said:

Adults are bigger and stronger and people treat them more seriously.

Willow and Hyder (1998, p. 60)

FUNDAMENTAL CHILD PROTECTION – THE RIGHT NOT TO BE ASSAULTED

A v UK is one of the most significant cases taken to the European Court of Human Rights concerning child protection. At the age of 6 years, child 'A' was hit with a cane by his stepfather. Child A's name was then placed on the child protection register (together with his brother's name), which was a central list held by each local authority (abolished in April 2008). The children were removed from the register the following year. However, less than 3 years later child A was examined by a consultant paediatrician who found he had injuries consistent with being beaten by a garden cane used 'with considerable force on more than one occasion'. The stepfather was charged with assault and relied on the 'reasonable chastisement' defence when he appeared in court. By a majority verdict, the jury found him not guilty.

The 'reasonable chastisement' defence originates from an 1860 case when the headteacher of a private boarding school in Eastbourne beat to death a teenager with learning difficulties. The judge told the jury:

By the law of England, a parent or a schoolmaster ... may for the purpose of correcting what is evil in the child, inflict moderate and reasonable corporal punishment, always, however, with the condition, that it is moderate and reasonable ... If his excessive violence caused the death find him guilty.

R v Hopley (1860)

The jury found the headteacher guilty and the 'reasonable chastisement' defence established by the case continued unchanged for parents until A v UK came before the European Court of Human Rights in 1998. The court found there had been a breach of Article 3 of the European Convention on Human Rights, which provides protection from inhuman and degrading treatment or punishment, and that UK law did not protect the boy because of the 'reasonable chastisement' defence. The boy was awarded damages by the court, and the UK Government was then obliged to amend the law to protect children.

Shamefully, the law in England was only amended to remove the availability of the 'reasonable punishment' defence (the new language used in the Children Act 2004) when a parent is charged with wounding and causing grievous bodily harm, assault occasioning actual bodily harm and child cruelty. The defence remains available for parental assault, meaning that children continue to be the only class of people in England who can be lawfully hit.

THE RIGHT TO BE HEARD AND TAKEN SERIOUSLY

Article 12 is probably the best known of all of the UNCRC's provisions. It grants every child who is able to form their own views the right to express these freely, and to have them given due weight in accordance with their age and maturity. Further, it entitles the child to be heard in all administrative and judicial proceedings, either directly or through a representative – an advocate or lawyer for example. Articles 6 and 8 of the ECHR require children's (and parents') active participation too; as noted above, this treaty has been made part of our domestic law, via the Human Rights Act 1998, which means breaches can be challenged through UK courts.

Despite clear obligations on practitioners working in child protection to seek out, understand and take seriously the child's feelings and perspective, research for the Children's Commissioner for England found that only 'a small minority' of children knew of the different ways their views could be presented at child protection meetings (Cossar et al., 2011, p.12). A triennial review of serious case reviews undertaken between 2011 and 2014 found that keeping children's needs and views central to investigations was a recurring theme of recommendations – meaning children's lives as experienced by them were too often eclipsed. The report highlights four learning points: the need to stay attuned to the 'silent' ways children communicate information about their lives, particularly noticing emotional and behavioural changes; the need for creativity in listening to and engaging with children; ensuring children always have the time and space to give their own perspectives; and remembering that children aged 16 and 17 are still vulnerable (Sidebotham et al., 2016, pp. 131–134).

A review of a child protection advocacy service in a London borough found that children's wishes and feelings became more central to decision-making through having an advocate. Both parents and professionals were able to appreciate aspects of children's lives and concerns hitherto invisible to them. With help from her advocate, one child was able to see her family at Christmas. Her social worker reflected:

You forget that kids at school are probably talking about it, and for me it's more clinical about how I'm going to sort out the taxi rather than the excitement and anticipation the child's having. I remember at the conference the advocate raised that and the team manager and the chair put that as a big decision we had to immediately sort out. I remember it focused all of us, to make sure we put a plan in place straight away.

Jelicic et al. (2013, p. 35)

When children and young people with experience of children's social care are asked what matters to them, they consistently hail the importance of being listened to and treated with respect, care and kindness (Butler and Williamson, 1994; Growney, 1998; Willow, 2003; Voice for the Child in Care and National Children's Bureau, 2004; Cossar et al., 2011, 2013). Interviews with 53 children and young people, aged 6 to 19 years, who had been sexually abused within their families elicited ten qualities they most valued in professionals: active listening; believing in what children say and feel; being caring and compassionate; facilitating choice and control (not rushing or pressurising children); enabling safety – in physical surroundings and in subjective feelings; exuding optimism and a sense of hope; acting as an advocate, through offering practical support and advice; being non-judgmental and countering shame, self-blame and stigma; and being trustworthy, honest and reliable (Warrington et al., 2017, pp. 112–114).

A study of 27 children's experiences of child protection investigations found that nearly every child (aged between 8 and 16 years) was able to name a social worker who had helped them. A 14-year-old girl reflected:

She listened and took me seriously and supported me. This stopped me being bad. [She] was a nice woman – she listened and cared.

Bell (2011, p. 144)

The emergence of 'contextual safeguarding' in recent years has championed the importance of reaching out and understanding the lived experiences of adolescents (Firmin, 2018); a children's rights approach demands this for all children.

It is often said that children don't tell of abuse. A more accurate statement would be that children are discerning in whom they confide in. One of the

CHILDREN'S RIGHT TO BE HEARD IN CHILD PROTECTION

WHEN FIRST HEARING FROM CHILDREN

Have you chosen a space which is private and comfortable for the child?

How do you introduce yourself and your role?

How do you let children know they have the right to be safe, and that their thoughts and feelings are incredibly important to deciding what help they and their families may need?

Have you enough time and space to proceed at the child's pace? What might you ask to discover what life is like for the child? Will you mostly elicit information through dialogue and conversation, will you use play and other forms of creative communication, will you ask them to draw or write about their lives?

How will you find out what (if anything) makes the child worried or afraid?

Has the child been led to believe they are to blame for their situation (by parents, carers or other professionals for example)? How will you counteract this?

How will you elicit what the child has done to date to try and protect themselves, their siblings and/or any other children? What do they believe would most help them and/or their family?

How will you check you have correctly understood the child's thoughts and feelings? How will you record what they have communicated to you?

How will you explain what happens next?

CHILD PROTECTION MEETINGS

Who has explained the purpose of this meeting to the child, and the roles of those attending? Has the child been asked whom they want to attend? Have they been offered help from an independent advocate?

Is the meeting space comfortable and inviting for the child (and their parents and others)?

Have basic courtesies been planned for – refreshments, everyone arrives on time, avoidance of 'small talk' between professionals, which can be excluding for those without these prior relationships?

Who explains, in accessible language, the rights of the child? What are the statutory duties and powers – including family support, education, mental health services, access to legal assistance – relevant to the child's recovery and prevention of future harm?

Have documents been prepared with the aim of encouraging genuine dialogue – respectful language, avoidance of jargon, as short as possible, appropriate use of graphics and easy-read formats when necessary?

Has the child (and their parents) been supported to contribute their own thoughts, feelings and ideas ahead of the meeting – setting out (in writing, short video or audio file for example) what they believe would help, what they want to stop and what they want to change (including in the conduct and help provided, or not provided, by the local authority and others)?

How are the child's views, wishes and feelings recorded in the notes of the meeting, and who is responsible for arranging time and space after the meeting for the child to reflect on the discussion and decisions made, to ask questions and raise any concerns?

CHILD PROTECTION PLANS AND ACTION

To what extent does this child protection plan reflect the child's concerns, priorities and proposals? What choice and control does the child have in how they are protected by others?

Is your involvement helping to make the child feel safer and stronger?

How do you know the action that is being taken is helping the child?

Who is responsible for ensuring promises made to this child (and their parents, family or other caregivers) will be fulfilled?

earliest analyses of children's calls to Childline found that friends were most likely to be told of sexual abuse (MacLeod, 1999). A decade later, a study of 60 young adults who had experienced abuse in childhood found their first abuse disclosures were most commonly made to friends and mothers; none were to social workers (Allnock and Miller, 2013, p. 23). An innovative, child-centred approach to child protection was launched in north London in 2018. Called the Lighthouse, it is based on Iceland's 'Child House' (Barnahus), a model pioneered two decades ago and then adopted in Sweden, Norway, Greenland and Denmark (Donovan, 2019). The Lighthouse is a multi-agency, safe space in which children and young people receive the support they need following sexual abuse, all under one roof. Achieving Best Evidence interviews take place there, and every child is offered an advocate. Even though there was no public awareness-raising during its first year, more than 20 children self-referred; this was across all four age categories (0 to 4, 5 to 12, 13 to 15 and 16 to 17 years) (The Lighthouse, 2020, p. 20).

Neither the UNCRC nor the Children Act 1989 prescribes a minimum age for children's right to be heard, and there is a large literature which refutes the assumed incapacity of young children (Alderson, 1993, 2000; Miller, 2003; Willow and Hyder, 1998; Clark and Moss, 2011; Winter, 2011). The very survival of babies and young children relies upon them being able to communicate their needs and feelings to parents and other caregivers. Astute, curious practitioners will be able to observe and elicit a very young child's important relationships, their preferences and their fears, through spending quality time with them and entering their world through play and skilful enquiry. Young children are extremely adept at showing rather than telling – an interested (and interesting) adult can elicit a multitude of information. The CRC gives this advice:

> To achieve the right of participation requires adults to adopt a child-centred attitude, listening to young children and respecting their dignity and their individual points of view. It also requires adults to show patience and creativity by adapting their expectations to a young child's interests, levels of understanding and preferred ways of communicating.
>
> *CRC (2006, para. 14)*

A man sought to appeal his conviction and sentence for the anal rape of a young child, by discrediting the testimony of his victim simply on the basis of her age. He claimed it was not acceptable to convict on the evidence of a 4-year-old child recounting events she said happened when she was just 2 years old. The Court of Appeal rejected this outright:

> *Many accreted suspicions and misunderstandings about children, and their capacity to understand the nature and purpose of an oath and to give truthful and accurate evidence at a trial, have been swept away ... the old misconceptions no longer apply... Unless we simply resuscitate the tired and outdated misconceptions about the evidence of children, there is no justifiable basis for interfering with the verdict.*
>
> *R v Barker (2010)*

There is similarly an abundance of evidence which supports the realisation of disabled children's right to be heard and taken seriously. The challenge is not that disabled children are unable to form or express views; it is the readiness of professionals to familiarise themselves with and respect each child's means of communication and access technologies and specialist assistance when required (Franklin, 2015, pp. 58–67).

RIGHT TO FAMILY LIFE

The right to respect for family life applies to everyone, adult and child, and is protected by both the Universal Declaration of Human Rights (UDHR) and the European Convention on Human Rights/the Human Rights Act 1998. The UNCRC goes much further. Building on the UDHR, its preamble describes the family 'as the fundamental group of society and the natural environment for the growth and well-being of all its members and particularly children'. Article 7 grants children the right, as far as possible, to know and be cared for by their parents. Fmily relationships are seen as integral to a child's identity in Article 8, and Article 9 provides that separation from parents must only occur when this is in the best interests of the child. Article 18 establishes that parents have the 'primary responsibility' for children's upbringing and development, and that the child's best interests are 'their basic concern'. It further requires states to provide 'appropriate assistance to parents and legal guardians in the performance of their child-rearing responsibilities'. Children have the right to a standard of living 'adequate for (their) physical, mental, spiritual, moral and social development' in Article 27; the UNCRC locates the 'primary responsibility' for realising this right with parents (or other caregivers). However, it also requires the state to 'provide material assistance and support programmes, particularly with regard to nutrition, clothing and housing' to families in need.

As a further marker of the importance of the family, Article 20 entitles children who are deprived of their family environment to 'special protection and assistance'. This recognises the impact on children of being separated from their families (parents, siblings and other family members), and the risks inherent in alternative settings, especially institutions.

THE RIGHT TO RECOVERY

Article 39 of the UNCRC grants children who have been abused the right to recover in environments where their health, self-respect and dignity are nurtured. This widens the lens of child protection from the act of physical rescue alone (transferring the child from an unsafe to a safe setting):

> For too long child protection has been concerned with rescuing and repairing the physical bodies of children and not enough attention has been paid to their inner feelings, thoughts and views: human rights protect the integrity and potential of the whole person.
>
> *Willow (2010, p. 6)*

Public policy increasingly acknowledges the wrench of women leaving violent partners; the enormous challenge this is psychologically and materially. In criminal law, there is a defence for serious crimes which recognises the drip, drip effect of domestic abuse. There is not the same level of public, professional or political understanding when it comes to the enduring effects of violence against children, particularly when teenage children are the victims. This was highlighted in a review of 161 serious case reviews between 2003

and 2005. Over a third of the children who had died or suffered serious harm were aged 11 and over. The review identified teenagers being perceived as 'hard to help' which resulted in agencies often neglecting their needs. It urged all organisations working with young people to proactively address 'the effects of early maltreatment and trauma' (Brandon et al., 2008, p. 110). Similarly, an age-based analysis of serious case reviews found that children aged 14 and over were too often treated as adults, rather than children in need of protection. Their behaviour was perceived as rebellious and challenging rather than demonstrative of suffering and turmoil (Ofsted, 2011). A serious case review undertaken after a 15-year-old hanged himself in prison powerfully shows the lack of connection with teenagers' pain:

> The severity of Child F's abuse in early childhood and the fact that it occurred in parallel with neglect and emotional abuse is likely to have had a lasting negative impact on all aspects of his emotional and behavioural development.
>
> *Ibbetson (2013, p. 11)*

The teenager had entered care at the age of 6 after medical examinations found he had been repeatedly raped over a substantial period of time. The serious case review continues:

> Increasingly Child F's behaviour began to reflect the very severe impact on him of the abuse that he had suffered, leading to more and more difficulties in controlling his emotions and his behaviour... gradually over the years detailed knowledge of the gravity of what had happened to Child F was lost.
>
> *Ibbetson (2013, p. 12)*

Research for the Youth Justice Board learned that the vast majority of children in custody – up to 92% – had experienced some form of maltreatment before incarceration (Day et al., 2008, p. 6). A review of the 'abuse of imprisonment' carried out by the author challenges societal attitudes, which inevitably soaks into practice:

> It is as if we would rather get them out of our sight altogether than deal with difficult and demanding

children – especially teenagers. It is Oliver Twist we are rooting for, not the Artful Dodger. All too late, thoughtful examinations of young offenders' lives, as occasionally happen after a child dies with a ligature around their neck, or when they have committed a particularly odious offence, bring forth biographies heaving with tragedy and hardship.

Willow (2015, p. 255)

A UK charity compiled testimonies of 23 people who had been sexually abused as children. Showing how sexual violence can invade the very core of a child's being, the authors summed up:

Many survivors wrote that their lives were not fully lived and that they felt as if a part of the self was missing, lost or broken.

One in Four (2015, p. 41)

A CHILD PROTECTION SYSTEM FIT FOR CHILDREN

Only a minority of children who endure serious, intimate rights violations are supported by the child protection system in England. As an illustration of this, the police recorded 54,168 child sexual abuse offences in the year ending March 2021 (Home Office, 2022), yet the number of children who were the subject of a child protection plan for sexual abuse on 31 March 2021 was 1,930 (Department for Education, 2021). Girls under the age of 16 were the victim of nearly a quarter (23%) of all female rapes last year, and boys under the age of 16 accounted for half (51%) of all male rape victims (Home Office, 2022). The Independent Inquiry into Child Sexual Abuse, the UK's largest ever public inquiry, has shone a bright light on devastating levels of sexual, physical and emotional violence against children in all parts of society – the family, residential schools, children's homes, child prisons, religious organisations and political networks and institutions. Asymmetrical power relationships between children and adults is the golden thread running through these investigations.

CONCLUSION

A children's rights approach starts with respecting every child as a person who has their own feelings, thoughts and views. Before any child protection practitioner enters their life, the vast majority of children will have taken steps to protect themselves – through, for example, trying to avoid certain individuals and situations, to confiding in friends, to changing their behaviour, to calling a helpline. Allnock and Miller's (2013, p. 10) interviews with 60 young adults who had been abused as children found that many 'couldn't use direct words so they tried to give clues with actions and indirect words'. Many children will have tried to protect younger siblings. Whatever has gone before, child protection practitioners must endeavour to see the child's life from their perspective. A pioneering study of 190 children's perspectives of harm and seeking help concluded that it is 'vitally necessary to establish what children themselves see as the primary causes of pain, distress and fear' (Butler and Williamson, 1994, p. 116). Investigations, inquiries and reviews repeatedly show meaning to children and young people's behaviour much too late. In Medomsley detention centre, young people would lie at the bottom of a staircase and allow others to jump down on them, so they could be taken to hospital to avoid further sexual assaults by prison officers. It is only through entering the child's world that adults can begin to understand how life feels and looks, and what they themselves believe would help.

Astrid Lindgren, the Swedish author and creator of Pippi Longstocking, was a staunch children's rights advocate. Upon accepting an international peace prize in 1978, she shared a story told to her by an older woman:

She was a young mother in the days when people still believed in the idea of 'Spare the rod and spoil the child' – or rather, she didn't really believe in it, but one day when her little boy did something naughty, she decided he had to have a good hiding, the first one of his life. She told him to go out and find a suitably supple stick or rod for her to use. The little boy was away for a long time. He eventually came back in tears and announced: 'I can't find a rod, but here's a stone you can throw at me'.

REFLECTIVE QUESTIONS

- How does understanding the Convention on the Rights of the Child, and adopting a children's rights approach, change how you relate to, and work with, children and young people?
- What does your team or organisation do to stay connected with the views and experiences of children and young people?
- How would our society have to change for children and young people to enjoy the same respect as adults?
- What are the consequences for children and young people of practitioners working in child protection not adopting a children's rights approach?

FURTHER READING

Convention on the Rights of the Child 1989

Allnock, D., Miller, P., 2013. No One Noticed, No One Heard: A Study of Disclosures of Childhood Abuse. NSPCC, London.

Butler, I., Williamson, H., 1994. Children Speak: Children. Trauma and Social Work, Longman, Essex.

REFERENCES

A and S (Children) v Lancashire County Council [2012] EWHC 1689 (Fam)

Adoption and Children Act 2002.

Alderson, P., 1993. Children's Consent to Surgery. Open University Press, Buckingham.

Alderson, P., 2000. Young Children's Rights. Jessica Kingsley Publishers Ltd, London.

Allnock, D., Miller, P., 2013. No One Noticed, No One Heard: A Study of Disclosures of Childhood Abuse. NSPCC, London.

Bell, M., 2011. Promoting Children's Rights in Social Work and Social Care: A Guide to Participatory Practice. Jessica Kingsley Publishers, London.

Brandon, M., Belderson, P., Warren, C., Howe, D., Gardner, R., Dodsworth, J., et al., 2008. Analysing Child Deaths and Serious Injury Through Abuse and Neglect: What Can We Learn?: A Biennial Analysis of Serious Case Reviews 2003–2005. Department for Children. Schools and Families, Nottingham.

Butler, I., Williamson, H., 1994. Children Speak: Children, Trauma and Social Work. Longman, Essex.

Butler-Sloss, E., 1988. Report of the Inquiry into Child Abuse in Cleveland 1987. HMSO, London.

Campbell, B., 2023. Secrets and Silence. Uncovering the Legacy of the Cleveland Child Sexual Abuse Case. Policy Press, Bristol.

Children Act 1989.

Children Act 2004.

Children and Social Work Act 2017.

Clark, A., Moss, P., 2011. Listening to Young Children: The Mosaic Approach, second ed. National Children's Bureau, London.

Cloke, C., Davies, M. (Eds.), 1995. Participation and Empowerment in Child Protection. Pitman Publishing, London.

Committee on the Rights of the Child (CRC), 2006. General comment no. 7. Implementing Child Rights in Early Childhood. United Nations, Geneva.

Committee on the Rights of the Child (CRC), 2011. General comment no. 13. The Right of the Child to Freedom From all Forms of Violence. United Nations, Geneva.

Committee on the Rights of the Child (CRC), 2013. General comment no. 14. The Right of the Child to Have His or Her Best Interests Taken as a Primary Consideration. United Nations, Geneva.

Committee on the Rights of the Child (CRC), 2016. Concluding Observations on the Fifth Periodic Report of the United Kingdom of Great Britain and Northern Ireland. United Nations, Geneva.

Committee on the Rights of the Child (CRC), 2023. Concluding Observations on the Combined Sixth and Seventh Reports of the United Kingdom of Great Britain and Northern Ireland. United Nations, Geneva.

Cossar, J., Brandon, M., Jordan, P., 2011. Don't Make Assumptions: Children and Young People's Views of the Child Protection System and Messages for Change. Office of the Children's Commissioner, London.

Cossar, J., Brandon, M., Bailey, S., Belderson, P., Biggart, L., 2013. It takes a lot to build trust'. Recognition and Telling: Developing Earlier Routes to Help for Children and Young People. Office of the Children's Commissioner, London.

Cunningham, H., 2005. Children and Childhood in Western Society Since 1500, second ed. Pearson Longman, Harlow, England.

Davies, L., Duckett, N., 2016. Proactive Child Protection and Social Work, second ed. Sage, London.

Day, C., Hibbert, P., Cadman, S., 2008. A Literature Review into Children Abused and/or Neglected Prior [to] Custody. Youth Justice Board, London.

Department for Education, 2021. Characteristics of Children in Need: 2020 to 2021.

Donovan, L., 2019. Into the Lighthouse: The UK's First Safe Space for Child Sexual Abuse Victims. Guardian Newspaper, 17 July 2019.

European Convention on Human Rights. https://www.echr.coe.int/european-convention-on-human-rights.

Farleys [online], https://www.farleys.com/9-6-million-awarded-to-brothers-following-local-authority-neglect/.

Ferguson, H., 2017. How children become invisible in child protection work: findings from research into day-to-day social work practice. Br. J. Soc. Work 47, 1007–1023.

Firmin, C., 2018. Contextual risk, individualised responses: an assessment of safeguarding responses to nine cases of peer-on-peer abuse. Child Abus. Rev. 27, 42–57.

Flegel, M., 2009. Conceptualizing Cruelty to Children in Nineteenth-Century England: Literature, Representation, and the NSPCC. Ashgate, Surrey.

Franklin, A., 2015. 'Voice' as more than words: Involving children and young people with communication needs in decision-making. In: Ivory, M. (Ed.), Voice of the Child: Meaningful

Engagement With Children and Young People. Research in Practice, Devon.

Freeman, M., 1989. Principles and processes of the law in child protection. In: Stainton Rogers, W., Hevey, D., Ash, E. (Eds.), Child Abuse and Neglect: Facing the Challenge. The Open University, London, pp. 129–134.

Growney, T. (Ed.), 1998. Sometimes You've Got to Shout to be Heard: Stories From Young People in Care. Voice for the Child in Care, London.

Hendrick, H., 2003. Child Welfare: Historical Dimensions, Contemporary Debate. Policy Press, Bristol.

Hindberg, B., 2001. Ending Corporal Punishment: Swedish Experience of Efforts to Prevent all Forms of Violence Against Children and the Results. Ministry of Health and Social Affairs and Ministry for Foreign Affairs, Stockholm.

Home Office, 2022. Police Recorded Crime and Outcomes Open Data Tables.

House of Commons Hansard, Cruelty to Children Prevention Bill, 19 June 1889, column 234.

Human Rights Act 1998. https://www.legislation.gov.uk/ukpga/1998/42/contents.

Ibbetson, K., 2013. Services provided for Child F June 2004 to January 2012. Tower Hamlets Local Safeguarding Children Board, London.

International Covenant on Civil and Political Rights (1966). https://www.ohchr.org/en/instruments-mechanisms/instruments/international-covenant-civil-and-political-rights.

Jelicic, H., Gibb, J., La Valle, I., Payne, L., 2013. Involved by Right: The Voice of the Child in the Child Protection Conferences. National Children's Bureau, London.

Lindgren, A., 1978. Never Violence!. Speech Reproduced by Swedish Book Review. 2007. https://www.swedishbookreview.com/article-2007-2-never-violence.asp.

MacLeod, M., 1999. 'Don't just do it'. Children's access to help and protection'. In: Parton, N., Wattam, C. (Eds.), Child Sexual Abuse. Responding to the Experiences of Children. Willey, West Sussex, pp. 141–158.

Marshall, K., 1997. Children's Rights in the Balance: The Participation-Protection Debate. The Stationery Office, Edinburgh.

Miller, J., 2003. Never too Young: How Young Children Can Take Responsibility and Make Decisions. Save the Children, London.

Morgan, R., 2003. Children's views from care and residential education on proposals. In the Green Paper 'Every Child Matters'. Report of the Children's Rights Director. National Care Standards Commission, London.

Munro, E., 2011. The Munro Review of Child Protection: Final Report, a Child-Centred System. The Stationery Office Limited, London.

Ofsted, 2011. Ages of Concern: Learning Lessons From Serious Case Reviews. A thematic report of Ofsted's evaluation of serious case reviews from 1 April 2007 to 31 March 2011. Ofsted, Manchester.

One in Four, 2015. Survivors' voices. Breaking the Silence on Living With the Impact of Child Sexual Abuse in the Family Environment. One in Four, London.

Qvortrup, J., 1985. Placing children in the division of labour. In: Close, P., Rosemary Collins, R. (Eds.), Family and Economy in Modern Society, pp. 129–145.

R v Barker [2010] EWCA Crim 4

R v Hopley [1860] EW Misc J73

Schofield, G., Thoburn, J., 1996. Child Protection: The Voice of the Child in Decision-Making. Institute for Public Policy Research, London.

Sidebotham, S., Brandon, M., Bailey, S., Belderson, P., Dodsworth, J., Garstang, J., et al., 2016. Pathways to Harm, Pathways to Protection: A Triennial Analysis of Serious Case Reviews 2011 to 2014. Department for Education.

Uddin, Baroness, 2004. House of Lords Debate on the Children Bill, Hansard volume 663 cc518–603.

United Nations Convention on the Rights of the Child 1989. https://www.unicef.org/child-rights-convention.

Universal Declaration of Human Rights 1948. https://www.un.org/en/about-us/universal-declaration-of-human-rights.

Voice for the Child in Care and National Children's Bureau, 2004. Start With the Child, Stay With the Child: A Blueprint for a Child-Centred Approach to Children and Young People in Public Care. Voice for the Child in Care, London.

Warrington, C., Beckett, H., Ackerley, E., Walker, M., Allnock, D., 2017. Making Noise: Children's Voices for Positive Change After Sexual Abuse. Children's Commissioner for England, London.

Willow, C., 2003. Let Them Have Their Childhood Again. Children's Rights Alliance for England, London.

Willow, C., 2009. Putting children and their rights at the heart of the safeguarding process. In: Cleaver, H., Cawson, P., Gorin, S., Walker, S. (Eds.), Safeguarding Children: A Shared Responsibility. Wiley-Blackwell, West Sussex, pp. 13–37.

Willow, C., 2010. Children's right to be heard and effective child protection. A Guide for Governments and Children's Rights Advocates on Involving Children and Young People in Ending all Forms of Violence. Save the Children Sweden, Thailand.

Willow, C., 2015. Children Behind Bars: Why the Abuse of Child Imprisonment Must End. Policy Press, Bristol.

Willow, C., 2021. United They Stand: Moving Beyond the Participation-Protection Divide. Discussion paper. Save the Children Sweden, Thailand.

Willow, C., Hyder, T., 1998. It Hurts You Inside: Children Talking About Smacking. National Children's Bureau, London.

Winter, K., 2011. Building Relationships and Communicating With Young Children: A Practical Guide for Social Workers. Routledge, Oxon.

ZH (Tanzania) v Secretary of State for the Home Department, 2011. UKSC 4.

3

HUMANE PRACTICE IN CHILD PROTECTION: THE STORY OF ONE PROJECT

JADWIGA LEIGH ■ CLARE WESTERN

KEY POINTS

- What is the meaning of humane practice and how can it be approached using group work and peer mentoring techniques?

- What impact can serious case reviews have on culture and practice of child protection work?

- Why are the concepts of time, space and narrative therapy important in social work practice?

INTRODUCTION

At the heart of humane social work practice is a range of informal, moral rationalities concerning care, trust, kindness and respect (Broadhurst et al., 2010), yet practitioners also need to be able to make sound judgements and decisions that bear the weight of retrospective and external scrutiny (Taylor and White, 2006). Serious case reviews and public inquiry reports demonstrate that humane practice is not always achieved, and as a result, a focus on ensuring practice and assessment is improved has become a dominant and important part of the current social work agenda (see Ingram and Smith, 2018). On the one hand, there is evidence that demonstrates that the number of families being investigated for concerns relating to abuse or neglect has risen significantly (Bilson and Martin, 2017), and on the other, there are a growing number of reports that demonstrate many parents and children encounter unpleasant and uncomfortable experiences when working with a child-protection social worker (Smithson and Gibson, 2016). So how can humane

practice be accomplished when there are concerns for the welfare of children? This chapter will attempt to answer this question by focusing on some of the challenges social workers can face in relational work with families.

Since 2018, the author has been part of a community outreach project called New Beginnings which has been working in partnership with parents and social work practitioners. The main aim of the project is to work with parents who have children on care orders or whose children are subject to the child protection process. For a period of 6 months, parents attend trauma informed group sessions where together, with the support of project facilitators, they explore how their past stories have not only affected their identity but also the way they parent their children. Using a participatory approach, the team work collaboratively with parents, with the aim of helping them reach their goals, fulfil their potential and reduce social care intervention. The main objective of the project is, therefore, to keep families together. At the end of the 6-month period, parents have the opportunity to carry out peer mentoring training so that they can help facilitate the next group. The project currently has eight peer mentors: women who have already completed the programme, carried out their peer mentoring training and have returned on a paid basis to run the groups.

Drawing on the experience of working on New Beginnings, this chapter will consider what it means to work relationally with children and families involved with child protection services. It will also consider some of the challenges parents and practitioners can face in relational work and make recommendations for how to overcome these challenges. It will also explore the views of a parent of two children who has been in the child protection system intermittently for 12 years. This parent now works at New Beginnings. Her role is to support parents who have been through the programme but still require ongoing practical support; she will share her story.

TIME, SPACE AND NARRATIVE THERAPY

Time, when working with families, is a concept which holds significant, but hidden, importance. In social work practice the majority of interactions that take place involve continuously talking about periods of time such as the past, present and futures of families (Hall et al., 2017). In assessments social workers often spend time exploring the 'current challenges' that parents face by discussing the 'past' events that have led to a referral being made. They then use the past to make decisions about what the 'future' will hold (Juhila et al., 2014). In addition to talking about the past, the present and the future, social workers spend a lot of time talking about 'time frames' or rather 'when time'. 'When time' forms an essential part of everyday social work whether we realise it or not.

For example, 'when time' can refer to a time 'when' a parent used drugs; 'when' she became a victim of abuse or 'when' the threshold for proceedings have been reached. What can be frustrating for parents is that they are often encouraged to relive their past moments, but they cannot reverse the actions that have already occurred which have often led to social workers becoming involved in their lives (Adam, 1995). In addition, social care professionals sometimes take it for granted that because parents have children they should mature and take responsibility for certain aspects of their life. However, what they sometimes overlook is that the transition and ability to mature from childhood to parenthood will take longer if a parent has suffered significant trauma.

One method used by New Beginnings is narrative therapy because it considers the 'story telling rights' of the parent whose story is being told (Epston and Madigan, 1995). Narrative therapy is a method that can be used effectively in social work as it acknowledges that

who we are and what we do is influenced by the stories that we tell about ourselves (White, 2007). It also recognises that we cannot always alter the stories that others tell about us and that all too often, the stories we believe about ourselves have been written by others (Denborough, 2014). Another advantage of narrative therapy is that it is a method which appreciates stories are not told in an empty space; it therefore can enable the storyteller to influence the story that is told about them.

On New Beginnings narrative therapy is used in the group work part of the project. It is recognised that many parents in the group have spent a lot of their *time* telling professionals their stories only to find these stories became distorted in the reports they later read. Parents tell of feeling 'stuck', unable to change or move forwards, often because they are frightened of what the desired change would bring as well as what it would force them to leave behind. This led staff at the project to realise that although professionals want to hear the history of a parent, offering the parent the time to tell their story in the way they wanted to was not always common place. Furthermore, when stories were being told, parents felt they were not properly being heard. Instead, parents said they were more likely to be blamed for the actions they had taken and, in turn, left feeling ashamed they had failed their children as well as unclear of what it was they needed to do to change the situation for the better.

An intrinsic part of New Beginnings is, therefore, to deepen the mothers' understanding of who they are and what they have been through from the telling and sharing of personal histories. This method is rooted in the recognition that if change is to occur in parenting practices, then individuals need to be able to articulate their perspectives on what has happened to them, be heard and also listened to. By creating safe spaces, and allowing enough time for parental change to take place, New Beginnings has evolved organically and taken on a dimension of its own. As the author of this chapter and a practitioner on the project, it is interesting to see how parents develop their stories by reflecting on what they have said or written as well as having the time to add to or edit their words. It is also apparent that although parents enjoy having the time and space to tell their stories, they also enjoy listening to the stories they are told. This not only brings the parents closer to one another but also provides a sense of solidarity by allowing them to see that they are not alone.

Serious Case Reviews and Risk Averse Practice

In recent years, high-profile cases of child abuse have provoked fervent reactions from the public with regard to the role social workers have played (Leigh et al., 2019). When a child dies, people want to know who is responsible, who is going to take the blame and what measures can be implemented in order that similar situations are avoided in future (Lonne and Parton, 2014; Leigh, 2017). Questions, which relate to accountability and prevention, therefore play a significant part in the social construction process of understanding what happened in order for lessons to be learned and future tragedies to be avoided (Leigh et al., 2019). This process of deconstruction tends to take place after a crisis has emerged. As it unfolds in the public eye it habitually demonstrates how societies react after a tragedy has occurred (von Scheve et al., 2016).

For example, in England, the serious case review (SCR) is one kind of social construction process that takes place after a child has been seriously harmed or died (Leigh et al., 2019). The purpose of such reviews is to identify how improvements can be made to protect the future welfare of children (Working Together, 2018). It is thought that by understanding the impact different organisations and agencies have had on a child's life, and on the lives of their family, professionals will learn whether or not different approaches or actions may have resulted in a different outcome (Working Together, 2018). One key theme that has arisen from the multi-analysis of SCR reports is the behaviour of parents and carers, particularly the way in which they are seen to have duped professionals into believing they are engaging with social work interventions when it later emerges they had no intention of doing so (see National Society for the Prevention of Cruelty to Children (NSPCC), 2014). However, what is rarely explored is the behaviour of the professionals involved, that is, the way in which they have interacted with the family or attempted (or not) to build relationships with the parents.

There is a wide range of literature that discusses the challenges of working with families who appear resistant to receiving support or intervention in research

and other relevant literature (see Turnell, 2006; Ferguson, 2009; Shemmings et al., 2012; Turney, 2012; Gibson, 2015). It has also been widely recognised that practitioners who miss signs of abuse or become too close to families are deemed responsible when a child has been harmed. The detailed accounts of, for example, Peter Connelly and Victoria Climbie documented the unsound judgments social workers were thought to have made as a result of being misled by the parents or carers (Leigh, 2017; Jones, 2014; Shoesmith, 2016; Warner, 2013). The more recent stories of Arthur Labinjo Hughes and Star Hobson have been reported on in the news. Social workers across the country would have all heard the words of Conservative Member of Parliament (MP) Tim Loughton, the former children's minister, who said that the reason why Arthur had not been removed is because 'it may be that the social workers here just didn't have the time to get over the threshold' (British Broadcasting Corporation (BBC) online, 4 December 2021).

Reactive and risk averse responses to tragedies, like those mentioned above, not only discretely shape the way future professional practices are developed but also the social interactions that take place between social care professionals and parents. However, one important factor that Tim Loughton acknowledges as crucial is 'time'. If social workers are to prevent harm, they need quality time to get to know families – with time, they will be able to know what is happening within a family, how it functions as a unit and how it affects children. With time, they will know if a child is in a seriously harmful situation from which they need to be removed or if they are in a situation where there is hope. With time, practitioners can reflect on the challenges they, and families, are presented with. With time, practitioners are more likely to adopt a humane manner when working with families so that they can remember that today's parents are yesterday's children (Crittenden, 2016). This means that if social workers are to protect children, then they need to consider the functioning and needs of their parents who may have themselves once been victims of abuse. High caseloads and reduced resources mean social workers have, if anything, limited time to make decisions about risk and safety.

In the next section of this chapter, a former parent on the programme who had been in the child protection system for 12 years before she began working with New Beginnings will share her story. She is now the Post Programme Support Worker for the organisation, and her role is to provide practical support to parents who have been through our 24-week intensive trauma informed programme.

She has chosen to talk about how parental learning needs impact upon the child protection process because one common theme that keeps reappearing with the families on New Beginnings is how many parents left school without any formal qualifications and furthermore, how many have an unidentified learning need or a neurodiverse condition that has gone undetected. This means that in many situations not only are parents unable to read the professionals' reports that are written about them, but those who can read are unable to understand what they mean – that is, what the concerns of professionals are. For those parents who the project later learns have autism or attention-deficit/hyperactivity disorder (ADHD), many have had to struggle for years with the misdiagnosis of a mental health disorder that has been more of a hindrance than a help, such as, for example, borderline personality disorder; emotionally unstable disorder; disorganised attachment disorder and so on. What is more, the project found that if parents are neurodiverse and/or do have learning needs, then it is highly likely that their children will have special educational needs too. Unfortunately, however, it has also found that this factor is being missed by schools and social care provision. Instead, their focus seems to be heavily placed on the parent's ability to parent their child rather than what school and social care providers can do to support both parent and child navigate a system which has been unintentionally designed to exclude those with additional needs.

REFLECTIVE QUESTIONS

Imagine you are the parent encountering a child protection social worker who has concerns about your parenting.

- How might you feel in that moment?
- How would you want a social worker to support and challenge you?

CONCLUSION

Humane practice is all about placing relationships at the heart of social work and valuing the stories of families. There is a wide range of compelling philosophical and practical rationale as to why practitioners should put relationships at the centre of practice. However, it is also apparent that current practice cultures, systems and external scrutiny processes make it difficult for social workers to act in truly relational ways. This cultural deficit means that families continue to feel the impact of environments which promote rising levels of social inequality and separation. If parents are to achieve personal goals and accomplish change, they require a healthy environment which encourages them to make connections and benefit from the support they are offered. Effective relationships are central to successful outcomes. New Beginnings offers a space in which each parent plays an integral role in creating a safe environment and where different group members learn to work together. This form of humane practice sees the group as 'a constellation' with all the members

GIVING TIME AND CREATING A SAFE SPACE FOR RELATIONSHIPS TO DEVELOP – ONE PARENT'S STORY

Recently I've come across a theme from parents who have been asking for help addressing the complex and additional needs of their children. It's a story that feels familiar to me, and every time I hear it, I recognise the reaction I see in the parent. This is because I remember the same words being thrown around when I was in the same situation. When parents are fighting a system that is not designed in their favour for help in identification and early intervention with marked, notable and complex additional needs in children, professionals seemingly tend to say the same thing: 'There is nothing wrong with your child, their behaviour is because of your treatment of them/experiences with them/neglect against them'. It's the same tune, same beat, differing lyrics that cut parents deeply all the same.

The parents I work with break as they recount this to me. Every ounce of strength drains from their faces, and I see a physical, visceral reaction akin to crumbling before my eyes. 'I've ruined my child. I've hurt my child. I've been horrible to my child'. It is then that I feel the white, hot anger inside of me; it is this that keeps me present in that moment. So, I grab their hand, I squeeze it, I pull it gently towards me so they'll look up at me; my song is confident, yet soft...

GIVING TIME AND CREATING A SAFE SPACE FOR RELATIONSHIPS TO DEVELOP – ONE PARENT'S STORY—cont'd

Without missing a beat it's always the same. I say, 'That is simply not true! You are not to blame. This is not your fault. It is not your child's fault. It is society's fault'. I pause, give them a moment to truly hear what I've just said. 'We haven't moved quickly enough with the times, we haven't recognised the prevalence of additional needs nor allocated the resources in time to meet that need. We didn't adapt, and it hurt you both. But nothing is beyond repair. I am here now, I will help you.'

I wonder, as I read reports filled with jargon, how long it has been since they've heard the words: 'I am here to help you'. One mother asks 'What is Speech and Language Therapy (SALT)? What does 'phonoically underdeveloped' mean? Why are they talking about percentiles? I don't understand any of this. I'm useless. I can't even understand a simple report about my daughter!' As a single mother to two children, both of whom have complex, identified and diagnosed additional needs I know the overwhelming strength, love, patience and compassion it takes to wake up every morning and keep going. I know all too well that crushing assumption that the needs of my child are a figment of my imagination I used to excuse my own behaviour. Sometimes, I was even told I was lying; in others, that I was deluded.

But I am lucky, few things in life give me strength to not take 'no' for an answer. My children have always been one of the few.

It still crushed me, but I was convinced that for my oldest child I was not wrong – she was neurodiverse, and I needed to prove it. So, convinced I did my homework, and I adapted to her needs. When the diagnosis came in, I was prepared, I was vindicated and I had the strength to continue fighting. Some parents are terrified and crushed by the power dynamic between professional and parent and then comply with the assumption for fear of what will happen if they do not. There is one result: their child suffers and so do they. I have seen children left unsupported; stigmatised as naughty, belligerent, non-compliant, violent, stupid, lazy or even school avoidant. This in turn gets flagged, reported and escalated when actually specialised early intervention would have worked and prevented all of the above. Furthermore, the parent is blamed, vilified and sent on a parenting course that teaches them what they already know, to develop skills

they already have, to address 'the wrong problem'. Without the proper knowledge, without the proper support, without the proper help, both child and parent alike develop maladaptive coping mechanisms that split, fracture and then compound their case, their progress and their lives.

Instead of asking 'What is wrong with you? What are you doing wrong? Why are you doing that wrong?' Start by asking: What has happened to you? How are you coping? What works for you? What doesn't? How can I help? A shift in language can fundamentally alter the social worker's role in the eyes of a family from aggressor to helper. A humane approach towards families places professionals in a unique position of never having to roll a boulder down a hill that then becomes impossible to stop for all but the privileged few.

I cannot help but think that a humane approach saves so much more, on so many levels. Ask yourselves how many times you or others have invested time, resources and money in the courts for a case where a push for Special Educational Needs investigation and advocacy would have intervened sooner and fixed the situation easier. For either the child, the parent or both. Ask yourselves if knowing then, what you are reading now, would have altered or eased, not just your workload and pressures, but that of the families you interacted with.

This isn't an easy revelation to have. It's uncomfortable, but that's because there is truth to it. How much truth there is will relate to the discomfort you're feeling now.

From a parent's perspective, being involved with the child protection system already carries the weight of intricately woven shame and guilt that then melds with the trauma of a parent's past. Akin to throwing petrol on a fire it amplifies destructive patterns and creates an intense barrier difficult for professionals or family alike to overcome. The stigma that we, as parents, are seen as 'less than deserving of our children' is beyond painful. It's crushing. We are each survivors of our own horrors, struggles, battles and trauma. Deep-seated wounds that will sometimes never show on an x-ray or magnetic resonance imaging (MRI), but yet these wounds are open, raw and take an incredibly long time to heal. Some may never do so, but we can learn to live with the pain in a productive and healthy manner. We just sometimes need your help, and we need it in a compassionate and humanely approached practice.

---

acting in solidarity rather than for the benefit of individual egotism (Benson, 2010, p. 129).

The project's form of humane practice is not exclusive; it allows practitioners and parents to spend 'time' appreciating that relationships are complex and require an awareness of 'self' that is, who we are as

professionals and how our presence can determine the future progress of a family. Practitioners also spend time appreciating that parents who are subject to the child protection process are often found in 'in-between' places, and their role is to root for them so that they can embrace and sustain change in a context that will do what it can to understand what is going on for that family. In relational work, narrative therapy is key, as spending time with and listening to the stories parents tell helps practitioners understand the difference between the past – the 'what was' – and the future – the 'what next' (Meyer and Land, 2003). That is, when practitioners take the time to hear where parents have been and where they want to be, they can then create a plan to help them reach those goals that they own and that they benefit from.

The New Beginnings project can be considered a humane form of practice as it is an approach that focuses on working with parents who have been stigmatised and marginalised as a result of their involvement in the child protection system. Creating a safe place for parents in similar situations to connect with one another and receive support, encouragement and inspiration can effect change for their families in a way that is empowering rather than stigmatising. The project not only offers its members an opportunity to select and engage with values that will assist and motivate change, but it also provides social workers with the opportunity to work humanely and compassionately with families.

REFLECTIVE QUESTIONS

- What kind of skills would you need to establish a group that could support families you work with?
- How might you connect parents you work with to one another?
- What benefits do you think this could bring to your practice and to the lives of those you are working with?
- What kind of ethical considerations would you have to contemplate before doing so?
- How humane is your own practice? What are the challenges to working in a humane way?

FURTHER READING

Benson, J., 2010. Working More Creatively With Groups, third ed. Routledge, London.

This updated new edition provides a comprehensive guide to group work and shows practitioners how they can move on from simple superficial engagement to more in depth and intensive work.

Denborough, D., 2014. Retelling the Stories of Our Lives: Everyday Narrative Therapy to Draw Inspiration and Transform Experience. W.W. Norton & Co., London.

Our lives and their pathways are not fixed in stone; instead they are shaped by story. The ways in which we understand and share the stories of our lives therefore make all the difference. If we tell stories that emphasise only desolation, then we become weaker. If we tell our stories in ways that make us stronger, we can soothe our losses and ease our sorrows. Learning how to re-envision the stories we tell about ourselves can make an enormous difference in the ways we live our lives. Drawing on wisdoms from the field of narrative therapy, this book is designed to help people rewrite and retell the stories of their lives.

Reber, D., 2018. Differently Wired: Raising an Exceptional Child in a Conventional World. Workman Publishing Company.

In this generous and urgent book, Deborah lets the light in. She helps parents see that they're not alone, and even better, delivers a positive action plan that will change lives. A valuable resource for parents, teachers, and family members of exceptional children of all types.

REFERENCES

Adam, B., 1995. Timewatch: The Social Analysis of Time. Polity Press, London.

BBC Online, 2021. Arthur Labinjo-Hughes: What Were the Opportunities Missed to Save Him? https://www.bbc.co.uk/news/uk-59519562.

Benson, J., 2010. Working More Creatively With Groups, third ed. Routledge, London.

Bilson, A., Martin, K., 2017. Referrals and child protection in England: one in five children referred to children's services and one in nineteen investigated before the age of five. Br. J. Soc. Work 47 (3), 793–811.

Broadhurst, K., Hall, C., Wastell, D., White, S., Pithouse, A., 2010. Risk, Instrumentalism and the humane project in social work: identifying the informal logics of risk management in children's statutory services. Br. J. Soc. Work 40, 1046–1064. https://doi.org/10.1093/bjsw/bcq011.

Crittenden, P., 2016. Raising Parents: Attachment, Representation and Treatment. Second Edition. Routledge: London.

Denborough, D., 2014. Retelling the Stories of our Lives: Everyday Narrative Therapy to Draw Inspiration and Transform Experience. W.W. Norton & Co., London.

Ferguson, H., 2009. Performing child protection: Home visiting, movement and the struggle to reach the abused child. Child Fam. Soc. Work 14, 471–480.

Gibson, M., 2015. Shame and guilt in child protection social work: new interpretations and opportunities for practice. Child and Family Social Work. 20 (3) p.333–343.

Hall, C., Morriss, L., Juhila, K., 2017. Negotiating risks, choice and progress in case- planning. In: Hall, C., Raitakari, S., Juhila, K. (Eds.), Responsibilisation at the Margins of Welfare Services. Routledge, Oxford.

HM Government, 2018. Working Together to Safeguard Children: A guide to inter-agency working to safeguard and promote the welfare of children. https://assets.publishing.service.gov.uk/government/uploads/system/uploads/attachment_data/file/942454/Working_together_to_safeguard_children_inter_agency_guidance.pdf

Ingram, R. and Smith, M., 2018. Relationship based practice: Emergent themes in social work literature. https://www.basw.co.uk/system/files/resources/basw_95107-2.pdf

Jones, R., 2014. The Story of Baby P: Setting the Record Straight. Policy Press, Bristol.

Juhila, K., Günther, K., Raitakari, S., 2014. Negotiating mental health rehabilitation plans: joint future talk and clashing time talk in professional client interaction. Time Soc. 24 (1), 5–26. https://doi.org/10.1177/0961463X14523925.

Leigh, J., 2017. Blame, Culture and Child Protection. Palgrave Macmillan, London.

Leigh, J., Beddoe, E., Keddell, E., 2019. Disguised compliance or undisguised nonsense? A critical discourse analysis of compliance and resistance in social work practice. Fam. Relatsh. Soc. 9 (2), 269–285.

Lonne, B., and Parton, N., 2014. Portrayals of child abuse scandals in the media in Australia and England: Impacts on practice, policy, and systems: Most media coverage distorts the public understandings of the nature of child maltreatment. Child Abuse and Neglect, 38(5), 822-836. https://doi.org/10.1016/j.chiabu.2014.04.020

Madigan, S. and Epston, D., 1995. 'From psychiatric gaze to communities of concern: From professional monologue to dialogue.' In S. Friedman (ed.), The Reflecting Team in Action. New York: Guilford Publications.

Meyer, J.H.F., Land, R., 2003. Threshold concepts and troublesome knowledge (1): linkages to ways of thinking and practicing. In: Rust, C. (Ed.), Improving Student Learning – Ten Years On. OCSLD, Oxford.

NSPCC, 2019. Disguised Compliance. https://learning.nspcc.org.uk/media/1334/learning-from-case-reviews_disguised-compliance.pdf

Shemmings, D., Shemmings, Y., Cook, A., 2012. Gaining the trust of 'highly resistant' families: Insights from attachment theory and research. Child Fam. Soc. Work 17 (2), 130–137. https://doi.org/10.1111/j.1365-2206.2012.00834.x.

Shoesmith, S., 2016. Learning from Baby P: The politics of blame fear and denial. JKP: London.

Smithson, R., Gibson, M., 2016. Less than human: a qualitative study into the experiences of parents involved in the child protection system. Child Fam. Soc. Work 22 (2), 565–574. https://onlinelibrary.wiley.com/doi/abs/10.1111/cfs.12270.

Taylor, C., White, S., 2006. Knowledge and reasoning in social work: educating for humane judgement. Br. J. Soc. Work 36 (6), 937–954.

Turney, D., 2012. A relationship-based approach to engaging involuntary clients: the contribution of recognition theory. Child Fam. Soc. Work 17 (2), 149–159. https://doi.org/10.1111/j.1365-2206.2012.00830.x.

Turnell, A., 2006. Constructive child protection practice: an oxymoron or news of difference? J. Syst. Ther. 25 (2), 3–12. https://doi.org/10.1521/jsyt.2006.25.2.3.

Van Gennep, A., 1960 [1909]. The Rites of Passage. University of Chicago Press, Chicago, IL.

von Scheve, C., Zink, V., Ismer, S., 2016. The blame game: economic crisis responsibility, discourse and affective framings. Sociology 50 (4), 635–651. https://doi.org/10.1177/0038038514545145.

Warner, J., 2013. Social work, class politics and risk in the moral panic over Baby P. Health Risk Soc. 15 (3), 217–233. https://doi.org/10.1080/13698575.2013.776018.

White, M., 2007. Maps of Narrative Practice. W.W. Norton and Co., New York.

4

POVERTY AND CHILD PROTECTION

ANNA GUPTA ■ BRID FEATHERSTONE

KEY POINTS

- The clear correlations between social deprivation and a child's chances of being subject to child protection plans and in care.

- The increasing research evidence indicating strong association between poverty, parenting, child abuse and neglect.

- The intrinsic links between poverty and other contributory factors, such as parental mental health or domestic abuse.

- Moving away from models of assessment that focus on individual blame and responsibility, to thinking in contextual, interactional and dynamic ways about families' lives.

- Considering how poverty intersects with other structural inequalities, such as race and gender.

- Poverty-aware practice and the requirement to understand poverty and the material and affective impacts.

- How policies and practices can address these to safeguard and promote the welfare of children.

Poverty is living day to day and making ends meet. The money you have is not enough to provide for your kids. My daughter was bullied at school for her clothes and not having the right fashions; she stopped attending school and I was threatened with prison. I don't like borrowing from family and friends so I asked for help from social services. Then a social worker came around, checked my cupboards and made me feel I had done the wrong thing by asking for help.

Gupta et al. (2016, p. 164)

This mother's experiences highlight the struggles millions of families living in poverty face daily trying to meet their children's most basic needs in the UK. It raises questions about the social protections provided by government, the social harms to children's development of living in poverty and the balance between risk and need, supportive and punitive state interventions. The associations between poverty, child abuse and neglect (CAN) and involvement with child protection and care systems have been subject to varied attention and contested debates in research, policy and practice arenas over the past decades. In the late 1980s, a study by Bebbington and Miles (1989) demonstrated how the cumulative effect of disadvantage dramatically increases a child's chances of coming into the care system. Since then, studies have suggested that poverty plays a causal role in parental problems and child maltreatment (Bywaters et al., 2022). But attention to poverty and its contribution to child protection issues has waxed and waned over the decades.

In this chapter, we explore shifting policy and practice contexts in England. We examine the evidence base on the relationship between poverty, CAN and child protection practices and discuss what constitutes poverty-aware practice.

POLICY AND PRACTICE CONTEXTS

When examining social problems, such as child abuse, neglect and societal responses, it is important to analyse what claims are made about the attribution of causality, blame and responsibility (Loseke, 2011). In 1985, Parton argued that the disease model of child abuse was the dominant perspective noting that:

> the pathology resides primarily in the parents but manifests itself in the relationship with the child. While allowing that in some cases it may be an expression of family stress, it is psychological or interpersonal family factors which are seen as of prime importance in the aetiology.
>
> Parton (1985, p. 132)

Whilst the individualising of risk and responsibility has been challenged over the years, child protection policy and practice continue to operate in a context 'where need is understood through a risk lens, and responsibility continues to be conflated with conscious intentionality' (Featherstone et al., 2018a, p. 13). The responsibilisation of parents has been a feature of all recent political administrations, although New Labour provided a supportive infrastructure to tackle child poverty.

The advent of a Conservative-led coalition government in 2010 resulted in stringent cuts to welfare benefits and support to families while their policy reforms to child protection were developed in the context of political and media responses to the death of a baby, Peter Connelly (Jones, 2014). Warner (2015) argues that the story of 'Baby P' was framed as a story of suffering, parental evil and catastrophic professional failings, fuelling media and political responses that perpetuated the demonisation and 'othering' of families living in poverty, thereby enabling more intensive moral regulation and social control of 'them'. Conservative politicians and government advisors promoted a newly invigorated child rescue project:

> We are leaving them to endure a life of soiled nappies and scummy baths, chaos and hunger, hopelessness and despair. These children need to be rescued, just as much as the victims of any other natural disaster.
>
> Gove (2012)

In the context of stringent cuts to family support services and welfare benefits, and a more authoritarian approach to child protection, the numbers of investigations, children on child protection plans, subject to care proceedings and in out of home care increased year on year for most of the second decade of the 20th century (Department for Education [DfE], 2022). Studies involving the perspectives of parents with experiences of child protection services repeatedly highlighted the shaming and blaming nature of child protection interventions and a shift from support to surveillance with their material hardship ignored (Gibson, 2015; Gupta et al., 2016; Smithson and Gibson, 2017). Morris et al.'s (2018) study of social work interventions found that poverty had become invisible in practice, not seen as the 'core business' of social work.

CAN continues today to be understood as resulting from the actions or inactions of their parents or carers with explanations usually located in either psychological dynamics or poor choices (Featherstone et al., 2018b). However, there have been increasing challenges to this framing from researchers, professionals and people with lived experience (Dettlaff et al., 2020; Hyslop and Keddell, 2018; Saar-Heiman, 2019).

The Child Welfare Inequalities Project (CWIP) has been instrumental in developing an evidence base about the relationship between deprivation and a child's chances of becoming subject to child protection systems and highlighted the existence of a social gradient in intervention rates (Bywaters, 2020). This research prompted serious questions about how policy makers and practitioners should respond to clear inequities, not just for those living in areas of high deprivation but across society.

The research raised questions about inequities in the proportion of children from different ethnic groups subject to child protection interventions and highlighted the need for an intersectional approach to understanding child welfare inequalities (Bywaters et al., 2019). Other studies in the UK and internationally have reinforced the need for an inequalities and intersectional approach to understanding child protection and welfare (Dettlaff et al., 2020; Keddell et al., 2019; Maguire-Jack, et al. 2015).

Anti-poverty organisations, such as ATD Fourth World (2019), and critical scholars, such as Lister (2013) and Krumer-Nevo (2016), have called for a multi-dimensional understanding of the impact of poverty. Featherstone et al. (2018b) argue for a need for a social model for protecting children and supporting families. This model moves away from individualised notions of risk to children of parents' actions or inactions, to recognising the social determinants of harm and the economic, social and cultural barriers faced by most of the families, as well as the protective capacities within families and communities and how these can be mobilised.

The imperative to address poverty and other structural inequalities in child protection policy and practice has become even more urgent in the third decade of the 20th century. COVID-19 laid bare the deeply entrenched structural inequalities in British society. Marmot et al. (2020) highlighted ways in which pre-existing socio-economic inequalities worsened the impact of the virus, due to overcrowded housing, precarious incomes and work in low-paid and low-status jobs through lockdowns. Families from Black, Asian and minority ethnic backgrounds were disproportionally impacted. Furthermore, there is currently a 'cost of living crisis', with rising inflation and huge rises in energy prices increasing the number of families unable to adequately feed their children and keep them warm (JRF, 2022).

THE RELATIONSHIP BETWEEN POVERTY AND CHILD ABUSE AND NEGLECT

In 2016, Bywaters and colleagues reviewed the international research evidence on the relationship between poverty and CAN. The review concluded that there was a strong association between families' socio-economic circumstances and the chances that their children would experience CAN (Bywaters et al., 2016). The review evidence suggests that the influence of poverty works directly and indirectly (through parental stress and neighbourhood conditions), and in interaction with other factors, such as domestic violence, mental health and substance abuse (Bywaters et al., 2016).

In 2022, this review was updated (Bywaters et al., 2022) and found that there was an even stronger evidence base than in 2016, of poverty as a key driver of harm to children. For example, 17 quasi-experimental studies found that changes in the economic circumstances of family life alone, without any other factors, impacted on rates of abuse and neglect, with increases in income reducing rates significantly. The importance of adequate social protection was noted as economic crises increased abuse and neglect rates, but compensatory policies (such as welfare payments) mitigated the effects.

THE INVESTMENT MODEL AND THE FAMILY STRESS MODEL

The investment model focuses on the capabilities of parents to provide resources for their children to thrive and succeed, that is dependent on the distribution of resources within societies. Bywaters et al. (2022, p. 34) suggest that the 'investment model also has the potential to explain why there is a social gradient in child outcomes generally and child maltreatment, in particular, because it points to a range of advantages that can be purchased with increasing family income and wealth'. This includes not just money but a range of human, social and cultural capital (Cooper and Stewart, 2020).

The family stress model focuses on the emotional and psychological consequences of poverty and lack of resources, with feelings of shame and stigma exacerbating stress. Living on low and insecure incomes creates psychological stress, which in turn can lead to mental health difficulties, substance misuse, relationship problems and disrupted parenting (Acquah et al., 2017; Masarik and Conger, 2017).

The review considered two main explanatory models for the relationship between poverty and CAN, the *investment model* (Duncan et al., 2014) and the *family stress model* (Conger et al., 2000).

An Early Intervention Foundation report (Acquah et al., 2017) concluded economic pressure placed parents at elevated risk for a variety of adverse psychological outcomes including anxiety and depression, which in turn are associated with problems in the inter-parental relationship including inter-parental conflict and reduced relationship satisfaction. The recent studies reviewed by Bywaters et al. (2022) found that neighbourhood level factors, such as social cohesion and availability of local services, also have an influence. Poverty is not a stand-alone factor, to be added to a list alongside others, but is intrinsic to other contributory factors, such as parental mental health or domestic abuse. When thinking about the relationship between poverty, parenting and CAN, an understanding of systemic causation requires us to move away from models of assessment that focus on individual blame and responsibility, to thinking in contextual, interactional and dynamic ways about families' lives (Featherstone et al., 2018b).

How families are identified as possibly abusing or neglecting their children and then responded to by social workers and other professionals are influenced by 'supply factors', including differential spending and service provision as well as the attitudes and behaviours of front-line managers and practitioners (Bywaters & Child Welfare Inequalities Project Team, 2020; Keddell et al., 2019). The evidence suggests that child protection systems and services too rarely engage effectively with the impact of income, employment and housing conditions on more commonly recognised parental problems, such as mental health difficulties.

A lack of recognition about the context of their lives can leave parents feeling shamed and humiliated, as explained by parents living in poverty who have experienced child protection interventions (Fig 4.1):

Alongside the developing knowledge base on the relationship between poverty and CAN, there has been increasing understanding about the multi-dimensional nature of poverty. Lister (2013, p. 112) describes poverty as not only being about material disadvantage and economic insecurity but also 'a shameful social relation, corrosive of human dignity and flourishing, which is experienced in interactions with the wider society and in the way people in poverty are talked about and treated by politicians, officials, professionals, the media, and sometimes academics'. A parent with experience of poverty and child protection services explains:

> *Social workers are perhaps one of the most intimate relationships [individuals] have with the state, and it's someone who has a lot of power over them... if that person is not treating them with recognition and respect, what it's doing to their self-esteem, their sense of themselves, regardless of the success of the social work relationship, is actually terribly damaging. It's reinforcing all the negative stuff they're seeing in the media or hear politicians talk.*
> **Gupta et al. (2018, p. 255)**

Poverty is implicated in innumerable ways in the lives of families and the decisions made every day by workers. A participatory research project with families living in poverty (ATD Fourth World, 2019) identified six inter-related dimensions:

- Disempowering systems, structures and policies
- Financial insecurity, financial exclusion and debt
- Damaged health and well-being

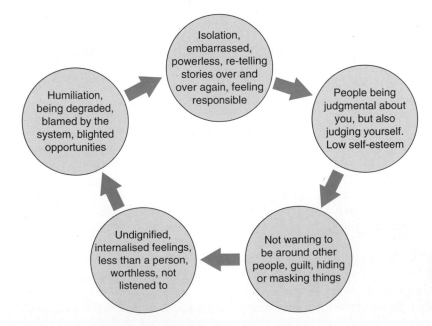

(Gupta, A., ATD Fourth World, 2015. Poverty and shame – Messages for social work. Crit. Radic. Soc. Work 3 (1), 131–139. Reprinted with permission of Bristol University Press and Policy Press.)

- Stigma, blame and judgment
- Lack of control over choices
- Unrecognised struggles, skills and contributions

Two of the participants describe what this means for their lives:

Poverty means being part of a system that leaves you waiting indefinitely in a state of fear and uncertainty. (p. 12)

Poverty is not being able to smell the flowers because the stress of life gets in the way. (p. 18)

REFLECTIVE QUESTIONS

- What are your values and beliefs about the relationship between poverty and child abuse and neglect?
- Where do these values and beliefs come from? How do these impact on your practice?

POVERTY-AWARE CHILD PROTECTION PRACTICE

A study by Morris et al. (2018, p. 371) of practitioners' approaches revealed the need for new conceptual frameworks to support practice to engage constructively with poverty as a child protection matter. The Poverty-Aware Paradigm (PAP) for social work aims to provide one such framework (Krumer-Nevo, 2020). It offers theoretical, ethical and practical principles for social work with families living in poverty. The application of PAP to child protection (PAPCP) has since been developed (Saar-Heiman and Gupta, 2020; Saar-Heiman, 2019).

PAP challenges the conservative paradigm that views 'poverty as the sum product of the psychological, moral, behavioural and cultural pathologies or deficits of poor people' (Krumer-Nevo, 2016, p. 1795). It builds on and extends a structural analysis of poverty and regards poverty as a violation of human rights. Drawing on the work of Lister (2004), Krumer-Nevo (2020) conceptualises poverty as a wheel comprised of three layers: the hub is lack of material capital; the second layer is lack of social capital (e.g. adequate housing, health care and education); and the outer layer lack of symbolic capital through dehumanising and 'othering' processes. The inclusion of relational/symbolic aspects in the definition of poverty sheds light on the everyday experiences of poor people.

People in poverty are perceived within the PAP as resisting poverty in their daily decision making, in explicit and implicit ways. Thus what can appear, when viewed from the outside, like a poor choice or decision may be rational or adaptive in the context of insufficient and precarious resources (Krumer-Nevo, 2020). Adopting a poverty lens can open possibilities for questioning taken-for-granted assumptions.

A PAP approach to child protection considers risks to children's well-being to include social harms, and policies and practices that contribute to such harms. Underpinning a PAP approach to child protection practice is an understanding of the multi-dimensional nature of poverty and the complex interactional relationship between poverty, parenting and child maltreatment (Bywaters et al., 2022). Saar-Heiman (2022) draws on a qualitative study with parents and social workers in Israel to construct a *child protection–poverty matrix* that assists professionals to better comprehend the complex relationships between social inequality, poverty and child maltreatment. The matrix consists of three dimensions of the material, the social and the relational–symbolic. Each dimension has three realms of influence: on the child, on the parents and on the parent–child relationship. For example, the material dimension includes inability to purchase concrete goods, i.e., rent, utilities, food or clothing, appliances, furniture or home repair, and the influence it has on children, parents and their relationships. The matrix is enveloped by an overarching experience of stress.

The relational–symbolic dimension highlights the affective impacts of poverty and inequality and helps explore the ways in which poverty influences professionals' interactions with parents and vice versa (Saar-Heiman, 2022). This requires critical reflection on workers' values and the practices and organisational processes that can perpetuate (and resist) discourses that encourage views of people in poverty as 'them – not like us' compounding shame and humiliation. It involves recognising and challenging 'micro-aggressions', often small, innocuous but shaming and 'othering' practices.

The PAP takes a critical constructivist approach which questions power relationships and knowledge construction (Krumer-Nevo, 2016). Workers need to reflect on how professional knowledge is valued above that of families living in poverty. This includes questioning how knowledge about risk is produced and the sources that shape it (Saar-Heiman and Gupta, 2020).

Engaging with families in local contextual interactions creates relationships-based knowledge (Saar-Heiman and Krumer-Nevo, 2020). This provides grounded understandings of families' lives in the contexts of their communities (Featherstone et al., 2018b).

PAP emphasises the ethics of solidarity, 'achieved through an active effort to include the other in the "we", based on the acknowledgement of the differences between us in terms of power, history and social position' (Krumer-Nevo, 2016, p. 1802). In the context of a risk-averse child protection system, creating solidarity with parents can be challenging and requires specific awareness of the effects of power and othering on professional practice. However, paradoxically, the ethics of solidarity and 'standing by' can make challenging parents more effective as service users feel cared about and the contexts of their lives better understood (Krumer-Nevo, 2016). As a parent from ATD Fourth World explains:

> *If actually you've got at least one person in authority that you feel is on your side and who does recognise you, that actually can be quite a turning point.*
> **Gupta et al. (2018, p. 254)**

CASE STUDY 4.1: TANYA'S STORY

Tanya is a mixed parentage woman recovering from problem drinking and heroin use. She is working towards her 3-year-old daughter (Susie) returning to her care. Tanya has supervised contact with Susie twice per week. She is allowed to take Susie out into the community. Whilst contact is generally going well, the social worker expressed her concern that Tanya was not taking her daughter to a local play centre. Tanya, however, receives £45 per week after rent, council tax and debt repayment. The play centre costs £6 per visit. She has never been asked by the social worker about the reason for not attending play centre, but also feels uncomfortable explaining why not because she feels ashamed and that it may jeopardise the return of her child.

This cases study highlights both the lack of attention to the economic circumstances and consequent pathologizing of parental actions on the part of the social worker, as well shame and fear felt by Tanya about being poor. Acknowledging the limited income she receives is difficult for anyone to survive on, alongside the provision of material support, at least for the contact sessions, would have been a more humane and socially just response.

Adapted from Gupta, 2017.

MESSAGES FOR CHILD PROTECTION POLICY AND PRACTICE

Child protection work that is poverty aware and practised within a social justice and human rights framework recognises the range of harms to children and families living in poverty. It moves away from a narrow focus on parental risk to focus on harmful contexts and ways of addressing the policies and practices needed to enable children and their families to flourish.

Featherstone et al. (2021) argue for robust social protections on a national level, to address welfare, housing, health, education and immigration policies, but also a focus on local, community-based support services, including anti-poverty strategies, co-produced with

CLOSER LOOK: POVERTY-AWARE PRACTICE

For individual practitioners, there is much they can do in their work within a poverty-aware practice framework. Some suggestions include:

- Recognition of the importance of values with social workers and other professionals asking themselves: What are my values and beliefs regarding poverty? How do I understand poverty? What are the implications for my practice?
- A nuanced multi-factorial analysis is necessary that questions how poverty and other inequalities impact on parental problems and children's development.
- Spending time in homes and communities, drawing on families' knowledge of their lives, constraints and opportunities; asking what is life like for this child, and this family, in this housing, on the income they have, and in this community?
- Providing practical help recognising the connections between the material and emotional: *'a washing machine for example would have made a big difference'* (birth parent) (Featherstone et al., 2018c, p. 23).
- Proactive right-based advocacy in relation to issues such as welfare benefits, housing and immigration, recognising the symbolic capital professionals bring to achieve positive benefits for families.
- Recognising and challenging 'micro-aggressions', shaming and 'othering' practices by self, others and organisational practices.
- Building alliances with local community and specialist organisations (e.g. supporting families with No Recourse to Public funds) who can provide additional support.

children, young people, families and communities. On an organisational level, one strategy is to undertake an audit, ideally with families, that aims to 'poverty-proof' policies and practices (see, e.g. poverty proofing in schools). This involves asking at each stage of the child protection process how a policy, for example, reimbursing fares to contact sessions, or holding on-line meetings, impacts on families. It would incorporate an intersectional approach, such as English language skills. Another initiative would ensure families have access to a specialist welfare rights advisor, and housing support if in insecure or unsuitable accommodation.

CONCLUSION

There is increasing evidence of the impact of poverty on rates of child maltreatment (Bywaters et al., 2022). The impact of poverty is not just one of material deprivation, but poverty is also about lack of social and symbolic capital, the latter impacting on how professionals view and treat families living in poverty. Whilst the structural causes of poverty and income inequality require action by government on national and local levels, there is also much social workers and other professionals can do to recognise and address the harmful social and economic contexts that blight the lives of many children and families involved with the child protection services.

REFLECTIVE QUESTIONS

- What are your views on poverty-aware practice as outlined above?
- Can you think of ways you incorporate or could incorporate these ideas in your practice?
- What might be some of the benefits/challenges of these be?

FURTHER READING

BASW – Anti-poverty guide for social work. https://www.basw.co.uk/what-we-do/policy-and-research/anti-poverty-practice-guide-social-work

The relationship between poverty, child abuse and neglect: an evidence review. https://www.jrf.org.uk/report/relationship-between-poverty-child-abuse-and-neglect-evidence-review

The relationship between poverty, child abuse and neglect: new evidence. https://www.hud.ac.uk/news/2022/march/poverty-links-to-child-abuse-report/

Using a Social Model for protecting children in supervision. https://practice-supervisors.rip.org.uk/wp-content/uploads/2019/11/Using-a-social-model-of-child-protection-in-supervision.pdf

REFERENCES

Acquah, D., Sellers, R., Stock, L., Harold, G., 2017. Inter-parental conflict and outcomes for children in the contexts of poverty and economic pressure. Early Intervention Foundation, UK. www.EIF.org.

ATD Fourth World, 2019. Understanding Poverty in All its Forms – 6 Dimensions: A Participatory Research Study into Poverty in the UK. https://atd-uk.org/projects-campaigns/understanding-poverty/.

Bebbington, A., Miles, J., 1989. The background of children who enter local authority care. Br. J. Soc. Work 19 (1), 349–368.

Bywaters, P., Bunting, L., Davidson, G., Hanratty, J., Mason, W., McCartan, C., et al., 2016. The Relationship between Poverty, Child Abuse and Neglect: An Evidence Review. Joseph Rowntree Foundation, York.

Bywaters, P., 2020. Child Welfare Inequalities Project Team. Child Welfare Inequalities Programme: Final Report https://research.hud.ac.uk/media/assets/document/research/cacyfr/CWIP-Overview-Final-V4.pdf.

Bywaters, P., Scourfield, J., Webb, C., Morris, K., Featherstone, B., Brady, G., et al., 2019. Paradoxical evidence on ethnic inequities in child welfare: Towards a research agenda. Child Youth Serv. Rev. 96, 145–154.

Bywaters, P., Skinner, G., Cooper, A., Kennedy, E., Malik, A., 2022. The Relationship Between Poverty and Child Abuse and Neglect: New Evidence. Nuffield Foundation/University of Huddersfield. https://research.hud.ac.uk/media/assets/document/hhs/RelationshipBetweenPovertyChildAbuseandNeglect_Report.pdf.

Conger, K.J., Rueter, M.A., Conger, R.D., 2000. The role of economic pressure in the lives of parents and their adolescents: The family stress model. In: Crockett, L.J., Silbereisen, R.K. (Eds.), Negotiating Adolescence in Times of Change. Cambridge University Press, Cambridge, pp. 201–223.

Cooper, K., Stewart, K., 2020. Does household income affect children's outcomes? A systematic review of the evidence. Child Indic. Res. 14, 981–1005.

Day, A.S., Gill, A.K., 2020. Applying intersectionality to partnerships between women's organizations and the criminal justice system in relation to domestic violence. Br. J. Criminol. 60 (4), 830–850.

Dettlaff, A.J., Weber, K., Pendleton, M., Boyd, R., Bettencourt, B., Burton, L., 2020. It is not a broken system, it is a system that needs to be broken: The upEND movement to abolish the child welfare system. J. Public Child Welf. 14 (5), 500–517.

Department for Education (DfE), 2022. Statistics: Children in Need and Child Protection. https://www.gov.uk/government/collections/statistics-children-in-need.

Duncan, G.J., Magnuson, K., Votruba-Drzal, E., 2014. Boosting family income to promote child development. Future Child 24 (1), 99–120.

Featherstone, B., Gupta, A., Morris, K., Warner, J., 2018a. Let's stop feeding the risk monster: towards a social model of' child protection. Fam. Relationsh. Soc. 7 (1), 7–22.

Featherstone, B., Gupta, A., Morris, K., White, S., 2018b. Protecting Children: A Social Model. Policy Press, Bristol.

Featherstone, B., Gupta, A., Mills, S., 2018c. The Role of the Social Worker in Adoption – Ethics and Human Rights: An Enquiry. www.basw.co.uk/adoption-enquiry.

Featherstone, B., Gupta, A., Morris, K., 2021. Post-pandemic: Moving on from 'child protection. Crit. Radic. Soc. Work 9 (2), 151–165.

Friedli, L., 2009. Mental Health, Resilience and Inequalities. WHO, Denmark.

Gibson, M., 2015. Shame and guilt in child protection social work: New interpretations and opportunities for practice. Child Fam. Soc. Work 20 (3), 333–343.

Gove, M., 2012. *The failure of child protection and the need for a fresh start*, Education Secretary speech on child protection. Institute for Public Policy Research, 19 November. https://www.gov.uk/government/speeches/the-failure-of-child- protection-and-the-need-for-a-fresh-start.

Gupta, A., 2017. Learning from others: An autoethnographic exploration of children and families social work, poverty and the capability approach. Qual. Soc. Work: Res. Pract. 16 (4), 449–464.

Gupta, A., ATD Fourth World, 2015. Poverty and shame – Messages for social work. Crit. Radic. Soc. Work 3 (1), 131–139.

Gupta, A., Blumhardt, H., ATD Fourth World, 2016. Giving poverty a voice: Families experiences of social work practice in a risk-averse system. Fam. Relationsh. Soc. 5 (1), 163–172.

Gupta, A., Blumhardt, H., ATD Fourth World, 2018. Poverty, exclusion and child protection practice: The contribution of the politics of recognition & respect. Eur. J. Soc. Work 21 (2), 247–259.

Hyslop, I., Keddell, E., 2018. Outing the elephants: Exploring a new paradigm for child protection social work. Soc. Sci. 7 (7), 105.

Jones, R., 2014. The Story of Baby P: Setting the Record Straight. Policy Press, Bristol.

JRF, 2022. Going Without: Deepening Poverty in the UK. https://www.jrf.org.uk/report/going-without-deepening-poverty-uk.

Keddell, E., Davie, G., Barson, D., 2019. Child protection inequalities in Aotearoa New Zealand: Social gradient and the 'inverse intervention law. Child. Youth Serv. Rev. 104:104383.

Krumer-Nevo, M., 2016. Poverty-aware social work: A paradigm for social work practice with people in poverty. Br. J. Soc. Work 46 (6), 1793–1808.

Krumer-Nevo, M., 2020. Radical Hope: Poverty-Aware Practice for Social Work. Policy Press, Bristol.

Lakoff, G., 2014. Don't Think of an Elephant: Know Your Values and Frame the *Debate*, second ed. Chelsea Green Publishing, Vermont.

Lister, R., 2004. Poverty. Polity Press, Cambridge.

Lister, R., 2013. 'Power, not pity': Poverty and human rights. Ethics Soc. Welf. 7 (2), 109–123.

Loseke, D.R., 2011. Thinking About Social Problems: An Introduction to Constructionist Perspectives. Transaction Publishers, Piscataway, NJ.

Maguire-Jack, K., Lanier, P., Johnson-Motoyama, M., Welch, H., Dineen, M., 2015. Geographic variation in racial disparities in child maltreatment: The influence of county poverty and population density. Child Abuse Negl 47, 1–13.

Marmot, M., Allen, J., Boyce, T., Goldblatt, P., Morrison, J., 2020. Build Back Fairer: the COVID-19 Marmot Review. www.health.org.uk/publications/build-back-fairer-the-covid-19-marmot-review.

Masarik, A.S., Conger, R.D., 2017. Stress and child development: A review of the Family Stress Model. Curr. Opin. Psychol. 13, 85–90.

Morris, K., Mason, W., Bywaters, P., Featherstone, B., Daniel, B., Brady, G., et al., 2018. Social work, poverty, and child welfare interventions. Child Fam. Soc. Work 23 (3), 364–372.

Parton, N., 1985. The Politics of Child Abuse. Macmillan, London.

Saar-Heiman, Y., 2019. Poverty–aware social work in the child protection system: A critical reflection on two single–case studies. Child Fam. Soc. Work 24 (4), 610–618.

Saar-Heiman, Y., 2022. Understanding the relationships among poverty, child maltreatment, and child protection involvement: Perspectives of service users and practitioners. J. Soc. Soc. Work Res. 13 (1), 117–141.

Saar-Heiman, Y., & Krumer-Nevo, M., 2020. 'You Decide': Relationship-Based Knowledge and Parents' Participation in High-Risk Child Protection Crisis Interventions. Br. J. Soc. Work, 50 (6), 1743–1757.

Smithson, R., Gibson, M., 2017. Less than human: A qualitative study into the experience of parents involved in the child protection system. Child Fam. Soc. Work 22 (2), 565–574.

Warner, J., 2015. The Emotional Politics of Child Protection. The Policy Press, Bristol.

5

CHILD PROTECTION AND THE FAMILY COURT: AN INTRODUCTION TO LEGISLATION, POLICY AND PRACTICE

ANN POTTER ■ SARAH DENNIS

KEY POINTS

- An introduction to legislation, policy and contemporary issues underpinning child protection.
- An overview of court orders in the Family Court.
- An overview of the legal processes in the Family Court.
- Court proceedings: people and processes in the Family Court.
- Being an effective professional witness.

INTRODUCTION

The aim of this chapter is to demystify the complex legal processes within the Family Court arena. The chapter begins with an introduction to legislation and policy underpinning child protection in England (and the devolved nations); following this, the chapter outlines key child protection court orders within the Family Court and provides an overview of the legal processes in child protection court proceedings. Attention is then paid to the various people and processes within the Family Court arena, before the chapter concludes by considering how to be an effective professional witness when providing written and oral evidence. Although the primary focus is on public law child protection, some attention throughout is paid to key private family law matters that may also involve child protection professionals.

PRIVATE LAW AND PUBLIC LAW

Private law cases are normally disputes between two parents about arrangements for their child(ren) following a separation. Private law cases generally involve parents who have separated, who cannot agree on arrangements for their children, and where other means to reach agreement have failed or are not suitable. Before applying to the court, parents are usually required to attend mediation to try to resolve disagreements (unless circumstances mean this is inappropriate, such as cases involving domestic abuse).

Public law cases are brought by the state (a local authority) when there are child protection concerns about a child, related to the care given by their parents and/or carers. These cases are usually dealt with via care proceedings, which is when a local authority makes an application for a care or supervision order under s.31 Children Act 1989 (known as 'issuing proceedings'). The local authority has a duty to notify the child's parents of their application in advance, except in cases where doing so might put the child at further risk.

The focus throughout the chapter is primarily on professional practice; however, we are mindful that these are high-stakes and life-changing processes for children and families. Throughout the chapter we therefore urge readers to keep families in mind and reflect on how this sensitive work can be undertaken in a humane and family-focussed way.

AN INTRODUCTION TO THE LEGISLATION AND POLICY UNDERPINNING CHILD PROTECTION

The Children Act 1989 has provided the legal framework for child protection court proceedings in England for over 30 years. A key aim of the Act was to 'rebalance' the relationship between the state, the courts, children and their parents (Department of Health (DH), 1993). The Children Act 1989 provides the key principles that continue to guide decisions made in the Family Court:

- **Child welfare is paramount.**
- Children are **best looked after within their own families.**
- Children should have **both parents playing a full part in their lives** where possible.
- Legal proceedings should be used **as little and as lightly as possible.** No legal order should be made, unless it is better for the child than no order at all. When an order is necessary, the **least draconian order** should be used.
- When legal action *is* necessary, **delay should be avoided** and decisions made as quickly as possible.

Other legislation has subsequently been introduced, albeit the Children Act 1989 remains the overarching legal framework for child protection in England. Subsequent legislation includes:

KEY LEGISLATION IN CHILD PROTECTION (ENGLAND)	
Adoption and Children Act 2002	Introduced to align adoption processes with the Children Act 1989, this act reaffirmed that child welfare is paramount in relation to decision making, attempted to address regional variation in practice (colloquially known as 'postcode lotteries'), matching processes and post-adoption support, and introduced special guardianship orders.
Children Act 2004	Introduced following the murder of Victoria Climbié, the act focussed on strengthening interagency communication and improving outcomes for all children. **s.10** duty on local authorities to make arrangements to promote co-operation between agencies—Local Safeguarding Children's Boards (LSCB). **s.11** duty for agencies who work with children to put safeguarding arrangements in place. **Note:** the Children Act 2004 **does NOT replace the Children Act 1989—both acts remain law and each act contains different provisions.**
Children and Social Work Act 2017	Introduced to reflect policy reforms in children's social care with a focus on safeguarding and promoting the welfare of looked after children, including new support for care leavers. It introduced new 'local partnership arrangements' (social care, health and police) and introduced a national child safeguarding practice review panel.

Alongside acts of parliament, statutory guidance provides more in-depth, specific processes to guide practice. Statutory guidance must be followed, unless there are exceptional circumstances.

KEY STATUTORY GUIDANCE (ENGLAND AND WALES)

Working Together 2018	This guidance outlines the processes for inter-agency family support and child protection practice prior to any legal proceedings, including inter-agency procedures for 'immediate protection'.
Court orders and pre-proceedings 2014	This sets out the procedures for local authority (social work) practice when care proceedings are being considered and issued. This includes pre-proceedings support and work with families (such as early help services and family group conferencing), which should normally be undertaken prior to issuing care proceedings, unless urgent action is needed.

Child protection systems and legislation differ between the countries making up the UK and devolution is likely to continue to evolve (Brabender et al., 2018). The key legal differences in family justice systems in Wales, Northern Ireland and Scotland are outlined here:

LEGAL DIFFERENCES BETWEEN ENGLAND, WALES, NORTHERN IRELAND AND SCOTLAND

Wales	England and Wales have a shared judicial system and most of the Children Act 1989 and Adoption and Children Act 2002 are also applicable in Wales. In April 2016, Part III of the Children Act 1989 was replaced by The Social Services and Well-Being (Wales) Act 2014. In Wales, Court Advisory and Support Service (CAFCASS) functions are devolved to Cafcass Cymru.
Northern Ireland	Northern Ireland has a separate judicial system to England, Wales and Scotland, although the law and legal processes are very similar to those in England and Wales. Key legislation includes The Children (Northern Ireland) Order 1995 and the Adoption (Northern Ireland) Order 1987. The policy framework for child protection, Co-Operating to Safeguard Children and Young People in Northern Ireland 2017, provides a helpful overview of legal orders.
	Northern Ireland does not have a single Family Court. Child protection cases are heard in the Family Proceedings Court, County Court or the High Court. In private law cases, instead of child arrangements orders, individuals can apply for residence and contact orders. Cafcass does not exist in Northern Ireland; instead, a similar service is provided by Nigala (the NI Guardian Ad Litem Agency).
Scotland	Scotland has a different legal system to England, Wales and Northern Ireland, although Scots law has been heavily influenced by legislation from the rest of the UK. The Children (Scotland) Act 1995 is the equivalent of the Children Act 1989. Other key acts include the Adoption and Children (Scotland) Act 2007; the Children and Young People (Scotland) Act 2014 and the Children (Scotland) Act 2020.

Most public and private law family cases are heard in the Sheriff Court, with some cases heard in the Court of Session (Scotland's supreme civil court). In 'private law' cases, under s. 11 Children (Scotland) Act 1995 the court may make orders including residence orders, contact orders and specific issue orders. In 'Section 11' cases, the court may appoint a child welfare reporter to undertake enquiries including children's views and best interests recommendations. Most child welfare reporters are solicitors; however, local authorities may also undertake child welfare reports.

In child protection cases in Scotland, a referral about children's welfare might be made to the Children's Reporter. Children's Reporters are employed by the Scottish Children's Reporter Administration and decide when a child needs to be referred to a Children's Hearing. Three lay panel members hear the cases. Children's Hearings can make compulsory supervision orders for children in need of protection, or those alleged to have committed a criminal offence. If matters are not agreed, the Children's Hearing can direct the children's reporter to apply to the Sheriff Court. Cafcass does not exist in Scotland. Other professionals (such as the Safeguarder) fulfil similar roles.

Contemporary Issues

The intention of the Children Act 1989 was for child protection court proceedings to be short – on average 12 weeks. However, concerns quickly grew about numbers of court proceedings, lengthy proceedings delaying decision-making, and increasing costs (Potter et al., 2015). A series of legal protocols were developed focussed on timescales, the first introduced a 40-week timescale (Lord Chancellor's Department (LCD), 2003), subsequently reduced to 26 weeks (PD12A). Initiatives to address persistent delays included guidance for local authorities about their pre-proceedings work and case management during proceedings, reflected in the Public Law Outline (PD12A). Other initiatives sought to standardise and improve written evidence, resulting in the (optional) Social Work Evidence Template (SWET) (ADCS, 2021).

Despite this range of system reviews and initiatives, over recent years, sector leaders and the judiciary have highlighted that the family justice system was at or near 'breaking point', with pressures exacerbated by sustained national increases in the numbers of care proceedings, along with rising numbers of children in state care (Munby, 2016). The 'Care Crisis Review' provided a sector-led overview of the worsening crisis in the court system (FRG, 2018; Thomas, 2018). The review highlighted the cumulative impacts of increasing poverty due to government austerity policies, including significantly reduced funding for local authority services, particularly in already disadvantaged areas. A growing body of research also demonstrates links between deprivation, inequalities (including between ethnic groups), and increasing numbers of referrals into children's social care, child protection plans and child protection court proceedings, including stark regional variations aligned with deprivation indicators (Featherstone et al., 2018; Mason and Broadhurst, 2020; Webb et al., 2020).

Whilst there are longstanding concerns about performance and effectiveness across the family justice system, initiatives and innovations have also been introduced. Some key examples include:

- **The Family Drug and Alcohol Court** (FDAC): a 'problem-solving' child protection court for cases where parents' problems are centred on alcohol and drug use. Piloted in 2008 and rolled out in 2013, FDAC currently has 16 projects across England. FDAC proceedings follow the same structure as 'ordinary' care proceedings, but with additional, integrated support features. An independent evaluation found more parents overcoming problems, more children remaining or reuniting with parents and lower rates of further abuse or neglect a year after (compared with 'ordinary') proceedings (Harwin et al., 2016).

■ **The Nuffield Family Justice Observatory:** a group of researchers are helping to address an identified need for improved co-ordination of research planning and data sources within the family justice system, resulting in the establishment of a Family Justice Observatory (FJO) in 2019. The FJO is funded by the Nuffield Foundation; its aim is to improve understanding of the family justice system through research, to form links between academia and frontline practitioners, and to ensure that children and families get the best possible evidence-based support. Research findings from the FJO and elsewhere are informing broader practice innovations relating to issues within Family Court proceedings, for example, in public law, a programme of research into recurrent care proceedings with mothers (and more recently fathers too) with the aim of reducing 'repeat removals' of children from parents (Ryan, 2021). For more regarding this issue, see Chapter 19d.

A final area to address briefly is the impact of COVID-19. During the pandemic, many child protection court hearings became *remote*, conducted over telephone or video call systems. As practice has developed, some have been *hybrid* hearings, where some of the parties and their legal representatives are present in the courtroom, and others are participating remotely. It seems likely that remote and hybrid hearings will remain in place for some cases; however, experience of these hearings has raised important issues for family members involved in proceedings, in relation to fairness and access to justice. Recent research (Nuffield Family Justice Observatory, 2020) highlights potential barriers to families' participation in remote hearings, including:

■ Access issues (including technology and Wi-Fi)
■ Confidentiality (particularly in relation to the location of all parties)
■ Appropriate support before, during and after court hearings (including understanding what is happening in the case)

Some groups such as disabled parents, or parties in need of an interpreter, may be particularly disadvantaged by remote hearings. Professionals must be mindful of potential accessibility issues and support families as best they can to understand and participate meaningfully in the legal process.

AN OVERVIEW OF COURT ORDERS IN THE FAMILY COURTS

There is a longstanding expectation that child protection professionals work in 'partnership' with parents (DH, 1995; Department for Education (DfE), 2018). The use of court proceedings by local authorities to acquire parental responsibility in relation to children, and to enable removal of children from their families, was always to be a 'last resort'. However, this section will now address the orders available in circumstances where no alternative option would effectively safeguard a child.

Public Law: Child Protection

Whilst an initial application in care proceedings will be for a care or supervision order, the court is entitled to make different types of orders, or no order at all, if the child's welfare requires it. At the start of care proceedings, the court may make *interim* (temporary) orders. At the end of care proceedings, depending on the long-term care plan for the child, the court may make a care order, a supervision order, a special guardianship order, a child arrangements order, another type of order or no order at all. Key orders made within and at the end of care proceedings are summarised below:

KEY ORDERS IN CARE PROCEEDINGS	
Name	**Key Points**
Interim Supervision Order/Supervision Order Children Act 1989 s.38/s.31	■ Places child/young person under *supervision* of the local authority ■ Parents retain parental responsibility and care of child/young person. Local authority *does not* acquire parental responsibility ■ Local authority must "advise, assist and befriend" the child/young person ■ Full supervision order can be granted for a year, or extended up to 3 years

Name	Key Points
Interim Care Order/ Care Order Children Act 1989 s.38/s.31	■ Places child/young person in the *care* of the local authority ■ Can only be made if child/ young person is suffering from, or likely to suffer, significant harm, linked with parental care ■ Local authority is given parental responsibility and can determine how far parents exercise their responsibility ■ An interim care order (ICO) is a temporary care order, pending the outcome of the full care proceedings process ■ Full care order lasts until child/young person is 18 (unless discharged earlier)
Special Guardianship Order Adoption and Children Act 2002 s.115	■ Grants parental responsibility to somebody other than the child/ young person's parents They become their *special guardian,* providing a home and long-term care ■ Special guardian can make most decisions without needing the parents' agreement, although parents retain parental responsibility. Local authority *does not* have parental responsibility ■ Usually lasts until child/ young person is 18. Can be discharged only if circumstances change significantly
Emergency Protection Order Children Act 1989 s.44	■ Grants the local authority power to remove a child from their home, or to keep them in a place of safety ■ Drastic intervention, and the evidence to the court must show that it is necessary and proportionate ■ Initially granted for up to 8 days, can be extended for up to 7 days, maximum length of an Emergency Protection Order (EPO) is 15 days ■ Local authority must return the child to their parents as soon as this is safe ■ EPO applications are not categorised as care proceedings, although they may lead on to a care proceedings application in some instances

In some circumstances, professionals may be so concerned about a child they may need to take more immediate action; this is covered in more depth in Chapter 16 but is also included briefly here for reference.

Other court proceedings may follow care proceedings, particularly if court orders are required for a child's long-term (permanence) care plan. For example, if the plan for a child is adoption, then an application for a *placement order* may be made towards the end of care proceedings. The same judge or magistrates will hear the placement order application and the care proceedings together, at the same time, even though they are different proceedings. Adoption proceedings are also separate – any court hearings relating to an adoption order application will be listed at a later date.

PROCEEDINGS/ORDERS THAT MAY BE MADE WHEN A CHILD'S PERMANENCE PLAN IS ADOPTION

Name	Key Points
Placement Order Adoption and Children Act 2002 s.21	■ Authorises a local authority to place a child/young person with prospective adopters ■ The court "must be satisfied that no other permanence option is appropriate and that only adoption will meet the needs of the child" (DfE, 2014, 25) ■ Local authority, birth parents and prospective adopters share parental responsibility, but in practice birth parents' responsibility is very limited ■ Lasts until an adoption order is granted (or the placement order is revoked/child or young person reaches 18)
Adoption Order Adoption and Children Act 2002 s.46	■ The most draconian order the Family Court can make ■ Permanently severs legal relationships between a child/young person and their birth parents ■ Mother and any other parent lose their parental responsibility ■ Parental responsibility is granted to the adoptive parents

Child protection proceedings can be complex and some may involve specific issues, requiring a particular legal response. Examples of other legal orders/powers/proceedings that you may come across, relating to child protection and the Family Court, are below (not an exhaustive list):

OTHER LEGAL ORDERS/POWERS/ PROCEEDINGS

Police Powers of Protection
Children Act 1989 s.46
■ These powers are not overseen by the court and there is no 'order'. Allow the police to remove a child/young person from home in an emergency. Last no longer than 72 hours. May precede an application by the local authority for an EPO, or care proceedings.

Recovery Order
Children Act 1989 s.50
■ Can direct that a child/young person who is 'in care' is produced, searched for, or removed from premises by the police.

Child Assessment Order
Children Act 1989 s.43
■ Enables assessment of a child/young person's health and development if their parents are not in agreement. These orders are used rarely.

Secure Accommodation Order
Children Act 1989 s.25
■ Child/young person can be placed or kept in accommodation provided to restrict their liberty. This is a draconian order and can only be granted under specific criteria. Note there is a severe shortage of approved secure accommodation, as highlighted in the judgment of *MacDonald J. in:* Lancashire CC v G (No3) (Continuing Unavailability of Secure Accommodation) [2020] EWHC 3280 (Fam).

Inherent Jurisdiction Proceedings
Children Act 1989 s.100(4)
■ Heard in the High Court. A way for the court to make decisions about a child/young person's circumstances when issues cannot be dealt with by existing legal frameworks. Cases might relate to medical treatment; child abduction; wardship (where important steps in a child's life need court consent); deprivation of liberty.

Forced Marriage Protection Order
Family Law Act 1996 s.63
■ Can help individuals who are being forced into marriage, or already in a forced marriage (see chapter 10e for more on forced marriage).

Female Genital Mutilation (FGM) Protection Orders

Female Genital Mutilation Act 2003 Schedule 2
■ Can help those at risk of FGM, or victims of FGM, to keep them safe or assist their return to the UK (see chapter 10f for more on FGM). Further details of these orders can be found within the relevant statute by searching https://www.legislation.gov.uk/.

In times of difficulty, parents may sometimes ask or agree for the local authority to temporarily care for their child. These 'Section 20 accommodation' arrangements are in regular use; however, they should only be used with the informed consent of those with parental responsibility (usually the parent/s). The Family Court is not involved, and there is no 'order'. Importantly, the local authority does **not** acquire parental responsibility within a Section 20 agreement – those with parental responsibility retain all their rights to make decisions about their child.

VOLUNTARY ACCOMMODATION

■ This is a section of the Children Act 1989 designed to provide temporary accommodation for children in agreement with parents. Those with parental responsibility must have given informed consent for any Section 20 agreement to be lawful.
■ Parental responsibility remains with the parent(s) and is not acquired by the local authority.
■ The use of Section 20's should be transparent; these should not be used to enable a 'swift' removal of children where there is no time to issue proceedings.
■ They should not be used for excessive periods of time.

Children Act 1989 s.20.

Private Law Proceedings

Private law cases make up a significant proportion of the work of the Family Court and regularly involve child protection issues (MoJ, 2020). Recent research provides a profile of private law cases in England and Wales (Cusworth et al., 2020, 2021):

■ Annually there are more than twice as many private law cases as public law cases.
■ Annually under 1% of families with dependent children make private law applications
■ About one fourth of these applications are made by someone involved in a previous application within the last 3 years
■ Most are brought by fathers who live apart from their children and concern a single child aged 1 to 9 years.
■ There is a clear link between social deprivation and private law applications.

Parents, or anybody with whom the child has lived for 3 years, can apply directly to the court requesting a Section 8 (s.8) order. Others (such as grandparents) need the permission of the court to apply. There are three main types of legal order (Table 5.1) that can be applied for under s.8 of the Children Act 1989:

An order made under s.8 usually lasts until a child is 16 and will always cease when the child reaches 18 years old. In private law cases, additional reports may be requested to supplement legal proceedings, including:

TABLE 5.1	
Legal Order	
Name	**Key Points**
Child arrangements order	States who the child lives with/spends time with. If the order states that a child will live with somebody, that person will be granted parental responsibility (if they do not already have it).
Prohibited steps order	Prevents somebody with parental responsibility undertaking certain action (e.g., moving abroad with child) without court consent.
Specific issue order	Determines a specific issue about a child (e.g., which school they should attend).

Section 7 reports (s.7 of the Children Act 1989): A Section 7 report is completed where parents disagree about the best plans for the child and there are concerns about the child's welfare, sometimes including safeguarding concerns or allegations. The court will usually specify which issues the report should focus on and will order completion by a date set by the court, ideally within 8 to 12 weeks, but more usually within several months given resource pressures within the system. In private law, these are undertaken by a Court Advisory and Support Service (CAFCASS) worker, or if there has been extensive or recent social work involvement with the family this will be undertaken by a social worker.

Section 37 reports (s.37 Children Act 1989): A Section 37 report is ordered when there are significant concerns about a child's welfare, which are so serious that a local authority application for a care or supervision order might be necessary. These are always completed by the local authority and are ordered to be completed by a date set by the court, ideally within 2 to 3 months, but more usually within several months given resource pressures within the system.

16.4 appointment (FPR, 2010): A '16.4 appointment' occurs when the court decides to make the child a party in private law proceedings. This is usually due to particularly complex issues within the case that require the child to be formally represented within the proceedings. A CAFCASS Children's Guardian will usually be appointed for the child. Alternatively, a caseworker from the National Youth Advocacy Service (NYAS) may be appointed to this role, supported by NYAS Legal Services.

REFLECTIVE QUESTION

What similarities/differences might exist for social workers involved in private law and public law cases?

AN OVERVIEW OF THE LEGAL PROCESSES IN CHILD PROTECTION COURT PROCEEDINGS

There are occasions where efforts to support parents are unsuccessful and social workers consider that to safeguard a child, it is necessary to ask the court for an order to acquire parental responsibility and to allow the removal of the child from the parents' care. For the court to approve this most severe intervention in family life, it must be satisfied that the local authority's (social work) evidence meets the threshold criteria for care proceedings:

(a) that the child concerned is suffering, or is likely to suffer, significant harm; **and**

(b) that the harm, or likelihood of harm, is attributable to —

   (i) *the care given to the child, or likely to be given to him if the order were not made, not being what it would be reasonable to expect a parent to give to him; or*

   (ii) *the child's being beyond parental control.*

(Children Act 1989 s.31(2))

Care proceedings are very sensitive, emotionally demanding work, and the long-term implications for children and their families are significant. It is also a difficult aspect of child protection work for professionals, which can be further compounded when navigating the complex legal stages involved. This section therefore focusses on simplifying these processes. Good reflective supervision (see Chapter 7) throughout this process should ensure decisions are made fairly and that families and social workers are emotionally supported in this work. Families should always be encouraged and helped to access independent legal advice and directed to family focussed resources to help them understand and navigate this process.

Pre-Proceedings Processes

Statutory guidance outlines the processes for inter-agency child protection practice prior to any legal proceedings in 'Working Together to Safeguard Children' (DfE, 2018) and 'Court orders and pre-proceedings for local authorities' (DfE, 2014). Key elements of the processes relating to care proceedings prior to court are summarised in Table 5.2.

Due to concern about the impact of delay on children's well-being, the law requires that care proceedings are concluded within 26 weeks from the date of issue. However, 'there will always be cases which are highly complex for which 26 weeks is not a realistic

TABLE 5.2
Key elements of the processes relating to care proceedings prior to court

Activity	Purpose	Who's Involved?
Management discussion	The social worker should discuss their concerns with their manager to consider whether a legal planning meeting is required, to decide whether care proceedings are necessary to safeguard the child.	**Social Worker** **Team Manager**
Legal planning meetings (*or legal gateway meetings*)	The aim is to conduct a professional discussion and analysis to decide if care proceedings should formally be considered. If it is agreed that care proceedings are being formally considered, the local authority (LA) must write to the parents to inform them (known as a **letter before proceedings**). This triggers an entitlement for parents to seek free legal advice.	**Social Worker** **Team Manager** **LA Lawyer**
Pre-proceedings meetings	Parents are normally invited (with their solicitor) to discuss the social worker's concerns and reasons for considering care proceedings. A pre-proceedings meeting may decide that care proceedings should be issued straight away, or that further (time limited) pre-proceedings support will be offered to resolve concerns and avoid care proceedings.	**Parent(s)** **Parent(s)' Solicitor(s)** **Social Worker** **Team Manager** **LA Lawyer**
Pre-proceedings support and work with families	If pre-proceedings work is an outcome of a pre-proceedings meeting, the agreed plan for support and work with the family must be focussed, involve a clear plan of support and include clear timescales for review and decision-making if the work proves ineffective. **Remember**: The aim of pre-proceedings work is to avoid care proceedings, support families to resolve issues and not simply gather further evidence.	**Family** **Social Worker** **Other agencies**
Applying to the court	If care proceedings are issued, the local authority solicitor completes the application form and sends this to the Family Court, accompanied by the social worker's written evidence and any other documents. **Following this:** *First*, CAFCASS is informed to allocate a Children's Guardian. *Second*, the application is reviewed by a judge who decides at which level of judiciary the case will be heard. *Third*, formal notice that care proceedings have been issued is sent to all parties. *Finally*, the timetable for the case is determined and all respondents are asked to provide written statements of evidence in advance of the first court hearing.	**LA Solicitor** **Social Worker** **CAFCASS** **Parent(s)** **Parent(s)' Solicitor(s)**

timeframe', and it is therefore possible for extensions to be granted for periods of up to 8 weeks at a time to 'resolve the proceedings justly' (DfE, 2014, 26). This section outlines the work that should be undertaken during the various court hearings included within this process. The Public Law Outline (PLO) is a legal protocol that sets out how care proceedings should be conducted in relation to judicial case management, within the mandatory 26-week time limit (PD12A). The PLO explains the types of court hearings to be held at each stage in the process. Parties to proceedings are normally required to attend court hearings, unless excused by the court. The exception to this is that children and young people do not normally attend child protection court hearings, as in most cases this is considered contrary to the child's welfare. The Children's Guardian and child's solicitor are the representatives of the child in court. Recent practice developments have focussed on providing ways for children and young people to participate in their care proceedings even when not present in court.

TYPES OF COURT HEARINGS

Case Management Hearing (CMH)
The first court hearing, involving consideration of the case court timetable, if additional evidence or further assessment is required, and whether parties agree the child's interim plans. If there is agreement between parties about interim plans, the hearing involves lawyers addressing the judge or magistrates and an agreed order is drawn up. The parties will be present in the courtroom, but no oral evidence is heard. If plans are not agreed, and agreement cannot be reached in discussions between parties outside the courtroom, then the judge or magistrates may hear oral witness evidence to decide interim plans. If there is insufficient time, an additional *contested hearing* may be listed at a later date, when oral evidence relating to the dispute about the interim plans is heard and a decision is made by the court.

Issues Resolution Hearing (IRH)
Takes place towards the end of care proceedings and involves consideration of the local authority's final care plan for the child. If the parties agree, then this may be the final hearing in the care proceedings. However, if any aspects of the care plan are not agreed, and if agreement cannot be reached by discussions between the parties outside the courtroom, then a final hearing will need to be listed for witness evidence to be heard and for the court to reach a decision.

Final hearing
Only required if any parties disagree with an aspect of the final care plan, and if evidence needs to be heard from witnesses to decide a particular issue(s). Only specific aspects of the care plan that are in dispute will be dealt with during final hearings, the length of any final hearing is determined by the range and complexity of issues to decide.

Whilst the formal aspects of planning and legal decision-making for children occur within the court room, important conversations between parties also occur outside of the formal court arena that can be useful and constructive in moving a case forward. Lawyers hold pre-hearing discussions with their own clients and other parties' representatives, seeking to explore if agreement can be reached in relation to proposed plans, or to signal that their client is not in agreement and the matter may need to be decided via a contested hearing. Discussions sometimes take place within meeting rooms in the court building, or even corridors. It is important to check with any lawyers whether they are happy with you talking directly to their client once you are in the court building. Post-hearing discussions are used to clarify what was agreed or not in court, to agree next steps and to receive constructive feedback on written and oral evidence to assist professional development. If a court hearing has resulted in an upsetting decision for a parent, then it is important also to consider how best they can be supported. If the hearing has involved you giving evidence that has been critical of them, then they may not want support from you, so alternative support should be considered. Children and young people may also need support after a hearing, even if they have not been present in court, to understand what has been decided and the implications for them.

CHILD PROTECTION COURT PROCEEDINGS: PEOPLE AND PROCESSES IN THE FAMILY COURT

The Family Court forms part of the wider civil justice system in England. Fig 5.1 summarises the overall courts structure (Judiciary UK, 2021).

The Family Court is a 'single court', established in its current form in 2014 (Potter et al., 2015). It is a national structure, made up of regional Family Court centres, each led by a senior circuit judge (Designated Family Judge). The administration of the family court is organised by HMCTS (His Majesty's Courts and Tribunal Service). The Family Court consists of different levels

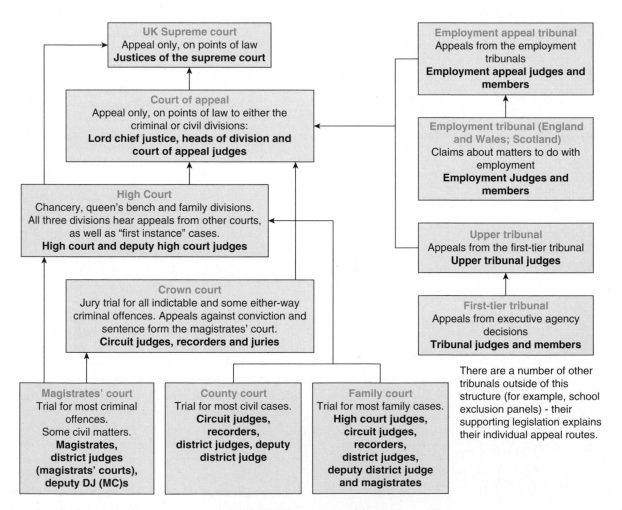

Fig. 5.1 ■ The structure of the courts.

of judiciary, to which cases are allocated according to complexity. Complexity in the Family Court does not neatly equate to 'seriousness'. A very 'serious' case may be heard by magistrates or a District Judge if it is less legally complex or has fewer witnesses. Cases allocated to higher levels of judiciary will have additional legal complexities (i.e. international elements or contentious expert opinions). The Family Court always hears cases 'in private' to ensure confidentiality. Recently, there have been developments to allow more transparency in relation to family court proceedings, to improve public trust. For example, limited press reporting of family court cases may now be permitted. Family Court work includes both private law and public law cases.

Who's Who in the Family Court?

The judiciary of the Family Court is comprised of magistrates and judges. *Magistrates* are 'lay' volunteers within the magistrates' level of the Family Court. Magistrates are drawn from the local community and have a range of life experience and/or professional qualifications. A legally qualified legal adviser assists magistrates in their decision-making. Magistrates deal with the least complex cases that come before the Family Court. All other judges who sit in the different levels of the Family Court are legally qualified and have previously practised as solicitors or barristers.

Deputy District Judges and District Judges will deal with cases that are considered too complex for magistrates but where the legal issues are not so complex that a Circuit Judge or High Court Judge is required. Circuit Judges deal with more complex cases. High Court Judges deal with the most complex cases. Recorders are practising lawyers, appointed as a part-time recorder (judge). They combine their usual job as a solicitor or barrister with several days per year *sitting* (working) in the Family Court, dealing with Family Court cases in the same way as a District Judge or Circuit Judge. Sometimes, if they are sufficiently experienced, Recorders will also sit as a judge in High Court family cases. It is important to understand that the 'complexity' of a case in the Family Court does not necessarily equate to the apparent 'seriousness' of the issues. Cases allocated to higher levels of judiciary in the Family Court will have additional *legal* complexities, for example international elements or contentious scientific or medical opinions.

HOW TO ADDRESS MAGISTRATES AND JUDGES IN THE FAMILY COURT

Level of Family Court judiciary	How to address directly (e.g. in court, whilst giving evidence)	How to address indirectly (e.g. in discussion with others)
Magistrates	Your worship(s) or Sir, Madam or Ma'am	Their worships
District Judge	Sir, Madam or Ma'am	District Judge [*surname*]
Circuit Judge	Your Honour	Her/His Honour Judge [*surname*]
High Court Judge	My Lady, My Lord	Ms/Mrs/ Mr Justice [*surname*]
Recorders	Your Honour	Recorder [*surname*]

Family members and local authorities who are directly involved in child protection court proceedings are known as *parties*. Parties to proceedings have access to all the court papers and are required to attend court hearings. In child protection cases, parties are either the *applicant* (the local authority) or a *respondent*. Parents and each child are always separate respondents. Parents and the child are entitled to free legal representation, publicly funded via the Legal Aid Agency. The child is also represented by their Children's Guardian (*see below*), who will usually be responsible for appointing the solicitor for the child. Parents or family members who represent themselves in court, communicating with the Judge directly instead of via a legal representative, are known as *litigants in person*.

There are two types of lawyers in the Family Court: solicitors and barristers. Both are legally qualified and may address the court during court hearings. The difference between solicitors and barristers relates to their professional training and legal role, although there are some overlaps. After acquiring a legal qualification, trainee lawyers specialise as a solicitor or barrister. Solicitors usually work in 'firms' and are usually the first point of contact for member of the public or professionals seeking legal advice. Barristers usually work in 'chambers' and are normally instructed by solicitors for court hearings, at which the barrister (not solicitor) will address the court. Within child protection proceedings, each party instructs a solicitor who will be involved throughout. In some cases, solicitors may instruct a barrister for specific court hearings, to avail of a barrister's specialist in-court advocacy skills, and/or to avoid the solicitor being tied into potentially lengthy court hearings. Within the Family Court, solicitors may address the court and ask questions of witnesses in court hearings at any level of the court, without restriction.

CLOSER LOOK: OTHER PEOPLE IN THE COURT ARENA

Ushers: Court staff who direct people to the relevant courtroom and attend to witnesses when they take their oath/affirm. Ushers usually wear court gowns and are normally outside the courtroom before hearings and by the witness box during hearings. You 'book in' with the usher when arriving at court.

Clerks: Court staff who provide administrative support to the judge. Clerks usually sit in front of the judge in the courtroom.

Legal advisor/clerk to the magistrates: Legally qualified court staff who provide legal advice to the magistrates. Legal advisors normally sit with the magistrates at the front of the court.

Non-legal advocate/intermediary: Advocates or intermediaries may assist vulnerable or disabled witnesses to understand the proceedings and communicate with the court.

Interpreters: Interpreters will assist witnesses for whom spoken English is not their first language.

CAFCASS, is a 'non-departmental government body' funded by central government. CAFCASS employs qualified social workers who provide independent, professional social work advice to the court, focusing on the child's welfare as paramount. The court must consider the advice of the CAFCASS worker, although the court is not required to agree or to follow the CAFCASS recommendation. CAFCASS involvement ends when a court case comes to an end. CAFCASS workers are involved in public law and private law proceedings.

In public law child protection proceedings, CAFCASS workers are appointed in the role of the Children's Guardian. The duties of the Children's Guardian include:

1. Appointing a solicitor for the child, who will act on the instructions of the Guardian, unless the child is old enough, able to and wishes to instruct their solicitor independently.
2. Analysing information from other professionals, identifying any gaps in evidence and discussing with the child's solicitor what additional evidence may be required to assist the court with its decision.
3. Spending time with the child and family to establish their views, circumstances and what support they might need. The Guardian must provide independent advice to the court about the expressed wishes and feelings of the child (as far as they are able to), and about the proposed plans of the local authority.
4. Making recommendations to the court (written and verbal) about the best plans for the child, based on their independent enquiries, including an analysis of the child's needs and whether the Guardian agrees with the local authority plans for the child.

In most private law cases, the CAFCASS worker is called a Family Court Adviser (FCA). The duties of the FCA include:

1. Screening all private law applications for safeguarding concerns.
2. Checking police and local authority information relating to the parties, which is sent to the court in a 'safeguarding letter'.
3. Undertaking Section 7 reports to advise on the welfare of the child when parents disagree about the details of a child arrangements order.
4. Acting as a Children's Guardian in 16.4 appointments.
5. Attending the first court hearing, known as a First Hearing Dispute Resolution Appointment (FHDRA) to assist discussions and see whether agreement can safely be reached about a child's circumstances.

REFLECTIVE QUESTIONS

■ There are several checks and balances included within the system, including a range of professionals independent from local authorities involved within proceedings (i.e. judges, family's solicitors and CAFCASS).
■ Why do you think it is important to have independent opinions?
■ Do you think this means families always get fair representation within the court arena?

BEING AN EFFECTIVE PROFESSIONAL WITNESS

Many professionals find court proceedings daunting, often due to a lack of familiarity with legal processes and courtroom etiquette. Understanding how court proceedings are conducted can help in developing as an effective professional witness. Child protection court proceedings have a mix of witnesses providing written and sometimes oral evidence, these include *ordinary*, *professional*, and *expert* witnesses:

- **Ordinary witnesses** may be a 'lay' person, such as a parent. They are only permitted to give factual evidence (not opinion-based) from direct experience about what they have seen or heard.
- **Professional witnesses** provide factual and *opinion-based* evidence and make recommendations about plans for children, based on their work with the family and their specific professional expertise. In care proceedings, the key professional witnesses are local authority social workers and Children's Guardians. Professional witnesses are not classed as 'expert' witnesses within the legal rules (see below) because they are parties to proceedings and therefore cannot be categorised as independent.
- **Expert witnesses** are professionals appointed by courts to provide *independent* opinion-based evidence, in relation to a specific issue requiring their specialist knowledge and expertise. For example, a consultant paediatrician may be appointed where a child has sustained serious inflicted injuries, and the cause is not clear or is disputed. Sometimes an Independent Social Worker (ISW) may be appointed as an expert witness if there is a conflict of interest or if the local authority cannot complete the social work assessments for a specific reason. Independent expert witnesses are only appointed in certain cases and only when 'necessary' (Children and Families Act 2014, s.13(6)).

Evidence in court is presented in two forms, written and oral. Being an effective professional witness involves creating a positive impression via your written evidence and in the courtroom. Child protection proceedings always start with and are based on written evidence (*except for some emergency applications, see Chapter 16*). In some cases,

proceedings will be dealt with via written evidence only. Written evidence must always include a signed 'statement of truth' and has the same legal status as oral evidence given in court 'under oath'. In care proceedings, written social work evidence forms part of the initial application by the local authority to the court. This should provide:

- a brief background,
- the reasons for the application,
- the proposed (interim) care plan for the child.

Written evidence should comply with required formats; however, professional witnesses should also ensure that they are able to communicate effectively to a legal 'audience', which means developing a good understanding of how the legal process works, and what judges and magistrates want and expect from professional witnesses. The social worker's written evidence may be provided in a standardised format known as the Social Work Evidence Template (SWET) (ADCS, 2021). There is a balance to be struck between providing enough detail to inform the court properly of the issues, the professional analysis and recommendation, whilst also being succinct and focussed on the issues that the court must decide on. In general, it is important to remember that at all stages in the legal process, the judge or magistrates need evidence as to:

- why they should grant this particular order,
- at this particular time.

This is especially important if there is an application at the start of (or during) the proceedings to remove a child from their parent(s) under an Interim Care Order.

At the end of proceedings, the court will also need succinct evidence that analyses and compares all *reasonable* options for the long-term care of the child, explaining why the recommendation is for a particular care plan and a particular order (or no order).

A common concern for professional witnesses is whether to include theory and research findings within their evidence. Theory and research can be useful. For example, it can be used to explain to the court why a particular model for practice with families is appropriate in general, or to illustrate general principles that are applied in care planning and placement decision-making. However, caution is advised if research findings are to be used to 'justify' a decision or recommendation about a particular child or family member. Attributing specific theory and/or research findings to individual characteristics, circumstances or potential outcomes for a child or family is likely to leave you open to challenge within cross-examination, as it is usually possible for lawyers to find alternative research or theory that can be applied or interpreted in different ways. For a helpful discussion of this issue, see Robertson and Broadhurst (2019).

Oral evidence is only required when an aspect of the case is *contested* (disputed) by one or more of the parties, and the court needs to hear oral evidence from witnesses to reach a decision. Oral evidence will be heard within a *contested hearing*, which may be one of the usual court hearings in the process, or it may be an additional hearing. Issues may be contested at any stage in the proceedings.

Being an effective professional witness is achieved with good quality, values-based professional practice with families, communicated effectively within written and oral evidence. However, it is important to understand and accept the adversarial nature of the legal process, which is most apparent in contested hearings (Welbourne, 2016; Potter, 2020). This requires lawyers to argue their client's case, and to seek to undermine their 'opponent's' case. Lawyers opposing the local authority's application in care proceedings will closely scrutinise all written evidence for potential lines of cross-examination, with a view to undermining the local authority's case. This can be challenging. However, it is important to remember that cross-examination is not necessarily a reflection of the merits of the application or the quality of the written evidence. Challenging cross-examination of a witness may be a strategy by a lawyer to undermine 'good' professional evidence, in order to pursue their client's case.

Research into how social work evidence in care proceedings is evaluated has identified aspects of communication and presentation within written and oral evidence that are likely to promote positive judicial evaluations of witness credibility and reliability. In both written and oral evidence, the crucial factors are thoroughness, focus, balance, clarity of expression, empathy and compassion; when giving oral evidence, confidence and emotional containment are also important (Potter, 2020).

Behavioural and presentational expectations for professional and other witnesses in court hearings,

described as 'court culture' and etiquette, emphasise formal dress, politeness and deference to authority (McCaul, 2011; Roach Anleu et al., 2014). Clarity about what the court expects of professional witnesses

---

CLOSER LOOK: PRACTICAL TIPS FOR MANAGING ORAL EVIDENCE AND CROSS-EXAMINATION

■ **Try always to address your answers to the judge or magistrates.** This means looking at the lawyer when they ask you a question but remembering to turn to look at the judge or magistrates to answer (even if they are not looking at you).

■ **Try always to remain calm and composed.** This means trying not to take 'critical' cross-examination questions personally, remembering that your role as a witness is to provide information to help the court, not to engage in a battle with a lawyer. It can help to remember and understand that lawyers must present their client's case, regardless of its merits.

■ **Remember that you can take a moment to think before answering a question** (but try not to pause too long!) and you can ask for a question to be repeated if required.

■ Try always to present **as a balanced, trustworthy professional who has compassion for the family members in the case.** Acknowledge parents' strengths and their love for their child, but also be clear about any concerns and your evidence for these. This will be easier if you have already used this approach in your written evidence.

---

and an informed understanding of legal processes can help professionals to be more effective and to feel more confident when preparing written evidence and giving oral evidence (Potter, 2020). Good quality court skills training and/or 'shadowing' other professional witnesses in court hearings, especially contested hearings involving oral evidence, can be particularly helpful.

CONCLUSION

Child protection proceedings in the Family Court are inter-disciplinary, involving legal and social work professionals, and often also health and other professionals. For non-legal professionals, the court environment, processes and terminology can feel unfamiliar and, at times, intimidating. The aim here has been to 'demystify' the legal and court processes, to develop positive professional practice in individual cases, with the potential to improve outcomes for children and families.

REFLECTIVE QUESTIONS

- How can you develop your practical understanding of legal structures and processes?
- How can you best prepare for being an effective professional witness in any particular case?
- How can you best support children and families as they navigate these legal processes?

FURTHER READING

Cafcass (Child and Family Court Advisory and Support Service): Cafcass represents children in family court cases in England and independently advises the family courts about what is safe for children and in their best interests. https://www.cafcass.gov.uk/

Cafcass Cymru: Cafcass service for Wales. https://gov.wales/cafcass-cymru

Family Rights Group: Accessible legal information for families involved in child protection court proceedings. https://frg.org.uk/

Family Procedure Rules 2010, SI 2010/2955 http://www.justice.gov.uk/courts/procedure-rules/family/rules_pd_menu

Legislation: UK government site containing electronic/searchable versions of all legislation enacted or amended. https://www.legislation.gov.uk/

NIGALA (NI Guardian Ad Litem Agency): NIGALA represents children in Northern Ireland who are subjects of public law and adoption proceedings before the courts. https://nigala.hscni.net/about-nigala/

Nuffield Family Justice Observatory: Research-based resources which aim to improve the lives of children and families by putting data and evidence at the heart of the family justice system. https://www.nuffieldfjo.org.uk/

Research in Practice: Supports evidence-informed practice with children and families, young people and adults, including parents' legal rights. https://supportingparents.researchinpractice.org.uk/

SCRA (Scottish Children's Reporter Administration): SCRA supports children who may require referral to the courts for compulsory supervision due to child protection or related concerns. https://www.scra.gov.uk/

Social Work Evidence Template (SWET): A resource developed by the Association of Directors of Children's Services to support social workers required to give evidence in the child and family courts. https://adcs.org.uk/care/article/SWET

REFERENCES

ADCS (Association of Directors of Children's Services), 2021. Social Work Evidence Template (SWET) Updates https://adcs.org.uk/care/article/SWET

Brabender, L., Verdan, A., Henke, R., 2018. A Handbook on Family Law Relating to Children in Scotland and in England & Wales. https://www.judiciary.uk.

Cusworth, L., Bedston, S., Trinder, L., Broadhurst, K., Pattinson, B., 2020. Uncovering Private Family Law: Who's Coming to Court in Wales? Nuffield Family Justice Observatory, London.

Cusworth, L., Bedston, S., Alrouh, B., Broadhurst, K., Johnson, R.D., Akbari, A., et al., 2021. Uncovering Private Family Law: Who's Coming to Court in England? Nuffield Family Justice Observatory, London.

Department for Education (DfE), 2014. Court Orders and Pre-Proceedings for Local Authorities. Department for Education, London.

Department for Education (DfE), 2018. Working Together to Safeguard Children: A Guide to Inter-Agency Working to Safeguard and Promote the Welfare of Children. HMSO, London.

Department of Health (DH), 1993. Children Act Report 1992. HMSO, London.

Department of Health (DH), 1995. The Challenge of Partnership in Child Protection: Practice Guide. HMSO, London.

Family Law Act, 1996. https://www.legislation.gov.uk/ukpga/1996/27/contents.

Featherstone, B., Gupta, A., Morris, K., White, S., 2018. Protecting Children: A Social Model. Policy Press, Bristol.

Female Genital Mutilation Act, 2003. https://www.legislation.gov.uk/ukpga/2003/31/contents.

FRG (Family Rights Group), 2018. Care Crisis Review: options for change, London: Family Rights Group.

Harwin, J., Alrouh, B., Ryan, M., McQuarrie, T., Golding, L., Broadhurst, K., et al., 2016. After FDAC: Outcomes 5 Years Later. Final Report. Lancaster University, Lancaster. http://wp.lancs.ac.uk/cfj-fdac/publications/.

Lord Chancellor's Department (LCD), 2003. Protocol for Judicial Case Management in Public Law Children Act Cases. Lord Chancellor's Department, London.

Mason, C., Broadhurst, K., 2020. Discussion paper: *What explains marked regional variations in infant care?* Nuffield Family Justice Observatory, London.

McCaul, K., 2011. Understanding courtroom communication through cultural Scripts. In: Watgner, A., Cheng, L. (Eds.), Exploring Courtroom Discourse: The Language of Power and Control. Ashgate, Farnham.

Ministry of Justice (MoJ), 2020. Assessing Risk of Harm to Children and Parents in Private Law Children Cases: Final Report. Crown Copyright, London.

Munby, J., 2016. 'View from the President's Chambers: care cases: the looming crisis' [2016]. Fam. Law. 1227.

Nuffield Family Justice Observatory, 2020. Remote Hearings in the Family Justice System: A Rapid Consultation. Nuffield Family Justice Observatory, London.

Potter, A., 2020. Local Authority Social Workers' Evidence in Care Proceedings: social work and legal evaluations of professional expertise [Online]. University of Bristol, Bristol. https://research-information.bris.ac.uk/ws/portalfiles/portal/251827612/Potter_Ann_PhD_THESIS_DEFINITIVE_COPY.pdf.

Potter, A., Newton, K., McLaughlin, H., 2015. 'It's good to talk'–judicial allocation decision making and the Family Court. J. Soc. Welf. Fam. Law 37 (2), 18–193.

Practice Direction 12a Care (PD12A), Supervision and Other Part 4 Proceedings: Guide to Case Management. The Public Law Outline. https://www.justice.gov.uk/downloads/protecting-the-vulnerable/care-proceeding-reform/pd12a.pdf.

Roach Anleu, S., Mack, K., Tutton, J., 2014. Judicial humour in the Australian courtroom. Melb. Univ. L. Rev. 38 (2), 621–665.

Robertson, L., Broadhurst, K., 2019. Introducing social science evidence in family court decision-making and adjudication: evidence from England and Wales. Int. J. Law Policy Fam. 33, 181–203.

Ryan, M., 2021. Recurrent Care Proceedings: Five Key Areas for Reflection From the Research. Spotlight Series. Nuffield Family Justice Observatory, London.

Adoption and Children Act 2002.

The Adoption (Northern Ireland) Order, 1987 No. 2203 (N.I. 22) https://www.legislation.gov.uk/nisi/1987/2203/contents/made.

The Children Act, 1989 c.41 https://www.legislation.gov.uk/ukpga/1989/41/contents.

The Children Act, 2004 c.31 https://www.legislation.gov.uk/ukpga/2004/31/contents.

The Children (Northern Ireland) Order, 1995 No. 755 (N.I. 2) https://www.legislation.gov.uk/nisi/1995/755/contents/made.

The Children (Scotland) Act 1995 c.36 https://www.legislation.gov.uk/ukpga/1995/36/contents.

The Adoption and Children (Scotland) Act, 2007 asp 4 https://www.legislation.gov.uk/asp/2007/4/contents.

The Children and Young People (Scotland) Act 2014 asp 8 https://www.legislation.gov.uk/asp/2014/8/contents/enacted.

The Social Services and Well-Being (Wales) Act 2014 anaw 4 https://www.legislation.gov.uk/anaw/2014/4/contents.

The Children (Scotland) Act 2020 asp 16 https://www.legislation.gov.uk/asp/2020/16/contents/enacted.

Children and Social Work Act, 2017.

Thomas, C., 2018. The Care Crisis Review: Factors Contributing to National Increases in Numbers of Looked After Children and Applications for Care Orders. Family Rights Group, London. https://frg.org.uk/images/Care_Crisis/Care-Crisis-Review-Factors-report-FINAL.pdf.

Webb, C., Bywaters, P., Scourfield, J., Davidson, G., Bunting, L., 2020. Cuts both ways: ethnicity, poverty, and the social gradient in child welfare interventions. Child. Youth Serv. Rev. 117, 105299.

Welbourne, P., 2016. Adversarial courts, therapeutic justice and protecting children in the family justice system. Fam. L.Q. 28 (3), 205–221.

6

INTER-AGENCY PRACTICE IN SAFEGUARDING CHILDREN

SARAH GOFF

KEY POINTS

- No individual agency can keep all children safe from harm at all times: effective child protection requires effective inter-agency working.

- Inter-agency working normally involves professionals with different training and different areas of knowledge.

- The *Working Together* guidance sets out how different agencies and different professionals should work together to safeguard children from harm.

- Reviews following the death or serious harm of a child have repeatedly highlighted difficulties with inter-agency practice.

- Clear communication and sharing of information are key aspects of inter-agency practice.

INTRODUCTION

The lives of children, young people and families who face harm, adversity or abuse can be complex, and they may need services and support from a range of different agencies including not only children's social care, but also health services (midwives, health visitors, general practitioners (GPs), hospitals and specialist services), education services (nurseries, schools, colleges), housing and police. Different agencies are staffed by people with different professional training and therefore different areas of expertise. All of these people and all of these organisations need to work together.

This chapter sets out the importance of inter-agency working. It will first provide an overview of the

legislation and policy which mandates inter-agency work. It will then move on to consider the safeguarding process, from early intervention services to child protection conferences, exploring the need for ways of working that cross professional and organisational boundaries. Following this, it will look at evidence from reviews following the death or serious harm of a child, many of which have highlighted failures of inter-agency practice. Finally, it examines the challenges of effective communication and information sharing.

WHAT IS INTER-AGENCY PRACTICE, AND WHY IS IT SO IMPORTANT?

Inter-agency practice refers to ways of working in which people employed in different organisations (or 'agencies') work together in order to achieve a shared goal. Inter-agency practice is a common feature of child protection. The agencies involved in protecting children from abuse and maltreatment may be from the public sector (e.g. local authority, National Health Service (NHS) and police), the private sector (e.g. a nursery run by a private company) or the voluntary sector. The voluntary sector is sometimes also referred to as the not-for-profit or 'third' sector and includes charities and academy schools, as well as not-for-profit companies which provide services to children and families.

Effective inter-agency practice is important because children, young people and their families may have contact with many different agencies, each familiar with different parts of their lives. For example, the child's school will know about their attendance, day-to-day appearance and educational attainment; the GP (family doctor) will know about their health and development; the police will have details relating to the property and those living there that have been brought to their attention. Each agency will know about different aspects of the child's life, but this information needs to be brought together in order to gain a holistic understanding of their situation.

Inter-agency working usually involves inter-professional working; this is the term used when people with different professional backgrounds work together. Inter-professional work can be challenging because different professionals not only have different knowledge and skills but also different priorities (Box 6.1). These different priorities have the potential to lead to misunderstandings or even conflict between the various agencies and professionals who need to work together in order to safeguard a child.

KEY LEGISLATION AND POLICY

Legislation and policy mandate inter-agency practices in relation to child safeguarding at both organisational and individual levels.

At an organisational level, the Children Act 2004 requires each local authority to 'promote co-operation' with other relevant organisations, including all those that work with children and young people, for the purpose of 'improving the wellbeing' of children and young people in their area. The Children and Social Work Act 2017 sets out in more detail the requirements for local arrangements for safeguarding and promoting the welfare of children. This Act identifies local authorities, police authorities and NHS

Integrated Commissioning Boards as being 'safeguarding partners' with shared responsibility for child safeguarding. The Act gives these partners a range of powers and duties in relation to the safeguarding of children and also establishes a legal requirement for other 'persons or bodies to supply (on request) information to the safeguarding partners for the purpose of enabling or assisting the performance of their functions' (Children and Social Work Act 2017, section 16H). These lead safeguarding partners are also required to develop local child safeguarding policies, procedures and guidelines for all local agencies who work with children, young people and their families.

At the level of individual cases, the overarching requirements for inter-agency practice are also established in Acts of parliament. The Children Act 1989 is the bedrock legislation for child protection in England and Wales and inter-agency practice is made relevant as part of the Act's key provisions. The Act places a duty on local authorities to promote and safeguard the welfare of children in need in their area. Section 17 makes local authorities responsible for determining what services should be provided to a child in need but does not require the local authority to provide the services directly. In many local authorities, children in need services which are provided by other agencies and this establishes a requirement for ongoing inter-agency practice. Similarly, the Act states that, where enquiries are conducted under Section 47 in order to decide whether action is necessary to safeguard or promote a child's welfare, then inter-agency cooperation is expected. Specifically, it is the duty of any local authority, any housing authority, and any National Health Service Commissioning Board, clinical commissioning group, Local Health Board, Special Health Authority, NHS trust or NHS foundation trust to assist with those enquiries, in particular by providing relevant information and advice. Similar legislation applies in other parts of the UK. In Scotland, the relevant legislation is the Children (Scotland) Act 1995 and in Northern Ireland the Children (Northern Ireland) Order 1995 is the principal statute.

Beyond the broad legal framework created by Acts of Parliament, statutory guidance provides more detailed information about how inter-agency practice should be undertaken in relation to individual cases. In England, the key guidance is called *Working Together to Safeguard Children* (HM Government, 2018a). Originally published in 1999, and since revised and updated on a regular basis, this guidance sets out the individual and collective

---

BOX 6.1
PROFESSIONAL PRIORITIES

Social worker: the welfare of the child is of paramount concern

GP, health visitor or other NHS professional: physical and mental health of the child and other family members is paramount

Police: ascertaining whether a crime has been committed and collecting evidence to prosecute those who may have committed an offence is paramount

School: the child or young person's educational attainment is paramount

responsibilities of different agencies and professionals. Its key message, as the title suggests, is that agencies must work together in order to safeguard children. An extract from the guidance is shown in Box 6.2

INTER-AGENCY PRACTICE FROM REFERRAL AND EARLY HELP TO CHILD PROTECTION CONFERENCES

Detailed guidance on inter-agency practice for all stages of the child protection process is provided in the *Working Together* (HM Government, 2018a), and this should always be the first source of advice for professionals from any agency. What follows is a brief summary of key issues, and this is not intended to replace reliance on statutory guidance.

Around half of all children who die or are seriously harmed as a result of abuse or neglect are known to children's social care services at the time of the incident (The Child Safeguarding Practice Review Panel, 2020). However, this means that around half of children were *not* known to children's social care services prior to the harm occurring. Some of these children may have been known to other services such as health services, nurseries or schools, housing authorities or police. In other cases, their parents may have been known to other services due to physical or mental health needs, domestic abuse, substance misuse, etc.

BOX 6.2
SAFEGUARDING IS EVERYONE'S RESPONSIBILITY

16. Everyone who works with children has a responsibility for keeping them safe. No single practitioner can have a full picture of a child's needs and circumstances and, if children and families are to receive the right help at the right time, everyone who comes into contact with them has a role to play in identifying concerns, sharing information and taking prompt action.
17. In order that organisations, agencies and practitioners collaborate effectively, it is vital that everyone working with children and families, including those who work with parents/carers, understands the role they should play and the role of other practitioners. They should be aware of, and comply with, the published arrangements set out by the local safeguarding partners.

From Working Together to Safeguard Children (HM Government, 2018a, p. 11).

Health, education and other services available for all children and young people are called 'universal' services. Children's social care is not a universal service; it is a targeted service which works with those identified as in need. This means that children will only become known to children's social care if someone makes a referral and provides information that a child may be at risk of harm. The person making that referral might be a professional working in another agency, a family member or a member of the general public. In this sense, all child protection activity requires an element of working together.

INTER-AGENCY PRACTICE AT THE POINT OF REFERRAL

Inter-agency practice starts at the point of referral. Information about the child or young person needs to be shared, including basic factual information (age, gender, ethnicity) as well as more complex and subjective information about the child's background and the reason for the referral. Risk and harm are not absolutes, they are professional judgements which may be challenged, confirmed or rebutted.

Practice cultures affect how referrals may be managed between agencies. Expectations that another agency will take responsibility for the needs of a child once a referral has been made, rather than seeing the referral as the starting point for working together can lead to poor outcomes. In order to help facilitate shared working from the start of the child protection process, many local authorities have Multi-Agency Safeguarding Hubs (often known as MASH teams) as the single point of contact to report safeguarding concerns about a child. MASH teams typically include social workers and police working alongside professionals from education and health. A key feature of the MASH approach is that professionals from different organisations are co-located so that right from the start of the child protection process a range of different agencies can be involved to reflect the specific needs of each child.

Regardless of whether or not services are structured around a MASH, having shared inter-agency and inter-professional understandings of the local referrals process is vital. This includes using shared language. For example, the word 'urgent' may have different meanings in different agencies. In health settings marking something as urgent may mean that an immediate response is expected – perhaps within the hour. In children's social care, an urgent child protection referral would normally expect a response within 24 hours. In an educational setting, an urgent referral might be interpreted as needing a response over a longer timeframe, perhaps a week or more. So rather than using the word 'urgent' it is better to state a time within which a response is needed.

Clarity within the referrals process is important. An effective referrals process will ensure:

- that the referral has reached the intended person or team;
- that information originating from one agency makes sense to another: different agencies may use different language;
- that the significance of the referral has been understood;
- that the referral has been responded to.

Box 6.3 contains a case study which addresses some of the challenges faced in making referrals.

BOX 6.3
CASE STUDY: THE REFERRAL

It is a Monday morning, and Shukhi is sitting alone in the sick room at school. The 13-year-old, who has mild learning difficulties, lives as part of a multi-generational British-Bangladeshi household in housing association property. She is the oldest of four children and is known to sometimes miss school to provide care for her younger siblings; her mother has diabetes and heart disease and is often unwell. During registration, Shukhi asked to speak to her teacher in private and once they were alone said 'I've got to stop him... he's done it to me for years, but I've got to stop him touching Maya'.

The teacher, Corinne, is shocked and unsure of what to do. She has never before had to make a referral to children's social care. She knows that two other staff have previously expressed concerns about what might be going on in this family, but she doesn't know whether their concerns were ever recorded. She is so worried about Shukhi and Maya that without waiting to check for any further information she phones the local authority Multi-Agency Safeguarding Hub (MASH) team.

You are working in the MASH team and receive Corrine's call:

- What information do you need to gather from Corrinne?
- What information do you need to give to Corrine?
- How can you work together to protect both Shukhi and Maya from further harm?
- Which other agencies might hold relevant information?
- What does Shukhi need right now, as she sits waiting?

The team receiving a referral should always inform the referrer of the outcome of the referral. This applies equally in cases when the referral results in a case becoming open to children's social care services or when the referral results in no further action and the case being closed. Confusion about decisions leaving the referrer unclear whether their information has been 'accepted' as a referral can leave children vulnerable (Social Care Institute for Excellence (SCIE), 2016).

Thresholds for accepting referrals can sometimes be a point of conflict between agencies. Each local authority publishes their own threshold criteria for different levels of service, and there is evidence of inconsistency and inequity in the application of these thresholds (Devaney, 2019). Differences in expectations and perception about whether thresholds have been reached can lead to conflict and frustration between agencies (Devaney, 2019). It is important that professionals in all agencies are clear about the thresholds which apply in the relevant local authority area. Thresholds should be publicly available on the website of the Local Safeguarding Children Partnership.

Working together effectively from the point of referral is important. Difficulties at this stage of the child protection system may reduce the confidence of professionals within universal services to refer other children, or to re-refer the same child if concerns re-emerge.

INTER-AGENCY PRACTICE: EARLY HELP

Early help can prevent harm from occurring or escalating. Effective early help relies on professionals in universal services identifying and referring children and families that may be in need of additional support. For newborns and infants, it is professionals in universal healthcare services – midwives, health visitors and GPs – who are most likely to identify need and make referrals. Once children are in nursery or attending school, it is education professionals who are most likely to identify need and make referrals.

Early help work covers a broad range of targeted support for the whole family and is carried out with the consent of the parent and child or young person. Engagement with early help services such as Children's Centres, parenting classes or other community-based services can help to safeguard children, but only where early help services are part of effective inter-agency practice networks. In 'Early Help, Whose Responsibility?' Ofsted (2015) highlighted that opportunities to provide early help for children and their families were missed by all statutory partners with a responsibility for this and that feedback on referrals was often neither sought nor offered. The report made a number of recommendations, including that Local Children's Safeguarding Boards should *'monitor and evaluate whether children's emerging needs are appropriately met elsewhere when referrals to children's social care do not meet the locally agreed threshold for statutory intervention'* and that *'all professionals working with families receive effective early help training'* and that *'Local Authorities should ensure that when a child is referred to local authority children's social care the referrer is consistently given good-quality feedback about the outcome of the referral'* (Ofsted, 2015, p. 8).

INTER-AGENCY PRACTICE: INITIAL STRATEGY MEETINGS

When initial inquiries suggest that a child may be at risk of significant harm, children's social care are responsible for coordinating an initial multi-agency strategy meeting. The purpose of this meeting is firstly to plan for the immediate safety of the child. Beyond that, the meeting should also determine when and how to speak to the child and relevant family members as well as considering what further enquiries are necessary, which other agencies need to be involved (e.g. police, education health, etc) and which professionals will take responsivity for what actions within the agreed timescales.

Ofsted (2020) highlights the importance of careful and thorough strategy meetings and the value of bringing professionals together at this early stage in the child protection process – particularly in complex cases. The important role of the police has also been emphasised, particularly where background information is needed about the adults involved in a child's life. At this stage, it may also be helpful to request a child health assessment which can provide important information, particularly where neglect may have caused health issues for the child. As with other stages of the child protection process, clear communication and timely sharing of relevant information are key.

INTER-AGENCY PRACTICE: CHILD PROTECTION CONFERENCES AND CHILD PROTECTION PLANNING

Child protection conferences provide a key opportunity for everyone involved in safeguarding a child to come together, including not only professionals from different agencies but also parents or carers and (where appropriate) the child. Research shows that families often have difficult experiences with child protection conferences (Gibson, 2020); it also reveals that critical practice issues can emerge where professional culture, language and behaviour combine to further marginalise and distress parents and family members.

Good inter-agency practice in the context of child protection conferences involves clear communication. Avoiding agency jargon and ensuring clarity of language is useful not only for parents but also for professionals. Respectful exploration of different views and enabling equal participation from all parties can present significant challenges but is vital to securing the best outcome for the child (Featherstone et al., 2016; SCIE, 2016).

LEARNING FROM CASE REVIEWS

Despite the existence of clear and detailed guidance on inter-agency working, children continue to experience harm even in situations where they are known to services. In many cases, these harms are attributable in part to poor inter-agency practice. Much of what we know about the shortcomings of inter-agency and inter-professional practices comes from Child Safeguarding Practice Reviews (previously known as Serious Case Reviews). These are statutory reviews which must take place when a child dies or is seriously harmed as a result of abuse or neglect. The key purposes of such reviews are (i) to explore what happened to the child, (ii) to identify things which could have been done differently or better and which could have prevented the abuse from occurring and (iii) to ensure the services learn lessons from what went wrong and do not repeat the same mistakes. The reviews seek to identify ways that organisations and professionals can improve how they work together to safeguard other children in the future. Box 6.4 contains the terminology in use for Serious Case Reviews across the four different jurisdictions of the UK.

BOX 6.4
CASE REVIEW TERMINOLOGY ACROSS THE UK

England: Child Safeguarding Practice Reviews https://www.gov.uk/government/organisations/child-safeguarding-practice-review-panel

Northern Ireland: Case Management Reviews https://www.safeguardingni.org/about-us/case-management-review

Scotland: Learning Reviews https://www.careinspectorate.com/index.php/notifications/learning-reviews-children-and-young-people

Wales: Child Practice Reviews https://www.northwalessafeguardingboard.wales/practice-reviews/child-practice-reviews/

Many individual case reviews have highlighted how problems with inter-agency safeguarding practice have contributed to the death or serious harm of a child. The outcomes from individual reviews can be further evaluated in order to draw attention to patterns of findings which may indicate systemic difficulties in inter-agency safeguarding work. Analyses of such reviews over time have revealed enduring patterns of inter-agency practice shortcomings. The last analysis of Serious Case Reviews in England prior to their being replaced by Child Safeguarding Practice Reviews highlighted a range of problems with inter-agency practice (Brandon et al., 2020), including gaps in how and when practitioners shared information and failures in understanding the meaning and significance of information which could have contributed to protecting the child. The authors call for '*greater rigour in information sharing, stronger assessment and planning at all stages of the process; and opportunities for building effective structures and promoting responsive cultures, even when constrained by limited resources*' (Brandon et al., 2020, p. 15).

With the introduction creation of the Child Safeguarding Practice Review Panel has come further evidence of the factors contributing to the death or serious harm of children. Serious Incident Notifications are made by local authorities where a child has died or is seriously harmed, and abuse or neglect is known or suspected. Between 2018 and 2019 the Child Safeguarding Practice Review Panel undertook a rapid review of 538 serious incidents of child abuse or neglect (The Child Safeguarding Practice Review Panel, 2020). It found patterns of weak assessments and poor decision-making, patterns of overly optimistic thinking without sound evidence and patterns of workers being overstretched, overwhelmed

and under pressure. Problems specifically linked to inter-agency practice were also noted, including poor sharing of information at critical and examples of poor practice when escalating concerns. Please see Box 6.5 which contains key learning with respect to Information sharing from the Child Safeguarding Practice Review Panel annual report 2020, published in 2021. This annual report also contains other key areas of learning significant to multi-agency practice.

These challenges remained when child protection practices changed during the COVID pandemic. The Child Safeguarding Practice Review Panel Annual Report 2020 noted the '*urgency of addressing what might be described as stubborn and perennial problems in multi-agency child protection practice. Issues such as weak information sharing, communication and risk assessment have, over decades, impeded our ability to protect children and to help families*' (The Child Safeguarding Practice Review Panel, 2021, p. 5).

BOX 6.5
KEY LEARNING FROM CASE REVIEWS

Thresholds for when to share information are not consistently understood and applied. Basic training for all practitioners needs to address a concern that General Data Protection Regulation (GDPR) and data protection regulations limit when information may be shared.

Lack of access by practitioners to IT systems outside their professional role limits sharing of information and can lead to a lack of accurate cross-service chronology. This is evidenced particularly in relation to health records held by GPs, health visiting, midwifery, Child and Adolescent Mental Health Services (CAMHS) and adult mental health services.

The development of information sharing capability between IT systems in partner agencies has the potential to offer a system-wide solution through the use of 'flags' and 'triggers' that prompt information sharing.

Poor quality recording, inaccurate and out-of-date information result in partial understanding of the needs of the child. Considerations of risk are based on circumstances that may no longer apply.

Timely circulation of minutes from multi-agency meetings provides reference points for chronology, decision-making, plans and evidence of progress to address safeguarding concerns.

Information in reports about the observed circumstances of children needs to be jargon-free and avoid using generic phrases such as 'children doing well'. Inaccurate use of language does not support critical thinking and can give false assurances when viewed by other practitioners.

From The Child Safeguarding Practice Review Panel, 2021, p. 31.

INFORMATION SHARING

Information sharing is recognised as one of the key elements of effective child protection but – as has been shown – is also often highlighted within case reviews as a problematic aspect of inter-agency practice. There are a number of reasons why information sharing is not as simple as might at first be assumed. The first relates to (unfounded) beliefs on the part of some professionals that data protection legislation prevents information sharing: as will be shown, this is not the case when information is being shared for purposes of child protection. The second relates to how (and what) information is recorded by different agencies. And the third relates to the shared use of language. Each of these issues will be considered in turn.

INFORMATION SHARING AND DATA PROTECTION LEGISLATION

Working Together states that 'fears about sharing information must not be allowed to stand in the way of the need to promote the welfare and protect the safety of children' (HM Government, 2018a, p. 18). Many of these fears stem from misunderstandings about data protection legislation. The truth is that no part of the Data Protection Act 2018 (also known as the General Data Protection Regulation or GDPR) prevents or limits the information which can be shared between relevant professionals for the purpose of protecting a child from harm. Moreover, such information can be legally shared without the consent of the child, their parent or guardian if it is shared for the purpose of safeguarding. This applies to information held by all agencies, including not only children's social care but also health, education, police, housing and third sector or private service providers.

In addition to the advice on sharing information which is provided within the Working Together guidance (HM Government, 2018a) additional guidance is provided in Information sharing: Advice for practitioners providing safeguarding services to children, young people, parents and carers (HM Government, 2018b). An extract from this guidance, setting out the 'seven golden rules to sharing information' is provided in Box 6.6.

BOX 6.6
THE SEVEN GOLDEN RULES TO SHARING INFORMATION

1. Remember that the General Data Protection Regulation (GDPR), Data Protection Act 2018 and human rights law are not barriers to justified information sharing, but provide a framework to ensure that personal information about living individuals is shared appropriately.
2. Be open and honest with the individual (and/or their family where appropriate) from the outset about why, what, how and with whom information will, or could be shared, and seek their agreement, unless it is unsafe or inappropriate to do so.
3. Seek advice from other practitioners, or your information governance lead, if you are in any doubt about sharing the information concerned, without disclosing the identity of the individual where possible.
4. Where possible, share information with consent, and where possible, respect the wishes of those who do not consent to having their information shared. Under the GDPR and Data Protection Act 2018 you may share information without consent if, in your judgement, there is a lawful basis to do so, such as where safety may be at risk. You will need to base your judgement on the facts of the case. When you are sharing or requesting personal information from someone, be clear about the basis upon which you are doing so. Where you do not have consent, be mindful that an individual might not expect information to be shared.
5. Consider safety and well-being: base your information sharing decisions on considerations of the safety and well-being of the individual and others who may be affected by their actions.
6. Necessary, proportionate, relevant, adequate, accurate, timely and secure: ensure that the information you share is necessary for the purpose for which you are sharing it, is shared only with those individuals who need to have it, is accurate and up-to-date, is shared in a timely fashion and is shared securely (see principles).
7. Keep a record of your decision and the reasons for it – whether it is to share information or not. If you decide to share, then record what you have shared, with whom and for what purpose.

From Information sharing: Advice for practitioners providing safeguarding services to children, young people, parents and carers (HM Government, 2018b).

The most important consideration when deciding whether information should be shared with another professional or another agency is whether that sharing information is likely to support the safeguarding and protection of a child. If information could help protect a child, then it should be shared and it is lawful for the information to be shared. This does not, however, mean that all and any information can or should be shared without careful consideration. Whenever information is shared, the following principles apply:

- *Necessary and proportionate*: any sharing of information must be proportionate to the level of risk. No more data than is strictly necessary should be shared. The impact of disclosing information (on both the subject of the information and on any third parties) should be considered.
- *Relevant*: only information that is relevant to protecting the child should be shared, and it should only be shared with people who need to know.
- *Adequate*: information which is shared should be adequate for its purpose, it should be able to be understood and relied upon.
- *Accurate*: information which is shared should be accurate, up-to-date and clearly distinguish between fact and opinion; where historical information is shared this should be clearly identified as such.
- *Timely*: information should be shared in a timely fashion: practitioners should always consider the urgency of requests for information as this can be vital in ensuring timely action to safeguard a child.
- *Secure*: information should be shared and stored securely, in accordance with agency guidelines.
- *Recorded*: decisions about whether or not information has been shared should be recorded, including the reason for the decision and who any information was shared with (summarised from HM Government, 2018b, p. 9–10).

RECORDING AND USING INFORMATION

Clear and accurate record-keeping on the part of all agencies can play a critical role in protecting children from harm. Records about not only the child and family but also the professionals and organisations they are engaged with needs to be maintained and regularly updated.

A case file should always include an up-to-date record of the names of the child's parents and carers, including all those with parental responsibility, and their siblings. Depending on the role of the agency, further information to enable equal opportunities monitoring should also be recorded including gender, ethnicity and disability. Children's social care records should include information on key family relationships and record who is living in the family home. Details of non-resident parents (often but not always the father) and of new partners moving in or out of the family home should also be recorded.

When carrying out child protection work, knowing exactly which practitioners are involved with a child and keeping up-to-date information about the work each person undertaking is important. Led by children's social care, agencies should maintain contact and share relevant information throughout the child protection process. Effective inter-agency practice within child protection, including sharing information, should be a continual process, not a one-off event. Staff turnover can present particular challenges. It is vital that practitioners in all agencies notify partner agencies if they leave their job; this includes when people are moving to take up a different role in the same agency. Before leaving, practitioners must ensure that they have clearly recorded all the work they have carried out with a child or family so that their replacement can take the work forward.

Information is of particular value when it can be brought together to provide a holistic picture of what may be happening to a child. This requires individual agencies to regularly review the information they hold in order to identify patterns of behaviour which could indicate a risk of harm. It also requires agencies to work together and to share information when concerns arise. This is sometimes likened to doing a jigsaw puzzle: each bit of information is a piece of the puzzle, and it is only when all the pieces are in place that the true picture of what may be happening to a child can be seen and understood. Please see Box 6.7 which illustrates some of the challenges in doing this and in making sense of the needs of a child.

In complex situations, it is necessary to not only share information, but also to actively use that information to create a picture of what is happening to a child.

BOX 6.7
CASE STUDY: COMPLETING THE JIGSAW TO GET THE FULL PICTURE

Kellyanne Davies is a 26-year-old mother of two children – Daniel aged 6 and Miranda aged 3. They have recently been rehoused in the Midlands. Kellyanne spent time in care as a child and was known to the care leaving team in the London borough where she grew up and where the children were born. Daniel and Miranda were known to children's social care in London due to witnessing domestic abuse perpetrated by their father. It was as a result of this abuse that Kellyanne ended her relationship with the children's father and the family were placed in temporary accommodation. The housing association flat in the Midlands is a huge improvement on their temporary accommodation in London, but the family have no social support network in their new area. Kellyanne is soon befriended by a neighbour, a man in his forties, and she begins a relationship with him.

***

Children's social care in London are aware of the family's history, but the case has been closed now that they have left the area.

The **care leaving team** in London have closed Kellyanne's case as she is past the age for ongoing care leaver's support.

Children's social care in the Midlands local authority have no information about Kellyanne or her children.

Daniel's **school** are aware that he often struggles to concentrate in class and his educational attainment is behind for his age. They have noticed that he is anxious around adult men.

Miranda's **nursery** are aware that she is small for her age and is not meeting her developmental milestones. They have noticed that she is anxious around adult men.

The **police** know that Kellyanne's new partner has previous convictions relating to domestic abuse.

The **housing association** knows that complaints have been made about noise from Kellyanne's property.

The **GP** knows that Kellyanne has asked for support with anxiety and depression.

***

DISCUSSION POINTS

- What conclusions might each agency come to if they were only aware of the information immediately available to them?
- What conclusion might be jointly reached if all the available information was shared to give a holistic picture of the family's life?

When many different agencies are involved with a family, having an accurate chronology of all the interactions which each agency has had with the child and their family can be vital. An accurate and detailed chronology can help to show how events have unfolded over time and can help to identify where closer inter-agency working may be needed.

Once created, a full chronology can be used to identify gaps, inconsistencies and missing information. It can be used to support effective inter-agency practice by providing an opportunity to note where and when decisions were made; an opportunity to ask for further explanations for key decisions; and an opportunity to consider what should happen next based on the fullest possible picture of what has happened up to that point.

SHARED LANGUAGE

Effective child protection practice requires communication and information sharing which is clear and unambiguous. This is true of communication with children and their families and of communication within agencies as well as communication between agencies. Communication with children and parents will be addressed in detail elsewhere in this volume where, amongst other things, consideration will be given to the particular needs of children and families from Black, Asian and ethnic minority backgrounds, children with disabilities, parents with learning disabilities and parents experiencing mental health difficulties. In this section, the focus is on inter-agency practice and ensuring clarity of communication between agencies.

Shared understanding is crucial for inter-agency work, but time pressures and hurried exchanges can lead to the use of acronyms and jargon which create misunderstandings. Communication may also be hampered by the use of euphemisms which unintentionally gloss over key issues. Language which is value-laden and which blames or shames may reduce trust between individuals or organisations and hinder effective inter-agency practice.

Acronyms are when letters are used as a shorthand for words. Sometimes acronyms are so commonplace that everyone understands them – for example, it is safe to assume that professionals in all agencies will know that the acronym NHS refers to the National Health Service. (Even here, however, some service users – particularly families who have recently arrived in the UK – may not know what the acronym NHS means.) However, the use of acronyms can lead to miscommunication, particularly where the same letters are used as shorthand for different things in different agencies. For example, in children's social care the letters CP are often used as shorthand for Child Protection, in health settings the letters CP would typically be used to refer to Cerebral Palsy (a type of disability), and in older police records the letters CP may sometimes still be used as an abbreviation for Child Pornography (though the more usual terminology is now 'child abuse images'). If a case file contains the acronym CP, this has the potential to cause serious miscommunication between these agencies. It is always better to spell words out in full rather than use acronyms.

Jargon is technical language, used within a particular organisation or a professional context, which may be poorly understood by people outside that setting. For example, 'child in need' has a particular (legal) meaning in the context of children's social care, but this phrase may not be understood in the same way by other professionals and is unlikely to be commonly understood by the general population. Professionals often slip into using jargon when communicating with one another, but this can create problems when there is a need for inter-agency work. It can also hinder effective working with the child or family, by leading them to feel excluded. The use of technical terms and jargon can be widespread in reports and during meetings. Some practitioners may lack the confidence to ask for jargon to be explained, and this can lead to misunderstandings or to missing the significance of key issues. Aim to avoid jargon whenever possible and remember that records and reports need to be understood by professionals in other agencies.

The use of acronyms and jargon can be an unwanted feature of communication in many professional contexts. However, within child protection, a third aspect of language can be equally problematic: the use of euphemisms. This is when 'milder' or less direct language is used to avoid saying something difficult. Some people use euphemisms to avoid embarrassment, particularly when referring to parts of the body or to sexual behaviours. Where there are concerns about possible sexual abuse, the use of euphemisms can create a lack of clarity about what has happened. Phrases such as 'inappropriate behaviour' or 'inappropriate touching' and 'sexualised behaviour' are often recorded in case notes (Brandon et al., 2020). However, these terms do not tell us what has happened to a child and may lead to risks being overlooked or misunderstood. It is important that factual information is recorded and shared. For example, instead of recording that a child was 'touched inappropriately by step-father' it would be better to accurately describe what was known to have happened, such as 'the stepfather touched the child's penis, both over and under their clothes'. Reluctance to use direct words may lead to information being lost.

Lastly, care needs to be taken across all inter-agency communications, written and verbal, to avoid terms or phrases that may imply blame or create mistrust. This may be phrases which blame the child – examples include phrases such as 'putting themselves at risk' or 'attention seeking' when all children and young people need emotional contact and attention. Or it may be phrases which seek to lay blame on other agencies or individual professionals – such as 'health were unresponsive' or 'children's social care failed to provide an update'. Language has the power to shape relationships, and positive professional relationships underpin effective inter-agency working.

CONCLUSION

Over recent decades, the importance of effective inter-agency working in child protection has increasingly been recognised in case review findings and reflected in Government policy and guidance. On the ground, however, good inter-agency practice in child protection can still be hard to achieve, particularly where resources are limited, and professionals are working under pressure.

Good inter-agency practice requires a recognition of the priorities and pressures in different organisations.

It requires relationships of trust between organisations as well as between individual professionals. It requires clear communication that avoids acronyms, jargon and euphemisms. This all takes time and thought. But, without this, children will not be protected as no single agency can adequately address the complex needs of all children at risk of harm.

FURTHER READING

Child Safeguarding Practice Review Panel, https://www.gov.uk/government/organisations/child-safeguarding-practice-review-panel.

Working Together to Safeguard Children, https://www.gov.uk/government/publications/working-together-to-safeguard-children-2.

REFERENCES

Brandon, M., Sidebotham, P., Belderson, P., Cleaver, H., Dickens, J., Garstang, J., Harris, J., Sorensen, P., Wate, R., 2020. Complexity and Challenge: A Triennial Analysis of SCRs 2014–2017. Department for Education, London.

Children Act 1989. https://www.legislation.gov.uk/ukpga/1989/41/contents.

Children Act 2004. https://www.legislation.gov.uk/ukpga/2004/31/contents.

Children and Social Work Act 2017. https://www.legislation.gov.uk/ukpga/2017/16/contents/enacted.

Children (Northern Ireland) Order 1995. https://www.legislation.gov.uk/nisi/1995/755/contents/made.

Children (Scotland) Act 1995. https://www.legislation.gov.uk/ukpga/1995/36/contents.

Data Protection Act 2018. https://www.legislation.gov.uk/ukpga/2018/12/contents/enacted.

Devaney, J., 2019. The Trouble with Thresholds: Rationing as a national choice in child and family social work. Child Fam. Soc. Work 24 (4), 458–466 Wiley.

Featherstone, B., Gupta, A., Morris, K., Warner, J., 2016. Let's stop feeding the risk monster: towards a social model of 'child protection'. Fam. Relatsh. Soc. 7 (1), 17–22.

Gibson, M., 2020. The shame and shaming of parents in the child protection process: findings from a case study of an English child protection service. Fam. Relatsh. Soc. 9 (2), 217–233.

Government, H.M., 2018a. Working Together to Safeguard Children: A Guide to Inter-Agency Working to Safeguard and Promote the Welfare of Children. Crown Copyright, London.

Government, H.M., 2018b. Information Sharing: Advice for Practitioners Providing Safeguarding Services to Children, Young People, Parents and Carers. Crown Copyright, London. https://assets.publishing.service.gov.uk/government/uploads/system/uploads/attachment_data/file/1062969/Information_sharing_advice_practitioners_safeguarding_services.pdf.

Ofsted, 2015. Early Help: Who's Responsibility? Crown Copyright, London.

Ofsted, 2020. The Multi-Agency Response to Child Sexual Abuse in the Family Environment; Prevention, Identification, Protection and Support. Crown Copyright, London.

SCIE, 2016. Practice Issues From Serious Case Reviews – Learning Into Practice. SCIE, London.

The Child Safeguarding Practice Review Panel, 2020. Annual Report 2018 to 2019: Patterns in Practice, Key Messages, and 2020 Work Programme. Crown Copyright, London.

The Child Safeguarding Practice Review Panel, 2021. Annual Report 2020: Patterns in Practice, Key Messages and 2021 Work Programme. Crown Copyright, London. https://assets.publishing.service.gov.uk/government/uploads/system/uploads/attachment_data/file/984767/The_Child_Safeguarding_Annual_Report_2020.pdf.

7

SUPPORTING SOCIAL WORKERS: THE ROLE OF SUPERVISION

ANGIE BARTOLI

KEY POINTS

- The functions, history and global perspectives of supervision.
- The emotional impact of child protection on practitioners.
- The benefits of reflective supervision for practitioners and practice.

INTRODUCTION

This chapter is divided into two sections. The first will start with a brief outline of what defines supervision, its history, functions and global perspectives. Through the use of a case study, the second section will go on to explore the impact of child protection on practitioners and will consider the importance of supervision in both supporting effective practice and protecting the well-being of practitioners. This chapter draws upon the author's significant experience of being a supervisor within child protection teams and of delivering supervisor training. The chapter is primarily concerned with supervision within a social work context; however, there are elements which relate to other professionals who receive supervision within a child protection context.

WHAT IS SUPERVISION?

Social work supervision has dominated the discourse of the profession, culminating in a situation where it

can be seen as 'the "fall guy" for all that is wrong in social work and, paradoxically, the all-encompassing "holy grail" to fix it' (Bartoli & Kennedy, 2015). Ask a group of social work practitioners, managers, students or academics how to ensure that practice is effective, reduce work-based stress, improve staff retention and morale and, inevitably, the provision of good-quality supervision is amongst their suggestions. Therefore it is somewhat surprising that a handbook on child protection has not, until this edition, had a chapter devoted to supervision. The art of supervision is a uniquely defining characteristic of the social work profession and particularly within child protection work.

Despite the emphasis of supervision within the practice and policy discourse surrounding social work, there is no universal definition as it is applied differently according to organisational and national contexts. Within the UK this can, at least in part, be attributed to the notion that supervision in social work serves an array of purposes. From a practitioner's perspective it can be a place of safety where emotions are contained and expressed (Ruch, 2007; Smith, 2000). Equally it can provide practitioners with time away from the fast-paced environment of practice by accommodating a reflective thinking space (Earle et al., 2017). For these reasons, it can be argued that supervision can be supportive and increase both job satisfaction and personal resilience (Beddoe & Davys, 2016; Collins, 2007). Wonnacott (2012) reminds us that defining supervision in terms of its functions alone has its limitations. Instead, supervision can be described as a process by which a practitioner is provided with support and guidance to talk through the impact of their work, explore decision making whilst providing the organisation with management oversight. At the heart of supervision is a relationship with the supervisee (Ruch et al., 2010; Wonnacott, 2012).

Despite all the changes to practice, the significance of supervision remains undisputed. History reveals that the development of the social work profession and supervision are parallel (Davys & Beddoe, 2010). It is considered to be highly likely that supervision evolved as a task fulfilled by managers to ensure administrative accountability and a monitoring of an unqualified workforce (Kadushin & Harkness, Supervision in Social Work, 2002; Tsui, 2005).

THE HISTORICAL DEVELOPMENT OF SUPERVISION

Kadushin developed a model of supervision which has become well-known, influential and refined over the decades (Kadushin, 1985; Kadushin & Harkness, 2002). His model defines supervision in terms of its three functions: administrative, educational and supportive. Kadushin (1985, p. 82) considers administrative supervision as the primary function within his model, perhaps unsurprising given that its evolutionary roots are located within an American context of 'vicarious liability'. The administrative function relates to the managerial discharging of responsibilities and procedural aspects of practice, where the manager ensures that the work is being carried out effectively and correctly according to the agency's policies and regulations. Educational supervision is considered by Kadushin (1985) as the second principal responsibility of the supervisor, where learning is extended, and professional knowledge questioned, debated and deepened. The supportive function is considered as both practical and emotional in

nature, with supervision affirming the practitioner's emotional involvement in the work to deal with the 'stubborn ambiguity in practice' (England, 1986, p. 40). This function also acknowledges the levels of stress associated with the profession and in particular child protection practice. To consider each function as a separate entity would be oversimplifying both the model and the art of supervision; instead the functions should be viewed as overlapping and interconnected (Davys & Beddoe, 2010; Kadushin & Harkness, 2002; Tsui, 2005).

TYPES OF SUPERVISION

ONE-TO-ONE SUPERVISION

Typically supervision is delivered in a one-to-one model which involves the supervisee and supervisor. Within a UK context, the supervisor tends to be the practice supervisor or manager and all functions of supervision will be included. Supervision is a formal arrangement and so will involve the drawing up of a contract or agreement and notes after each session.

GROUP SUPERVISION

Group supervision can be peer or supervisor led and is often used effectively for case discussion or for a practitioner to present a complex dilemma. Group supervision complements rather than replaces one-to-one supervision. Whilst group supervision can be effective to gain many perspectives to a situation, it may not be appropriate for exploring more personal or emotional issues.

Earle, F., Fox, J., Webb, C., Bowyer, S., 2017. Reflective Supervision: Resource Pack. Research in Practice (RiP), Dartington.

Over time supervision has become enmeshed within the fabric of social work agencies and subsequently is both structurally and professionally situated (Tsui, 2005). This is reflected somewhat in the Morrison and Wonnacott (2010) 4×4×4 supervision model as a response to the dominance of the administrative function of supervision. They introduced a fourth function – mediation, which locates the individual (the practitioner/supervisee) within the organisation and so providing a context in which they practice (Wonnacott, 2012).

4×4×4 SUPERVISION MODEL

This is a popular model used within many local authorities in England and based on Morrison's (2005) framework. Much of the model's popularity is due to its practical application that promotes reflective supervision and locates supervision within the context that it is practised. It is an integrative model, bringing together:

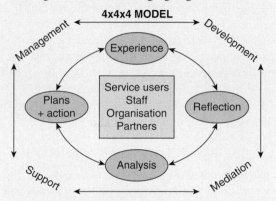

4x4x4 MODEL

Management — Development — Support — Mediation

Experience → Reflection → Analysis → Plans + action

Service users
Staff
Organisation
Partners

The model is based on the following principles:

- All elements are interdependent
- Dynamic in nature
- Relationships are at the heart of the process
- Uses the reflective cycle to fulfil the four functions
- The four elements are based on Kolb's model of experiential learning (1988)

Morrison, T. (2005). Staff Supervision in Social Care (3rd edition). Pavilion Publishing and Media, Brighton.

Theoretical frameworks of practice used in supervision have historically mirrored social work practice. The literature indicates that originally psychoanalytical supervisory approaches were utilised within supervision to reflect the traditional case work model of social work practice (Kadushin, 1985; Tsui, 2005). A combination of factors and working practices have influenced and reshaped supervision styles. Newer models of working such as task centred and solution focussed are reflected in supervision as well as practice. Such models have moved away from longer-term therapeutic and relationship-based working to shorter-term, goal-orientated approaches (Ruch et al., 2010). As a result of this, supervision has been criticised for being dominated by the administrative function and being too managerialist in focus. Jack and Donnellan's (2010) study explores the experiences of newly qualified social workers and managers in England. They highlight the dominance of supervision being focussed upon practitioners' skills and procedural knowledge with less time devoted to thoughts and feelings of the impact of practice on the individual. There are signs of a commitment towards a revival of relationship-based practice and a move away from bureaucratic procedures (Murphy et al., 2013).

GLOBAL PERSPECTIVES

The importance and significance of supervision within the social work profession are globally acknowledged. From a global perspective, there is a growing interest in the value and purpose of social work supervision. For example, in China where social work is relatively young as a profession, supervision is considered critical for its development (Mo et al., 2019). Similarly, in Malta, supervision is regarded as a 'specialism in the making' (Cole, 2019, p. 1). An extensive review of the literature conducted by O' Donoghue et al. (2018) highlights an international commonality of the functions of supervision as administrative, educational and supportive. However, they go on to draw attention to the fact that these functions are influenced by context which might relate to a number of factors including geographical location, organisational and practice setting, and diversity amongst supervisees. This leads to what they describe as a 'plurality of supervision arrangements internationally' (O'Donoghue et al., 2018, p. 354).

Supervision has been a topic of increasing interest throughout the past 2 decades, generating a large body of research and literature. A review of this literature by McPherson et al. (2016) has highlighted two key areas of focus including:

- The significance of the relationship between the supervisor and supervisee
- Supervision as a response to anxiety and vicarious trauma which addresses the emotional impact of practice.

This review involved interviewing social workers and supervisors who highlighted eight core themes in relation to supervision which include:

1. Safety
2. Responding to the emotional impact of the work

3. Learning and growth
4. Leadership
5. Integrity and justice
6. Balancing supervision functions
7. Organisational processes
8. Community understanding and valuing practice

A number of these core themes will resonate through the case study below and demonstrate that simply concentrating on organisational processes is failing to consider the emotional impact of practice and potentially limiting the learning and growth of both the practitioner and supervisor.

BACK TO REFLECTION

Within a UK context, the growth of managerialism in the 1980s with an emphasis on accountability and performance management changed the style of practice and in turn of supervision. This shifted the focus from reflective supervision to one of adherence and compliance to audit, underpinned with a proliferation of national government targets based on budgets and efficiency (Wonnacott, 2012). Managerialism has had a significant impact on public sector organisational reforms, social work practice and the manager's role, with supervisors managing budgets as well as overseeing practice (Pritchard, 1995). The managerial model prevailed for a significant period of time, but more recently, Munro (2011), in her review of the child protection process, promoted a more flexible and adaptable social work practice that is child-centred rather than prescriptive in response. Hence there is much more emphasis on the reflective nature of both social work and supervisory practice. The literature indicates a shift of emphasis on supervision to become more reflective in style (Wonnacott, 2012) and more proactive rather than reactive in nature (Shohet, 2011).

There is a strong argument for a reflective approach to supervision shifting focus from the task to the emotions experienced by practitioners. Reforms in social work practice within the UK have provided an opportunity to refocus supervision practices. A number of models promoting reflective supervision have been proposed with an emphasis on learning (Rankine, 2017; Wonnacott, 2012), a systemic approach (Dugmore et al., 2018) and outcome focussed practice (Johnstone & Miller, 2010). The word 'reflection' is frequently referred to within social work practice and supervision, but it is not always a well-defined term (Wonnacott, 2012). Reflective supervision can be described as 'above all a learning process' (Earle et al., 2017, p. 11). This enables practitioners to explore their practice and factors which might influence it and take into consideration the emotional impact of the work (Jennings, 2017; Wonnacott, 2014).

In other words, reflective supervision adopts a holistic approach where it considers both a reflection upon the practice interventions and the impact this has on the practitioner (Fook & Gardner, 2007).

Using a case study, this second section will consider the benefits of a reflective supervisory approach.

REFLECTIVE SUPERVISION

Reflective supervision is facilitated on an individual basis or in groups. According to Jennings (2017), reflective supervision provides a safe space for practitioners 'to go beneath the surface of their work, to consider the emotional impact of the work, the unquestioned assumptions and biases they bring, varying perspectives (including theoretical perspectives) and ethical dilemmas inherent in social work practice'. To gain the full benefit of reflective practice, it is useful for both the supervisor and supervisee to adopt a position of professional curiosity rather than rush to provide solutions to the dilemma.

REFLECTIVE SUPERVISION IN ACTION

The following case study is offered as a means to gaining an insight to how reflective supervision can be applied in practice by considering the dilemmas posed by a practitioner involved in working with a young baby to her supervisor. The case study is useful in considering the emotions that child protection work evokes in practitioners and how a supervisor might contain these feelings. Reflective supervision will also be applied to consider how risk and uncertainty are balanced and the benefits and challenges in adopting a strengths-based approach to practice.

CASE STUDY 7.1: REFLECTIVE SUPERVISION IN PRACTICE

When asked at the start of a supervision session, Kate, a social worker, says that she is feeling fine. She later discusses a contact visit that she has recently supervised. The contact visit involved Mr and Mrs Jasper, the parents of baby Alice who is 6 weeks old. Mrs Jasper has a history of depression, which means that she tends to isolate herself and neglect her own basic needs. During her pregnancy with Alice, Mr and Mrs Jasper move in with Mrs Green (Mr Jasper's mother and baby Alice's paternal grandmother). Mrs Green is known to Children's Services and had her own children (including Mr Jasper) removed from her care due to concerns around neglect. As a child, Mrs Jasper has also been placed in foster care and then later in a residential children's home.

Kate was involved in the prebirth assessment, which Mr and Mrs Jasper engaged positively with. Kate's work formed part of the evidence to recommend that Alice was made subject to a child protection plan and to remain in the care of her parents. For the first 4 weeks, all the professionals involved noted how Alice was thriving and that there were no safeguarding concerns.

Last week, the police were called by neighbours who had heard shouting and screaming coming from the house and a baby crying incessantly. Mr and Mrs Jasper had an argument, each accusing the other of hitting one another, both had sustained injuries – cuts and bruises to the face and arms. Mrs Green was under the influence of alcohol at the time and could not recall what happened. All the adults in the household insisted that Alice was asleep when the argument occurred.

The local authority made the decision to place Alice in a foster placement (under section 20 of Children Act 1989). Kate was supervising the first contact between Alice and her parents. Kate explained in supervision how Mr and Mrs Jasper appeared nervous about holding Alice and that Kate had to show them how to do this safely. Kate talked of feeling confused as she observed that Mr and Mrs Jasper appeared to take little notice of Alice and instead were preoccupied separately with their mobile phones. Mr and Mrs Jasper did talk about their past experiences of being in foster care, recalling this as a positive and happy time in their own childhood. Kate was surprised that after 20 min Mr Jasper chose to end the contact session because Alice was asleep. Although appearing reluctant to leave, Mrs Jasper was persuaded by her husband that there was 'little point staying'.

Kate, who has recently returned from maternity leave, explains that immediately after the contact session she was left with feeling an overwhelming sense of sadness, and that now during supervision she is also feeling angry and cannot identify anything positive in the relationship between Alice and her parents. As a new mother herself, Kate had assumed that Mrs Jasper would be distressed during contact and would be eager to spend as much time as possible with her baby. Kate says that she is at a loss to know what to do next.

PAUSE AND REFLECT

It would be tempting for a practice supervisor to listen empathetically and then respond to Kate by focusing upon the task in hand offering her procedural solutions to her dilemma. Practitioners can present unthinkable situations in supervision, and supervisors often feel compelled to provide a 'quick fix', simple answer. However, in doing so, the practice supervisor would be at risk of mirroring the fast-paced practice of child protection that propels practitioners and managers into intuitive decision-making rather than taking time to pause and reflect during supervision (Saltiel, 2017). At this point, it is useful to apply the four elements of the 4×4×4 supervision model, with the supervisor slowing down the process by taking the practitioner around the cycle: starting with their *experience*, moving onto *reflection*, then onto *analysis* to understand the meaning and finally onto *action planning*. There can be a tendency to miss out the reflection and analysis stages and move from experience to action planning in an attempt to provide a 'quick fix' (Wonnacott, 2012, p. 57).

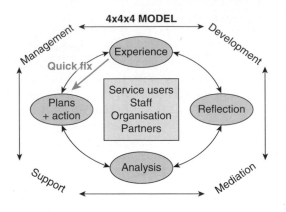

Taking a step back to pause and reflect upon the feelings provoked by the contact session will inevitably take more time on the part of the supervisor and supervisee. However, it will also provide an opportunity for supervision to slow down thinking, using supervision as a means to interrupt and punctuate practice (Ryan, 2004). According to Shohet (2011) reflection is bound closely to mindfulness, being attentive, perceptive and adopting an emotional focus.

By its very nature, child protection work is about balancing risk and uncertainty, and practitioners are working with families where violence, poverty and vulnerabilities are key features as illustrated by the case study. Through their day-to-day work, social workers like Kate can become overwhelmed by what they see and hear, and they need a safe and reliable place to share and deposit such feelings (Ruch, 2007). It can be difficult for practitioners to share feelings associated with shame, blame and inadequacy (Shohet, 2011). The case study suggests a positive relationship between Kate and her supervisor, and she appears to be using supervision as a place where she can formally 'off load' and have her emotions contained (Ferguson, 2018). Similarly, in this situation, supervision can serve a number of purposes. It would appear that within the contact session, Kate has absorbed the feelings surrounding her in the room and it has evoked inner feelings connected to her own separation and loss. Kate's own feelings appear to have become bound up with those of Mrs Jasper like a tangled ball of wool, and supervision could help here in safely allowing Kate to share and unravel these feelings. Reflective supervision can also contain Kate's emotions in an empathetic manner, while at the same time the supervisor can help

Kate explore Mr and Mrs Jasper's role as 'containers' for their daughter (Ruch, 2007).

CONTAINMENT: CONTAINING THE CONTAINER

Containment is a complex concept, and put simply it is a term developed by Bion (1962), a psychoanalyst, to describe primitive feelings engendered by complex situations and the disruptive effect that they can have on thought processes. In order to manage our feelings and be able to integrate both thinking and feeling, Bion developed the concept of 'contained-container', where within a therapeutic relationship, the therapist acts as the container for overwhelming feelings. Within child development, the primary carer's role is to contain their infant's insecurities.

Within the context of supervision, if practitioners are not emotionally contained by their supervisors, there is a strong possibility that they will feel overwhelmed, and this will have a negative impact on their practice. Whereas when social workers are effectively supervised and have their emotions contained in a supportive manner, they in turn are able to connect with children and their families and develop meaningful relationships (Research in Practice (RiP), 2019). Patterson (2019, p. 51) suggests that 'while supervision does not seek to infantilise or to rescue a practitioner, the ability to listen and contain feelings of vulnerabilty, loss, anger or frustrations without being overwhelmed allows these to be processed' and so making the work more manageable.

At the beginning of the supervision session, Kate describes herself as feeling fine, but as the session progresses, Kate shares feelings of sadness, pessimism, helplessness and anger. It is not unusual for practice supervisors to 'check in' at the start of a supervision session asking about the social worker's general well-being, but as illustrated by the case study, it is through storytelling—telling of the experience—that the practitioner's true feelings unfold. This is echoed in research of Wilkins et al. (2017, p. 946) based on 34 supervisory recordings. They found that managers did ask how the practitioner was, but that the case discussions between supervisor and supervisee did not include emotions associated with the practitioner, children or families. 'This is not to say managers were uncaring once the discussion focussed on particular families, emotional references were largely absent' (Wilkins et al., 2017, p. 946). A model of emotionally inclusive supervision could be adopted as proposed by Ingram (2013), which could encompass the exploration of Kate's emotions and feelings.

Kate ends her discussion with a sense of pessimism, struggling to find any positives in the situation and uncertain what to do next. A strengths-based approach to supervision might help in this situation. Collins (2007) reminds us of the benefits of positive reappraisal, which involves utilising cognitive strategies for reframing a situation. In other words, to appraise a challenging situation or event more positively. Supervision can play a pivotal role in positive reappraisal by considering the situation from an alternative position and offering possible solutions from a strengths-based approach. The supervisor could support Kate to explore options for the family, what the parents' behaviour and conversations might mean, how this might impact on the child. The supervisor can also adopt what Edwards and Chen (1999, p. 353) refer to a 'competence focus', where the supervisor models what they want from the practitioner, shifting the focus to successful interventions and so reinforce Kate's competence so that she in turn might consider the strengths of the family and the positive aspects of the contact session. Supervision could support Kate in looking beyond the contact session and explore Mr and Mrs Jaspers' personal histories as the answers to the present can sometimes lie in the past.

A possible drawback of a strengths-based approach is that perceptions, if unchecked, can become skewed and practitioners might become overly optimistic and potentially lose sight of the child and safeguarding concerns. This is reminiscent of the term the 'rule of optimism,' which was first highlighted by Dingwall et al. (1983). They suggested that social workers tend to adopt an optimistic lens when working with families. It has been suggested that to endorse this position exclusively can potentially put children in further

danger and remains a central concept within child protection discourse (Kettle & Jackson, 2017). Revell and Burton (2016) hypothesise that the 'rule of optimism' that exists in practice can also play out within the supervisory relationship where the likelihood of the supervisor exercising professional curiosity of the supervisee is reduced. Within supervision, it is therefore imperative that the supervisor is inquisitive and considers the complexity of practice from all angles, whilst maintaining the child's needs central to these conversations.

CONCLUSION

Despite the evidence base linking supervision with positive outcomes for children and their families (Carpenter et al., 2013; Wilkins et al., 2017) studies have confirmed that social workers benefit from effective supervision. It has shown to enhance practitioners' performance, job satisfaction and strengthen the social work workforce (Akesson & Canavera, 2018; Roby, 2016). Supervision is also seen as a source of support, identification of stress and burnout (Bradbury-Jones, 2013) and a space in which to develop skills and knowledge (Bradbury-Jones, 2013; Chiller & Crisp, 2012).

Lack of time is often highlighted as the reason that reflective supervision is frequently not provided and instead the procedural check list approach is somehow quicker and easier (Manthorpe et al., 2015; Rushton & Nathan, 1996). However, rather than seeing supervision as onerous and time consuming, it could be seen as an investment in practitioners and so in turn an investment in the protection of children. Reflective supervision needs to be seen as one term rather than two separate words, reflection is not a bolt on to supervision; instead it needs to become an intrinsic part of the process and relationship. One supervisor recently suggested that offering the lack of time as a reason not to engage in reflective supervision is a myth. Instead she suggests reflective supervision is like riding a bike: once you understand what it is and learn how to do it, you do it without thinking. In other words, reflectiveness becomes an unconscious part of the fabric woven into supervision.

Supervision serves a number of purposes, including a vehicle for practitioners to learn about reflection, become more reflective and engage in mindful practice. The supervisor is bestowed with the responsibility to model good practice. To demonstrate a calm, reflective and considered response to complex situations which can be passed on to their supervisees to emulate in their practice. In this sense, supervision can be compared to the well-known children's game of 'tag'. The game involves one person being 'it', and their role is to touch someone else, who in turn immediately becomes 'it' and goes on to tag someone else. In a supervisory context 'it' is good reflective practice characterised by empathetic listening, positive reappraisal and curiosity, which the supervisor models and in turn is practised by the supervisee with children and their families.

There are a number of negative impacts to the practitioner, organisation and most worryingly to children and their families if reflective supervision is not provided. This includes less effective practice, poor levels of job satisfaction, high turnover of staff and levels of sickness due to high levels of stress and burnout. Effective supervision is a two-way process and happens within the context of a relationship. Practitioners are not passive recipients of supervision, and they can adopt strategies to try and get the most from supervision. This can be summarised by adopting three principles:

1. *Prioritisation* – avoid cancelling and/or postponing supervision. Supervision is about professional and personal needs, and so it is important that the best possible service for children and families is provided.
2. *Preparation* – make time to prepare for supervision by re-reading the notes from the previous session, identifying tasks that have been completed (or not).
3. *Proactiveness* – contribute to the supervision agenda by identifying (in advance) particular children/young people and families that you would like to discuss.

It is highly important that both supervisor and supervisee are congruent within the supervisory relationship. The delivery and quality of supervision are often challenged by pressures relating to resources and time (Earle et al., 2017). If this arises, it will need addressing in an open and transparent manner. In addition, as mentioned previously, there are other forms of reflective supervision such as group supervision which can also be helpful to complement one-to-one supervision.

Social work supervision has been instrumental, and continues to be, in highlighting the issues and debates pertinent to practice. The role of the practice supervisor is multi-faceted. It provides the conduit through which practitioners can access a safe space for reflection, support, resources and learning. Reflective supervision creates a safe space where the supervisor acts as a facilitator that encourages practitioners to discuss emotions associated with the intricacies of child protection work. Given the emotionally disturbing nature and complexity of child protection work, it is important that social workers have the opportunity to pause and reflect upon their practice and the impact this work has on their emotions and well-being. Supervision could provide practitioners the space they need to feel 'replenished and fortified' (Weatherston et al., 2010, p. 3).

REFLECTIVE QUESTIONS

- As a practitioner, how can you best benefit from supervision?
- As a supervisor, how can you ensure that your supervision is characterised by empathetic listening, positive appraisal and curiosity?
- Supervision is a two-way process. What can you do to ensure that reflection is embedded into your supervision?

FURTHER READING

Davys, A., Beddoe, L., 2010. Chapter 8: Communication and emotion in supervision. Best Practice in Professional Supervision: A Guide for the Helping Professions. Jessica Kingsley, London, pp. 158–176.

Research in Practice, 2017. Reflective supervision resource pack. https://www.rip.org.uk/resources/publications/practice-tools-and-guides/reflective-supervision-resource-pack-2017/.

Ruch, G., 2007. Reflective practice in contemporary child-care social work: the role of containment. British Journal of Social Work 37, 659–680.

REFERENCES

Akesson, B., Canavera, M., 2018. Expert understandings of supervision as a means to strengthen the social service workforce: results from global Delphi study. Eur. J. Soc. Work 21 (3), 333–347.

Bartoli, A., Kennedy, S., 2015. Tick if applicable: a critique of a National UK Social Work Supervision Policy. Practice 27 (4), 239–250.

Beddoe, L., Davys, A., 2016. Challenges in Professional Supervision – Current Themes and Models of Practice. Jessica Kingsley, London.

Bion, W., 1962. Learning from Experience. Heinemann, London.

Bradbury-Jones, C., 2013. Refocusing child protection supervision: an innovative approach to supporting practitioners. Child Care Pract 19 (3), 253–266.

Carpenter, J.W., Webb, C.M., Bostock, L., 2013. The surprisingly weak evidence base for supervision: findings from a systematic review of research in child welfare practice. Child. Youth Serv. Rev. 35 (11), 1843–1853.

Chiller, P., Crisp, B.R., 2012. Professional supervision: a workforce retention strategy for social work? Aust. Soc. Work 65 (2), 232–242.

Cole, M., 2019. Social work supervision in Malta: a specialism in the making. Clin. Soc. Work 38, 1–19.

Collins, S., 2007. Social workers, resilience, positive emotions and optimism. Practice 19, 255–269.

Davys, A., Beddoe, L., 2010. Best Practice in Professional Supervision: A Guide for the Helping Professions. Jessica Kingsley, London.

Dingwall, R., Eekelar, J., Murray, T., 1983. The Protection of Children: State Intervention and Family Life. Blackwell, Oxford.

Dugmore, P., Partridge, K., Sethi, I., Krupa-Flashinska, M., 2018. Systemic supervision in statutory social work in the UK: systemic rucksacks and bells that ring. Eur. J. Soc. Work 21 (3), 400–414.

Earle, F., Fox, J., Webb, C., Bowyer, S., 2017. Reflective Supervision: Resource Pack. Research in Practice (RiP), Dartington.

Edwards, J.K., Chen, M.W., 1999. Strength-based supervision: frameworks, current practice and future directions. Fam. J. 7 (4), 349–357.

England, H., 1986. Social Work as Art: Making Sense for Good Practice. Allen and Unwin, London.

Ferguson, H., 2018. How social workers reflect in action and when and why they don't: the possibilities and limits to reflective practice in social work. Soc. Work Educ 47 (4), 415–427.

Fook, J., Gardner, F., 2007. Practicing Critical Reflection: A Resource Handbook. Open University Press, London.

Ingram, R., 2013. Emotions, social work practice and supervision: an uneasy alliance? J. Soc. Work Pract 27 (1), 5–19.

Jack, G., Donnellan, H., 2010. Recognising the person within the developing professional: tracking the early careers of newly qualified child care social workers in three local authorities in England. Soc. Work Educ 29 (3), 305–318.

Jennings, S., 2017, 5 September. How do you manage the reflective supervision juggling act? Community Care. https://www.communitycare.co.uk/2017/09/05/manage-reflective-supervision-juggling-act/.

Johnstone, J., Miller, E., 2010, October. Staff support and supervision for outcomes based working. https://personaloutcomes.files.wordpress.com/2014/03/staff_support_and_supervision_for_outcomes-11.pdf.

Kadushin, A., 1985. Supervision in Social Work, second ed. Columbia University Press, New York.

Kadushin, A., Harkness, D., 2002. Supervision in Social Work, fourth ed. Columbia University Press, New York.

Kettle, M., Jackson, S., 2017. Revisiting the Rule of Optimism. Br. J. Soc. Work 47, 1624–1640.

Kolb, D., 1988. Experience as the Source of Learning and Development. Prentice Hall, London.

Manthorpe, J., Moriarty, J., Hussein, S., Stevens, M., Sharpe, E., 2015. Content and purpose of supervision in social work practice in England: views of newly qualified social workers, managers and directors. Br. J. Soc. Work 45 (1), 52–68.

McPherson, L., Frederico, M., McNamara, P., 2016. Safety as a fifth dimension in supervision: stories from the frontline. Aust. Soc. Work 69 (1), 67–79.

Mo, Y.H., Leung, T.L., Tsui, M.S., 2019. Chaos in order: the evaluation of social work supervision practice in the Chinese Mainland. Clin. Superv. https://doi.org/10.1080/07325223.2019.1610681.

Morrison, T., 2005. Staff Supervision in Social Care (3rd edition). Pavilion Publishing and Media, Brighton.

Morrison, T., Wonnacott, J., 2010. Supervision: now or never – reclaiming reflective supervision in social work.

Munro, E., 2011. The Munro Review of Child Protection: Final Report A Child-Centered System. Department for Education, The Stationery Office Ltd.

Murphy, D., Duggan, M., Joseph, S., 2013. Relationship-based social work and its compatibility with the person-centred approach: principles versus instrumental perspectives. Br. J. Soc. Work 43, 703–719.

O'Donoghue, K., Wong Yuh Ju, P., Tsui, M.S., 2018. Constructing an evidence-informed social work supervision model. Eur. J. Soc. Work 21 (3), 348–358.

Patterson, F., 2019. Supervising the supervisors: what support do first-line managers need to be more effective in their supervisory role? Aotearoa N. Z. Soc. Work 31 (3), 46–57.

Pritchard, J., 1995. Good Practice in Supervision Statutory and Voluntary Organisations. Jessica Kingsley, London.

Rankine, M., 2017. Making the connections: a practice model for supervision. Aotearoa N. Z. Soc. Work 29 (3), 66–78.

Research in Practice (RiP), 2019. Containing Difficult. Research in Practice. https://practice-supervisors.rip.org.uk/wp-content/uploads/2019/11/Containing-difficult-emotions-in-supervision.pdf.

Revell, L., Burton, V., 2016. Supervision and the dynamics of collusion: a rule of optimism? Br. J. Soc. Work 46 (6), 1587–1601.

Roby, J., 2016. The evidence base on the social service workforce: current knowledge, gaps and future research direction. Global Social Service Workforce Alliance, Washington, DC. http://www.socialserviceworkforce.org/system/files/resource/files/Evidence%20Base%20on%20the%20Social%20Service%20Workforce_0.pdf.

Ruch, G., 2007. Reflective practice in contemporary child-care social work: the role of containment. Br. J. Soc. Work 37, 659–680.

Ruch, G., Turney, D., Ward, A. (Eds.), 2010. Relationship-Based Social Work: Getting to the Heart of Practice. Jessica Kingsley, London.

Rushton, A., Nathan, J., 1996. The supervision of child protection work. Br. J. Soc. Work 26 (3), 357–374.

Ryan, S., 2004. Vital Practice Stories From the Healing Arts: The Homeopathic and Supervisory Way. Sea Change, Portland.

Saltiel, D., 2017. Supervision: a contested space for learning and decision making. Qual. Soc. Work 16 (4), 533–549.

Shohet, R. (Ed.), 2011. Supervision as Transformation: A Passion for Learning. Jessica Kingsley, London.

Smith, M., 2000. Supervision of fear in social work. A re-evaluation of reassurance. J. Soc. Work Pract 14 (1), 17–26.

Tsui, M.-S., 2005. Social Work Supervision – Contexts and Concepts. Sage, London.

Weatherston, D., Weigand, R.F., Weigand, B., 2010. November. Reflective Supervision: Supporting Regulation as a Cornerstone for Competency. Arizona.

Wilkins, D., Forrester, D., Grant, L., 2017. What happens in child and family social work supervision? Child Fam. Soc. Work 22 (2), 942–951.

Wonnacott, J., 2012. Mastering Social Work Supervision. Jessica Kingsley, London.

Wonnacott, J., 2014. Developing and Supporting Effective Staff Supervision. Pavilion, Hove.

PART 2 Key Issues in Child Safeguarding

8

CUMULATIVE RISK OF HARM

SARAH-JO LEE ■ HELEN WOODS

KEY POINTS

- The individual and cumulative risk of parental domestic abuse, substance misuse and mental health on children and families.
- Current statistics on prevalence.
- Examples from practice to encourage reflection and explore the complexities in practice of working with these issues.
- Challenges facing parents and children seeking change.

INTRODUCTION

Domestic abuse, substance misuse and mental health issues continue to be prevalent factors in families who receive social care services and are notable in data from serious case reviews (Sidebotham et al., 2016; HM Gov, 2018). Often referred to as the 'toxic trio' (Featherstone et al., 2018, p. 11; Morris et al., 2017), the co-presence of these factors continues to present practitioners with significant challenges in how they understand, unpick the issues and respond. The latest data on serious case reviews (Sidebotham et al., 2016) reveal that domestic abuse was found in 54% of cases, mental distress in 53% of cases and parental substance misuse (PSM) in 47% of cases, with all three factors present in 22% of cases. However, as there were 27% of cases where only one of the three factors was present, it is important to be able to address each factor in its own right. As parental mental health is discussed in more detail elsewhere in (Chapter 19b) of this volume, the

main focus of this chapter will be domestic abuse and substance misuse.

While understanding the impact of domestic abuse, substance misuse and mental health difficulties on children is our imperative, it is not possible to do so without considering the experiences and difficulties faced by parents and carers. In recent years, concerns have been raised about a trend towards approaches in child protection which seek to individualise children and demonise parents, rather than recognising the interdependence of family life (Featherstone et al., 2014; Leigh, 2016). This may be particularly the case with issues such as substance misuse and domestic abuse, which are often associated with poor life choices and personal 'fecklessness' (Houston, 2016, p. 533). Ultimately, however, it is the adults who will need to make the changes where required, though children can also benefit enormously from accessing support. When planning with parents, recognising strengths and opportunities for change is key, while also being realistic about our expectations and timescales.

CUMULATIVE RISK AND THE 'TOXIC TRIO'

The term 'toxic trio' has become a catch-all in social care for cases where domestic abuse, substance misuse and mental health issues co-exist. However, this phrase has been criticised as reductionist, conflating these three issues without sufficiently representing their significance for individuals and families and without consideration of other factors that might be impactful (Morris et al., 2017; Featherstone et al., 2018; Skinner et al., 2021). Cumulative risk of harm is defined as 'the effects of multiple adverse circumstances and events on a child's life' (Bromfield et al., 2007, p. 35). The cumulative risk of domestic abuse, substance misuse and mental ill-health has been examined in depth elsewhere (Cleaver, Unell and Aldgate, 2011; Stanley et al., 2010). Whilst these can create significant risks for children, it is not the assumption here that adversity resulting from these factors in childhood always leads to a lifetime of disadvantage.

In this chapter, we encourage practitioners to carefully assess how different presenting factors relate to one another uniquely within families and, most importantly, to reflect on the barriers which their own practice may present for families. It can be tempting to try and make such complexity more manageable by imagining that once referrals to appropriate services are made the risks will reduce, when in fact this can present new challenges. Furthermore, in the current era of austerity and economic recession, it is vital to acknowledge the often severe limitations on service provision for domestic abuse, substance misuse and mental health. Within this context, it is vital to recognise the central importance for social work and social care practitioners in facilitating change. Research shows that the quality of relationships between practitioners working in the safeguarding field and children and their parents/carers are key to the outcomes that are achieved for children (Ruch, 2005; Hingley-Jones and Ruch, 2016), and therefore echo calls for practitioners to be given the time to focus on building and engaging in effective relationship-based practice (BASW, 2020).

DOMESTIC ABUSE

In this chapter, domestic abuse is considered in the context of *men's* abuse towards *women* as *mothers;* this reflects much of the day-to-day experience of child protection worker's involvement with families, wherein it is *mothers* and their children who are most frequently the victims of *men's* violence, abuse and coercive control. This was echoed in an analysis of serious case reviews from 2011 to 2014 (Sidebotham et al., 2016), which found that many identified multiple reports of domestic abuse, often involving vulnerable mothers with multiple abusive partners. Incidents of severe physical violence

against mothers were often recorded in cases where children died, but this was not always the case, and the presence and importance of being alert to coercive control were highlighted:

A picture emerged of women living with aggressively controlling men, who would isolate these women, impose restrictions on them, and control many aspects of their lives

Sidebotham et al., (2016, p. 78)

Research shows that concerns about the risks to children of living in such environments often result in social work practice that focuses on requiring women to leave their partners. When they do not, concerns for children's safety and well-being often escalate; women are viewed as 'failing to protect' their children and may be threatened with care proceedings (Stanley, 2011).

At the time of writing, the Domestic Abuse Bill 2020 is nearing enactment. This sets out a statutory definition of domestic abuse that recognises that abuse can include violent, threatening, controlling or coercive behaviour as well as physical, sexual, economic, psychological, emotional and/or 'other' abuse, and that 'it does not matter whether the behaviour comprises a single incident or a course of conduct' (Domestic Abuse Bill, 2021, p. 2).

It is easy to read this list of behaviours without engaging with what these might mean for its 'victims'; yet understanding the nature of domestic abuse and its harmful and debilitating effects is critical for effective child safeguarding practice. Significantly, the proposed legislation also recognises children who 'see, hear or experience the effects of domestic abuse' as 'victims' in their own right and requires locally commissioned services to consider and address the needs of child 'victims' (HM Gov, 2020). However, whilst this recognition aligns with the Children Act's (1989) amended definition of 'harm' to include the 'impairment suffered from seeing or hearing the ill-treatment of another' (Adoption and Children Act 2002, s120), both fail to adequately capture the complex ways that children may be harmed through their experiences of domestic abuse.

This chapter therefore considers the nature of domestic abuse and its effects on adult *and* child 'victims', paying attention to some of the *specific* practice issues and challenges. Whilst there are often no easy answers, readers will be encouraged to critically reflect on the extent to which their practice with children and families in the context of domestic abuse is safe, effective and aligned with the aims and values of social work.

Research shows that both men and women may perpetrate and be victims of domestic abuse, and that this can be present in both heterosexual and same sex relationships (Turrell, 2000; Stonewall, 2018).

Domestic abuse also occurs in the context of forced marriage and so-called 'honour crimes', both of which might involve women family members as perpetrators and men as victims (Home Office, 2020).

However, different contexts of domestic abuse elicit a range of different issues and complexities that practitioners need to be aware of, but which there is insufficient space to them consider here. We have therefore identified some resources at the end of this chapter which you might find helpful.

REFLECTIVE QUESTION

Revisit the definition of domestic abuse together with the 'picture' that emerged from the analysis of serious case reviews:

- How reasonable/realistic do you think it is for social work practice to expect abused women to protect themselves and their children from 'aggressively controlling men'?

DOMESTIC ABUSE AND HARM TO CHILDREN

Exposure to domestic abuse is commonly associated with children experiencing fear, anxiety, guilt and shame, which, in turn, might have a range of negative consequences for their emotional, behavioural, social and educational development. Research has identified the many ways that these might unfold and present differently according to factors such as the age and gender of children, the degree of exposure to, and 'seriousness' of, the abuse and the presence of other 'adversities' and/or 'protective factors' in the children's lives (Holt et al., 2008; Cleaver et al., 2011).

The legal definition of harm has provided a lens through which practitioners have tended to view, and work with, children's experiences of domestic abuse. This lens has focused attention on children witnessing or hearing discrete *incidents* of domestic abuse and conceptualised it as a 'parental problem' that emotionally harms children. It is recognised, too, that children can be injured if they get caught up in incidents and/or try to intervene, and that domestic abuse can impact parenting capacity such that children might also experience neglect (Stanley et al., 2010). This is reflected in child protection plans wherein harm caused by domestic abuse is most often identified within the categories of emotional abuse and/or neglect.

However, a closer look at the research points to the need for practitioners to broaden their conceptual lens when seeking to understand the ways that children may be harmed through domestic abuse. Whilst the concept of 'coercive control' has only recently gained currency, the controlling aims and functions of men's domestic abuse, and ways that children might be used, abused and effected within this context, have long been understood (Pence and Paymar, 1984) and documented in research. For example, Hester and Radford (1996) identified that children may be abused as part of the abuse of their mother and vice versa, whilst McCloskey et al. (1995) cited in Holt et al., 2008, p.800 concluded from their research that a father's relationship with his children was secondary to his use of them to abuse their mother. The tragic consequences of this are seen when abusers kill children – sometimes with their mothers and sometimes without – as a means of asserting their ultimate act of control over partners or ex-partners and/or as a form of punishment and revenge. Whilst such outcomes represent the most extreme consequences of domestic abuse, they also underline the importance of recognising the inter-related nature of the harm caused to mothers and children through domestic abuse.

More recent research (Katz, 2016) draws on the concept of coercive control to document ways that harm to mothers and children is intertwined. For example, abusers' control over women's time, money, movement and relationships can isolate both mothers and children by restricting their access to social activities and relationships with wider family members and within the community. The research also shows how perpetrators use coercive control to create an environment of fear such that children conform to expectations and demands around behaviour. In Katz's (2016) study, this extended to how much time and attention women were 'allowed' to give to their children, further illustrating that domestic abuse can serve to undermine and damage relationships between mothers and their children (Bancroft et al., 2012; Morris, 2009). The significance and importance of understanding and responding to this form of harm has led to calls for domestic abuse to be viewed as an attack on the mother-child relationship (Humphreys and Bradbury-Jones, 2015).

COERCIVE CONTROL

'Not only is coercive control the most common context in which women are abused, it is also the most dangerous'

Stark (2007), p.276.

The Serious Crimes Act 2015 made controlling or coercive behaviour within intimate or familial relationships a criminal offence. Statutory guidance (Home Office, 2015) explains that:

■ Controlling behaviour is: a range of acts designed to make a person subordinate and/or dependent by isolating them from sources of support, exploiting their resources and capacities for personal gain, depriving them of the means needed for independence, resistance and escape and regulating their everyday behaviour.

■ Coercive behaviour is: a continuing act or a pattern of acts of assault, threats, humiliation and intimidation or other abuse that is used to harm, punish or frighten their victim.

The multi-faceted nature of children's experiences of domestic abuse and the development in our understanding about the dynamics of harm they experience point to the fact that some of our assumptions about the *cause* of harm might be misplaced (Holt et al., 2008; Katz, 2016). It is vital that we reflect this within our practice if we are to effectively protect and support children's recovery from harm.

DOMESTIC ABUSE AND PRACTICE ISSUES

An understanding of coercive control is critical for safe and effective social work assessment and intervention.

Crucially, practitioners should be aware that separation from abusers does not necessarily bring about safety for women and children and should be neither the aim, nor the endpoint, of social work involvement (Stanley et al., 2012). Conversely, research has shown that women and children may be at *increased* risk of experiencing serious and lethal violence at the point of separation and post-separation (Holt et al., 2008; Stanley, 2011).

Fathers will often use the family courts and child contact as a means of continuing to abuse their ex-partners, which occurs through the ongoing use and abuse of children. Quizzing of children, use of them to pass on threatening messages and continuing to seek to undermine their relationships with their mothers, as well as more direct forms of abuse, are all reported as occurring within the context of child contact (Stanley, 2011).

Identifying the Perpetrator and How Coercive Control Is Operating

Identifying how coercive control is used and functions in a family is often far more complex than it first appears, and there may be a range of barriers to practitioners seeking to understand this.

One of the first and foremost often relates to women's shame and fear of acknowledging and talking about domestic abuse with professionals; abusers often make women feel that they are 'unfit mothers' and instil fear that social care will remove their children from their care (Lapierre, 2010). This becomes a powerful method of silencing women, particularly when we consider the ways in which domestic abuse might impact women's parenting capacity. Practitioners – whether aware of the domestic abuse or not – can therefore become another very powerful weapon in the abuser's armoury and another person for the woman to fear.

It is perhaps not surprising then that abusers will often seek to capitalise on this new weapon by framing their partners as 'the problem'. Social work tends to make this easy for perpetrators since the effects of domestic abuse might indeed be viewed as 'problematic' when using an assessment framework that focuses on parenting capacity. For example, the depression and anxiety that many abused women experience as a result of abuse can impede their ability to be emotionally present and available for their children (Holt et al., 2008);

mental ill-health as well as the effects of physical injuries might affect their ability to undertake basic household tasks; whilst feelings of shame and the need to hide visible injuries might mean mothers feel unable to undertake day-to-day tasks like taking their children to school and shopping. Whilst some men might not consider or respond to the 'gap' that this leaves in children's care, others might 'step in' and take on these tasks making their ongoing involvement and role within the family seem essential to the care and well-being of the children. Practitioners taking a positive view of those aspects of childcare that are undertaken by perpetrators can inadvertently support them to tighten their net of coercive control.

It is also critical that we understand, and take into account, the ways that coercive control might impact children and their relationships within the family. Children also often feel the shaming and silencing effects of domestic abuse and might fear the consequences of social care involvement (Stanley et al., 2012). Practitioners are required to be 'child-focused' and to take children's wishes and feelings into account in decision-making (HM Gov, 2018). However, what might this mean in the context of coercive control?

CLOSER LOOK: CHILDREN'S WISHES AND FEELINGS IN THE CONTEXT OF THEIR EXPERIENCES OF COERCIVE CONTROL

Imagine for a moment that you have grown up listening to your mother being told she is stupid; that she can't look after her own children; that she's a drunk; that you would have been 'taken away' if it wasn't for your father being there. Imagine that it has been your father who has taken you to school on those mornings when your mother has not got out of bed; that he has been the one to go out and buy food when there was nothing to eat; that he has been the one to occasionally treat you with a trip to the cinema or suchlike. How would these experiences shape your relationships with your mother and father? What might you wish for, and how might you feel about social workers being involved?

Whilst there are no easy answers as to how to identify how coercive control operates in domestic abuse situations, practitioners need to be alert to the ways that social work involvement in domestic abuse situations can shore up men's power, abuse and control over their partners and children, compound women's and children's oppression and increase the risks to their safety and well-being. With this in mind we turn to consider some key principles when working with domestic abuse.

GOOD PRACTICE PRINCIPLES

Risk Sensitive Practice

Given the potentially serious consequences for some children of living with domestic abuse, practitioners should be conscious of risk. However, many 'domestic abuse referrals' into Children's Social Care will not reach the threshold of 'significant harm', and there will be wide variation in children's experiences and their levels of resilience (Stanley, 2011). Therefore, whilst it is crucial to attend to any immediate child safeguarding issues, a 'risk-sensitive', as opposed to a risk-averse, approach is encouraged (see resource list at the end of this chapter for guidance and resources that can help).

A Compassionate and Non-Blaming Approach

Practitioners need to:

- Move away from blaming women for failing to protect their children and for neglecting to meet their needs.
- Recognise the fear stigma, shame and embarrassment that act as barriers to people disclosing and talking about domestic abuse. This is true for perpetrators as well as for women and children (Stanley et al., 2012).

Practitioners need to build empathic relationships with men, women and children that enable them to feel heard and which acknowledge them. Emotional *and* practical support for fathers, especially following separation, will be important in trying to reduce risk and furthermore might provide opportunity for building an effective working relationship that can facilitate change. This is crucial if we hope to prevent men from going on to be abusive in future relationships *and* when we consider the high rates of post-separation violence and abuse to women and children (Coy et al., 2012).

Women and children will also experience a range of, potentially mixed, emotions relating to the ending of their relationships, which they are likely to need support with. These can include heightened levels of fear related to their safety; feelings of sadness and loss; and anxiety about the future. Women and children often have to leave their homes, belongings, schools and support networks, which can be extremely isolating. Women themselves identify that they would like social workers to provide a range of practical support and advice at this point, such as support to settle in and to develop or retain support networks (Stanley et al., 2012).

The emotional and practical consequences of separation can place further strain on potentially already damaged relationships between children and their mothers. Research shows a correlation between children experiencing domestic abuse and subsequently using violence and abuse against their mothers themselves (Kennair and Mellor, 2007). It is crucial that women are supported to strengthen their relationships with children, particularly as it has been argued that the mother/child relationship is key to children's ability to recover from trauma caused by domestic abuse (Leung, 2015 cited in Robbins and Cook, 2018, p. 1669).

SUBSTANCE MISUSE AND PARENTING

The Scale of Substance Misuse

Substance abuse or misuse refers to 'the harmful or hazardous use of psychoactive substances, including alcohol and illicit drugs' (World Health Organisation, 2020). Since the publication of *Hidden Harm* by the Advisory Council on the Misuse of Drugs (ACMD, 2003), estimating that there were between 250,000 and 350,000 children living with PSM in the UK, there has been greater professional awareness of the impact on children. Turning Point also published 'Bottling It Up' (2006, 2011), reporting on the impact of alcohol use on children and families. According to the National Drug Treatment Monitoring Service (NDTMS) data (HM Gov, 2018):

- 25,593 people started drug treatment.
- 20% of this group said they lived with a total of 46,109 children under 18.
- This includes parents living with their biological children and those living with children of a partner or another member of their household.

- People in treatment for opiates were most likely not to live with their children (39%), compared to those in alcohol-only treatment (26%).
- 69% of those in treatment said their children were *not* in receipt of early help services, as defined in Working Together to Safeguard Children 2018, or engaged with children's social care services.
- Eight percent (4409) of parents or people living with children said that a child protection plan was in place. A further 5% (2688) were looked after children and 3% (1845) were engaged with child in need services with a further 3% (1699) receiving early help services.

We can see therefore that a significant number of children are affected by parent and carer substance misuse. While it continues to be an important factor for children in care (HM Gov, 2018), there are a substantial number of children receiving no specific support around this issue. The impact of substance misuse on families is now featured in the National Drugs Strategy (HM Gov, 2017). However, recent research shows that there remains a lack of early intervention in social care services for families experiencing PSM, and that, particularly given the relapsing nature of PSM, families are likely to be repeatedly referred (Roy, 2021). It is also worth noting in a child protection context that, like domestic abuse, the impact of parental drug or alcohol use is likely to be listed under the category of neglect (Roy, 2021).

Hidden Harm

It is to be expected that alcohol use is more prevalent than Class A drugs such as heroin, and that a higher portion of problematic alcohol use will remain hidden. Approximately 2.6 million children are living with a parent who is drinking at hazardous levels, and Turning Point noted that nearly 50% of their service users in alcohol treatment were parents:

- The average alcohol consumption in this group was 30 units per day, 24 for mothers and 33 for fathers, well in excess (nearly 10 times) of the amount recommended by the Department of Health (Turning Point, 2011).

■ It is likely that parents drinking at this volume will also experience a degree of mental ill health due to the depressant nature of alcohol.

It is estimated in terms of illicit drug use that approximately 70% of drug users in treatment also experience mental health difficulties (NDTMS, 2017/18), and the significant overlap between domestic abuse and substance misuse has been noted in repeat research findings, particularly in relation to the impact on women (Humphreys et al., 2005; Holland et al., 2014). The Standing Conference on Drug Abuse published guidelines for inter-agency working (1997), referred to as 'The SCODA Guidelines', which remain helpful in assessing the potential impact of PSM on children and families. (See the link to the CAFCASS assessment tool at the end of this chapter.)

Of particular note is the risk of 'silo working', as child protection, drug treatment, domestic abuse and mental health agencies often prioritise their own area of provision, which can reduce holistic care for adults and more effective outcomes for children (Humphreys et al., 2005). Multi-agency collaboration often remains too dependent on the initiative of individual staff and managers (please see chapter 6 on Interagency practice in safeguarding children). It is also worth bearing in mind that parents may be susceptible to violence from others, such as drug dealers or other family members (Holland et al., 2014), and that in instances of domestic abuse, drug dependency can be a point of control of the victim.

The Impact on Children: Perinatal Considerations

The extent of harm generated by PSM depends on a range of factors, as detailed in the SCODA assessment guidelines (1997), including the substance(s) of choice, length, extent and nature of substance use (e.g. whether heroin is smoked or injected), and the wider support available to children and their parents. It can be of tremendous benefit if there is a non-substance-using parent or carer. In seeking to reduce the impact of drug use in pregnancy, it is important that parents seek support early on from both maternity and drug or alcohol treatment services. Illicit and controlled drugs, including alcohol, tobacco and cannabis, have been shown to have an adverse impact pre-birth. It is difficult to gauge specific impact, as many people engage

in multiple substance use, and the impact of different substances depends on the severity of use and stage of pregnancy (Forray and Foster, 2015). However, certain features are common to various substances. Tobacco impacts on foetal growth, leading to reduced birth weight. Alcohol also can lead to low birth weight and developmental abnormalities such as foetal alcohol syndrome (FAS). However, there is little evidence regarding the extent of alcohol use and FAS (Prentice, 2010). Babies may also suffer from alcohol withdrawal which will need specialist care. The picture regarding cocaine and crack cocaine use is less clear; while there is a connection to reduced birth weight, premature labour and a higher risk of miscarriage (Cleaver et al., 2011), the risk of reduced growth could be caused by co-occurring factors such as poverty and tobacco use (Prentice, 2010). In the case of intravenous drug use, it is also important to be mindful of the risk of blood-borne viruses. Children born with neo-natal abstinence syndrome due to opiate withdrawal are more likely to suffer irritability and require specialist care (Cleaver et al., 2011).

If a parent or parents have withdrawn from a substance or made significant changes to their drug use during pregnancy, it is worth considering that they are facing parenthood without a substance which may have previously supported their coping ability and provided a source of routine. Aftercare from treatment services at this time can therefore be important in addition to post-natal care.

Protecting Against Impact During Pregnancy

From a social care perspective, it is important to bear in mind that achieving greater stability and working towards achievable treatment goals are *more important* than abstinence (Prentice, 2010). In this regard taking a harm minimisation approach will be crucial, alongside working to clearly defined treatment goals and the management of any risk of harm to both parents and children. Sudden withdrawal from a substance could pose a greater risk of both mental and physical harm to mother and physical harm to the unborn child. The potential impact on their pregnancy, and indeed older children, is often a serious concern to women accessing treatment (ACMD, 2003; Turning Point, 2006) and can be a great source of motivation. Some authorities retain substance misuse specialist midwives who can assess a woman's substance use in conjunction with treatment services. It is important to know what support is available in your locality and to address any anxieties parents will hold early on.

THE IMPACT OF PARENTAL SUBSTANCE MISUSE ON CHILDREN AND YOUNG PEOPLE

Physical Health

While there is no need for social workers and others working in a child protection capacity to be experts in substance misuse, it certainly helps to have a basic knowledge of the effects of different stimulants, depressant and other types of substances, and be aware of any available drug or alcohol treatment in your locality. In families where substance misuse is having a significant financial impact, it may mean children's basic needs are not met due to a lack of food, material resources, heating or adequate accommodation (Cleaver et al., 2011). Substances such as alcohol and stimulant drugs such as amphetamine can reduce a parent's appetite meaning they may be less in tune with the need for regular mealtimes or have limited funds for food and basic necessities. This may also lead to older children taking on excessive caring responsibilities for young ones or other family members stepping in (Stanley et al., 2010; Cleaver et al., 2011). Prolonged Class A or alcohol misuse can lead to overall decline in a parent's physical and mental well-being and ability to cope, and at times this can be linked to physical abuse of children (Holland et al., 2014).

It is common for parents accessing treatment services to be given a 'safe storage box' for prescribed medication. However, in cases of heroin use and prescribed opiate substitutes, it is important to be mindful of instances where children have been given methadone or other substitute medication as a 'calmer', or to induce sleep, or have taken the medication accidentally, leading to dependence, overdose or death (Alotaibi et al., 2012; Ramesh, 2014). Regardless of whether child protection practitioners think a parent is likely to harm their child in this way, it is worth making sure parents are aware of the risks of giving prescribed, particularly opiate, medication

to children. It is also important to consider how the introduction of new prescribed medication may interact with any existing prescriptions, and check this with the parent and their general practitioner (GP), if concerned.

Emotional Well-being

In cases of prolonged substance misuse, children are likely to feel acutely aware that they are not their parents first priority, or even their second priority, as their parents' primary relationship will be with the substance(s). This can clearly impact self-esteem, and children can be helped enormously by explaining the nature of dependency and the cycle of change, i.e. that giving up is very hard and does not reflect the worth of the child or other family members. Children also feel a sense of shame and isolation and may perceive that they and their family are different from other children's (Wangensteen et al., 2019). Indeed, where substance misuse and domestic abuse combine, families are likely to experience 'double the stigma' (Policy worker cited in Humphreys et al., 2005, p. 1312). It is very helpful to inform children that they are not alone and that substance misuse *is common* in families. It may be worth exploring how children manage this stigma, and who they do, or can, confide in. Due to the consuming nature of drug or alcohol dependency and the impact of intermittent withdrawal, children may experience their parent(s) as inconsistent in mood, time, attention and warmth (ACMD, 2003; Kroll, 2004; Turning Point, 2006, 2011).

There may also be a lack of routine, such as mealtimes and bedtimes, which creates anxiety and impacts on other areas of the child's well-being. Some parents do manage their drug use routine around childcare, for example, drinking after the children are in bed and sourcing drugs around school hours, and it is worth exploring how parents manage their drug use in this respect and recognising they may be taking steps to reduce the harm to their children in ways which can be built on.

EDUCATION AND FUTURE LIFE OUTCOMES

Particularly chaotic substance use can impact on school attendance and a child's social presentation, concentration and ability to learn. Children will worry about their parents, which can make it hard to engage with other children, or concentrate on school work, and many experience social isolation and stigma (ACMD, 2003; Mentor-ADEPSIS & ADFAM, 2020). One aspect of cumulative risk is that substance misuse can be more likely among these children in adolescence and adulthood (Public Health England, 2019). It is helpful to think about what might help a child manage their anxiety in the context of parental substance use, and to understand what their worries are, bearing in mind that their parents may underestimate the extent to which their children are aware of their use of substances (ACMD, 2003).

CLOSER LOOK: BARRIERS TO ACCESSING TREATMENT

Gender

While there has been an improvement in professional awareness of substance misuse since the publication of ACMD, 2003, treatment services have been remiss in responding to the needs of parents, particularly *mothers,* accessing treatment. The provision of childcare would potentially improve the accessibility of treatment for women (Fountain, 2009). It is important that community treatment and children's services recognise the need for women to manage their drug treatment around childcare and school routines. Many service users struggle with the drug treatment waiting room, as it can place them in the company of people they would wish to avoid. This can be compounded for women, who see the treatment service as an undesirable location to bring children. Additionally, Turning Point (2011) found a driver for female alcohol misuse was feeling the need to be a 'perfect mother' who often lacked support from male partners. It is important that services do not add to such pressures in creating extra demands if this can be avoided.

Ethnicity and Treatment Access

In addition to gender, consideration of the impact of ethnicity is also important. For example, research on the experience of help seeking among Black Caribbean drug users found that there was a lack of awareness of service provision and basic drug information compared to White drug users. A concern to avoid stigma and stereotyping, a perceived lack of cultural understanding within treatment services, and a lack of consideration for the needs of families and carers were also barriers to accessing services (Fountain, 2009). In addition, there were links between Black male drug use and wider experiences of social exclusion, which may be compounded for the children of drug users (Fountain, 2009). The gendered, classed, racial and ethnic dimensions of treatment access therefore need consideration in relation to our expectations.

Service Provision and Multi-Agency Working

While Public Health England advocates a 'whole family approach' with regards to PSM, research repeatedly shows gaps in information sharing between specialist workers in both mental health and substance misuse services (Turning Point, 2006; Humphreys et al., 2005). There is also a lack of in-depth inquiry about children, or being aware of their presence particularly if an individual is not listed as living with children (Humphreys et al., 2005; Galvani et al., 2014). Professionals may have an anxiety that raising the subject of any impact on children may cause parents to disengage with either mental health or substance misuse treatment. Both substance misuse and adult mental health services can be adult focused, and understandably, they are often more preoccupied with their adult client's engagement and progress in treatment than potential child welfare concerns, or the impact of any such treatment on an individual's parenting ability. For example, while it is obviously desirable for a parent to be on substitute prescribing programme, changes to an opioid prescription or alternatively medication for a mental health disorder can have a significant impact on a parent or carers mood or energy levels and this may need planning around. Children will be very sensitive to any changes in parental mood or well-being, and this may impact on their sense of anxiety or vigilance (ACMD, 2003).

GOOD PRACTICE PRINCIPLES

If children's exposure to violence and substance abuse is to be reduced, we have to acknowledge the gaps in service provision and ask ourselves how a child might experience being brought into the spaces offered. For example, are local treatment services child friendly? Do they offer parent-only treatment times? Are parents able to access outreach services, for example, via their local GP practice, instead? A lack of attention to the impact of any treatment provision upon children also misses an opportunity to build on a parent's motivation for accessing services. Many drug-using parents cite a desire to be a better parent as a reason for addressing their problems (Forray and Foster, 2015), and reflecting on success in this area may be more productive

seen as an understandable response to feelings of shame (Gibson, 2015). From this perspective, we promote relationship-based practice as a method of tackling complexity and overcoming interpersonal barriers to change.

ADDITIONAL RESOURCES

Websites

http://safelives.org.uk
https://adfam.org.uk/files/docs/adepis_psu_schools.pdf
https://rightsofwomen.org.uk
https://www.cafcass.gov.uk/grown-ups/professionals/ciaf/resources-for-assessing-other-forms-of-harmful-parenting/
https://www.communitycare.co.uk/2017/10/02/identify-perpetrators-domestic-abuse-coercive-control/
https://equation.org.uk/best-practice-library/supporting-survivors/
https://equation.org.uk/product/guidelines-for-working-with-men-perpetrating-domestic-abuse/
https://www.iriss.org.uk/resources/insights/domestic-abuse-and-child-protection-womens-experience-social-work-intervention
https://www.nspcc.org.uk/keeping-children-safe/child-protection-system/parental-substance-alcohol-drug-misuse/
https://www.tommys.org/pregnancy-information/im-pregnant/drugs-and-medicines/illegal-drugs-and-pregnancy
https://www.womensaid.org.uk/information-support/downloads-and-resources/

REFERENCES

Adoption and Children Act, 2002. https://www.legislation.gov.uk/ukpga/2002/38/contents.
Advisory Council on the Misuse of Drugs (ACMD), 2003. Hidden Harm. ACMD, Great Britain.
Aldridge, J.B., 2006. The experiences of children living with and caring for parents with mental illness. Child Abuse Rev 15 (2), 79–88.
Alotaibi, N., Sammons, H., Choonara, I., 2012. Methadone toxicity in children. Arch. Dis. Childh. 97, e1.
Bancroft, L., Silverman, J.G., Ritchie, D., 2012. The Batterer as Parent: Addressing the Impact of Domestic Violence on Family Dynamics, second ed. Sage, London.
BASW, 2020. Relationship based practice campaign information. https://www.basw.co.uk/what-we-do/campaigns/relationship-based-practice. (Accessed March 2020).
Beddoes, D., Sheikh, S., Khanna, M., Francis, R., 2010. The Impact of Drugs on Different Minority Groups: A Review of the UK Literature. UKDP, London.
Bromfield, L.M., Gillingham, P., Higgins, D.J., 2007. Cumulative harm and chronic child maltreatment, developing practice. Child Youth Fam. Work J. 19, 34–42.
Cafcass. SCODA: Risk assessment with parental drug use. https://www.cafcass.gov.uk/grown-ups/professionals/ciaf/resources-for-assessing-other-forms-of-harmful-parenting/. (Accessed February 2020).
Children Act's, 1989. https://www.legislation.gov.uk/ukpga/1989/41/contents.
Children's Commissioner, 2019. Pass the Parcel. Children Posted Around the Care System. https://www.childrenscommissioner.gov.uk/wp-content/uploads/2019/12/cco-pass-the-parcel-children-posted-around-the-care-system.pdf. (Accessed March 2020).
Chisnell, C., Kelly, C., 2019. Safeguarding in Social Work Practice. A Lifespan Approach. Sage, London.
Cleaver, H., Unell, I., Aldgate, J., 1999. Children's Needs - Parenting Capacity. The Impact of Parental Mental Illness, Problem Alcohol and Drug Use, And Domestic Violence on Children's Development. The Stationary Office, London.
Cleaver, H., Unell, I., Aldgate, J., 2011. Children's Needs - Parenting Capacity. Child abuse: Parental mental illness, learning disability, substance misuse and domestic violence. The Stationary Office, London.
Copello, A., Templeton, L., Powell, J., 2009. Adult family members and carers of dependent drug users: prevalence, social cost, resource savings and treatment responses. UK Drug Policy Commission.
Coy, M., Perks, K., Scott, E., Tweedle, R., 2012. 'Picking up the Pieces': Domestic Violence and Child Contact. Research Report. Rights of Women. https://rightsofwomen.org.uk/wp-content/uploads/2014/10/Picking_Up_the_Pieces_Report-2012l.pdf.
Domestic Abuse Bill, 2021. Parliament: House of Lords. Bill No. 171. The Stationary Office, London.
Featherstone, B., Gupta, A., Morris, K., White, S., 2018. Protecting Children: A Social Model. Policy Press, Bristol.
Featherstone, B., White, S., Morris, K., 2014. Re-Imagining Child Protection: Towards Humane Social Work With Families. Policy Press, Bristol.
Forray, A., Foster, D., 2015. Substance use in the perinatal period. Curr. Psychiatry Rep. 17, 91.
Fountain, J., 2009. Issues surrounding drug use and drug services among the Black Caribbean communities in England. National Treatment Agency/UCLAN, London.
Galvani, S., Hutchinson, A., Dance, C., 2014. Identifying and assessing substance use: findings from a National Survey of Social Work and Social Care Professionals. Br. J. Soc. Work 44 (7), 1895–1913.
Ghaffar, W., Manby, M., Race, T., 2012. Exploring the experiences of parents and carers whose children have been subject to child protection plans. Br. J. Soc. Work. 42, 887–905.
Gibson, M., 2015. Shame and guilt in child protection social work: new interpretations and opportunities for practice. Child Fam. Soc. Work 20, 333–343.
Hester, M., Radford, L., 1996. Domestic Violence and Child Contact Arrangements in England and Denmark. Bristol: The Policy Press.
Hingley-Jones, H., & Gillian Ruch, 2016. 'Stumbling through'? Relationship-based social work practice in austere times, J. Soc. Work Pract., 30:3, 235–248.
HM GOV, 2017. Drug Strategy. https://assets.publishing.service.gov.uk/government/uploads/system/uploads/attachment_data/file/628148/Drug_strategy_2017.PDF. (Accessed February 2020).
HM GOV, 2017–2018. Substance Misuse Treatment for Adults report 2017–2018. HM Government. (NDTMS - National Drug Treatment Monitoring System). https://www.gov.uk/government/statistics/substance-misuse-treatment-for-adults-statistics-2017-to-2018/alcohol-and-drug-treatment-for-adults-statistics-summary-2017-to-2018

HM GOV, 2018. Working Together to Safeguard Children: a Guide to Inter-agency Working to Safeguard and Promote the Welfare of Children. https://assets.publishing.service.gov.uk/government/uploads/system/uploads/attachment_data/file/779401/Working_Together_to_Safeguard-Children.pdf.

HM GOV, 2019a. Adult Substance Misuse Treatment Statistics 2018-2019: Report. https://www.gov.uk/government/publications/substance-misuse-treatment-for-adults-statistics-2018-to-2019/adult-substance-misuse-treatment-statistics-2018-to-2019-report. (Accessed March 2020).

HM GOV, 2019b. Transforming the Response to Domestic Abuse: Consultation Responses and Draft Bill. https://assets.publishing.service.gov.uk/government/uploads/system/uploads/attachment_data/file/772202/CCS1218158068-Web_Accessible.pdf. (Accessed March 2020).

HM GOV, 2020. Statutory Definition of Domestic Abuse Factsheet (updated August 2020). https://www.gov.uk/government/publications/domestic-abuse-bill-2020-factsheets/statutory-definition-of-domestic-abuse-factsheet. (Accessed March 2021).

Holland, S., Forrester, D., Williams, A., Copello, A., 2014. Parenting and substance misuse: understanding accounts and realities in child protection contexts. Br. J. Soc. Work 44, 1491–1507.

Holt, S., Buckley, H., Whelan, S., 2008. The impact of exposure to domestic violence on children and young people: a review of the literature. Child Abuse Negl. 32, 797–810.

Home Office, 2015. Controlling or Coercive Behaviour in an Intimate or Familial Relationship: Statutory Guidance Framework. https://assets.publishing.service.gov.uk/government/uploads/system/uploads/attachment_data/file/482528/Controlling_or_coercive_behaviour_-_statutory_guidance.pdf. (Accessed March 2021).

Home Office, 2020. Statistics on So Called 'Honour-Based' Abuse Offences Recorded by the Police. https://www.gov.uk/government/statistics/statistics-on-so-called-honour-based-abuse-offences-england-and-wales-2019-to-2020/statistics-on-so-called-honour-based-abuse-offences-recorded-by-the-police.

Houston, S., 2016. Beyond Individualism. Social Work and Social Identity. Br. J. Soc. Work 46, 532–548.

Humphreys, C., Bradbury-Jones, C., 2015. Domestic abuse and safeguarding children: focus, response and intervention. Child Abuse Rev. 24, 231–234.

Humphreys, C., Regan, D., Thiara, R.K., 2005. Domestic violence and substance use: tackling complexity. Br. J. Soc. Work 35, 1303–1320.

Katz, E., 2016. Beyond the physical incident model: how children living with domestic abuse are harmed by and resist regimes of coercive control. Child Abuse Rev. 25, 46–59.

Kennair, N., Mellor, D., 2007. 'Parent abuse': a review. Child Psychiatry Hum. Dev. 38, 203–219.

Kroll, B., 2004. Living with an elephant: growing up with parental substance misuse. Child Fam. Soc. Work 12 (1), 84–93.

Lapierre, S., 2010. More responsibilities, less control: understanding the challenges and difficulties involved in mothering in the context of domestic violence. Br. J. Soc. Work 40, 1434–1451.

Leigh, J., 2016. The story of the PPO queen: The development and acceptance of a spoiled identity in child protection social work. Child Fam. Soc. Work, 21: 412–420.

Mentor-ADEPIS.org/ADFAM, 2020. Identifying and Supporting Children Affected by Parental Substance Use. https://adfam.org.uk/files/docs/adepis_psu_schools.pdf.

Morris, A., 2009. Gendered dynamics of abuse and violence in families: considering the abusive household gendered regime. Child Abuse Rev. 18 (6), 414–487.

Morris, K., Mason, W., Featherstone, B., Bywaters, P., 2017. We need to rethink use of 'the toxic trio'. Professional Social Work Magazine. BASW.

Pence, E., Paymar, M., 1984. Power and control: tactics of men who batter. Domestic Violence Intervention Project, Duluth, Minnesota.

Prentice, S., 2010. Substance misuse in pregnancy: case based learning. Obstet. Gyanaecol. Reprod. Med. 20 (9), 278–283.

Public Health England, 2019. National Statistics: Young people's substance misuse treatment statistics 2018 to 2019: report. https://www.gov.uk/government/publications/substance-misuse-treatment-for-young-people-statistics-2018-to-2019/young-peoples-substance-misuse-treatment-statistics-2018-to-2019-report. (Accessed February 2020).

Radford, L., Aitken, R., Miller, P., Ellis, J., Roberts, J., Firkic, A., 2011. Meeting the Needs of Children Living With Domestic Violence in London. Refuge/NSPCC Research report. https://www.nspcc.org.uk/globalassets/documents/research-reports/meeting-needs-children-living-domestic-violence-london-report.pdf. (Accessed March 2020).

Ramesh, R., 2014. Parents using methadone to pacify children, charity warns. The Guardian. https://www.theguardian.com/uk-news/2014/apr/29/parents-methadone-pacify-children-deaths-adfam. (Accessed March 2021).

Robbins, R., Cook, K., 2018. Don't even get us started on social workers': domestic violence, social work and trust—an anecdote from research. Br. J. Soc. Work 48 (6), 1664–1681.

Roy, J., 2021. Children living with parental sybstance misuse. A cross sectional profile of children and families referred to children's social care. Child Fam. Soc. Work 122–131.

Ruch, G., 2005. Relationship-based practice and reflective practice: holistic approaches to contemporary child care social work. Child Fam. Soc. Work, 10: 111–123.

Sidebotham, P., Brandon, M., Bailey, S., Belderson, P., Dodsworth, J., Garstang, J., et al., 2016. Pathways to Harm, Pathways to Protection: A Triennial Analysis of Serious Case Reviews 2011-2014. Final Report. Department of Education. https://assets.publishing.service.gov.uk/government/uploads/system/uploads/attachment_data/file/533826/Triennial_Analysis_of_SCRs_2011-2014_-__Pathways_to_harm_and_protection.pdf. (Accessed March 2020).

Skinner, G.C.M., Bywaters, P.W.B., Bilson, A., Duschinsky, R., Clements, K., Hutchinson, D., 2021. 'The 'toxic trio' (domestic violence, substance misuse and mental ill-health): How good is the evidence base?' Child. Youth Serv. Rev. 120, 1–11.

Stanley, N., 2011. Children Experiencing Domestic Violence: A Research Review. Research in Practice, Totnes.

Stanley, N., Cleaver, H., Hart, D., 2010. The impact of domestic violence, parental mental health problems, substance misuse and learning disability on parenting capacity. In: Howarth,

J. (Ed.), The Child's World. The Comprehensive Guide to Assessing Children in Need. Jessica Kingsley, London.

Stanley, N., Miller, P., Richardson Foster, H., 2012. Engaging with children's and parent's perspectives on domestic violence. Child Fam. Soc. Work 17, 192–201.

Stanley, N., Fell, B., Miller, B., Thomson, G., Watson, J., 2013. Men's talk: men's understandings of violence against women and motivations for change. Violence Against Women. 18 (11), 1300–1318.

Stark, E., 2007. Coercive Control. How Men Entrap Women in Personal Life. Oxford University Press, New York.

Stonewall, 2018. LGBT in Britain: home and communities. https://www.stonewall.org.uk/sites/default/files/lgbt_in_britain_home_and_communities.pdf. (Accessed March 2021).

Thiara, R.K., 2010. Continuing control: child contact and post-separation violence. In: Thiara, R.K., Gill, A. (Eds.), Violence Against Women in South Asian Communities: Issues for Policy and Practice. Jessica Kingsley Publishers, London.

Turning Point, 2006. Bottling It Up: The Next Generation. The effects of alcohol use on children, parents and families.

https://www.turning-point.co.uk/turning-point-reports.html. (Accessed February 2020).

Turning Point, 2011. Bottling It Up: The Next Generation. The effects of alcohol use on children, parents and families. https://www.turning-point.co.uk/turning-point-reports.html. (Accessed February 2020).

Turrell, S., 2000. A descriptive analysis of same-sex relationship violence for a diverse sample. J. Fam. Violence 15, 281–293.

Velleman, R., Templeton, L.J., 2016. Impact of parents' substance misuse on children: an update. Br. J. Psychiatry Adv. 22, 108–117.

Wangensteen, T., Bramness, J.G., Halsa, A., 2019. Growing up with parental substance use disorder: The struggle with complex emotions, regulation of contact, and lack of professional support. Child Fam. Soc Work 24, 201–208.

World Health Organisation (WHO), 2020. Health Topics – Substance Abuse. https://www.who.int/topics/substance_abuse/en/. (Accessed February 2020).

9

ENDURING FORMS OF CHILD ABUSE (NEGLECT, SEXUAL, PHYSICAL, EMOTIONAL AND FUTURE HARM)

DIANA BENTLEY

KEY POINTS

- An understanding of child abuse – language and definitions.
- Prevalence of child abuse.
- The identification of child abuse.

INTRODUCTION

On average 26 to 28 children are killed each year as a direct result of abuse (Sturt, 2020), and on 31st March 2020, 51,510 children were assessed as being at risk of harm and the subject of a child protection plan (Department for Education, 2020).

The identification of child abuse and harm to children can be complex and daunting. Practitioners working with children and families can worry about wrongly accusing a parent or carer of abusing their child whilst at the same time being conscious that not identifying abuse and taking decisive action could lead to a child being harmed or even killed.

Contemporary research shows there is unequal use of statutory interventions used to investigate child abuse and what practitioners recognise as abuse is changing. Families with children growing up in deprived areas are more likely to have a welfare intervention, and despite a reduction in the number of children who are the subject of a child protection plan, there are increasing numbers of plans in the categories risk of neglect and risk of emotional abuse (Department for Education, 2020; Nuffield Foundation, 2021).

In all communities, there will be children (from pre-birth to adulthood) who have or who are experiencing abuse. Sometimes the indicators will appear to be obvious, and at other times there will be few explicit signs. Practitioners will recognise multiple indicators of child abuse and multiple parental vulnerabilities for some families who will need minimal support and intervention, whereas other children will be at risk of significant harm and immediate statutory intervention will be needed.

Keeping children safe is not a linear process. Children who live in different environments who experience similar events will not all need the same interventions. Practitioners familiar with the indicators of child abuse must use this knowledge to have open and honest conversations with colleagues, other practitioners, children, and their families, to achieve a balanced understanding of the child and family context and particular aspects of culture and values which could influence decision making and outcomes.

This chapter will explore clear explanations and definitions of child abuse which practitioners can use to support the balanced, unbiased and evidence-informed identification of children and families who need additional help and support, through statutory interventions, universal services or support from the wider community and family.

Terminology Over Time: Defining Child Abuse

There is no one legal or procedural definition of the term **Child Abuse**. The Metropolitan police have a simple and useful definition, which can be used as a starting point:

> *Child abuse is when anyone under the age of 18 is either being harmed or not properly looked after. There are four main categories of child abuse: physical abuse, emotional abuse, sexual abuse and neglect.*
>
> *Police, UK (2019)*

The National Society for the Prevention of Cruelty to Children (NSPCC, 2019a) defines child abuse as 'when a child is intentionally harmed by an adult or another child – it can be over a period of time but can also be a one-off action. It can be physical, sexual or emotional and it can happen in person or online. It can also be a lack of love, care and attention – this is neglect'.

In general, physical and sexual abuse definitions refer to (often deliberate) acts of commission, where something is done to a child, while neglect refers to acts of omission where there has been a failure to act, which can either be a deliberate act or circumstantial. Emotional abuse can happen as an act of commission (where something is done to the child) or by omission where something is not done (Schrader-McMillan, 2014).

Working Together to Safeguard Children (HM Government, 2018) is statutory guidance for local authorities and other agencies or organisations who work with children and their families. It details their legal responsibilities for safeguarding and promoting the welfare of children in England. The statutory guidance is issued under Section 7 of the Local Authority Social Services Act 1970; local authorities are expected to follow the guidance unless they can prove a good reason for not doing so (Mitchell, 2018; Legislation.gov.uk, 2019). It states there should be a coordinated approach to protecting children; everyone who works with children has a responsibility for keeping them safe.

The statutory guidance expands the definition of child abuse to include neglect, abuse and exploitation, which can be perpetrated (by an adult, adults or another child) within the family and in an institutional or community setting by those known to the child or, by people not known to them. A child can be abused in person, but abuse can also be 'partially or wholly' online, with the use of social media and digital technology. *'Abuse can take a variety of different forms, including: sexual, physical and emotional abuse; neglect; exploitation by criminal gangs and organised crime groups; trafficking; online abuse; sexual exploitation and the influences of extremism leading to radicalisation'* (HM Government, 2018).

Practitioners need to be aware that perceptions and definitions of what constitutes child abuse will differ between agency professionals, individuals and communities depending on lived experience, training, values and social and cultural norms. The legal and social definitions of child abuse are not static; they change and adapt over time. For example, it was once a social norm and accepted that children worked in harsh conditions and were beaten, the concept of 'childhood' or children's rights was not yet established, and children were seen as income earners. The 1880 Education Act made school attendance in the UK compulsory between the ages of five and ten, increasing to thirteen years of age in 1889. In 1889 parliament passed the first act for the 'prevention of cruelty to children', which for the first time gave the police the ability to intervene if a child was being 'ill-treated' (Ferguson, 2011; Parliament.uk, 2021).

Until the 1960's the language used was that of child ill-treatment or child cruelty. This changed in the late 1960s when C. Henry Kempe, a pioneering paediatric radiologist working at the University of Colorado (USA), coined the phrase 'battered child syndrome'. It is suggested that until this point society found it too difficult to recognise that parents and people who care for children do sometimes deliberately hurt or even kill them (Ferguson, 2011; Oliver, 2017). During the 1970s and 1980s public knowledge of child abuse and neglect increased, when tragedies such as the death of Maria Colwell (1973) and Tyra Henry (1984) were reported and formal reviews of professional practice were undertaken leading to legislative and system change (Timmins, 1994; Bentovim 2009).

The term **'Child Abuse'** entered the vocabulary of child protection practitioners in the 1980s as a generic term which covered physical, sexual and emotional abuse and neglect (Ferguson, 2011; Kemp and Kemp, 1978).

CLOSER LOOK: IDENTIFYING AND UNPICKING SIGNIFICANT HARM

There is often some confusion about how 'child abuse' differs from the commonly used terms **Child Maltreatment, Safeguarding Children, Child Protection** and **Significant Harm**.

Child Maltreatment is an alternative term used for child abuse, often used in medical literature, research or when talking about an international context.

Safeguarding is a generic, umbrella term introduced in the early 2000s, it is used to cover all aspects of how statutory and non-statutory organisations work with families in the UK to promote the welfare of children, ensuring that children grow up with safe care and are able to achieve their best outcomes. The term safeguarding covers a spectrum of interventions from early help services to the use of statutory powers to ensure the immediate protection of children who are being abused.

Child protection is a specific function of safeguarding children, which focusses on protecting children who are suffering, or likely to suffer, significant harm.

Significant harm is the legal term used in the Children Act (1989) to describe and measure the actual or likely harm to a child who has experienced child abuse.

Significant harm is defined in section 31(9) of the Children Act 1989 as *'ill treatment'* which includes sexual abuse or physical abuse *'or the impairment of health or development'* which includes harm caused to a child's physical or mental health, or their physical, intellectual, emotional, social or behavioural development (Legislation.gov.uk, 2019). This definition was widened in section 120 of the Adoption and Children Act 2002 to include *'impairment suffered from seeing or hearing the ill-treatment of another'* such as emotional harm suffered by children who witness domestic violence or are aware of domestic abuse within their home environment (Legislation.gov.uk, 2020).

Section 47 (1) (b) of the Children Act (1989) states that when there is 'reasonable cause to suspect' that a child 'is suffering, or is likely to suffer, significant harm' the Local Authority children services (or Children Services Trust) has a duty to investigate and to make 'enquiries' so they can decide whether they need to take any action to 'safeguard or promote the child's welfare' (Legislation.gov.uk, 2019).

When considering whether a child has or is likely to suffer 'significant harm', practitioners must ensure they are very clear about the harm (child abuse) which has been experienced and how this harm has (or is likely to) impact on the health and development of the child and their ability to achieve their best outcomes.

REFLECTIVE QUESTIONS

- Make a list of the safeguarding activities which are undertaken in different settings (e.g. Children's Services, schools, GP surgeries, hospitals and youth clubs). How and why might understandings of child abuse differ across professional groups?
- Think about two forms of child abuse which could be classified as 'significant harm'. How confident do you feel about recognising child abuse? How are you supported to increase your understanding?

PREVALENCE

Children and young people can be abused at different ages and stages of development, and for different reasons including a variety of parental vulnerabilities, poverty and unique family circumstances (Wilkinson and Bowyer, 2017; Bywaters, 2020). However, the probability of being referred to children's services is not the same for all children and families. Children are more likely to be considered 'at risk of significant harm' if they live in poorer areas, and within some ethnic groups (Nuffield Foundation, 2021). The impact of child abuse can have devastating consequences.

The triennial analysis of serious case reviews undertaken between 2014 and 2017 reports that the number of child deaths which are the direct result of child abuse has not increased in recent years, averaging at 26 to 28 per year (Sturt, 2020). Research by the NSPCC also suggests that overall rates of child abuse may be less prevalent than 20 years ago (NSPCC Learning 2020). It is therefore interesting that despite this, more children and families are being referred to children's services because of concerns about child abuse and neglect - and a growing proportion of young children have been subject to children services interventions over the last 10 to 15 years (Nuffield Foundation, 2021). Bilson and Munro (2019) suggest that the current wide interpretation of 'risk' of significant harm has led to the 'investigative turn' and an increasing number of invasive assessments being completed. They found that of all children born 2010/11 it is estimated 17% were assessed by children services before the age of 5.

A study completed by Radford et al. (2011) for the NSPCC looked at the actual prevalence of child abuse and neglect in the UK. It estimated that 6% of children aged under 11 years, 19% of children aged 11 to 17 years and 25% of those aged 18 to 24 years had experienced severe abuse at some point during childhood. Disabled children are more likely to be abused than their peers who are not disabled; children with particular impairments, including communication difficulties, sensory impairments, learning disabilities and disorders, appear to be at greater risk (Wilkinson and Bowyer, 2017). The Office for National Statistics (2019) report that adults aged 18 to 74 years with a disability were significantly more likely to have experienced abuse before the age of 16 years than those without a disability, at 32% compared with 19%.

A lack of data makes it impossible to know if the increases in child protection investigations are because of actual increases in abuse and neglect, more reporting, more risk-averse practice or cuts to preventative services, but it is likely to be a combination of all of these (Nuffield Foundation, 2021).

ENDURING FORMS OF ABUSE

All practitioners working with children and their families have legal duties and responsibilities to identify and protect children who might be at risk of significant harm (child abuse). The Working Together to Safeguard Children statutory guidance makes it clear that 'Everyone who comes into contact with children and families has a role to play' and 'practitioners will be clear about what

is required of them individually, and how they need to work together in partnership with others' (Working Together to Safeguard Children 2018, p. 6).

It is vital therefore that all practitioners have a good understanding of the different forms abuse can take. Child protection work is multi-agency in nature, and it is vital that all practitioners working with children understand their own roles and responsibilities and signs of abuse. The following sections will describe and explore the key forms of abuse outlined in Working Together to Safeguard Children (2018).

Neglect

The persistent failure to meet a child's basic physical and/or psychological needs, likely to result in the serious impairment of the child's health or development. Neglect may occur during pregnancy as a result of maternal substance abuse. Once a child is born, neglect may involve a parent or carer failing to: (a) provide adequate food, clothing and shelter (including exclusion from home or abandonment) (b) protect a child from physical and emotional harm or danger (c) ensure adequate supervision (including the use of inadequate caregivers) (d) ensure access to appropriate medical care or treatment It may also include neglect of, or unresponsiveness to, a child's basic emotional needs.

HM Government (2018)

Children and young people of any age can be neglected. A child can be subjected to neglect in utero (before they are born) up until their 18th birthday (and beyond). Children and young people are more likely to experience neglect at home than any other form of child abuse (The Children's Society, 2018). Neglect is an ongoing and pervasive form of child abuse; practitioners who have regular contact with a child or young person who is being neglected can become used to their presentation and therefore not recognise the extent or impact of the abuse. The 2019 Triennial Analysis of Serious Case Reviews identified that neglect is consistently a factor in the lives of children who die or are seriously harmed as the result of abuse (Sturt, 2020). Practitioners can often underestimate the impact of neglect on a child or young person. In the most extreme cases, neglect can lead to grave harm and even to death (The Children's Society, 2018).

There might not be any obvious signs that a child is being neglected. Younger children particularly may not be aware that their life at home is different to their friends and peers and that they are being neglected. Unlike physical abuse, there is rarely an incident or crisis which needs to be responded to. There is evidence that professionals struggle to identify neglect in young people and are unsure what to do when they come across it (The Children's Society, 2018).

There are many physical features which can indicate a child is being neglected. A list of some of the common features is given below; however, this is not an exhaustive list, and other signs may be found.

- Clothing and shoes are dirty, too small or worn out. The child may wear the same items of clothing on repeated days or does not have the right clothing for the weather conditions. Children at secondary school may not have school uniforms and shoes.
- Babies do not have nappies changed when needed.
- Being left alone or inappropriately in the care of other children
- Not being provided with adequate food, children stealing food because they are hungry, eating more than usual at meal times or saving food for later or to take home to share with other family members.
- A child does not get medical, dental, or mental health care, or medical advice is ignored.
- Inconsistent school attendance and missing school. Children may bring themselves to school at an age when peers are brought to school by a carer.
- Poor weight gain and growth.
- Poor language skills.
- Poor personal hygiene; in the home the child or young person may not have a toothbrush or basic toiletries and there is no routine for bathing and washing.
- Basic need for shelter is not being met, which can include home conditions which are dirty, smelly and in a poor state of repair, no heating, lack of clean and comfortable bedding.
- Child does not have their own special possessions or toys (NSPCC, 2016c; Wilkinson and Bowyer, 2017; The Children's Society, 2018).

Neglect has been linked to a variety of additional problems for older children, including violence and aggression and increased risk-taking. It can lead to poor physical health, difficulties with relationships, low levels of well-being or mental ill health (The Children's Society, 2018).

Children's needs can become neglected due to poor parenting. This is usually unintentional and is the result of the child's parent or carer lacking knowledge, having their own vulnerabilities or other problems (Wilkinson and Bowyer, 2017; The Children's Society, 2018). A family may face a significant event or change in circumstances such as an eviction from a property, separation, bereavement or new partner entering the family which can lead to neglect. Child neglect is more often associated with poverty than other forms of child abuse (Wilkinson and Bowyer, 2017). It is absolutely crucial however that practitioners do not conflate poverty and neglect. Poverty is a risk factor for neglect as it can lead to high levels of stress, which can make it difficult for parents to cope with the demands of parenting. However, poverty in and of itself does not equate to neglect. The majority of parents experiencing poverty love and care for their children and have the capacity to meet their needs; many are disempowered by poverty which in turn can lead to higher levels of scrutiny over their parenting ability.

Early identification of neglect can result in support services being offered and the cause of the neglect being dealt with. The Department for Education recommends that all practitioners, including those in universal services and those providing services to adults with children, should share information with other practitioners to support early identification and assessment (HM Government, 2018). Where a child and family would benefit from co-ordinated support from more than one organisation or agency (e.g. education, health, housing, police) a lead practitioner should undertake the assessment, provide help to the child and family, act as an advocate on their behalf and coordinate the delivery of support services. A lead practitioner could be a practitioner from any of the agencies who know the family; a decision about who should be the lead practitioner should be taken on a case-by-case basis and should be informed by the child and their family.

Emotional Abuse

The persistent emotional maltreatment of a child such as to cause severe and persistent adverse effects on the child's emotional development. It may involve conveying to a child that they are worthless or unloved, inadequate, or valued only insofar as they meet the needs of another person. It may include not giving the child opportunities to express their views, deliberately silencing them or 'making fun' of what they say or how they communicate. It may feature age or developmentally inappropriate expectations being imposed on children. These may include interactions that are beyond a child's developmental capability, as well as overprotection and limitation of exploration and learning, or preventing the child participating in normal social interaction. It may involve seeing or hearing the ill-treatment of another. It may involve serious bullying (including cyberbullying), causing children frequently to feel frightened or in danger, or the exploitation or corruption of children. Some level of emotional abuse is involved in all types of maltreatment of a child, though it may occur alone.

HM Government (2018)

Emotional abuse does not have a single identifiable event but will happen over a period of time; it is persistent and pervasive. Emotional abuse is a feature of all forms of child abuse, but can also happen when there is no physical abuse, sexual abuse or neglect. Carers may specifically target one child in the family who has different experiences to their siblings and half-siblings, or a whole sibling group can experience emotional abuse.

Children of any age can be emotionally abused, but living in a more affluent family has been seen as a link to experiencing more emotional abuse (The Children's Society, 2018). A study for the City of London in 2017 looking at factors arising when responding to abuse in affluent families found that parents who have busy careers and can afford to have their own hobbies and interests away from the family home can spend less quality time with their children and be less emotionally available for them. Affluent parents are more likely to put extreme pressure on their children to be high achievers and conform, in their academic work, sport, music or other areas. Because of the status society gives to financially successful and practitioners' unconscious bias, emotional abuse of children in middle-class families will often go undetected (Bernard, 2017).

There might not be any obvious signs that a child is being emotionally abused. A child might not be aware that their life at home is different to their friends and peers and may not feel able to talk to anyone about how they feel. Practitioners need to be alert to the child and their behaviour and, rather than seeing the behaviour as the presenting problem and blaming the child, should try to see it instead as a form of communication and understand why the child acts in the way they do.

Children who are being emotionally abused might:

■ seem unconfident or lack self-esteem (worthless, unloved, unlovable, only value themselves in terms of what they can do to please others);
■ struggle to control their emotions;
■ have difficulty making or maintaining relationships; and
■ act in a way that's inappropriate for their age (CELCIS, 2012; NSPCC, 2016a)

Carers who emotionally abuse their children may demonstrate some of the following characteristics or behaviours towards the child:

■ Emotionally unavailable and unresponsive, i.e. does not comfort the child when they are hurt, upset or in distress
■ Gives negative feedback and little positive encouragement
■ See the child as 'irritating and demanding' and blames the child for things, which are outside of their control
■ Is verbally aggressive when disciplining the child and is strict and controlling
■ Has expectations for the child which are not consistent with their age, understanding or stage of development or giving a child responsibilities which the carer should be fulfilling
■ Not seeing the child as an individual with their own needs and personality.
■ Isolating the child, not encouraging them to form friendships and relationships, or actively encouraging the child to form inappropriate

relationships or behaviours, such as involving a child in criminal activity

■ Causing the child to feel frightened or in danger (such as children who are living in an environment where they see or hear domestic abuse) (NSPCC, 2016a; Royal College of Paediatrics and Child Health (RCPCH), 2017b)

Early identification is important both because the abuse can have a lasting impact and in many cases, parents can be supported to change their behaviours. Evidence informs us that many parents do have the capacity to change and are able to prove that they can change their behaviour or external factors that would otherwise have a severe impact on the child's welfare (Platt and Riches, 2016). How different parents or carers engage with support offered by their own network or professional agencies and how they change their behaviour will differ from person to person the ability to make changes must be measured according to the child's timescale.

Children and young people can experience emotional abuse at any age. There are specific factors that can intensify the impact of emotional abuse such as poverty and social isolation. If a carer is experiencing mental ill health, is living in a violent relationship, or is misusing substances, they can be offered support and interventions, which will enable them to be more responsive to the needs of their children.

Physical Abuse

A form of abuse which may involve hitting, shaking, throwing, poisoning, burning or scalding, drowning, suffocating or otherwise causing physical harm to a child. Physical harm may also be caused when a parent or carer fabricates the symptoms of, or deliberately induces, illness in a child.

HM Government (2018)

When a child is seen with a physical injury, it is often not easy to determine the exact cause and therefore not easy to establish whether the injury is the result of physical abuse, an avoidable accident caused by neglectful care or whether the injury is the result of an accident or unavoidable trauma.

Practitioners working with children and their families must keep an open mind about how a child has sustained an injury and be alert to *'unsuitable explanations'* for an injury which are implausible, inadequate or inconsistent (National Institute for Health and Care Excellence (NICE), 2017). To make these judgements, practitioners must take into consideration the presentation of the child, their age and stage of development, the child's mobility and normal activities and any existing medical conditions or needs. Alongside the physical presentation, it is vital to listen to the explanation given by the child and to observe their appearance and reactions. The practitioner should contrast this with the presentation and information given by parents and carers, and how this may differ or change.

Wilkinson and Bowyer (2017) identified that practitioners may be reluctant or lack the confidence to make judgements about parental behaviour, particularly when these are thought to be culturally rooted, linked with social disadvantages such as poverty or when the parent is a victim in their own right. Practitioners must also be alert to the risk of accepting accounts based on perceived religious or cultural traditions or gender-based stereotypes about what others do. Children who have been physically abused may present with an isolated injury or a number of different injuries; features of physical abuse are included below (NICE, 2017; RCPCH, 2019).

CULTURAL COMPETENCY

Cultural competence is the ability to understand and interact effectively with people from other cultures.

A 2020 Serious Case Review (Duncan, 2020) identified that a 'gap in the knowledge and understanding of culture and beliefs' within Traveller communities led to practitioners from a number of agencies downplaying the concerns about domestic abuse, learning disability and neglect.

Practitioners did not focus on the clear evidence of harm but allowed implicit associations influence their judgements that everything would fall into place if the family were found suitable housing. This proved not to be the case and a 2-and-a-half-year-old child was eventually admitted to the hospital suffering from severe malnutrition.

Professionals and managers did not support and challenge one another to gain a better understanding of the situation and lived experience for the child.

REFLECTIVE QUESTIONS

It is difficult to understand another's culture if you are not familiar with your own.

- Think about your own culture, and make a list of assumptions you have within your family about where families with children should live.
- List how cultural assumptions about looking after children might be different for relatives from different generations.
- What cultural assumptions have you challenged within your own family?

For many professionals, working with families from different communities for the first time means working within a new culture and context. This can be challenging and difficult to navigate, and it is normal to have questions.

SOFT TISSUE INJURIES INCLUDING BRUISES, CUTS OR HEALED SCARS

Bruising can be the first visible indicator of abuse. Practitioners need to know the importance of recognising and recording unusual or abnormal patterns of bruising (RCPCH, 2019).

In mobile children bruising that suggests physical child abuse include:

- bruises that are seen away from bony prominences;
- bruises to the face, back, abdomen, arms, buttocks, ears and hands;
- multiple bruises in clusters;
- multiple bruises of uniform shape;
- bruises that carry an imprint of an implement; or
- bruises with petechiae (dots of blood under the skin) around them

Practitioners should suspect child abuse if a child has cuts, grazes or scars with no suitable explanation:

- On a child who is not independently mobile
- Numerous (different locations)
- Have a symmetrical distribution (in the same place on both right and left side of body)
- On areas usually protected by clothing
- On the eyes, ears and sides of face
- On the neck, ankles and wrists that look like ligature marks (NICE, 2019)

BITES

Practitioners should be conscious that a child may have been physically abused if they have bites which look human and unlikely to have been caused by a child. Practitioners should also consider if the child is being neglected if there is an animal bite on a child who has not had proper adult supervision (NICE, 2017).

HEAT INJURIES EITHER BURNS OR SCALDS

Burns and scalds are damage caused by heat. A burn is caused by dry heat such as a cigarette, iron or fire. A scald is caused by something wet, such as hot water or steam (National Health Service (NHS) Inform, 2019). Scalds are the most common burn type in children who have been abused, and the most common cause is tap water (RCPCH, 2017a).

Abusive scalds tend to be seen on the buttocks, genital area, hands and feet will often have a clear or straight edge (glove or stocking distribution) where the limb has been put or held in the hot water.

Contact burns caused by physical abuse tend to be seen on parts of the body which would not normally be exposed such as the back, shoulders, and buttocks, with a shape and edges often matching the object used, such as an iron, cigarette, hair straighteners etc. (NICE, 2017; RCPCH, 2017a).

Children with abusive burns tend to be significantly younger than those with accidental burns and are almost always under the age of 10 (RCPCH, 2017a).

FRACTURED OR BROKEN BONES

It is not uncommon for children to have falls and non-avoidable accidents which result in broken bones or fractures. When children present with a fracture where there is no plausible explanation, underlying bone disease that can cause 'fragile bones' must be explored (NICE, 2019).

Some indicators that a fracture could be the result of physical abuse include:

- fractures of different ages;
- occult (hidden) fractures identified on x-rays that were not initially identified;

■ intracranial (scull) injuries, when there is no know major trauma or medical explanation;

■ rib fractures, when there is no known major trauma (multiple rib fractures are more commonly abusive than non-abusive);

■ fractures of the femur (thigh bone) in children who are not yet walking; and

■ fractures of the humerus (upper arm bone) in children under 18 months of age (RCPCH, 2018; NICE, 2019)

The identification of fractures which have been caused by physical abuse is complex. Practitioners who suspect that a child has been physically abused and may have sustained a fracture need to work closely with clinical experts with access to the latest research.

HEAD, BRAIN, EYE AND ORAL INJURY (ABUSIVE HEAD TRAUMA)

The head is the most common place to be injured when a child is physically abused, with 43% of abusive injuries occurring to the face and neck, with brain and head injuries being the most common cause of death and disability of children who are less than 2 years of age (RCPCH, 2013; Joyce and Huecker, 2019).

A torn [labial] frenulum (the soft tissue in the front of the mouth, between the upper lip and the upper gum and between the lower lip and the lower gum) is frequently described as a specific sign of child abuse. Whilst it is true that this injury can be caused by an abusive act such as force-feeding or a slap/punch to the face, studies have found that this injury can also be caused accidentally if a child falls or gets an accidental blow to the head (Teece, 2005). There is no clinical evidence that a torn frenulum as an isolated injury can substantiate a suspicion that a child has been physically abused (Teece, 2005).

FABRICATED OR INDUCED ILLNESS (FORMERLY KNOWN AS MUNCHHAUSEN'S SYNDROME BY PROXY)

Fabricated or induced illness happens when a parent or carer exaggerates or deliberately causes symptoms of illness in the child or restricts a child's activity to convince doctors that their health is impaired or more impaired than is actually the case (Hardy, 2019; NHS Choices, 2020i; RCPCH, 2021). Fabricated or induced illness is not a category of abuse on its own and can be emotional abuse, neglect, or physical abuse, depending on the circumstances.

This is arguably the most difficult form of child abuse to identify, with a healthy debate about its prevalence and causes. In 2021 the RCPCH introduced the term 'Perplexing Presentations' to describe possible fabricated or induced illness where there is no perceived risk of immediate serious harm to the child's physical health or life (RCPCH, 2021). The over- and under-identification of fabricated or induced illness can have a profound impact on children and their families. Bilson (2021) argues that there should be more flexibility in the approach taken, and rather than entering a formal child protection process, medical practitioners should be able to explore perplexing presentations in a more open and sensitive way with parents, carers and children.

In around 85% of reported cases of fabricated or induced illness, the child's mother is responsible for the abuse (NICE, 2017); however, other carers such as a child's father, foster carer, grandparent or a childcare professional can also be responsible. There is currently no data on same-sex parental couples (RCPCH, 2021). People who fabricate or induce illness in children are often seen as trusted people, and their descriptions of illness are initially plausible.

Boys and girls are equally likely to be abused, except in cases where the perpetrator is male. In this instance, boys are far more likely to be abused than girls (Precey, 2018).

Behaviours in carers which can be suggestive of fabricated or induced illness include:

■ reports symptoms of an illness which are only seen by one person;

■ persuades healthcare professionals that their child is ill, which can result in unnecessary medical investigations or procedures;

■ reports new illnesses once the symptoms of the first one has gone;

■ exaggerates or lies about their child's current symptoms and past history;

■ manipulates evidence;

■ manipulates test results to suggest illness;

■ deliberately induces symptoms of illness; and

■ despite a medical opinion that a child does not have an illness, they continue to seek opinions from multiple practitioners (Precey, 2018; NHS Choices, 2020a).

For disabled children detection of fabricated or induced illness can be particularly challenging. A carer may have genuine concerns for the child and may be struggling to care for a child and therefore exaggerate or induce symptoms so that more help or support is offered. Practitioners may find it more challenging to consider that parents of disabled children may be capable of harming their child in this way.

REFLECTIVE QUESTIONS

- Is fabricated or induced illness physical abuse?
- Why might a mother fabricate illness?
- When would it be okay for a parent to repeatedly take their child to a doctor?

Sexual Abuse

Involves forcing or enticing a child or young person to take part in sexual activities, not necessarily involving a high level of violence, whether or not the child is aware of what is happening. The activities may involve physical contact, including assault by penetration (for example, rape or oral sex) or non-penetrative acts such as masturbation, kissing, rubbing and touching outside of clothing. They may also include non-contact activities, such as involving children in looking at, or in the production of, sexual images, watching sexual activities, encouraging children to behave in sexually inappropriate ways, or grooming a child in preparation for abuse. Sexual abuse can take place online, and technology can be used to facilitate offline abuse. Sexual abuse is not solely perpetrated by adult males. Women can also commit acts of sexual abuse, as can other children.

HM Government (2018)

In the United Kingdom, the age at which someone can legally consent to having a sexual relationship is 16 years. This is the same for all young people irrespective of their gender, sexual identity or the age of their partner(s). The Sexual Offences Act 2003 sets out the law on sexual offences committed by those in positions of trust. It is illegal for a person in a 'position of trust' (for example a teacher, police officer, doctor, social worker or care worker) to have a sexual relationship with a young person under the age of 18 who is in the care of their organisation.

Sexual abuse is any act that involves the child or young person in any activity for the sexual gratification of another person, whether or not it is claimed that the child or young person consented or allowed this to happen. The Office for National Statistics (2019) estimates that in England and Wales, 3.1 million people (7.5% of adults) experienced sexual abuse as children.

NSPCC (2019b) research shows that recorded sexual offences against children in the UK between April 2017 and March 2019 reached an all-time high. There were 76,204 recorded sexual offences against children in the UK in 2018/19, a rise of over 60% since 2014/15. It however should be noted that higher recorded sex offences do not necessarily indicate an increase in sexual abuse crimes, but could be due to better recording, greater awareness of what abuse is, and survivors feeling more confident in coming forward. Sexual abuse as a child can have an impact throughout adulthood resulting in problematic and failed relationships, involvement in crime, depression and suicide (Symonds, 2000).

Sexually abusive behaviours include (again, not an exhaustive list):

Contact abuse (where an abuser makes physical contact with a child):

- Sexual touching of any part of the body, whether the child is wearing clothes or not
- Forcing or encouraging a child to take part in sexual activity
- Making a child take their clothes off or touch someone else's genitals
- Rape or penetration by putting an object or body part inside a child's mouth, vagina or anus.

Non-contact abuse (where there is no physical contact):

- Flashing at a child
- Encouraging or forcing a child to watch or hear sexual acts
- Not taking proper measures to prevent a child being exposed to sexual activities by others
- Making a child masturbate while others watch
- Persuading a child to make, view or distribute child abuse images (such as performing sexual acts over the internet, sexting or showing pornography to a child)
- Making, viewing or distributing child abuse images
- Allowing someone else to make, view or distribute child abuse images
- Meeting a child following grooming with the intent of abusing them (even if abuse did not take place). Sexually exploiting a child for money, power or status (child sexual exploitation) (NSPCC, 2019c).

Research undertaken for the Centre of Expertise on Child Sexual Abuse showed that most children who have or are being sexually abused do not tell anyone what is or has happened. Children however explained that they tried to disclose their abuse by showing signs or act in ways that they hope adults will notice and react to (Allnock et al., 2019).

There are a range of reasons why children do not disclose; these include shame and guilt, embarrassment, and fear about what others will think about them. Children might also be frightened about the consequences of telling; they might have been threatened or told that they must keep the secret or may not want to get the perpetrator into trouble. For some younger children, they may not have an awareness that they have been or are being sexually abused because it is the norm within their household and could be seen as a game or something which always happens. Girls are often more confident talking about sex and sexual relationships. Evidence tells us that girls who experience sexual abuse are more likely than boys to tell someone about their abuse during childhood (Allnock et al., 2019). It is possible that masculine stereotypes and gender assumptions of independence, sexual assertiveness and denying emotion can inhibit the ability of some boys to talk about their abuse during childhood or in later life.

Disabled children may be more likely than others to exhibit behaviours as signs, particularly where they do not have access to an adult who understands their means of communication. It is important that these behaviours are recognised and understood, and not simply attributed to the child's disability (Allnock et al., 2019).

Children and young people can display a number of physical and/or emotional signs when they are being sexually abused which can include:

- having sexual knowledge or behaviour, which they would not be expected to have;
- avoiding being alone with or frightened of people or a person they know;
- having nightmares or bed-wetting;
- changes in eating habits or developing an eating problem, starting to self-harm or misusing alcohol or drugs;
- bruises (particularly where a child might have been grabbed or held);

- genital or anal injury (bruising, cuts or swelling) with no explanation, or one that is not consistent with the injury;
- persistent or recurrent genital or anal symptom (for example, bleeding or discharge) that has no medical explanation;
- discomfort on passing urine or discomfort in the genital or anus areas that is continual or keeps coming back and does not have a medical explanation;
- child or young person with a sexually transmitted infection where there is no known mother-to-child transmission during birth or transmission of the infection; and
- pregnancy in children and young women under the age of 16 and pregnancy in young people over 17 years of age where there is a clear difference in power or mental capacity between the young woman and the putative father (NSPCC, 2016b; NICE, 2017).

Practitioners working with children must provide positive conditions to encourage and enable children to feel able to tell them about their experiences of being sexually abused. Practitioners should appear friendly, approachable and caring and recognise that many children need to feel believed when they disclose, and they should not act surprised or shocked at what the child says (Allnock et al., 2019). Practitioners must ensure that they have knowledge of the local and national safeguarding policies, and do not ask children questions or offer to support in a way that might prejudice any evidence or ability to safeguard and protect the child.

Contextual Safeguarding

As well as threats to the welfare of children from within their families, children may be vulnerable to abuse or exploitation from outside their families. These extra-familial threats might arise at school and other educational establishments, from within peer groups, or more widely from within the wider community and/or online. These threats can take a variety of different forms and children can be vulnerable to multiple threats, including: exploitation by criminal gangs and organised crime groups such as county lines; trafficking, online abuse; sexual exploitation and the influences of extremism leading to radicalisation. Extremist groups make use of the internet to radicalise and recruit and to promote extremist materials. Any potential harmful effects to individuals identified as vulnerable to extremist ideologies or being drawn into terrorism should also be considered.

HM Government (2018).

In addition to the more broadly understood categories of abuse, Working Together to Safeguard Children also outlines 'Contextual Safeguarding'. This is an approach to understanding, and responding to, young people's experiences of significant harm (or abuse) *'beyond their families'* (Contextual Safeguarding Network, 2019). Contextual Safeguarding is not a single entity; it is a generic term used regarding risks to young people which they experience in their communities and places where young people 'hang out' (i.e. parks, leisure centres, shopping centres), schools and online. These situations are outside of the family and are new and emerging forms of abuse such as:

- Child sexual exploitation (CSE)
- Child criminal exploitation (CCE) occurs where an individual or group takes advantage of an imbalance of power to coerce, control, manipulate or deceive a child or young person under the age of 18 into any criminal activity. Child criminal exploitation can involve children and young people carrying drugs on behalf of dealers and gangs and is closely associated with human trafficking and modern-day slavery
- Radicalisation, where a young person comes to support or be involved in extremist ideologies
- Harmful sexual behaviour (HSB)
- Online grooming/exploitation
- Human trafficking and modern slavery

It is not within the remit of this chapter to explore each of these issues in any depth. Readers can learn more about child protection in each of these areas in corresponding chapters elsewhere in this book. Practitioners need to be alert to harm and abuse which occurs outside the home and must remain vigilant in terms of 'new' forms of abuse and harm.

CONCLUSION

Children (and their families) must be treated with respect, dignity and with fair process and given access to the correct help, support and/or statutory intervention they need to be safe and to achieve.

REFLECTIVE QUESTIONS

Consider your own personal perceptions of the following questions:

- What stereotypes are common in society about parents or carers who harm or abuse their children? What are your own personal beliefs, and how do they impact on your practice?
- Why might some communities have higher or lower incidents of child abuse?
- Why are disabled children particularly vulnerable to abuse?
- What are your views about physical punishment? How does this influence your professional practice?
- Are you confident in understanding how to share information in a language that describes the risks, vulnerabilities and experience of a child?
- When it comes to child abuse, is the state intervening too little or too much? How does this influence your professional practice?

FURTHER READING

What to do if you're worried a child is being abused. Advice for practitioners (HM Government, 2015), https://assets. publishing.service.gov.uk/government/uploads/system/ uploads/attachment_data/file/419604/What_to_do_if_you_re_ worried_a_child_is_being_abused.pdf.

Working Together to Safeguard Children: A guide to inter-agency working to safeguard and promote the welfare of children (HM Government, 2018), https://assets.publishing.service.gov. uk/government/uploads/system/uploads/attachment_data/ file/779401/Working_Together_to_Safeguard-Children.pdf.

NSPCC – What is child abuse?, https://www.nspcc.org.uk/what-is- child-abuse/.

Child abuse and neglect (National Institute for Health and Care Excellence), https://www.nice.org.uk/guidance/qs179.

Neglect

Neglect (childline), https://www.childline.org.uk/info-advice/ bullying-abuse-safety/abuse-safety/neglect/.

NSPCC, Neglect (NSPCC), https://www.childline.org.uk/info- advice/bullying-abuse-safety/abuse-safety/neglect/.

Emotional Abuse

Emotional Abuse (NSPCC), https://www.nspcc.org.uk/what-is-child-abuse/types-of-abuse/emotional-abuse/.

Domestic Abuse: How to Get Help (HM Government), https://www.gov.uk/guidance/domestic-abuse-how-to-get-help.

Physical Abuse

Physical Abuse (NSPCC), https://www.nspcc.org.uk/what-is-child-abuse/types-of-abuse/physical-abuse/.

Fabricated or Induced Illness (NHS), https://www.nhs.uk/conditions/fabricated-or-induced-illness/symptoms/.

Perplexing Presentations (PP)/Fabricated or Induced Illness (FII) in Children Guidance, https://childprotection.rcpch.ac.uk/resources/perplexing-presentations-and-fii.

Sexual Abuse

Centre of Expertise on Child Sexual Abuse, https://www.csacentre.org.uk/.

Contextual Safeguarding

Safeguarding Network, Contextual, https://www.contextualsafeguarding.org.uk/about/what-is-contextual-safeguarding.

Criminal Exploitation and Gangs (NSPCC), https://www.nspcc.org.uk/what-is-child-abuse/types-of-abuse/gangs-criminal-exploitation/.

Digital Dangers (Barnardo's), https://b.barnardos.org.uk/what_we_do/our_work/sexual_exploitation/about-cse/digital-dangers.htm.

Radicalisation, N.S.P.C.C., https://learning.nspcc.org.uk/safeguarding-child-protection/radicalisation/.

Modern Slavery (HM Government), https://www.gov.uk/government/collections/modern-slavery.

Protecting Children from Harmful Sexual Behaviour (NSPCC), https://learning.nspcc.org.uk/child-abuse-and-neglect/harmful-sexual-behaviour/.

REFERENCES

Adoption and Children Act, 2002. https://www.legislation.gov.uk/ukpga/2002/38/contents.

Allnock, D., Miller, P., Baker, H., 2019. Key Messages From Research on Identifying and Responding to Disclosures of Child Sexual Abuse. https://www.csacentre.org.uk/resources/key-messages/disclosures-csa/. (Accessed 12 January 2020).

Barnardos, 2015. Digital Dangers | Impact of Technology. https://b.barnardos.org.uk/what_we_do/our_work/sexual_exploitation/about-cse/digital-dangers.htm. (Accessed 12 January 2020).

Barnardos, 2019. Cut Them Free. https://b.barnardos.org.uk/what_we_do/our_work/sexual_exploitation/about-cse/cse-spot-the-signs.htm. (Accessed 24 January 2020).

Belfer, R.A., Klein, B.L., Orr, L., 2001. Use of the skeletal survey in the evaluation of child maltreatment. Am. J. Emerg. Med. 19 (2), 122–124. https://www.ncbi.nlm.nih.gov/pubmed/11239255. (Accessed 12 January 2020).

Bentovim, B., 2009. Safeguarding Children Living With Trauma and Family Violence: Evidence-Based Assessment, Analysis and Planning Interventions. Jessica Kingsley Publishers, London, Philadelphia.

Bernard, C., 2017. An Exploration of How Social Worker Engage Neglectful Parents From Affluent Backgrounds in the Child Protection System. University of London, Goldsmiths.

Bilson, A., 2021. Response to RCPCH Draft Guidance on FII. https://bilson.org.uk/home/response-on-fii/?doing_wp_cron=1617124298.9121849536895751953125. (Accessed 30 March 2021).

Bilson, A., Munro, E.H., 2019. Adoption and child protection trends for children aged under five in England: increasing investigations and hidden separation of children from their parents. Child Youth Serv. Rev. 96, 204–211.

Bywaters, P., 2020. The Child Welfare Inequalities Project: Final Report. University of Huddersfield.

CELCIS, 2012. Emotional Abuse. Celcis.org. https://www.celcis.org/index.php?cID=1827. (Accessed 22 January 2020).

Children Act, 1989. https://www.legislation.gov.uk/ukpga/1989/41/contents.

Contextual Safeguarding Network, 2019. What is Contextual Safeguarding? https://www.contextualsafeguarding.org.uk/about/what-is-contextual-safeguarding. (Accessed 22 January 2020).

Department for Education, 2019. Characteristics of Children in Need: 2018 to 2019. GOV, UK. https://www.gov.uk/government/statistics/characteristics-of-children-in-need-2018-to-2019. (Accessed 2 December 2019).

Department for Education, 2020. Characteristics of Children in Need: Headline Facts and Figures – 2020. GOV, UK. https://explore-education-statistics.service.gov.uk/find-statistics/characteristics-of-children-in-need/2020. (Accessed 30 March 2021).

Duncan, A., 2020. Report of the Serious Case Review regarding Child AG. Norfolk Safeguarding Children Partnership.

Featherstone, B., Morris, K., White, S., 2014. Re-Imagining Child Protection: Towards Humane Social Work With Families. Policy Press, Bristol.

Ferguson, H., 2011. Child Protection Practice. Palgrave Macmillan, New York.

Fowler, J., 2003. A Practitioner's Tool for Child Protection and the Assessment of Parents. Jessica Kingsley Publishers, New York.

Hardy, R., 2019. Fabricated or Induced Illness: What it is and What the Signs Are. Community Care. https://www.communitycare.co.uk/2019/02/25/fabricated-induced-illness-signs/. (Accessed 18 January 2020).

HM Government, 2018. Working Together to Safeguard Children: A Guide to Inter-Agency Working to Safeguard and Promote the Welfare of Children. https://assets.publishing.service.gov.uk/government/uploads/system/uploads/attachment_data/file/779401/Working_Together_to_Safeguard-Children.pdf. (Accessed 18 December 2019).

Johnson, S., 2019. The Prefrontal Cortex, Cerebellum and Reward Systems. Big Think. https://bigthink.com/mind-brain/adult-brain?rebelltitem=2#rebelltitem2. (Accessed 31 December 2019).

Jones, A., 2009. Serious Case Review: Child A. Local Safeguarding Children Board Haringey. http://media.education.gov.uk/assets/files/pdf/s/second%20serious%20case%20overview%20report%20relating%20to%20peter%20connelly%20dated%20march%202009.pdf. (Accessed 11 January 2020).

Joyce, T., Huecker, M.R., 2019. Pediatric Abusive Head Trauma (Shaken Baby Syndrome). Nih.govhttps://www.ncbi.nlm.nih.gov/books/NBK499836/. (Accessed 18 January 2020).

Kemp, A., Maguire, S.A., Sibert, J., Frost, R., Adams, C., Mann, M., 2006. Can we identify abusive bites on children? Arch. Dis. Child. 91 (11). 951–951 https://www.ncbi.nlm.nih.gov/pmc/articles/PMC2082944/. (Accessed 11 January 2020).

Kemp, R.S., Kemp, C.H., 1978. Child Abuse – The Developing Child. Fontana/Open Books Publishing Ltd, London.

Laming, H., 2003. The Victoria Climbié Inquiry: Report of an Inquiry by Lord Laming. TSO, Norwich.

Legislation.gov.uk, 2019. Children Act 1989. https://www.legislation.gov.uk/ukpga/1989/41/contents. (Accessed 22 January 2020).

Legislation.gov.uk, 2020. Adoption and Children Act 2002. http://www.legislation.gov.uk/ukpga/2002/38/section/120. (Accessed 22 January 2020).

McNeish, D., Scott, S., 2018. Key Messages From Research on Intra-Familial Child Sexual Abuse. Centre of Expertise on Child Sexual Abuse, Essex.

Ministry of Housing, Communities & Local Government, 2019. English Indices of Deprivation 2019. GOV.UK. https://www.gov.uk/government/statistics/english-indices-of-deprivation-2019. (Accessed 22 January 2020).

Mitchell, E., 2018. Working Together 2018: How It Affects Your Social Work Role – Childrens. https://www.ccinform.co.uk/practice-guidance/working-together-2018/?practice_guidance=working-together-2018#038. (Accessed 31 December 2019).

National Collaborating Centre for Women's and Children's Health (UK), 2009. Physical Features. Nih.govhttps://www.ncbi.nlm.nih.gov/books/NBK57169/. (Accessed 22 January 2020).

NHS Choices, 2020a. Fabricated or Induced Illness. https://www.nhs.uk/conditions/fabricated-or-induced-illness/. (Accessed 18 January 2020).

NHS Choices, 2020b. Dealing With Child Sex Abuse. Department of Health. https://www.nhs.uk/video/Pages/child-abuse.aspx. (Accessed 19 January 2020).

NHS Choices, 2020c. Subdural Haematoma. https://www.nhs.uk/conditions/subdural-haematoma/. (Accessed 18 January 2020).

NHS Inform, 2019. Burns and Scalds. https://www.nhsinform.scot/illnesses-and-conditions/injuries/skin-injuries/burns-and-scalds. (Accessed 18 January 2020).

NICE, 2017. Child Maltreatment: When to Suspect Maltreatment in Under 18s | Guidance NICE. https://www.nice.org.uk/Guidance/CG89. (Accessed 20 December 2019).

NICE, 2019. When to Suspect Child Maltreatment. RCOG Press, London. https://www.nice.org.uk/guidance/cg89/evidence/full-guideline-pdf-243694625. (Accessed 11 January 2020).

Nicolas, J., 2015. Conducting the Home Visit in Child Protection. Open Univ Press, Maidenhead.

Nuffield Foundation, 2021. Protecting Young Children at Risk of Abuse and Neglect Summary. https://mk0nuffieldfounpg9ee. kinstacdn.com/wp-content/uploads/2022/01/Summary-Protecting-young-children-at-risk-of-abuse-and-neglect-Nuffield-Foundation.pdf. (Accessed 28 March 2021).

NSPCC, 2016a. Emotional Abuse. NSPCC. https://www.nspcc.org.uk/what-is-child-abuse/types-of-abuse/emotional-abuse/. (Accessed 18 December 2019).

NSPCC, 2016b. Sexual Abuse. NSPCC. https://www.nspcc.org.uk/what-is-child-abuse/types-of-abuse/child-sexual-abuse/. (Accessed 18 December 2019).

NSPCC, 2016c. Neglect. NSPCC. https://www.nspcc.org.uk/what-is-child-abuse/types-of-abuse/neglect/ (Accessed 18 December 2019).

NSPCC, 2019a. What is Child Abuse? NSPCC. https://www.nspcc.org.uk/what-is-child-abuse/. (Accessed 15 November 2019).

NSPCC, 2019b. Child Abuse Offence Recorded Every 7 Minutes in UK. NSPCC. https://www.nspcc.org.uk/what-we-do/news-opinion/7-minutes-child-abuse-image-offence/. (Accessed 22 January 2020).

NSPCC, 2019c. Statistics Briefing: Child Deaths Due to Abuse or Neglect. https://learning.nspcc.org.uk/media/1652/statistics-briefing-child-deaths-abuse-neglect.pdf. (Accessed 22 January 2020).

NSPCC, Learning, 2019. Protecting Children From Sexual Abuse | NSPCC Learning. https://learning.nspcc.org.uk/child-abuse-and-neglect/child-sexual-abuse/. (Accessed 15 November 2019).

NSPCC, Learning, 2020. Statistics Briefing: Child Deaths Due to Abuse or Neglect. https://learning.nspcc.org.uk/media/1652/statistics-briefing-child-deaths-abuse-neglect.pdf. (Accessed 28 March 2021).

Office for National Statistics, 2019. Child Abuse Extent and Nature. Office for National Statistics, England and Wales. https://www.ons.gov.uk/peoplepopulationandcommunity/crimeandjustice/articles/childabuseextentandnatureenglandandwales/yearendingmarch2019. (Accessed 22 January 2020).

Oliver, C., 2017. Strengths-Based Child Protection – Firm, Fair and Friendly. University of Toronto Press, Toronto.

Parliament.uk, 2021. The 1870 Education Act. https://www.parliament.uk/about/living-heritage/transformingsociety/livinglearning/school/overview/1870educationact/. (Accessed 28 March 2021).

Platt, D., Riches, K., 2016. C-Change, Capacity to Change. University of Bristol, Bristol.

Police, UK, 2019. What is Child Abuse?. https://www.met.police.uk/advice/advice-and-information/caa/child-abuse/what-is-child-abuse/. (Accessed 31 December 2019).

Precey, G., 2018. Fabricated or Induced Illness: Understanding the Risks to Children. https://www.ccinform.co.uk/practice-guidance/guide-to-understanding-the-risk-to-children-in-whom-illness-is-fabricated-or-induced/. (Accessed 18 January 2020).

Radford, L., Corral, S., Bradley, C., Fisher, H., Bassett, C., Howat, N., Collishaw, S., 2011. Child Abuse and Neglect in the UK Today. NSPCC, London. https://learning.nspcc.org.uk/media/1042/child-abuse-neglect-uk-today-research-report.pdf. (Accessed 22 January 2020).

RCPCH, 2013. Abusive Head Trauma and the Eye in Infancy. The Royal College of Paediatrics and Child Health and The Royal College of Ophthalmologists, London. https://www.rcophth.ac.uk/wp-content/uploads/2014/12/2013-SCI-292-ABUSIVE-HEAD-TRAUMA-AND-THE-EYE-FINAL-at-June-2013.pdf. (Accessed 18 December 2019).

RCPCH, 2017a. Child Protection Evidence Systematic Review on Bite. The Royal College of Paediatrics and Child Health. https://www.rcpch.ac.uk/sites/default/files/2019-09/child_protection_evidence_-_bites.pdf. (Accessed 18 December 2019).

RCPCH, 2017b. Child Protection Evidence Systematic Review on Burns. The Royal College of Paediatrics and Child Health. https://www.rcpch.ac.uk/sites/default/files/2019-09/child_protection_evidence_-_burns.pdf. (Accessed 18 December 2019).

RCPCH, 2017c. Child Protection Evidence Systematic Review on Parent/Child Interaction. The Royal College of Paediatrics and Child Health. https://www.rcpch.ac.uk/sites/default/files/2019-09/child_protection_evidence_-_parent-child_interaction.pdf. (Accessed 10 January 2020).

RCPCH, 2018. Child Protection Evidence Systematic Review on Fractures. The Royal College of Paediatrics and Child Health. https://www.rcpch.ac.uk/sites/default/files/2019-02/child_protection_evidence_-_fractures.pdf. (Accessed 18 December 2019).

RCPCH, 2019. Child Protection Evidence – Bruising. https://www.rcpch.ac.uk/resources/child-protection-evidence-bruising. (Accessed 10 January 2020).

RCPCH, 2021. Perplexing Presentations (PP)/Fabricated or Induced Illness (FII) in Children Guidance – RCPCH Child Protection Portal. https://childprotection.rcpch.ac.uk/resources/perplexing-presentations-and-fii/. (Accessed 29 March 2021).

Schrader-McMillan, A., 2014. Emotional Abuse and Neglect: Identifying and Responding in Practice With Families. Research in Practice, Dartington.

Scie.org.uk., 2012. SCIE: Introduction to...Children's Social Care – Child Protection Procedures. https://www.scie.org.uk/publications/introductionto/childrenssocialcare/childprotection.asp. (Accessed 15 December 2019).

Sexual Offences Act, 2003. https://www.legislation.gov.uk/ukpga/2003/42/contents.

Sturt, P., 2020. 2019 Triennial Analysis of Serious Case Reviews: Children's Social Care. Research in Practice, Dartington.

Symonds, T., 2000. One in Five Adults Experienced Abuse as Children. BBC. https://www.bbc.co.uk/news/uk-51105266. (Accessed 18 January 2020).

Teece, S., 2005. Torn frenulum and non-accidental injury in children. Emerg. Med. J. 22 (2). 125–125 https://emj.bmj.com/content/22/2/125. (Accessed 12 January 2020).

The Children's Society, 2018. Adolescent Neglect Briefing for Professionals. https://www.childrenssociety.org.uk/sites/default/files/thinking_about_adolescent_neglect_practitioners_briefing.pdf. (Accessed 18 December 2019).

Timmins, N., 1994. Maria Colwell Death Led to Legislation Over Two Decades. Independent. https://www.independent.co.uk/news/uk/maria-colwell-death-led-to-legislation-over-two-decades-1431158.html. (Accessed 18 December 2019).

Wilkinson, J., Bowyer, S., 2017. The impacts of abuse and neglect on children; and comparison of different placement options. Department for Education, London.

World Health Organization (WHO), 2016. Child Maltreatment. Who.int. https://www.who.int/news-room/fact-sheets/detail/child-maltreatment. (Accessed 15 January 2020).

10

'NEW' FORMS OF CHILD ABUSE (EDITORS' INTRODUCTION)

RACHEL FYSON ■ LISA WARWICK ■ RACHAEL CLAWSON

Child abuse has always existed and probably always will. Chapters 8 and 9 have outlined those elements of child abuse which persist across the generations and which can be found in societies across the globe: neglect, physical abuse, sexual abuse, emotional and future harm. This chapter will explore 'new' forms of child abuse, which have come to public and professional attention in the UK more recently and with which some readers may therefore be less familiar.

It should be noted that in addressing 'new' forms of child abuse the use of quotation marks is intentional, for it could be argued that these forms of child abuse are not new in any meaningful sense – they are merely thought of as new because they are facilitated by new technologies or associated with recent global trends in migration. It may be better to think of these 'new' forms of abuse as merely the most recent manifestations of enduring forms of child abuse. Certainly, when these practices are dissected in detail, they reveal themselves to consist of the enduring forms of abuse which were addressed in Chapter 9, exacerbated by the risks of harm discussed in Chapter 8, and often intensified by both poverty and other characteristics which accentuate vulnerability (Chapter 11). Setting aside the debate about whether or not these are new forms of child abuse, each of the issues addressed in this chapter reflect the experiences of children living in the UK today and highlight areas in the vanguard of child protection practice.

The forms of child abuse discussed in this chapter are those which are considered 'new' at the time of writing, but child abuse is not a static concept. As societies change, so do the ways in which child abuse is understood and the ways in which it may manifest itself. There are a number of reasons why these changes occur. Firstly, gradual changes in social attitudes and behaviours occur in all societies over time. This results in things which were once regarded as ordinary aspects of childhood experience or child rearing practice gradually coming to be seen as dangerous, damaging to the child or otherwise socially unacceptable. In Victorian England it was usual for working class families to send their children to work from a young age so that everyone could afford to eat; children worked in factories and down coal mines. It is now unlawful in the UK to employ a child aged under 13 for any work except acting or modelling, and there are strict limits on working hours and types of employment. It would be regarded as a form of child abuse to break these laws. Although child labour still exists in some parts of the world, the United Nations Sustainable Development Goals aim to end child labour in all its forms by 2025. On a more mundane level, most people born in the 1940s or 1950s (today's pensioners) would have walked to school by themselves, often from the age of 5 or 6. Today, few infant or junior school children walk to school by themselves, and it would likely be regarded as neglect to allow a child of 5 or 6 to walk to school alone. This change in attitude can be traced to a number of other social changes: rise in car use has made crossing roads more dangerous; more children now live in families where both parents work and it is quicker and easier to drop a child at school in the car, which in turn creates more traffic and increases the dangers for children who walk.

The second way in which 'new' forms of abuse may emerge is when enduring forms of abuse are facilitated or enabled by advances in technology. In particular, the internet age and mobile phones have provided opportunities for communication at speed and across local or international borders. This has enabled would-be criminals and child abusers to connect with like-minded others in ways which would have been impossible before the existence of these technologies. The section by Amanda Taylor-Beswick on *Technology Assisted Child Sexual Abuse* shows how sexual abuse – an enduring form of child abuse – is now being facilitated via online grooming and sharing of child abuse images. And the section by Donna Peach on *Child Sexual Exploitation* notes the use of text and social media to groom children. Other 'new' forms of child abuse can similarly be understood as emerging and expanding in response to available technologies. In the section on *Gangs and Criminal Exploitation*, Grace Robinson notes phenomena such as county lines drug dealing which are facilitated by mobile phone communication before going on to take a closer look at child criminal exploitation within a gang context; and in the section on *Radicalisation* Lisa Curtis and Nigel Bromage demonstrate how internet memes can be used to recruit children to extremist and hate-filled ideologies.

Thirdly, some 'new' forms of child abuse may arise in response to wider social changes and linked to patterns of global migration. These forms of abuse may be associated with cultural norms, beliefs and expectations which are prevalent in some part of the globe and which have become apparent in the UK following migration from those areas. For the most part, such 'new' forms of abuse may have grown in incidence and prevalence owing to patterns of migration, but in fact already existed in White British communities. As Rachael Clawson discusses in the section on *Forced Marriage of Children and Young People*, child marriage remains lawful in some parts of the UK and forced child marriage is not limited to ethnic minority communities. Leethen Bartholomew sets out how *Female Genital Mutilation,* which remains commonplace in some parts of the world, has recently been criminalised in the UK. And in the section on *Child Abuse Linked to Faith or Belief,* Mor Dioum and Stephanie Yorath demonstrate how beliefs in spirit possession persist across all faiths, ethnicities and cultures.

Over time, these 'new' form of child abuse may change, and their prevalence may increase or decrease as new social and cultural norms emerge. It is important for all those involved in child protection to be aware of and begin to understand these 'new' forms of abuse – and any other forms of abuse which may begin to emerge in the future – in order to equip themselves to identify and respond confidently to the needs of all children.

10a

TECHNOLOGY-ASSISTED CHILD SEXUAL ABUSE: AS A FRAME THROUGH WHICH TO DEVELOP AND BROADEN UNDERSTANDINGS OF ABUSE INVOLVING TECHNOLOGIES AND THE ONLINE

AMANDA M.L. TAYLOR-BESWICK

KEY POINTS

- How the rapidly shifting sociotechnical context can exacerbate risk for children or young people.
- Navigating explanations, definitions and the emergent nature of technology involved abuse.
- The complexities of estimating and managing the scale of abuse when technologies and the online are involved.
- The need to engage in critical digital assessment and analysis, to inform professional digital practices.

INTRODUCTION

Fundamental to 21st century child protection practices are practitioners with an appreciation of the emergent social world. As Horwath (2001 p. 24) points out 'the needs of the child cannot be met without a consideration of the world in which the child lives'. In current terms, understanding a child or young person in context requires a robust appreciation of technologies, the online and how the two are inextricably enmeshed. Within this enmeshed context, whilst considerable opportunities await, the potential for considerable harm lies in wait too, and this knowledge is significant to keeping children safe. Although abuse involving technologies takes many forms, for example, bullying, sexting, radicalisation and criminal

exploitation, this chapter focuses on Technology-Assisted Child Sexual Abuse (TA-CSA).

TECHNOLOGY-ASSISTED CHILD SEXUAL ABUSE: A DEFINITION

The use of the internet and other digital communications technology (collectively 'the internet') to facilitate child sexual abuse, including by way of sharing indecent images of children; viewing or directing the abuse of children via online streaming or video conferencing; grooming or otherwise coordinating contact offences against children; or by any other means (Independent Inquiry into Child Sexual Abuse (IICSA, 2019a, np).

It does so for two reasons. Firstly, in recognition of the fact that 'no issue is more pressing for contemporary child protection than the role of the internet in facilitating child sexual abuse' (IICSA, 2016a, np); and secondly, due to how understandings acquired through examining TA-CSA are transferable to the range of online harms to which children can be exposed. Given the vastness of the subject matter, where space constraints or elaboration would be helpful, readers will be signposted to supplementary resources, including open access web-based content and immersive experiential material, to augment an exploration of this issue. The overarching aim of this chapter is to support professionals to develop understandings at the intersection of technologies and child protection.

A FAMILIAR SOCIAL PROBLEM IN A RAPIDLY EVOLVING SOCIOTECHNICAL WORLD

Whilst TA-CSA is an urgent social and professional matter, the use of technology to assist abuse is not a new phenomenon: 'perpetrators of online-facilitated CSA have been using information and communication technology (ICT) to commit child abuse since the late 1980s' (DeMarco et al., 2018, p. 9). What makes recent manifestations different is how 'developments in technology have created new opportunities for offending against children...' (IICSA, 2016a, np). These newer opportunities have been persistently difficult to identify and manage, due to the sophisticated digital strategies and tactics employed by perpetrators to prey on children (Dance and Keller, 2020). Adding to the insidious nature of this technological manipulation is an uncontained and unregulated digital environment (DCMS, 2020) that is largely beset by irreconcilable differences. 'Potentials' and 'perversities' is how LaMendola (2010, p. 115) describes the contradictions associated with the use of technologies and the online. Therefore an appreciation of the intricacies and dynamics of this complex and unwieldy sociotechnical system is vital for human service practitioners, particularly now when practice involves getting much closer to it (Ballantyne, 2015; 5Rights Foundation, 2020).

SOCIOTECHNICAL

A term used to describe the interaction and relationship between people, the environment and things. In this work, the term sociotechnical is used to describe the interaction and relationship between children, the internet, and the range of platforms, devices or technologies that are widely available.

NAVIGATING DESCRIPTIONS, TERMS AND DEFINITIONS

Similar to any other social phenomenon there is variation across the literature in how child sexual abuse involving technologies and the online is described and defined (ECPAT, 2018). Whilst, 'Online-facilitated Child Sexual Abuse' (O-fCSA) (May-Chahal et al.,

2018) and 'Technology-facilitated sexual violence' (TFSV) (Henry and Powell, 2016, p. 195) are two of the more frequent terms in use, TA-CSA is the term preferred for this work. This is because it captures how the internet and the platforms that run on it are both technologies and because these technologies are typically used in tandem to assist a human actor to craft and carry out abuse of this kind (Hamilton-Giachritsis et al., 2017).

In moving on towards developing a robust understanding of both what TA-CSA is and what it involves, 'The Internet and Child Sexual Abuse Inquiry: An inquiry into institutional responses to child sexual abuse and exploitation facilitated by the internet' is clarifying (IICSA, 2016a, 2016b, 2019a). The 'Internet Investigation' is just one of 15 strands of investigation within a broader UK Inquiry, the 'Independent Inquiry into Child Sexual Abuse' (IICSA) (IICSA, 2015a, 2015b) that was established as a statutory inquiry on 12 March 2015 to consider the growing evidence of institutional failures to protect children from child sexual abuse, and to make recommendations to ensure the best possible protection for children in future (IICSA, 2016b, np).

The internet strand was introduced to gain insights into 'the nature and extent of the use of the internet and other digital communications technology to facilitate CSA' (DeMarco et al., 2018, p. 13), owing to gaps in understandings about the involvement of technologies in child sexual abuse and if or how this involvement exacerbates and intensifies an abuse experience. In addition, the 'Learning about online sexual harm' report commissioned by the IICSA Inquiry is also significant, because of how the forms of manipulation associated with TA-CSA are made clear:

> *Online grooming and receiving sexual requests; being exposed to pornography; some sexting activities; online-facilitated child sexual exploitation (e.g. offering gifts, money or affection in return for sexual activities taking place or orchestrated online, but enacted during an offline meeting with the perpetrator or others); engaging with online images of child sexual abuse (including searching, viewing, downloading,*

exchanging, producing and commissioning of indecent images).

Beckett et al. (2019, p. 13)

SEXTING

The sending, sharing or receiving of explicit and intimate photographs from one mobile device to another via the internet. Sexting images can be in the form of a still image or in video format and can include nudity and sexual acts. There is no guarantee as to where the sexted content will end up. Whilst sexting can be manipulated and associated with grooming, it can also be part of young people's exploration of relationship intimacy.

What must be held in mind when considering descriptions, terms and definitions is the rapid and fluid nature of technological change. Platforms, devices and online spaces are easy to infiltrate, to manipulate, and to repurpose for the intention of causing harm (Elliot and Beech, 2009). Ultimately, it is the relentlessness of unregulated technological innovation that enables perpetrators to continue to lurk, to continue to lie in wait and to continue to find ways to carry out abuse through and in the online. It is again vital that practitioners working with children and young people can hold both the opportunities and perils of the online world simultaneously in mind.

ESTIMATES OF SCALE

Understandings of a social problem would be incomplete without reference to scale. Estimates of scale (how often an issue occurs, the likelihood of it reoccurring and the numbers of reported incidents, individual and social costs) are often what prompts an appraisal of professional practices and methods, particularly when a new social problem arises or an existing problem requires a modified or customised response. Specific to TA-CSA, a 'Rapid Evidence Assessment' (REA), commissioned by the IICSA Inquiry, aimed at 'Quantifying the Extent of Online-Facilitated Child Sexual Abuse' outlined four aspects thought to be useful for measuring the scale of abuse of this nature. They include 'counting the number of offences committed, the number of perpetrators, the number of victims and the number of images that have been viewed documented, downloaded and exchanged' (Wager et al., 2018, p. 11).

The Office of National Statistics (ONS), on the other hand, employed the following 'indicators' in their attempts to estimate scale:

- adults' self-reported experiences of child sexual abuse,
- child sexual abuse offences recorded by the police,
- children who come to the attention of children's services, and
- contact with support services (Office of National Statistics (ONS (2020, p. 4).

Despite the robustness of both sets of measurements, similar to abuse that does not involve digital technologies and the online, the 'true extent of... [TA-CSA] remains difficult to ascertain' (Wager et al., 2018, p. 13). An unsurprising conclusion when factors such as:

- the potential hiddenness of activity on digital social platforms,
- the increased use of the dark web,
- the rapidity of technological change,
- the threat and fear of the scale of exposure possible through the online,
- the lack of public digital awareness and reporting, and
- the unavailability of digital data and data inaccuracies

are taken into account. Each of these layers hinder the identification of TA-CSA, but serve to highlight the magnitude of the prevention, the reduction and the management task.

DARK WEB

The dark web forms part of the deep web, a section of web not searchable or indexed. The dark web is not visible, nor is it accessible without the downloading and use of specific software.

A brief look at UK data and statistics provides insights into the scale of TA-CSA at this time. For example, the information collated by the National Crime Agency (NCA) found that 'at least 80,000 people in the UK are believed to pose a sexual threat to children online' (Quinn, 2018, np), and that out of the '450 child sex offenders' apprehended and arrested in the UK 'each month' (National Crime Agency (NCA), 2018, np) a significant percentage are categorised as TA-CSA. Associated with this are recent reports that evidence a 700% increase in the volume of child abuse images being created, shared and sold online, and that 'a child abuse image offence [is] recorded every seven minutes [in] the UK' (NSPCC, 2019a, np). Furthermore, data drawn from the ONS details that during the period spanning October 2017 to September 2018 police, in England and Wales alone, had registered 'thousands of incidents of the internet being used to commit child sexual offences' (NSPCC, 2019b, np). Furthermore, 'The Crime Survey for England and Wales' (CSEW) survey estimates that 'approximately 3.1 million adults, aged 18 to 74 years experienced sexual abuse before the age of 18 years'; this they go on to point out is 'equivalent to 7.5% of the population' of that age group (ONS, 2020, p. 4).

It is important to bear in mind that a significant amount of child sexual abuse goes 'unreported' or is 'hidden' (NCA, 2018, p. 26) and that current data provides little more than a 'best estimate' (Kelly and Karsna, 2017, p. 4). The scale of incidents of abuse and attempts to abuse in and through technologies and the online remains worryingly high (EPACT, 2018; INTERPOL, 2018), exacerbated further by the significant increase in internet usage during the current global coronavirus pandemic (Europoll, 2022). However, in the absence of robust governance and appropriate levels of regulation, platform designers, those who built these more social-type technologies, will continue to fall short on the protections needed to keep children and young people safe online. In my view, we social care actors have a role in campaigning for regulatory change.

VOICES OF EXPERIENCE

Significant to developing appropriate practice responses is listening to and learning from people with experience (Tanner et al., 2017). Distinct in more recent abuse disclosures is how unable some people feel to share the abuse experience, meaning that they often carry their mistreatment for long periods (Moors and Webber, 2013). Issues such as sextortion and non-consensual image sharing add another dimension to this, given the fear and humiliation associated with the threat of wide-scale exposure, compounded even further by a glaring disparity in the lack of prosecutions when people find the courage to come forward (Ellison, 2018; Law Commission, 2018).

SEXTORTION

The term used to explain a form of revenge employed to coerce people into engaging in further sexual activity, or to blackmail for financial gain. The threat of exposure has resulted in a large number of deaths due to fear of humiliation that having images or videos made public evokes.

The following subsection of the chapter provides two distinctly different examples of how technologies and the online can be manipulated and exploited to assist child sexual abuse. These examples are again drawn from the IICSA Internet Inquiry. Opportunities to engage in a more immersive type learning experience – including guidance on how to access these – are set out in the closer look box activities.

PERSONAL ACCOUNTS OF TA-CSA; EVIDENCE PROVIDED TO THE INTERNET STRAND OF THE IICSA INQUIRY

IN-A3

IN-A3 confirms that she was 14 years old when groomed and sexually abused by a male in his early 60's. The exploitation and sexual harm IN-A3 explains began when she secured a part-time job in a Bed & Breakfast owned by Laurence Glynn. IN-A3 describes how Glynn manufactured circumstances and constructed connections, both in the online and in the physical world, which assisted him to abuse. Glynn's grooming, amongst many other activities, included: taking pictures of IN-A3, alleging them to be for his business website; infiltrating her personal social media networks to persistently flatter and charm her; providing the funds to purchase clothes of his choosing; and the installation of a camera in the staff toilet. Ultimately, Glynn used his power, position, and knowledge of the internet and social media platforms to support his grooming and abusive intentions and behaviours. The sexual abuse that occurred was both virtual and physical in nature. The lasting impacts recounted by IN-A3 are unsurprisingly extensive and include anxieties about surveillance, privacy and safety in personal digital spaces. It is important to note how non-specialist digital knowledge and skills are largely sufficient for using the internet and technologies to groom, manipulate and sexually abuse children in the way that IN-A3 describes.

> ## CLOSER LOOK: IICSA INTERNET INQUIRY: IN-A3 INTERVIEW EVIDENCE
>
> IN-A3's audio/video transcript of evidence can be accessed by typing the following URL into an internet browser: https://www.youtube.com/watch?v=7I-jomc0 e3A&list=PLQrDHIqFcNWFQRXe4pIAK4pnTEWn16IM R&index=27
>
> IN-A3's oral evidence can be read by typing the following URL into an internet browser: https://www. iicsa.org.uk/key-documents/11365/view/public-hearing-transcript-13-may-2019.pdf
>
> Reading and or listening to IN-A3's evidence offers an opportunity to engage in additional depth with the nuances of TA-CSA. It provides a detailed and authentic learning experience, in that it draws out the detail of the grooming and abuse, and the possible responses of the professional self as related to professional practice or when engaged in work of this nature.

IN-A1 & IN-A2

The evidence provided to the Internet Inquiry regarding the sibling group IN-A1, IN-A2, a 13-year-old girl and a 12-year-old boy at the time of the incidents, details how they were manipulated, groomed and sexually abused in and through the online. This sibling group were abused by 57-year-old Anthony O'Connor. O'Connor posed as a 22-year-old female on the social media website Bearshare, a peer-to-peer file-sharing platform, purposively chosen by O'Connor due to its children and young people population or orientation.

O'Connor's grooming and exploitation, initially of IN-A1, progressed to include manipulation that led IN-A1 to introduce O'Connor to IN-A2, her younger brother. The non-contact abuse that took place was scripted and directed virtually by O'Connor and involved both siblings, individually and as a pair. Distinct about this abuse experience is that it occurred and was orchestrated by O'Connor using audio/video technology, in and through the online.

> ## NON-CONTACT INTERNET MEDIATED CHILD SEXUAL ABUSE
>
> Sexual abuse that involves being forced to engage in sexual talk, sexual acts, and the watching of explicit material. The exchange of graphic photographs or live or recorded video material – including material that a child has been instructed to create by an adult can also feature. As can exposure of body parts by the adult and encouragement to touch oneself, and or others intimately for the adult's gratification.

The type of sexual abuse these children experienced, non-contact internet and technology-assisted abuse, is no less harmful and or damaging than any other type of sexual abuse.

> ## CLOSER LOOK: IICSA INTERNET INQUIRY: IN-A1 & IN-A2 EVIDENCE
>
> Statements given by IN-A1 & IN-A2, read at the IICSA Internet Inquiry, can be heard by typing the following URL into an internet browser: https://www.iicsa.org.uk/ video/iicsa-internet-investigation-day-1-13052019-pm2-trim
>
> IN-A1 & IN-A2's mothers' evidence can be heard by typing the following URL into an internet browser: https://www.iicsa.org.uk/video/iicsa-internet-investigation-day-2-14052019-am1
>
> Both IN-A1, IN-A2 (https://www.iicsa.org.uk/key-documents/11365/view/public-hearing-transcript-13-may-2019.pdf) and the account of their mother (https://www.iicsa.org.uk/key-documents/11407/view/ iicsa140519opensessionamd1.pdf) can be read by typing the attached URL's into an internet browser.
>
> As noted in the previous closer look box, listening to and reading evidence from voices of experience adds an additional dimension to learning about how abuse using technologies and the online can and does occur. It is worth thinking about the knowledge, skills and values needed to be alert and equipped to identify and engage in work of the nature described. To ask: 'How might I engage with children and young people at risk of non-contact sexual abuse' or 'How might I work with children and young people who have experienced abuse of this nature'?

The above two examples outline contact and non-contact abuse. They provide insights into child sexual abuse that occur solely in and through technologies and the online, and abuse that involves both the online and in offline spaces – in physical and digital environments, places or spaces. As far back as the 1990s Durkin (1997, p. 14) posited four character-istics of perpetrators of TA-CSA, those who intend 'to traffic child pornography, to locate children to molest, to engage in inappropriate sexual communi-cation with children, and to communicate with other paedophiles'. As is evident in the above accounts these typologies continue to hold true.

CLOSER LOOK: IICSA INTERNET INQUIRY

A more detailed and broader exploration of the 'Internet Inquiry', the timetable of the hearings, to include web links to the audio/video and written transcripts, can be found by typing the following URL into an internet browser: https://www.iicsa.org.uk/investigations/child-sexual-abuse-facilitated-by-the-internet?tab=hearing. This internet search will take you to the IICSA Internet Inquiry Timetable of Hearings.

This archive of hearings includes transcripts from the evidence given by a number of relevant stakeholders. As a resource it offers insights into what is known about internet abuse to date, about issues of governance, the rationale of technology companies regarding safety and design, and accounts from various professionals and professional groupings responsible for keeping children safe.

In addition, the Internet Inquiry has culminated in the following report: The Internet Investigation Report (IICSA, 2020). Here too we have a robust learning and reference resource, relevant for examining our knowledge and practice abilities relating to an effective, timely and appropriate professional response to TA-CSA experiences.

Given the unwieldy nature of the internet as an institution, environment or part of the practice land-scape, preparedness to practice in this area needs to be viewed as both urgent and ongoing.

EQUIPPED TO RESPOND?

Even though it is broadly accepted that 'new digital technologies are reconfiguring professional practice and responsibility... the education of professionals has yet to adequately reflect this' (Fenwick and Edwards, 2016, p. 117). An issue further hindered by profes-sional standards and educational programmes that remain largely unchanged (Hamilton-Giachritsis et al., 2017; Taylor, 2017; Lough, 2019). Evidence provided,

again, in the recent IICSA Inquiry corroborates this, where it is outlined how the lack of standardisation in professional education, in regards to TA-CSA, has con-tributed to the rise of an unregulated training environ-ment; one that is described as 'congested, competitive and confused' (IICSA, 2019b, np).

CLOSER LOOK: IICSA INQUIRY: EDUCATION AND TRAINING INTERVIEW EVIDENCE

The following content is the evidence of Mr Jim Gamble outlining his experiences of establishing and leading the 'Child Exploitation Operation Unit' (CEOP), and latterly his development of the independent safeguarding company (INEQE). He makes comment on what he believes is needed, in terms of the regulation, education and training of professionals, to manage and contain TA-CSA.

The audio/video and written transcripts can be accessed by typing the following URLs into an internet browser:

Oral Transcript https://www.youtube.com/watch?v=9voadhw5ZLA&list=PLQrDHIqFcNWFQRXe4pIAK4pnTEWn16IMR&index=31

Typed Transcript https://webarchive.nationalarchives.gov.uk/ukgwa/20221215001807/https://www.iicsa.org.uk/key-documents/11365/view/public-hearing-transcript-13-may-2019.pdf

In terms of progressing understandings of TA-CSA what isn't required, necessary, or particularly help-ful is another elaborate practice model or convoluted intervention (Hunter, 2011), that often complicates, obstructs or distracts from what is fundamentally a case of seeing a child within the context of their lived experience (Ferguson, 2017). Indeed, the professional response to TA-CSA remains the same as it would be to any other issue of this nature. The divergence relates to a robust understanding of the range of possibilities and or problems that can arise when the social, technical and child or children converge. A convergence that can be best understood through the 'Four properties – persistence, searchability, replicability, and scalability – and three dynamics – invisible audiences, collapsed contexts, and the blurring of public and private' (Boyd, 2008, p. 2), of the internet and online spaces.

FOUR PROPERTIES OF THE INTERNET

Persistence: Digital expressions are automatically recorded and archived

Searchability: Digital content is often accessible through search engines

Replicability: Digital content is easily duplicated

Scalability: The potential visibility of digital content is great

A starting point for reviewing understandings of these four properties and three dynamics of the internet is engaging in a review of one's own presence, choices and behaviours online. This should include an analysis of implicit and explicit audiences and publics, when active online contexts collapse, and where boundaries are difficult to maintain. A useful method for reflective analysis of this kind is the Digital Professionalism Mapping Tool (Fig. 10a.1) as a device to unlock insights into one's professional digital knowledge, digital values, and digital skills.

Completing an analysis of this nature is helpful to developing insights into the experiences of children and young people and can evolve understandings that capture the context of the other in relation to the self and or another's points of view. An online and interactive version of the tool is in the additional information and resources section below.

THE POTENTIALITIES

Whilst this chapter has centred on the problems associated with 'digitalisation' (Beer, 2005, np), the term used to explain 'the integration of digital technologies into everyday life' (Taylor-Beswick, 2019, p. 32), the benefits must too be acknowledged, given the distinct opportunities that being online can offer to children (London School of Economics (LSE), 2020). These opportunities have evolved traditional methods of living and learning, given how they traverse conventional geographic boundaries. In doing so they provide a

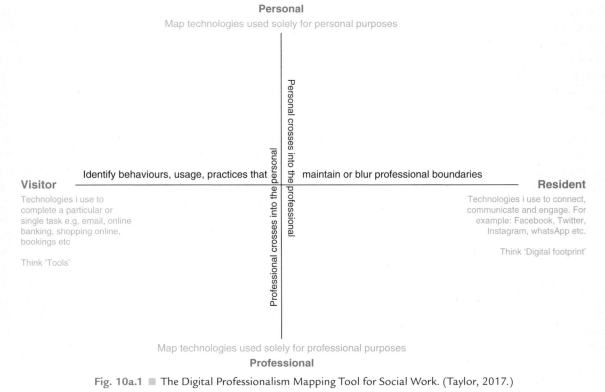

Fig. 10a.1 ■ The Digital Professionalism Mapping Tool for Social Work. (Taylor, 2017.)

gateway to information and global citizenship, in ways that were previously less possible. Supporting access, and cultivating children's digital capabilities and digital mindedness, is therefore central to how they become informed and participatory digital citizens (Ofcom, 2020). Key to fostering these abilities are digitally minded and digitally capable professionals. Professionals aware of the nuances of digitalisation; those with a grasp on how the online and offline are melded, or 'enmeshed' as Jurgenson (2012, p. 83) explains it, are much better equipped to keep children safe.

Whilst digital criticality and vigilance is vital to keeping children safe, professional practices should not be overly restrictive, or limiting, because of how important it is that children are supported to explore and move around in 'this brave new world of digital space' (Turner, 2015, np). As noted by Livingstone (2019, np), 'the digital has become the terrain on which we are negotiating who we are – our identities, our relationships, our values, and our children's life chances'. It is therefore essential that professionals are discerning and balanced regarding the differences between actual and possible risks and harms; and that they are professionally prepared, equipped and willing to support children to navigate online social spaces, as they would previously, offline social spaces. In research designed to examine 'Children's online activities, risks and safety' Livingstone et al. (2017 p. 3) contextualise the variables associated with assessing the risk/harm paradigm, explaining how:

> A host of risk/vulnerability factors are likely to shape children's online experiences, and this is mediated by the ways in which children develop emotionally, cognitively, in terms of their identity needs, social relationships and need for support, and their peer cultures; however, it remains difficult except in retrospect to pinpoint the moment when children succumb to specific online risks.

Even though exposure to the digital environment is significant to a children's overall development, what also must be borne in mind is that the responsibility and burden of safety should never be located solely with the child. Keeping children safe is a collective activity, involving parents, caregivers, carers, professionals, groups, communities and children themselves. Furthermore, it is a societal task that requires an appropriate degree of attention because the digital landscape is, to a greater extent, out of control, and policy-level directives are long overdue (5Rights Foundation, 2020; Garland et al., 2019; DCMS, 2020).

CONCLUSION

The development of the internet, the worldwide web and the platforms that run upon it has not resulted in the 'egalitarian paradise' that was initially imagined (Lomas, 2017, np). Indeed, there can be little doubt about the challenges and dilemmas that the online has and continues to present - to individuals, to groups, to communities, and to societies. The internet is an institution of gargantuan dimensions, populated by unmoderated, untested and unregulated platforms and people, some of which, as drawn out in this chapter, pose a considerable risk to the safety of our children. As outlined by the chairman of Google, 'the internet is the first thing that humanity has built that humanity doesn't understand' (Schmidt, E., 1999, np). It is worth keeping in mind that is not the internet, the world wide web and the platforms per se that are the problem, it is the misappropriation and manipulation of this environment and these tools that 'mirror, magnify and make visible... the bad, and ugly' (Boyd, 2014, p. 24) of the human condition, and human life.

Until, and beyond such times as the internet, and the platforms that run on it, are better understood, and regulation, legislation and legal protections are put in place, methods of identifying, preventing, and intervening in cases of TA-CSA, indeed all forms of technology involved abuse, must be kept under review. What must be avoided is a repeat of the '70s and 80s', a time when child abuse reached 'epidemic' proportions, a time from which incidents of abuse continue to be exposed and revealed (Dodd, 2020, np). There can be little doubt, as Naughton (2012, p. 10) points out, that the majority of the populace have 'become critically dependant on a technology that is poorly understood'. We, the professionals, must make it our business to change this.

REFLECTIVE QUESTIONS

- How would you describe the shifting sociological context of a child or young person's lived experience?
- How would you describe abuse that involves technologies and the internet?
- What would alert you to abuse involving technologies and or the online?
- What issues has this chapter raised in terms of your continuing professional development?
- What would you suggest as a way forward for addressing understandings of TA-CSA and online harms within qualifying and post-qualifying education structures?
- How might you influence understandings of TA-CSA in your professional area?

I am grateful to have the opportunity to acknowledge the influence that Pamela Beswick had on the writing of this chapter. Pamela was determined that the voices informing the Truth Project should be clearly heard and that they should be used to shape practice in meaningful ways. Pamela's commitment to the work of the Truth Project and her value of it shaped my decision to situate this chapter in the learning taken from the Internet Investigation. I will be forever grateful for her thinking and steering in the writing of this work. She was a champion of children and social care work. On a more personal note, I was honoured to have Pamela as my mother-in-law, and I do hope that I have done her and the voices informing the Internet aspect of the Truth Project justice.

ADDITIONAL RESOURCES

Websites

Independent Inquiry into Child Sexual Abuse (IICSA) [https://www.iicsa.org.uk/].

Internet Watch Foundation (IWF) [https://www.iwf.org.uk/].

London School of Economics (LSE) EU Kids Online Project [http://www.lse.ac.uk/media-and-communications/research/research-projects/eu-kids-online/reports-and-findings].

National Crime Agency (NCA). Child sexual abuse and exploitation [https://www.nationalcrimeagency.gov.uk/what-we-do/crime-threats/child-sexual-abuse-and-exploitation].

Sexual Offences Definitive Guideline [https://www.sentencingcouncil.org.uk/wp-content/uploads/Aug-2015-Sexual-Offences-Definitive-Guideline-web.pdf].

UK Council for Internet Safety (UKCIS) [https://www.gov.uk/government/organisations/uk-council-for-internet-safety].

We Protect Global Alliance: End Child Sexual Exploitation Online [https://www.weprotect.org/]

Blogs

Parenting for a Digital Future. Professor Sonia Livingstone [blog] space.

The Interactive Digital Professionalism in Social Work [Mapping Tool].

My Moves to Becoming a Digital Odds Changer. Dr Amanda M L Taylor-Beswick for BoingBoing [blog] post.

Ordinary Magic and the New Beginnings Maternal Commons. New Beginnings [blog] post.

Podcasts

IICSA Internet Facilitated Child Sexual Abuse [hearings].

Virginia Eubank [talk] at The Berkman Klein Centre for Internet & Society on Automating Inequality and Predictive Risk Modelling.

Moving Groupwork online during Covid19. Dr Amanda M L Taylor-Beswick for New Beginnings [vlog] post.

REFERENCES

Aiken, M., 2016. The Cyber Effect: An Expert in Cyberpsychology Explains How Technology Is Shaping Our Children, Our Behavior, and Our Values – and What We Can Do About It. Murray Publishers, London.

Alaggia, R., Collin-Vézina, D., Lateef, R., 2019. Facilitators and barriers to child sexual abuse (CSA) disclosures: A research update (2000–2016). Trauma Violence Abuse 20 (2), 260–283.

Ballantyne, N., 2015. Human service technology and the theory of the actor network. J. Technol. Hum. Serv. 33 (1), 104–117.

Beckett, H., Warrington, C., Devlin, J.M., 2019. 'Learning about online sexual harm': Independent Inquiry into Child Sexual Abuse. http://uobrep.openrepository.com/uobrep/handle/10547/623588. (Accessed 17 January 2020).

Beer, D., 2005. Sooner or later we will melt together: Framing the digital in the everyday. First Monday 10 (8), https://firstmonday.org/ojs/index.php/fm/article/view/1268 online OA journal.

Bingham, A., Delap, L., Jackson, L., Settle, L., 2016. Historical child sexual abuse in England and Wales: the role of historians. Hist. Educ. 45 (4), 411–429.

Boyd, D., 2008. Taken Out of Context: American Teen Sociality in Networked Publics. [thesis] https://www.danah.org/papers/TakenOutOfContext.pdf. (Accessed 17 May 2020).

Boyd, D., 2014. Its Complicated. The Social Lives of Networked Teens. Yale University Press, New Haven.

Dance, G.J.X., Keller, M.H., 2020. Tech Companies Detect a Surge in Online Videos of Child Sexual Abuse. https://www.nytimes.com/2020/02/07/us/online-child-sexual-abuse.html. (Accessed 17 January 2020).

DCMS, 2020. Online Harms White Paper. https://www.gov.uk/government/consultations/online-harms-white-paper/online-harms-white-paper#the-harms-in-scope. (Accessed 17 February 2020).

DeMarco, J., Sharrock, S., Crowther, T., Barnard, M., 2018. Behaviour and Characteristics of Perpetrators of Online-

Facilitated Child Sexual Abuse and Exploitation. Independent Inquiry into Child Sexual Abuse, London.

Dodd, V., 2020. Police uncovering 'epidemic of child abuse' in 1970s and 80s. https://www.theguardian.com/uk-news/2020/feb/05/police-uncovering-epidemic-of-child-abuse-in-1970s-and-80s

Durkin, K.F., 1997. Misuse of the Internet by pedophiles: Implications for law enforcement and probation practice. Fed. Probat. 61 (14), 14–18.

Elliot, I. A., & Beech, A. R., 2009. Understanding online child pornography use: Apply-ing sexual offense theory to internet offenders. Aggression and Violent Behavior, 14,180–193

Ellison, M., 2018. Less than half revenge porn cases passed to prosecutors. BBC. https://www.bbc.co.uk/news/uk-scotland-42689607. (Accessed 17 February 2020).

Eric Schmidt, 1999. At Internet World Trade Show, New York, 18 November 1999. https://www.oxfordreference.com/display/10.1093/acref/9780191826719.001.0001/q-oro-ed4-00017947;jsessionid=B56E8223A7B52EB9328087291109F930

Europol, 2022. Exploiting Isolation: Offenders and victims of online child sexual abuse during the COVID-19 pandemic. https://www.europol.europa.eu/publications-events/publications/exploiting-isolation-offenders-and-victims-of-online-child-sexual-abuse-during-covid-19-pandemic

Fenwick, T., Edwards, R., 2016. Exploring the impact of digital technologies on professional responsibilities and education. Eur. Educ. Res. J. 15 (1), 117–131.

Ferguson, H., 2017. How children become invisible in child protection work: Evidence from day-to-day social work practice. Br. J. Soc. Work. 47 (4), 1007–1023.

Freeman, H., 2019. 'He was a master manipulator': abducted in plain sight and the truth about abuse. Guardian. https://www.theguardian.com/society/2019/feb/06/he-was-a-master-manipulator-abducted-in-plain-sight-and-the-truth-about-abuse. (Accessed 30 January 2020).

Garland, J., Armstrong, H., Wyatt, D., Roberts, J., 2019. Radical overhaul of tech regulation is overdue. Guardian. https://www.theguardian.com/media/2019/feb/19/radical-overhaul-tech-regulation-overdue-letters. (Accessed 30 January 2020).

Goodman, E., Livingstone, S., 2018. Protection of children online: does current regulation deliver? LSE. https://blogs.lse.ac.uk/medialse/2018/11/27/protection-of-children-online-does-current-regulation-deliver/. (Accessed 30 January 2020).

Hamilton-Giachritsis, C., Hanson, E., Whittle, H., Beech, A., 2017. "Everyone Deserves to Be Happy and Safe": A Mixed Methods Study Exploring How Online and Offline Child Sexual Abuse Impact Young People and How Professionals Respond to It. NSPCC, London.

Henry, N., & Powell, A. (2016). Sexual Violence in the Digital Age: The Scope and Limits of Criminal Law. Social & Legal Studies, 25(4), 397–418. https://doi.org/10.1177/0964663915624273 https://journals.sagepub.com/doi/abs/10.1177/0964663915624273

Horwath, J.A., 2001. The Child's World: Assessing Children in Need. Jessica Kingsley Publishers, London.

Hunter, S., 2011. Munro debate: Social workers need time not new interventions. Community Care. https://www.communitycare.co.uk/2011/04/01/munro-debate-social-workers-need-time-not-new-interventions/. (Accessed 19 December 2019).

IICSA, 2015a. Statement by the Chair of the Independent Inquiry into Child Sexual Abuse. https://www.iicsa.org.uk/key-documents/275/view/update-statement-november-2015.pdf. (Accessed 19 December 2019).

IICSA, 2015b. The Scope of the Investigation. Independent Inquiry into Child Sexual Abuse. https://www.iicsa.org.uk/key-documents/269/view/internet-child-sexual-abuse.pdf. (Accessed 17 December 2019).

IICSA, 2016a. The Internet and Child Sexual Abuse: SUMMARY. Independent Inquiry into Child Sexual Abuse. https://www.iicsa.org.uk/search?keyword=internet%20&en=1&o=da. (Accessed 17 December 2019).

IICSA, 2016b. The Internet and Child Sexual Abuse: Background. Independent Inquiry into Child Sexual Abuse. https://www.iicsa.org.uk/background. (Accessed 17 December 2019).

IICSA, 2019a. The Internet and Child Sexual Abuse: An inquiry into institutional responses to child sexual abuse and exploitation facilitated by the internet – Scope of Investigation. https://www.iicsa.org.uk/sites/default/files/the-internet-and-child-sexual-abuse.pdf. (Accessed 31 October 2019).

IICSA, 2019b. Investigation – The Internet. [YouTube] https://www.youtube.com/playlist?list=PLQrDHIqFcNWFQRXe4pIAK4pnTEWn16IMR. (Accessed 29 October 2019).

IICSA, 2019c. IICSA – Internet Investigation – transcriptions. https://www.iicsa.org.uk/search?keyword=IICSA%20-%20internet%20investigation&en=1&o=re. (Accessed 29 October 2019).

IICSA, 2020. The Internet Investigation Report March 2020. https://www.iicsa.org.uk/document/internet-investigation-report-march-2020. (Accessed 28 April 2020).

Internet Watch Foundation (IWF), 2019. IWF launches 'Once Upon a Year' and vows to tackle the demand for images of child rape. https://www.iwf.org.uk/news/iwf-launches-once-upon-a-year-and-vows-to-tackle-demand-for-images-of-child-rape. (Accessed 31 October 2019).

INTERPOL, 2018. Towards a Global Indicator: On Unidentified Victims in Child Sexual Abuse Material. https://www.interpol.int/en/Crimes/Crimes-against-children/International-Child-Sexual-Exploitation-database. (Accessed 17 January 2020).

Jurgenson, N., 2012. When atoms meet bits: Social media, the mobile web and augmented revolution. Fut. Int. 4 (1), 83–91.

Kelly, L., Karsna, K., 2017. Measuring the scale and changing nature of child sexual abuse and child sexual exploitation. Scoping report. CSA Centre. https://www.csacentre.org.uk/documents/scale-and-nature-scoping-report-2018/ (Accessed 31 November 2019).

LaMendola, W., 2010. Social work and social presence in an online world. J. Technol. Hum. Serv. 28 (1–2), 108–119.

Law Commission, 2018. Abusive and Offensive Online Communications: A Scoping Report. https://s3-eu-west-2.amazonaws.com/lawcom-prod-storage-11jsxou24uy7q/uploads/2018/10/6_5039_LC_Online_Comms_Report_FINAL_291018_WEB.pdf. (Accessed 31 January 2020).

Livingstone, S., 2019. Parenting in the Digital Age. https://www.ted.com/talks/sonia_livingstone_parenting_in_the_digital_age#t-180008. (Accessed 31 November 2019).

Livingstone, S., Haddon, L. (Eds.), 2009. Kids Online: Opportunities and Risks for Children. Policy Press, Bristol.

Livingstone, S., Haddon, L. (Eds.), 2012. Children, Risk and Safety on the Internet: Research and Policy Challenges in Comparative Perspective. Policy Press, Bristol.

Livingstone, S., Davidson, J., Bryce, J., Batool, S., Haughton, C., Nandi, A., 2017. Children's online activities, risks and safety: a literature review by the UKCCIS evidence group. UKCCIS evidence group Technical Report http://www.lse.ac.uk/business-and-consultancy/consulting/assets/documents/childrens-online-activities-risks-and-safety.pdf. (Accessed 31 January 2020).

London School of Economics (LSE), 2020. EU Kinds Online: Reports and Findings [online]. http://www.lse.ac.uk/media-and-communications/research/research-projects/eu-kids-online/reports-and-findings. (Accessed 31 October 2019).

Lough, C., 2019. Teachers 'need more training' to combat sexual abuse. TES. https://www.tes.com/news/teachers-need-more-training-combat-sexual-abuse. (Accessed 31 December 2019).

May-Chahal, C., Palmer, E., Dodds, S., Milan, S., 2018. Rapid Evidence Assessment: Characteristics and Vulnerabilities of Victims of Online-Facilitated Child Sexual Abuse and Exploitation. Independent Inquiry into Child Sexual Abuse. https://www.researchgate.net/publication/324013936_Rapid_Evidence_Assessment_Characteristics_And_Vulnerabilities_Of_Victims_Of_Online_Facilitated_Child_Sexual_Abuse_And_Exploitation#fullTextFileContent

Megele, C., 2017. Safeguarding Children and Young People Online: A Guide for Practitioners. Policy Press, Bristol.

Moors, R., Webber, R., 2013. The dance of disclosure: Online self-disclosure of sexual assault. Qual. Soc. Work 12 (6), 799–815.

National Crime Agency (NCA), 2018. National Strategic Assessment of Serious and Organised Crime. https://www.nationalcrimeagency.gov.uk/who-we-are/publications/173-national-strategic-assessment-of-serious-and-organised-crime-2018/file. (Accessed 18 December 2019).

Naughton, J. 2012. From Gutenberg to Zuckerberg: What you really need to know about the Internet. London: Quercus.

NSPCC, 2019a. Child abuse offence recorded every 7 minutes in UK. https://www.nspcc.org.uk/what-we-do/news-opinion/7-minutes-child-abuse-image-offence/. (Accessed 24 December 2019).

NSPCC, 2019b. Over 9,000 police-recorded online child sexual abuse offences. https://www.nspcc.org.uk/what-we-do/news-opinion/web-exploited-by-child-sex-offenders/. (Accessed 18 December 2019).

Ofcom, 2020. Parents more concerned about their children online. https://www.ofcom.org.uk/about-ofcom/latest/features-and-news/parents-more-concerned-about-their-children-online. (Accessed 31 January 2020).

ONS, 2020. Child abuse in England and Wales: January 2020: Statistics and research on child abuse in England and Wales, bringing together a range of different data sources from across government and the voluntary sector. https://www.ons.gov.uk/peoplepopulationandcommunity/crimeandjustice/bulletins/childabuseinenglandandwales/january2020. (Accessed 14 February 2020).

Pearce, J. (Ed.), 2019. Child Sexual Exploitation: Why Theory Matters. Policy Press, Bristol.

Quinn, 2018. Call for tech firms to act as 80,000 in UK pose sexual threat to children. https://www.theguardian.com/uk-news/2018/sep/03/google-facebook-tech-firms-do-more-combat-child-sex-abuse-sajid-javid

Rogers, C., 2018. Perceptions of victims of historically reported sexual offences: Insights from England and Wales. Salus J. 6 (2), 3–20.

Staksrud, E., 2016. Children in the Online World: Risk, Regulation, Rights. Routledge, Oxon.

Tanner, D., Littlechild, R., Duffy, J., Hayes, D., 2017. 'Making it real': Evaluating the impact of service user and carer involvement in social work education. Br. J. Soc. Work 47 (2), 467–468.

Taylor, A.M.L., 2017. The Unintended Impacts of I Daniel Blake [Blog]. https://amltaylor66.wordpress.com/2017/06/02/the-unintended-impacts-of-i-daniel-blake/. (Accessed 14 February 2020).

Taylor-Beswick, A.M.L., 2019. Examining the contribution of social work education to the digital professionalism of students for practice in the connected age. EThOS. https://ethos.bl.uk/OrderDetails.do?uin=uk.bl.ethos.784597. (Accessed 20 January 2020).

Turner, D., 2015. Lack of clear social media guidance is creating 'anxiety' and 'alienation'. Community Care. http://www.communitycare.co.uk/2015/04/29/lack-clear-social-media-guidance-creating-anxiety-alienation/. (Accessed 20 January 2020).

Wager, N., Armitage, R., Christmann, K., Gallagher, B., Ioannou, M., Parkinson, S., et al., 2018. Rapid Evidence Assessment: Quantifying the Extent of Online-facilitated Child Sexual Abuse. A report for the Independent Inquiry into Child Sexual Abuse (IICSA). IICSA, London.

10b CHILD SEXUAL EXPLOITATION

DONNA PEACH

KEY POINTS

- Defining child sexual exploitation (CSE).
- Outlining the prevalence of CSE in the UK.
- Examining the relevant legal and policy framework regarding CSE.
- Considering the needs of children victimised by CSE.

INTRODUCTION

The criminal enterprise of sexually abusing children for profit and cloaked behind concepts such as prostitution and slavery has occurred across the ages (Clarkson, 1939; Hepburn and Simon, 2013). It is a crime of significant magnitude, often hidden and underreported but also not consistently recorded by the state. In the UK, the launch of the national referral mechanism to record incidents of suspected exploitation in 2016, has shown thousands of children are victims of child sexual exploitation (CSE). The profiteering nature of this criminal activity provides a reason for some to conceive CSE as different from child sexual abuse that occurs within familial relationships. Thus those victimised can be perceived as participating in their abuse, leading to concepts such as 'exchange' becoming commonplace and preventing both the victim and protective agencies from recognising victimhood (Tennent, 2019). Historically, the term 'child prostitution' was embedded within our legislation, until campaigners argued for it to be replaced by CSE by the enactment of the Serious Crime Act 2015 (O'Hara, 2019). Those changes present the term CSE as a new concept in the UK. However, usage of the term CSE is longstanding in the USA (Ennew, 1986).

There are multiple challenges to achieving a shared understanding of CSE. In the UK, the term child sexual exploitation can be portrayed as a 'new' form of child abuse, using the public 'scandals' in towns such as Oxford, Rotherham and Rochdale as a catalyst for inquiry (Brown and Barrett, 2002). It is important to understand the manifestation of CSE in those towns and the learning it generates (Beckett et al., 2012; Ringrose et al., 2012; Dodsworth, 2014; Peach et al., 2015; Hallett, 2017). This chapter will explore how we define and respond to CSE and how these have changed in recent years. It will critique the use of language predominantly developed to define criminal activity and reflect on the effect of the discursive construct of victimhood on those who experience exploitation. Any examination of CSE should keep those who are victimised central to its focus. As practitioners, we should consistently work to co-produce our service provision to ensure victims and survivors of CSE are empowered. The chapter will introduce a communication model developed with children, young people and survivors of CSE from a project they named 'Not Just a Thought…'; it will end with a focus on a serious care review and questions to assist your interrogation of the concerns.

What Is Child Sexual Exploitation?

The Department for Education (2017) defines CSE for practitioners and community leaders who are working to protect children, as part of its non-statutory advice.

131

It recognised sexual exploitation as a criminal activity which can have devastating effects not only on those who are victimised but also their families. This government advice details the nature of the sexual activity that might constitute a crime which includes a range of physical touching, producing sexual images or watching sexual activity. The guidance notes these criminal activities can occur in person, via technology and online.

The specific definition of CSE is as follows:

> *Child sexual exploitation is a form of child sexual abuse. It occurs where an individual or group takes advantage of an imbalance of power to coerce, manipulate or deceive a child or young person under the age of 18 into sexual activity (a) in exchange for something the victim needs or wants, and/or (b) for the financial advantage or increased status of the perpetrator or facilitator. The victim may have been sexually exploited even if the sexual activity appears consensual. Child sexual exploitation does not always involve physical contact; it can also occur through the use of technology.*
>
> **Department for Education (2017, p. 5)**

Importantly, the Department for Education (2017, p. 6) guidance makes specific note that 'Child sexual exploitation is never the victim's fault, even if there is some form of exchange: all children and young people under the age of 18 have a right to be safe and should be protected from harm'.

As we can see from the above definition, the concept of exchange is explicit in its suggestion of the victim being rewarded by having their needs or wants met. It is worth pausing to think about that. Although the terminology has changed from prostitution to CSE, the underpinning assumptions of the participatory relationship in this criminal activity remain. It minimises the threat behind what is often a child being raped. That distinction is inherent in positioning CSE as *a form of* child sexual abuse rather than it being considered the same. If a father rapes his daughter and then buys her a gift, or promises not to rape her younger sister, would we consider that exchange in quite the same way? The Department for Education (2017, p. 9) provides a list of potential indicators of children and young people who might be victims of sexual exploitation (see Table 10b.1). These potential indicators are used

TABLE 10B.1
Potential Indicators of Child Sexual Exploitation

- Acquisition of money, clothes, mobile phones etc. without plausible explanation;
- Gang association and/or isolation from peers/social networks;
- Exclusion or unexplained absences from school, college or work;
- Leaving home/care without explanation and persistently going missing or returning late;
- Excessive receipt of texts/phone calls;
- Returning home under the influence of drugs/alcohol;
- Inappropriate sexualised behaviour for age/sexually transmitted infections;
- Evidence of/suspicions of physical or sexual assault;
- Relationships with controlling or significantly older individuals or groups;
- Multiple callers (unknown adults or peers);
- Frequenting areas known for sex work;
- Concerning use of internet or other social media;
- Increasing secretiveness around behaviours; and
- Self-harm or significant changes in emotional well-being

Department for Education (2017, p. 9).

by practitioners in the form of checklists that have been developed to identify children at risk of sexual exploitation (Franklin et al., 2018).

PREVALENCE OF CSE IN THE UK

Separate from the UK parliament's recent decision to withdraw from the Economic European Commission (EEC), we remain a member of the Council of Europe (CoE). The UK is 1 of 12 Council of Europe countries that collate and report on the incidence of human trafficking via the previously discussed National Referral Mechanism. The Council of Europe (Council of Europe (CoE), 2018) estimate up to 18 million children are subjected to child sexual abuse and exploitation across European countries. The majority of victims of CSE identified originate from the UK and Albania (Home Office, 2019a). Since 2009, the UK has recorded multiple incidences of children and young people who are exploited via the National Referral Mechanism and Duty to Notify protocols. Those recording processes have been adapted to improve data collection and decision making, which are now governed centrally by a dedicated Home Office-based unit. The Home Office compile quarterly reports from the data collated, which continue to show a rise in the number of potential victims of modern slavery. The number of potential victims identified in 2019 showed a 61% increase in those reported in 2018 (Home Office, 2019a). As shown in Fig. 10b.1 there has been a sharp increase in recorded cases since 2016, largely due to improved identification of victims. The number of victims has grown each subsequent year, with 561 children were identified in 2017, 628 in 2018, and 718 in 2019.

Additionally, slavery has become more visible as a domestic crime in the UK, leading to the enactment of the Modern Slavery Act 2015, which was primarily initiated due to concerns of the trafficking of persons for sexual exploitation (Craig, 2017). The Modern Slavery Act 2015 provides the legal structure to address the criminality of human trafficking and exploitation. Broad and Turnbull (2019) note the relevance of terminology in policies moving from human trafficking to slavery and its emergence as an internationally adopted concept. However, they sound a cautionary note about the void between elite top-down dominated policy responses and the need for an effective response to the criminality that is modern slavery, the

exploitation of children and adults. It defines slavery as 'knowingly holding a person in slavery or servitude or knowingly requiring a person to perform forced or compulsory labour'. This Act can be used to respond to any exploitation when there is an arrangement made to travel or to facilitate travel with a view to child exploitation. The challenge remains to provide evidence for that intent and disrupting this form of criminality before the sexual assault of a child.

The UK government has continued to develop its response to online CSE and has more recently adopted the term child sexual exploitation and abuse (CSEA). Its strategy includes tackling the sexual exploitation and abuse of children that occurs both in-person and online. This is a mammoth task with the National Crime Agency (NCA) reporting that approximately 144,000 accounts that are engaged in harmful child sexual abuse using encrypted internet content (often known as the dark web that is not linked to mainstream search engines) are registered in the UK. The global estimated figure of such harmful online accounts is 2.88 million (Home Office, 2019b). The live streaming of CSEA is a major concern for which the government has identified an increased budget of £30 million to target the most dangerous and prolific offenders (Home Office, 2019b). Home Office (2019a) estimates that 80,000

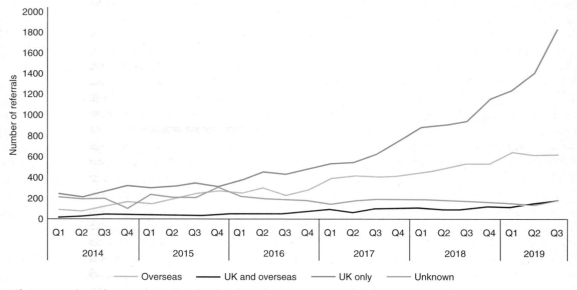

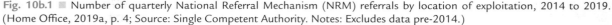

Fig. 10b.1 ■ Number of quarterly National Referral Mechanism (NRM) referrals by location of exploitation, 2014 to 2019. (Home Office, 2019a, p. 4; Source: Single Competent Authority. Notes: Excludes data pre-2014.)

individuals in the UK are a sexual threat to children via online activities. Children can become a victim of online CSE within a matter of minutes. The Children's Commissioner has developed digital safety and well-being kits for children and their parents which can be accessed via https://www.childrenscommissioner.gov.uk/coronavirus/digital-safety-and-wellbeing-kit/.

Despite efforts to promote awareness and identification of victims, often we are all aware of the exploitation until children have become adults (Leishman, 2007). In the UK and across the globe, sexual assault remains underreported, which indicates we are failing to safeguard many vulnerable children (Leishman, 2007). It is important to note that the backdrop to CSE is male-dominated violence. Repertoires that protect patriarchal figures serve to perpetuate misogynistic narratives. These ideologies are challenged by feminist voices who have been building a foundation of critique to interrogate concepts of morality, blame and choice (Brown & Barrett, 2002; Outshoorn, 2004; Butler, 2015). However, this activity is an uphill battle against a relentless tide of inequality, abuse, and exploitation (Núñez Puente and Gámez Fuentes, 2017). A simple but profound example remains in the UK Sexual Offences Act 2003 which continues to make the distinction between children aged 13 years and above. This is important, as it permits an alleged abuser a defence of a reasonable belief that a child aged 13 years or over was believed to be 18 years of age.

> **CLOSER LOOK: SEXUAL OFFENCES ACT 2003**
>
> (Also of note: The Sexual Offences (Northern Ireland) Order 2008; Sexual Offences (Scotland) Act 2009).
>
> In England since 1885, the age of consent to heterosexual activity has been 16 years of age. Despite that fact, the Sexual Offences Act 2003 distinguishes between children who are aged 13 years and above, and 12 years and under. Arguably, this distinction is reminiscent of the 19th century acceptance in England that girls aged 12 years could be legally married (Peach, 2019). The issue of consent remains legally complex (Sjölin, 2015). However, in the UK children under the age of 18 years cannot consent to their abuse through exploitation. The Act also makes 'grooming' an offence, defined as to befriend a child on the internet or by other online means

and meet or intend to meet the child to abuse them. A Risk of Sexual Harm Order can be imposed on adults to prevent them from engaging in inappropriate sexual behaviour such as having sexual conversations with children online. The police can apply for such orders if they believe that someone poses a risk to young people under 16 years of age.

VULNERABILITIES, VICTIMHOOD AND SURVIVORS

The Children Act 1989 remains the UK's substantive legislation that aims to protect children from both the likelihood of and actual significant harm. It also embeds the importance of decisions being made in a child's best interests and with the consideration of their wishes and feelings. The prolific nature of CSE suggests all children have some vulnerability. However, some children may have additional vulnerabilities, or less protective factors such as originating from families where parents have a history of depression and other mental health needs (Levine, 2017). Other vulnerable factors can include poverty, homelessness and poor education (Naramore et al., 2017). Importantly, whether prior vulnerabilities are evidenced, or not, the experience of sexual exploitation can create significant needs (Greenbaum and Crawford-Jakubiak, 2015). The needs of those who are victimised do not end with the cessation of abuse. The experience of legal proceedings to gain justice brings its stress and challenges that we are only beginning to understand (Ahern, 2018).

Unsurprisingly, the repeated experience of sexual violence and the associated physical and emotional abuse can have long-term effects on children's physical and psychological well-being (Oram et al., 2015). Sexual exploitation can lead to forced pregnancy and premature childbearing, in addition to the risk of contracting sexually transmitted diseases (ECPAT, 2015). Failure to meet the needs of children traumatised by their experience of CSE can cause long-term health needs and even lead to death by suicide (Powell et al., 2018; Laser-Maira et al., 2019). Welfare, health and public services must ensure the development, flexibility and sustainability of prevention and post-exploitation resources (McIntyre, 2014; Laser-Maira et al., 2019). Additionally, service providers must be sensitive to the ethnic and cultural needs of children who have experienced CSE (Ijadi-Maghsoodi et al., 2018). In particular, children who have been illegally brought into the UK to be exploited may face further vulnerabilities if deported (Polaris, 2010).

The United Nations Convention on the Rights of the Child (UNCRC), with 54 articles detailing how governments should ensure all children have access to their rights, was introduced in 1989 and ratified by the UK in 1991. Article 34 of the convention provides for governments to have a duty to protect children from sexual abuse and exploitation. In practice, we must use supervision and critical reflection to examine how our laws and social policies both facilitate and inhibit our ability to protect children.

This chapter has considered how age can factor into perceptions of victimhood, and the same is also true of gender. CSE is experienced by both boys and girls, but it remains a largely gendered crime with victims overwhelmingly being female. In a study, collating data in 2015 to 2016 from local authorities in England (albeit without a shared definition of identification), it was estimated that as many as 17,600 children were at risk of sexual exploitation (Kelly and Karsna, 2017). That study estimated 15% of girls were victims compared to 5% of boys. However, those figures are not in keeping with international estimates of 30% of girls and 23% of boys (Kelly and Karsna, 2017). A study by Cockbain et al. (2017) demonstrates that more boys than girls have been found likely to be sexually abused in extra-familial rather than intra-familial contexts and a slightly higher proportion of boys than girls are sexually abused by female offenders. Cockbain et al. (2017, p. 661) argue that considerable knowledge gaps persist in respect to 'the interplay between victim gender and their individual characteristics, the abuse process, and official responses to them'. Additionally, most service provision in the UK is geared towards meeting the needs of young women, meaning the needs of male victims may be unmet or even unidentified. There remains much we do not understand about the incidence of CSE. Too often, our understanding of victim experience is retrospectively understood; therefore, the method by which they were historically exploited could have changed for children

who are currently subject to sexual assault. Importantly, Brown (2019) explored the concept of vulnerability with survivors of childhood sexual exploitation and argued there is a need to move beyond concepts of risk to critically examine the complexity of social divisions and their impact on young people. We are aided in this pursuit by survivors who have forfeited their right to anonymity in order to raise public awareness (Peach, 2019).

No discussion of CSE should occur without including the voice of those who have been victimised by this form of criminality; their knowledge is essential to the construction of the development of our informed response (Peach, 2019). Those who have been exploited need to be empowered to realise their survivorhood and ability to thrive beyond their experience of abuse (Laser-Maira et al., 2019).

One of the important messages from children and young people in the Not Just A Thought... project (http://notjustathought.org.uk/) was that they wanted practitioners to have direct conversations and not to go *all around the houses* to ask a question. The children and young people made the point that it is important that they understand what it is you need to know, and that you tell them that you are willing to hear anything they have to share. The project provides questions created with children and young people that practitioners can use (https://www.researchgate.net/publication/332734916_Not_just_a_thought). There are additional resources created specifically with and for Asian and Muslim children.

Using the Not Just A Thought... resources and/or those detailed in the section below, consider the following Serious Case Report and accompanying questions. It is important to remember to use critical analytic skills to interrogate assumptions and stereotypes that can undermine our ability to safeguard children and young people.

CONCLUSION

This chapter has examined the prevalence of CSE in the UK and highlighted the voracity of those who perpetrate these crimes. There remains much we do not understand about the prevalence and the experience of CSE, which will continue our ability to effectively respond to the needs of victims. The sexual abuse and

---

CASE STUDY 10B.1: KATIE'S STORY

Read the full Serious Case Review Report about Katie https://library.nspcc.org.uk

In brief, Katie was 14 years old, her life was fragmented and the Serious Case Review reflects the involvement of family members, state actors and agencies who collectively failed to protect her from experiencing sexual exploitation. The focus of the report is on the incidence of sexual exploitation, but there are multiple issues not addressed by that perspective. For example, becoming a looked-after child is a risk factor for CSE, as in not engaging in education. Often we are encouraged to individualise problems, but what structural changes could be made within a child protection plan to ameliorate those risks and accentuate their protective nature?

When you read the report, examine:

- What other aspects of Katie's life are a concern?
- What relationships could be supported to enable greater care and a sense of safety and belongingness for Katie?
- What form of advocacy would Katie have benefitted from and where could this be sourced?
- Consider the Welfare Checklist – who was responsible for ensuring that decisions were in Katie's best interests?
- How would you do things differently if you were a practitioner involved in Katie's life?

---

enslavement of children for profit is a longstanding form of abuse, and the laws created to protect children can also position them as having agency in their abuse. Those matters create conflict in the positioning of victims as having participated for the purpose of some exchange to meet their needs and wants. That issue coupled with the distinction made regarding the age of the victim serves to compromise the application of the legal concept of consent. Amid these legal complexities, the local authority provision for victims can also create risk, leaving practitioners with a quandary of how to meet complex needs with provisions that could create additional harm.

FURTHER READING

UK Government 2017 – Child sexual exploitation: definition and guide for practitioners: Definition of child sexual exploitation, potential vulnerabilities and indicators of abuse and appropriate action to take in response. https://www.gov.uk/government/publications/child-sexual-exploitation-definition-and-guide-for-practitioners.

Department for Education 2017 – Child sexual exploitation Definition and a guide for practitioners, local leaders and decision-makers working to protect children from child sexual exploitation. https://assets.publishing.service.gov.uk/government/uploads/system/uploads/attachment_data/file/591903/CSE_Guidance_Core_Document_13.02.2017.pdf.

North Pennine NHS England North, University of Salford & The Pennine Acute Hospitals NHS Trust, 2017 Practitioner resources co-produced with children and young people. https://www.researchgate.net/publication/332734916_Not_just_a_thought.

National Working Group Network 2017 – Mapping UK national initiatives on CSE. https://www.nwgnetwork.org/national-reports/.

NSPCC 2019 – Protecting children from sexual exploitation. https://learning.nspcc.org.uk/child-abuse-and-neglect/child-sexual-exploitation/.

National Police Chiefs Council in association with the Children's Society and Victim Support and National Working Group – Appropriate language: child sexual and/or criminal exploitation guidance for professionals. https://www.csepoliceandprevention.org.uk/sites/default/files/Guidance%20App%20Language%20Toolkit.pdf

REFERENCES

Ahern, E., Kowalski, M., Lamb, M., 2018. A case study perspective: The experiences of young persons testifying to child sexual exploitation in British criminal court. J. Child Sex. Abus 27 (3), 321–334.

Beckett, H., Brodie, I., Factor, F., Melrose, M., Pearce, J., Pitts, J., et al., 2012. Research into Gang-associated Sexual Exploitation and Sexual Violence: Interim Report. University of Bedfordshire, Luton.

Broad, R., Turnbull, N., 2019. From human trafficking to modern slavery: the development of anti-trafficking policy in the UK. Eur. J. Crim. Policy Res. 25 (2), 119–133.

Brown, K., 2019. Vulnerability and child sexual exploitation: Towards an approach grounded in life experiences. Crit. Soc. Policy 39 (4), 622–642.

Brown, A., Barrett, D., 2002. Knowledge of Evil Child Prostitution and Child Sexual Abuse in Twentieth-Century England. Cullompton, Devon, UK.

Butler, C., 2015. A critical race feminist perspective on prostitution & sex trafficking in America. Yale J. L. Feminism. 27 (1), 95–139.

Children Act, 1989. https://www.legislation.gov.uk/ukpga/1989/41/contents.

Clarkson, F., 1939. History of prostitution. Can. Med. Assoc. J 41 (3), 296–301.

Cockbain, E., Ashby, M., Brayley, H., 2017. Immaterial Boys? A large-scale exploration of gender-based differences in child sexual exploitation service users. Sex. Abus 29 (7), 658–684.

COE (Council of Europe), 2018. Action Against Trafficking in Human Beings: Monitoring Mechanism. https://rm.coe.int/8th-/168094b073.

Craig, G., 2017. The UK's modern slavery legislation: an early assessment of progress. Soc. Incl 5 (2), 16.

Department for Education, 2017. Child sexual exploitation Definition and a guide for practitioners, local leaders and decision makers working to protect children from child sexual exploitation. https://assets.publishing.service.gov.uk/government/uploads/system/uploads/attachment_data/file/591903/CSE_Guidance_Core_Document_13.02.2017.pdf.

Dodsworth, J., 2014. Sexual exploitation, selling and swapping sex: victimhood and agency. Child Abus. Rev. 23 (3), 185–199.

ECPAT International, 2015. Unrecognized sexual abuse and exploitation of children in child, early and forced marriage. https://ecpat.org/search-our-library/

Ennew, J., 1986. Selling children's sexuality. N. Soc. 77 (1234), 9.

Franklin, A., Brown, S., Brady, G., 2018. The use of tools and checklists to assess the risk of child sexual exploitation: lessons from UK practice. J. Child Sex. Abus 27 (8), 978–997.

Greenbaum, J., Crawford-Jakubiak, J., Committee on Child Abuse and Neglect, 2015. Child sex trafficking and commercial sexual exploitation: Health care needs of victims. Pediatrics 135 (3), 566–574. https://doi.org/10.1542/peds.2014-4138.

Hallett, S., 2017. Making Sense of Child Sexual Exploitation: Exchange. Abuse and Young People. Policy Press, Bristol.

Hepburn, S., Simon, R., 2013. Human Trafficking Around the World: Hidden in Plain Sight. Columbia University Press, New York.

Home Office, 2019a. National Referral Mechanism Statistics, UK, Quarter 3 2019 – July to September 2019. https://assets.publishing.service.gov.uk/government/uploads/system/uploads/attachment_data/file/850824/national-referral-mechanism-statistics-quarter-3-2019-july-to-september.pdf.

Home Office, 2019b. Factsheet: Child Sexual Exploitation and Abuse. https://homeofficemedia.blog.gov.uk/2019/11/05/factsheet-child-sexual-exploitation-and-abuse/.

Ijadi-Maghsoodi, R., Bath, E., Cook, M., Textor, L., Barnert, E., 2018. Commercially sexually exploited youths' health care experiences, barriers, and recommendations: A qualitative analysis. Child Abus. Negl 76, 334–341.

Kelly, L., Karsna, K., 2017. Measuring the Scale and Changing Nature of Child Sexual Abuse and Child Sexual Exploitation. Scoping Report. Centre of Expertise on Child Sexual Abuse. Barnardos, Essex. https://www.csacentre.org.uk/research-publications/scale-and-nature-of-child-sexual-abuse-and-exploitation-report/scoping-report/.

Laser-Maira, J.A., Peach, D., Hounmenou, C.E., 2019. Moving towards self-actualization: A trauma-informed and needs-focused approach to the mental health needs of survivors of commercial child sexual exploitation. Int. J. Soc. Work 6 (2), 27. https://doi.org/10.5296/ijsw.v6i2.15198.

Leishman, M., 2007. Human trafficking and sexual slavery: Australia's response. Aust. Fem. Law J. 27 (27), 193–208.

Levine, J., 2017. Mental health issues in survivors of sex trafficking. Cogent Med 4, 1278841.

McIntyre, B.L., 2014. More than just rescue: Thinking beyond exploitation to creating assessment strategies for child survivors of commercial sexual exploitation. Int. Soc. Work 57 (1), 39–63. https://doi.org/10.1177/0020872813505629.

Modern Slavery Act, 2015. https://www.legislation.gov.uk/ukpga/2015/30/contents/enacted.

Naramore, R., Bright, M.A., Epps, N., Hardt, N.S., 2017. Youth arrested for trading sex have the highest rates of childhood adversity: A statewide study of juvenile offenders. Sex. Abus 29 (4), 396–410.

Núñez Puente, S., Gámez Fuentes, M., 2017. Spanish feminism, popular misogyny and the place of the victim. Fem. Media Stud 17 (5), 902–906.

O'Hara, M., 2019. Making pimps and sex buyers visible: Recognising the commercial nexus in 'child sexual exploitation'. Crit. Soc. Policy 39 (1), 108–126. https://doi.org/10.1177/0261018318764758.

Oram, S., Khondoker, M., Abas, M., Broadbent, M., Howard, L.M., 2015. Characteristics of trafficked adults and children with severe mental illness: a historical cohort study. Lancet Psychiatry 2 (12), 1084–1091.

Outshoorn, J., 2004. The Politics of Prostitution Women's Movements, Democratic States, and the Globalisation of Sex Commerce. Cambridge University Press, Cambridge, UK; New York.

Peach, D. (2019). Child Sexual Abuse and Exploitation. In S. Pollock, K. Parkinson, & I. Cummins (Eds.), Social Work and Society: Political and Ideological Perspectives (pp. 185-199). Bristol University Press. doi:10.46692/9781447344735.016.

Peach, D., Allen, D., Brown, P., 2015. Needs Analysis Report following the Sexual Exploitation of Children in Rotherham. University of Salford. https://moderngov.rotherham.gov.uk/documents/s103693/APPROVED%20FINAL%20RMBC%20CSE%20Needs%20Analysis%20report%20-%20Salford.pdf.

Polaris, 2010. Identifying Victims of Human Trafficking: What to look for during a medical exam/consultation. https://humantraffickinghotline.org/resources/what-look-healthcare-setting.

Powell, C., Asbill, M., Louis, E., Stoklosa, H., 2018. Identifying gaps in human trafficking mental health service provision. J. Hum. Traffick 4 (3), 256–269.

Ringrose, J., Gill, R., Livingstone, S., Harvey, L., 2012. A qualitative study of children, young people and 'sexting': a report prepared for the NSPCC. NSPCC. London.

Serious Crime Act, 2015. https://www.legislation.gov.uk/ukpga/2015/9/contents/enacted.

Sexual Offences Act, 2003. https://www.legislation.gov.uk/ukpga/2003/42/contents.

Sexual Offences (Northern Ireland) Order, 2008. https://www.legislation.gov.uk/nisi/2008/1769/contents.

Sexual Offences (Scotland) Act, 2009. https://www.legislation.gov.uk/asp/2009/9/contents.

Sjölin, C., 2015. Ten years on: Consent under the Sexual Offences Act 2003. J. Crim. Law 79 (1), 20–35.

Tennent, E., 2019. 'Do you think it's a crime?' Building joint understanding of victimisation in calls for help. Discourse Soc. 30 (6), 636–652.

10c

GANGS AND CHILD CRIMINAL EXPLOITATION

GRACE ELLEN ROBINSON

KEY POINTS

- While county lines drug supply has become the dominant form of child criminal exploitation (CCE), children and young people are commonly exploited into a wide range of criminal acts.

- Victims of CCE come from a wide variety of backgrounds, both deprived and affluent. Most victims have experienced some form of adversity.

- School exclusion, mental health and learning difficulties make young people more susceptible to criminal exploitation.

- Victims of CCE rarely acknowledge their exploitation and/or accept victim status. Exploited young people will often present with 'challenging' behaviours rather than stereotypical victim attributes.

- A trauma-informed approach to working with victims of CCE is necessary for safeguarding professionals in avoiding retraumatising children and young people.

INTRODUCTION

The criminal exploitation of children and young people presents itself as a challenging issue for law enforcement and child protection agencies to both understand and work with. The problem is complex and often rooted in inconsistent conceptualisations of young people involved in gangs and drug supply, and compounded by tensions between punishment and welfare, or keeping children safe from harm.

In 2019, Anne Longfield, the Children's Commissioner for England, warned of the potential for child criminal exploitation (CCE) to become the next major 'grooming scandal', urging the United Kingdom (UK) Government to make it a national priority (Children's Commissioner, 2019). Yet CCE is not new, and the abuse of young people through coerced or forced participation in criminality, particularly in international contexts (Elechi et al., 2007), has a lengthy history.

While CCE has become a cause for concern for practitioners, a historical lack of research and literature on the topic means understandings of the issue are emerging at a much slower pace than experiences of it are arising. However, CCE shares many similarities with child sexual exploitation (CSE) (Hallett, 2015), and it is useful to draw upon research and serious case reviews from this area of practice to help inform understandings. Similarities include the vulnerabilities of its victims and the role of grooming. High profile cases of CSE, including Rotherham and Rochdale, and the growing body of literature that has followed (Firmin et al., 2016; Firmin and Hancock, 2018; Hallett, 2017) can supplement practitioners' understanding of CCE.

Discussion of CCE to date has focused primarily on county lines drug supply – with the disruption of county lines gangs becoming the primary focus of law enforcement and child protection agencies (National Crime Agency, 2016; 2017; 2019). For example, stories of 'county lines dealers' or 'county lines drugs gangs' have appeared in abundance in the mainstream media, with news reports featuring almost daily. Other forms of criminal exploitation have subsequently remained unnoticed.

This chapter will focus on exploring CCE within a gang context, encouraging professionals to look beyond the complex behaviours that many victims of exploitation present with. Drawing on the serious case review of Chris, the chapter will demonstrate what lessons can be learned in order to prevent more children and young people losing their lives to gangs and CCE. The chapter concludes by demonstrating the importance of trauma-informed practice when working with gang-involved young people and victims of exploitation. This approach to child protection work moves away from victim-blaming and toward an holistic approach of exploring what has led to the offending behaviour.

CLOSER LOOK: CHILD CRIMINAL EXPLOITATION (CCE) IN MERSEYSIDE

Robinson (2019) conducted interviews with 18 gang-involved young people and victims of CCE in Merseyside.[1] She found that criminal exploitation existed on a continuum, ranging from subtle hints of coercion to outright force. For example, a small number of children in her study reported being forced to engage in drug supply, where their noncompliance would have resulted in victimisation through serious violence. However, the majority of children demonstrated agency in their involvement in illicit activity, acknowledging that they had been 'used' by drug dealers, yet accepting this to be part and parcel of the worlds in which they are involved. She also found that 'the challenge with any form of exploitation is that victims seldom see themselves as such' (Robinson et al., 2019, p. 706). The grooming that permeates cases of exploitation, in which victims are provided with luxurious items and other intangible goods, seeks to deceive victims into believing that the perpetrators are their friends.

Perpetrators capitalised on young males' need to belong and their desire for significance and respect by promising friendship, comradery and security. Professionals (N=26) in this research were often faced with confrontational and complex behaviours from young males who rejected any notion of victimhood and professed that engaging in criminality was their choice, and in exchange for high financial return (of which, in reality, they saw very little).

She also found 'the challenge with any form of exploitation is that victims seldom see themselves as such' (Robinson et al., 2019, p. 706). Both males and females are subjected to criminal exploitation; however, males are disproportionately affected and are rarely accepting of victim status due to feelings of shame and the stigma associated with the victim label which 'may draw blame, derogation, [and] weakness' (Fohring, 2018, p. 2). This is explored further under the heading 'Addressing criminal exploitation in the safeguarding arena'.

SERIOUS CASE REVIEW: CHRIS

The following information is taken from a serious case review commissioned by Newham Local Safeguarding Children's Board (Hill, 2018) and describes the life course of 14-year-old Chris, who was tragically shot and killed in 2017, following an 18-month period of involvement in gang-related activity.

Chris experienced a turbulent start to life, growing up with his mother and sister following reported domestic violence between his parents. He ceased contact with his father in 2012, reporting to others that he was dead.

Chris spent years in temporary accommodation which meant that he was regularly moved from one address to another. Already experiencing a lack of identity, Chris struggled with his diagnosis of attention-deficit/hyperactivity disorder (ADHD) and conduct disorder with reports that it made him feel different to his peers. Reluctant to take his medication, Chris presented with challenging behaviour throughout school, receiving a permanent exclusion by the age of 13 years. In January 2016, Chris was enrolled at a pupil referral unit in Newham. It was from this point that concerns began growing around gang activity. Seven months after entering the pupil referral unit, Chris was referred to a youth offending team for purchasing a knife. He had also ordered a knife and bullet proof vest to his grandfather's house, where he was living prior to his death. During November 2016, Chris went missing from home on two separate occasions, refusing to disclose any information upon his return. Shortly after,

---

[1] All young people in this research were male, had been excluded from mainstream school and had been raised – or were residing in – deprived areas.

and upon trying to stop him leaving the house, Chris assaulted his mother, later claiming that the assault was a form of self-defence.

On multiple occasions, there were reports of Chris expressing concerns that his life was in danger. In December 2016, he revealed to his mum that he was being pressured by drug dealers into the supply of drugs, after his mum found and disposed of Class A drugs with a reported value of £600. Police later recovered a mobile phone stolen in an armed robbery at Chris' address, and in April 2017 they arrested and convicted Chris for possession of a knife. In a police interview, Chris stated that he carried the weapon for protection, disclosing that he had been receiving threats on social media and had grown fearful over his safety. Chris was again arrested in August 2017 for possession of acid, to which he again stated that it was for his protection. While awaiting trial, Chris was out with a group of four young people on 4th September 2017, when he was passed by an unknown attacker in a stolen vehicle. The individual fired multiple shots into the group, hitting Chris with a bullet wound to the head. He died the following day at the age of 14 years.

The details of Chris' death points to a lengthy period of trauma, isolation and consequent criminal exploitation. From a young age, Chris had been subjected to a range of painful experiences in the form of domestic violence, victimisation, exclusion and rejection. Chris' lack of identity was compounded by learning disabilities and disrupted friendships that were exacerbated by living in temporary accommodation. At every stage of his educational life, Chris was met with punishment rather than compassion. As such Chris found comfort in gangs, identifying with individuals facing similar adversity to himself. He rapidly found himself involved in drug supply where he was coerced, manipulated and forced into paying off a drug debt that he had become trapped in. Chris' story is not an isolated account, but rather, indicative of the experiences of many young people associated with gangs and drug supply.

1. With regard to the given information, what factors made Chris susceptible to grooming and exploitation?
2. How could Chris' case study be used to identify and respond to victims of exploitation earlier?

There were clear signs of adversity and vulnerability in Chris' life, making him susceptible to CCE. Chris had a turbulent upbringing, being exposed to domestic violence and family breakdown from a young age. Living in temporary accommodation exacerbated his need to belong, and his ability to manage his emotions was compounded by his ADHD diagnosis. There were numerous opportunities for intervention; however, as stated in the serious case review, Chris faced punitive measures rather than compassion and understanding. As such, perpetrators were able to take advantage of his vulnerabilities and use coercion, manipulation and violence (Berelowitz et al., 2013) to secure his compliance.

In light of Chris' experience, practitioners may want to ask the following questions:

■ have you come across similar cases to Chris' in your organisation?
■ how were they responded to?
■ what behaviours would you expect Chris to present with upon first meeting him? and
■ how could a trauma-informed approach have helped Chris?

These questions may be useful for informing a more effective approach to dealing with vulnerable young people.

In acknowledging the many adversities that young people face, in addition to an increased awareness of what they may have been subjected to before reaching the criminal justice system, it is suggested here that professionals incorporate a trauma-informed approach (Hickle, 2016) to working with children and young people who have offended. Bateson et al. (2019, p. 3) argues that for professionals, a trauma-informed approach encourages a shift in thinking from 'What's wrong with you?' to 'What's happened to you?' and for service users a shift from 'There's something wrong about me' to 'I'm not a bad person, I'm like this because bad things happened to me'. Importantly, this approach also emphasises the need to spot the signs of trauma and actively avoid retraumatising children and young people. Taken together, these components have the ability to avoid victim-blaming, promote confidence, build trust and reduce the tensions between 'us' and 'them'.

DEFINING CHILD CRIMINAL EXPLOITATION

In the absence of a universal definition, child criminal exploitation involves the coercion, control, manipulation and force of a child or young person into any criminal activity, by an individual or group (HM Government, 2018, p. 8) who exploit vulnerability. According to the National Crime Agency (2017; 2019), the UK's lead law enforcement organisation in the fight against organised crime, cases of CCE are growing across the UK. Cross border drug supply (or county lines) is cited as the most prevalent form of CCE. Entangled with county lines narratives, understandings of CCE have been reduced to local and national media reports which do little other than distort and amplify the problem, creating a new 'moral panic' (Cohen, 1972) and encouraging reactive, short-term policies that seldom address the underlying issues. Research shows that overly punitive sentencing and increased police powers have, to some extent, encouraged the criminal exploitation of children and young people, earmarking them as useful scapegoats – by organised criminals – for maximising profits and reducing risk of detection by law enforcement (Brewster et al., 2023). For example, the use of stop and search powers have resulted in more 'innocent' children and young people, or those without criminal records (also known as 'clean skins') (National Crime Agency, 2017), being tasked with possessing and moving illicit items (Robinson, 2019).

CCE is an umbrella concept encompassing a wide range of criminal activities. Such activities include – but are not limited to – the distribution and retrieval of illicit drugs and money, the possession and concealment of weapons such as knives and firearms, perpetrating violence, harbouring offenders and providing false alibies. While these activities vary in terms of level of involvement and severity of offence, the individuals at the root of criminally exploiting children and young people are organised criminals (individuals), criminal gangs/groups and, contentiously, current or previous victims of criminal exploitation. Essential to exploitation is the 'element of exchange' and 'meeting ... of unmet needs' (Hallett, 2017, p. 2). The exchange of a child's services in criminality is usually met with rewards such as affection, 'friendship', belonging, money and drugs. Perpetrators can identify the unmet needs of children and seek to fill them to encourage their services in return. For example, children in precarious living situations (i.e. those in the care system) might be vulnerable to the offer of accommodation by exploiters who, after providing the child with somewhere to live, then force their involvement in criminality as a form of rent. The subsequent harms that those involved are subject to are significant, increasing the risk of illness, physical harm and death, mental ill health and involvement with the criminal justice system.

Emerging trends reveal that children and young people from more affluent backgrounds are increasingly becoming involved in CCE (Brewster et al., 2023; Robinson, 2019; Turner et al., 2019). However, most victims have been exposed to adversity, or adverse childhood experiences. For example, family dysfunction, mental illness, drug misuse, experiences of victimisation and violence school exclusion, and marginalisation (Bakkali, 2019) are among some of the traumatic situations faced by children and young people involved in CCE. Children and young people with learning disabilities and conditions such as ADHD are also much more likely to be victimised (Spicer et al., 2019) and/or engage in criminal activity (Fletcher and Wolfe, 2009).

THE RELATIONSHIP BETWEEN GANGS AND CRIMINAL EXPLOITATION

According to the Children's Society (2019), there are upwards of 46,000 children and young people entrenched in gangs and more than 313,000 children and young people on the periphery. These estimates are modest, and there is much controversy around the proper definition of 'gangs' (Esbensen et al., 2001). Debates on what constitutes a 'gang' frequently centre around the level of organisation (Harding et al., 2019) and the characteristics and structural makeup. These debates can make discussions of what a gang *is* or *is not* laborious and, at times, counterproductive. For the purpose of this chapter, it is more constructive to situate gangs in their role in the criminal exploitation of children and young people. Gangs are described by the

Eurogang network[2], a joint American and European initiative of leading gang researchers, as any:

durable, street-oriented youth group whose involvement in illegal activity is part of its group identity

Weerman et al. (2009, p. 20)

The past few decades have given rise to a growing gang problem in the UK, particularly in marginalised communities (McLean, 2020). Austerity measures implemented by the 2010 UK Coalition Government have exacerbated the conditions of poverty, inequality and social exclusion which many children are living in. Some isolated and disenfranchised young people have found solace in associating with like-minded individuals, in the form of criminal groups. Indeed, previous violent victimisation and anti-social behaviour are key predictors of gang involvement (Medina et al., 2012). However, many children and young people living in gang-affected communities also experience – and fear – victimization; this itself is a significant driver of gang-involvement with 'protection' featuring highly among motivations for young people joining gangs (Smithson et al., 2009). Yet research demonstrates that gang members are more likely to be victimised than non-gang members (Young et al., 2013).

Gangs in the UK have extended beyond traditional involvement in petty crime, becoming involved in more organised aspects of criminality, particularly drug supply (McLean, 2020). The area in which we have seen the most rapid evolution is the establishment of 'county lines'. Commonly referred to by those involved as 'going country' or 'OT' (out there) (Robinson, 2019), county lines is a term used by the police to explain a process whereby:

A [criminal] group ... establishes a network between an urban hub and county location, into which drugs ... are supplied. A branded mobile phone line is established ... to which orders are placed ... the group exploits young or vulnerable persons ... [whom] regularly travel between the urban hub and the county market, to replenish stock and deliver cash ...

National Crime Agency (2017, p. 2)

The use of children in these operations offers distance and anonymity for county lines dealers who manage the supply from their local areas without having to travel to the destinations themselves (National Crime Agency, 2016). In a 2017 report, the National Crime Agency noted that 65% of police forces in England and Wales reported gangs exploiting children and young people (National Crime Agency, 2017). However, not all victims of criminal exploitation are lured into county lines activity; most will have been coerced or forced into local drug supply and other drug-related activities by local drug networks. In such cases, the criminally exploited child would usually return home each night without perpetrators arranging hotels, B&Bs, or cuckooed properties. The accessibility of drugs and ease of becoming involved in the trade has provided children and young people with what they deem to be a legitimate substitute for lawful work. Aspirations, status and the need to belong – encouraged by excessive consumerism and reinforced by the media through images of celebrity culture – have increased to heights that far exceed the level of income that any legitimate work could meet for most marginalised young people. The result has meant that involvement in drug supply, or 'grafting', has become one of the most accessible ways in which many young people can achieve and meet their expectations (Hesketh and Robinson, 2019).

It is important for practitioners to understand the cultural and socioeconomic dynamics that may lie behind the behaviours of the young people they encounter. Professionals should be on notice for signs that young people might be engaged in gang-driven activity, such as county lines. Prolonged, frequent, or unexplained absences are one sign. It may be useful for practitioners to have some knowledge of the means of their young people's families: such background information may assist in identifying unexplained purchases and cash in the possession of exploited young people. It is also vital that the professional workforce has an understanding of the wider community and the existing barriers to engagement that those living within these communities face. This can be achieved by ensuring a culturally competent workforce in which services users are able to 'see themselves reflected in the services on offer and have confidence that they will be understood' (Williams et al., 2020, p. 3).

---

[2]More information about the Eurogang network can be found by accessing the following link https://eurogangproject.com

WHAT CAN HAPPEN TO CHILDREN AND YOUNG PEOPLE INVOLVED IN CRIMINAL EXPLOITATION?

The policy of austerity and spending cuts, including the reduction in welfare and state intervention, has disproportionately impacted young people. Many will have experienced the shrinkage in youth services and the closure of youth clubs, both highly visible public sector cuts. School exclusion is a significant feature in the lives of many criminally exploited young people (Robinson, 2019); for those still in education, beyond the school gates there is little in the way of opportunities. Simultaneously, there has been a significant increase in the production and use of cannabis in the UK, which has driven the normalisation and social acceptance of consuming the drug (Aldridge et al., 2011) – not solely by young people but across the wider population in general. In part, this has meant that some young people have been exposed to the drug from a young age through peers, siblings and even parents. Smoking cannabis now forms part of the landscape, curing the boredom and perceived monotony of everyday life and helping young people deal with marginalisation and pain (Bakkali, 2019). Young people who are prolonged cannabis users experience regular contact with drug dealers, some of whom secure their compliance in criminality through the promise of 'free' cannabis. Robinson (2019) suggests that rather than being a gateway to further drug use, cannabis has become a gateway into criminality.

The NSPCC (2023) have highlighted a non-exhaustive list of risk factors and possible signs of victimisation through criminal exploitation, including 'alcohol or drug misuse, self harm and changes in mood'. Such issues are also typical of the offending population. Less attention has been given to the role of cannabis in the lives of young people. Indeed, findings drawn from interviews with youth justice practitioners have revealed that cannabis was at the crux of involvement in coerced or forced drug supply (Robinson, 2019). Due to the hierarchical structure of gangs, money from drug supply is not evenly distributed to those working at maximum capacity to secure profit for others. Instead, cannabis has become the primary method of payment for completion of criminal tasks, with the intention being to promote addiction and increase the availability pool of young people to exploit.

To encourage the development of debts, drug dealers have allowed, and encouraged, children and young people to purchase drugs on credit (Coomber and Moyle, 2018) through a process known as 'strapping' or 'tick'. This practice allows trusted individuals to purchase drugs on the spot without payment. Once the young person has accrued a large enough debt, they will be coerced into drug supply or face violent repurcussions for breaking their credit agreement (Moeller and Sandberg, 2017). Other debt-building methods have included 'staged' thefts and robberies, whereby drug dealers instruct other individuals to rob money and drugs from young people. These practices come under the broad umbrella of 'debt-bondage' (Harding, 2020), in which victims are trapped in a cycle of exploitation.

As we can see from our case study, Chris revealed to his mother that he was being pressured by drug dealers to supply drugs, after his mother disposed of a quantity of Class A drugs with an estimated value of £600. The loss of drugs, whether due to a genuine loss, being subjected to a robbery, or as a result of seizures by police, would have left Chris in debt to the drug dealers and in a situation of having to offer his labour in exchange for paying off the debt. Children in these situations need intense intervention from professionals who can seek to make the child as inaccessible to the drug dealers as possible.

CLOSER LOOK: OUTCOMES FOR VICTIMS OF CHILD CRIMINAL EXPLOITATION (CCE)

There are a plethora of harms that children and young people are exposed to during their criminal exploitation pathway. Experiences of violence through gang-involvement; risks to physical health from drug concealment; introduction to intravenous drug use(rs) and paraphernalia, and the witnessing of overdoses and death are common (Robinson, 2019). In recent years, violent retaliations have extended beyond the individual and been directed towards their family members with threats of, or actual violence being carried out on siblings, partners and parents (Densley, 2013; Robinson, 2019). It is this which often secures the compliance, and silence, of children and young people and ensures their participation in the gang and all of its activities. Outcomes for victims of CCE usually include (but are not limited to):

1. Continued involvement in the gang and participation in criminality (mostly drug supply), using cannabis to manage emotions and adding to their debt. Moving up the hierarchy is possible but not probable and will depend upon levels of social capital

(Harding, 2020). Interaction with police which may cease upon receiving punitive criminal justice intervention (Robinson, 2019);

2. Going missing from home out of fear for their own and their family's safety, escaping the gang and cumulative debt for short periods of time. More often than not they will encounter equally exploitative situations in new locations, later being picked up by law enforcement (Windle and Briggs, 2015);

3. Becoming the repeated target of violent assaults for noncompliance and nonrepayment of debt. The perceived lack of respect and disloyalty to the gang will usually result in life-changing injury or death (Pitts, 2007; Robinson, 2019).

Instances of young people exiting the gang without retaliation are rare (Decker et al., 2014), particularly where they owe money to an individual or group. And while law enforcement, media and political narratives succeed in portraying some young people as 'vulnerable victims of exploitation, in reality they are frequently met with the full force of the law' (Densley et al., 2020, p. 5).

ADDRESSING CRIMINAL EXPLOITATION IN THE SAFEGUARDING ARENA

Widespread acknowledgement of CCE in addition to county lines remaining a national priority (Home Office, 2018) has encouraged shifts in attitudes towards children and young people who offend from perpetrator/offender to complete – or part – victim status. Yet this chapter highlights that there are challenges for safeguarding professionals in recognising the exploitative nature at the heart of much offending behaviour. Attitudes towards victims of CCE vary, often depending upon the professional's role and the victim's appearance (Christie, 1996). Indeed, how victims present themselves when arrested can determine the way in which they are perceived and their subsequent treatment. Research demonstrates that experiences of trauma (of which many of these victims have faced), particularly in males, is re-enacted through anger and aggression (Ford et al., 2012). Such behaviour both undermines cooperation with law enforcement (the consequences of which are described later) and acts as a barrier to victims accessing care. These behaviours are also pertinent in considering the relationship between trauma and posttraumatic stress disorder (PTSD) (Beresford and Wood, 2016)

and, if taken at face value, have the potential to skew the perceived level of vulnerability of a victim. Whether a victim of CCE is perceived by the professional dealing with them as a victim or an offender is influenced by the presentation of the victim at the point of contact. The classic example of this is arrest by a police officer. Victims of CCE may respond with behaviours that are perceived by the arresting officers as dismissive, aggressive, and confrontational. Without training in trauma-induced behaviours, professionals, such as police officers, may regard such a response to arrest as an indication of offending rather than victimhood. Despite levels of fear of their exploiters and potential reprisals resulting from assisting in police investigations, a failure to cooperate during police interview is often used to the detriment of victims of CCE. An example of this is more punitive sentences at the conclusion of the court process. Such uncooperative behaviours may appear as assertive and confrontational, but are often adopted to mask fear and suffering.

Haines and Case (2015) 'children first, offenders second' model emphasises the importance of listening to the voices of young people (Creaney, 2018) and ensuring that interventions are child-friendly, diversionary and inclusive (Maynard et al., 2019). Children and young people should be recognised as stakeholders within their communities and special attention should be paid to the skills that they have to offer. Young people in gangs share similar merits with others, qualities such as loyalty, respect and brotherhood (Harding, 2020) are what binds the gang together. Yet these traits become misplaced and distorted, taken advantage of by perpetrators of criminal exploitation. Channelling these traits into positive activities could be the difference between life and death, but there needs to be more opportunities for young people first.

Returning to the case study, Chris faced exclusion in different capacities. Firstly he was living in temporary accommodation, and later he was excluded from mainstream school. Efforts by professionals working with children in these situations should focus on encouraging inclusion and activities that allow children to be children, whilst also promoting self-esteem building and environments where children can formulate an identity.

Agencies need to work together in a concerted approach to address social exclusion and disenfranchisement, shifting attitudes towards children and young people who break the law and offering an understanding of the difficulties that they experience. The key to making significant improvements to outcomes is joined-up thinking and responses. Ideally, public authorities and nongovernmental organisations would 'speak with one voice' to each child and young person. Consistency is key to forging relationships, which in turn enable children and young people to open up about their experiences to responsible professionals.

CONCLUSION

With this in mind, there are a number of practical points that professionals may wish to take away from the findings presented in this chapter. These practice points are:

1. Use appropriate language. There are resources to aid in developing best practices in your workplace with respect to language.[3]
2. In terms of personal conduct, listen to young people intently, communicating that you are listening, and adopt a compassionate response to every young person during every interaction.
3. Be informed about the latest research in trauma studies by engaging in training and continuing professional development. This may seem obvious, but it is vital. This is a growing field, and our understanding of trauma in victims of CCE is becoming ever more sophisticated. It is important to make a conscious effort to remain up to date with the latest research. This will help inform points (1) and (2).
4. Adopt a policy of 'one worker, one child/young person'. Children in the system are typically dealt with by numerous different workers. They then find it difficult to open up and trust professionals, because they learn that professionals' involvement in their life will ultimately come to an end, and they will have to once again recount traumatic experiences. As such, they do not see the point in opening up and lose faith in the system.

5. Engage in basic equality law practices: 'include not exclude'. Equip yourself and your colleagues with training in the latest best practices in equality and inclusion. This is a field rich with training providers and resources. Equality training will supplement your trauma-focused training and inform your approach to points (1), (2), and (6).
6. Ensure you have a culturally competent workforce, whose members understand and can relate to the individuals with whom they are working.[4]

To achieve the maximum benefit, these suggestions should be (a) taken together, not individually, and (b) interpreted generously, not narrowly. In terms of the former, it should be clear from the list that some of these proposals have direct benefits for the enactment of other proposals (e.g. point (5)). Regarding the latter, it is important not to regard these proposals as cursory tick-box exercises. Sustained immersion in equality training, for instance, can lead to more sophisticated cultural literacy and sharper critical thinking skills. In this way, deep engagement with point (5), to take one example, can have meaningful and practical knock-on benefits for fulfilling proposals (1), (2), and (6).

It is important to recognise that there is no easy fix to the problems in the CCE sector. The issues touched on in this chapter are themselves the outgrowths of entrenched socioeconomic structures. It is beyond the capabilities of CCE professionals to get to the root of these structural issues in the course of their everyday work – to do so would likely require system-wide fiscal responses. However, there is much that can be done to improve the responses to CCE and, in doing so, to improve materially the many lives that CCE professionals encounter in the course of their work. CCE professionals perform an invaluable role in improving the outcomes for children and young people who have been the victims of exploitation or otherwise trapped in the criminal justice system. It is hoped this chapter may be of practical use in furthering these efforts to improve outcomes for young people.

---

[3]For one resource on language best practice, see: https://www.childrenssociety.org.uk/information/professionals/resources/child-exploitation-language-guide?utm_source=Twitter&utm_medium=Social&utm_campaign=TwitterSocial_SexualAbuseAwareness_Feb22.

[4]For more information on how to develop a culturally competent workforce, see: https://www.powerthefight.org.uk/wp-content/uploads/2021/11/tip-pilot.pdf.

FURTHER READING

Children's Commissioner, 2019. Keeping Kids Safe: Improving Safeguarding Responses to Gang Violence and Criminal Exploitation. Children's Commissioner, London.

Densley, J., 2013. How Gangs Work: an Ethnography of Youth Violence. Palgrave Macmillan, New York.

Hill, N., 2018. Serious Case Review – Chris. Newham Local Safeguarding Children Board [online]. https://www.newhamscp.org.uk/wp-content/uploads/2018/10/Serious-Case-Review-Chris-.pdf.

McLean, R., Robinson, G., Densley, J., 2019. County Lines: Criminal Networks and Evolving Drug Markets in Britain, first ed. Springer, New York. https://doi.org/10.1007/978-3-030-33362-1_3.

National Crime Agency, 2019. County Lines Drug Supply, Vulnerability and Harm 2018. Intelligence Assessment. National Crime Agency, London.

Robinson, G., McLean, R., Densley, J., 2019. Working county lines: Child criminal exploitation and illicit drug dealing in Glasgow and Merseyside. Int. J. Offender Ther. Comp. Criminol. 63, 694–711.

REFERENCES

Aldridge, J., Measham, F., Williams, L., 2011. Illegal Leisure Revisited: Changing Patterns of Alcohol and Drug Use in Adolescents and Young Adults. Routledge, London.

Bakkali, Y., 2019. Dying to live: Youth violence and the munpain. Sociol. Rev. 1–16. https://doi.org/10.1177/0038026119842012.

Bateson, K., McManus, M., Johnson, G., 2019. Understanding the use, and misuse, of adverse childhood experiences (ACEs) in trauma-informed policing. Police J. 93 (3). https://doi.org/10.1177/0032258X19841409.

Berelowitz, S., Clifton, J., Firimin, C., Gulyurtlu, S., Edwards, G., 2013. "If only someone had listened": Office of the Children's Commissioner's Inquiry into Child Sexual Exploitation in Gangs and Groups, Final Report. Office of the Children's Commissioner, London.

Beresford, H., Wood, J.L., 2016. Patients or perpetrators? The effects of trauma exposure on gang members' mental health: a review of the literature. J. Criminol. Res. Policy Pract. 2 (2), 148–159.

Brewster, B., Robinson, G., Silverman, B., Walsh, D., 2023. Covid-19 and child criminal exploitation in the UK: Implications of the pandemic for county lines. Trends Organ. Crime 26 (2), 156–179. https://doi.org/10.1007/s12117-021-09442-x.

Children's Commissioner, 2019. Keeping kids safe: Improving safeguarding responses to gang violence and criminal exploitation. Children's Commissioner, London.

Christie, N., 1986. The Ideal Victim. In: Fattah, E. (Ed.), From Crime Policy to Victim Policy. Palgrave MacMillan, London.

Cohen, S., 1972. Folk Devils and Moral Panics: The Creation of the Mods and Rockers. Martin Robertson, Oxford.

Coomber, R., Moyle, L., 2017. The changing shape of street-level heroin and crack supply in England: Commuting, holidaying and cuckooing drug dealers across 'county lines. Brit. J. Criminol. 58 (6), 1323–1342. https://doi.org/10.1093/bjc/azx068.

Creaney, S., 2018. Children's voices – are we listening? Progressing peer mentoring in the youth justice system. Child Care Pract. 26 (1), 22–37. https://doi.org/10.1080/13575279.2018.1521381.

Decker, S., Pyrooz, D.C., Moule, R.K., 2014. Disengagement from gangs as role transitions. J. Adolesc. Res. 24 (2), 268–283.

Densley, J., 2013. How Gangs Work: An Ethnography of Youth Violence. Palgrave MacMillan, New York.

Densley, J., Deuchar, R., Harding, S., 2020. An introduction to gangs and serious youth violence in the United Kingdom. Youth Justice 20 (1–2), 3–10. https://doi.org/10.1177/1473225420902848.

Elechi, O., Okosun, T., Ngwe, J., 2007. Factors vitiating against the effectiveness of the Nigeria police in combating the criminal exploitation of children and women. Afr. J. Int. Crim. Justice 3 (1), 1–49.

Esbenson, F., Winfree, L., He, N., Taylor, T., 2001. Youth gangs and definitional issues: When is a gang a gang, and why does it matter? Crime Delinq. 47 (1), 105–130.

Firmin, C., Hancock, D., 2018. Profiling CSE: Building a contextual picture of a local problem. In: Beckett, H., Pearce, J. (Eds.), Understanding and Responding to Child Sexual Exploitation. Routledge, Abingdon, pp. 107–120.

Firmin, C., Warrington, C., Pearce, J., 2016. Sexual exploitation and its impact on developing sexualities and sexual relationships: The need for contextual social work intervention. Br. J. Soc. Work 46 (8), 2318–2337.

Fletcher, J., Wolfe, B., 2009. Long-term consequences of childhood ADHD on criminal activities. J. Ment. Health Policy Econ. 12 (3), 119–138.

Fohring, S. 2018. What's in a word? Victims on 'victim'. Int. Rev. Vict. 24 (2), https://doi.org/ 10.1177/0269758018755154

Ford, J.D., Chapman, J., Connor, D.F., Cruise, K.R., 2012. Complex trauma and aggression in secure juvenile justice settings. Crim. Justice Behav. 39 (6), 694–724.

Haines, K., Case, S., 2015. Positive Youth Justice. Children First, Offenders Second. University of Bristol: Policy Press.

Hallett, S., 2015. 'An uncomfortable comfortableness': 'Care', child protection and child sexual exploitation. Br. J. Soc. Work 46 (7), 2137–2152.

Hallett, S., 2017. Making Sense of Child Sexual Exploitation: Exchange, Abuse and Young People. Policy Press, Bristol.

Harding, S., 2020. County Lines: Exploitation and Drug Dealing Among Urban Street Gangs. Bristol University Press, Bristol.

Harding, S., Deuchar, R., Densley, J., McLean, R., 2019. A typology of street robbery and gang organization: Insights from qualitative research in Scotland. Brit. J. Criminol. 59, 879–897.

Hesketh, R.F., Robinson, G., 2019. Grafting: "the boyz" just doing business? Deviant entrepreneurship in street gangs. Safer Communities 18 (2), 54–63. https://doi.org/10.1108/SC-05-2019-0016. 18.

Hickle, K., 2016. A Trauma-informed Approach: Policing Responses to Child Sexual Exploitation. Briefing Report. University of Sussex, UK.

Hill, N., 2018. Serious case review – Chris. Newham Local Safeguarding Children Board [online]. https://www.newhamscp.org.uk/wp-content/uploads/2018/10/Serious-Case-Review-Chris-.pdf.

HM Government, 2018. Serious Violence Strategy. [online]. https://assets.publishing.service.gov.uk/government/uploads/system/uploads/attachment_data/file/698009/serious-violence-strategy.pdf.

Home Office, 2018. National County Lines Coordination Centre to Crack Down on Drug Gangs. Gov.uk [online]. https://www.gov.uk/government/news/national-county-lines-coordination-centre-to-crack-down-on-drug-gangs.

Medina-Ariza, J., Cebulla, A., Ross, A., Shute, J., Aldridge, J.A., 2013. Children and young people in gangs: a longitudinal analysis. London: Nuffield Foundation, p. 6.

Maynard, E., Pycroft, A., Spiers, J., 2019. "They say 'yes, I'm doing it...and I'm fine'": The lived experience of supporting teenagers who misuse drugs. J. Soc. Work Pract. 35 (2), 1–15. https://doi.org/10.1080/02650533.2019.1697868.

McLean, R., 2020. Understanding and Policing Gangs Report. Cumberland Lodge, Berkshire.

Moeller, K., Sandberg, S., 2017. Debts and threats: Managing inability to repay credits in illicit drug distribution. Justice Q. 34 (2), 272–296.

National Crime Agency, 2016. County Lines Gang Violence, Exploitation & Drug Supply. National Briefing Report. National Crime Agency, London.

National Crime Agency, 2017. County Lines Violence, Exploitation & Drug Supply 2017. National Briefing Report. National Crime Agency, London.

National Crime Agency, 2019. County Lines Drug Supply, Vulnerability and Harm 2018. Intelligence Assessment. National Crime Agency, London.

NSPCC, 2023. Child Sexual Exploitation: Who Is Affected. NSPCC [online]. https://www.nspcc.org.uk/what-is-child-abuse/types-of-abuse/child-sexual-abuse/.

Pitts, J., 2007. 'Reluctant gangsters: Youth gangs in Waltham Forest'. Report for the Waltham Forest Crime and Community Safety Partnership. University of Bedfordshire, UK.

Robinson, G., 2019. Gangs, county lines and child criminal exploitation: A case study of Merseyside. Unpublished PhD thesis, Edge Hill University.

Robinson, G., McLean, R., Densley, J., 2019. Working county lines: Child criminal exploitation and illicit drug dealing in Glasgow and Merseyside. Int. J. Offender Ther. Comp. Criminol. 63, 694–711.

Smithson, H., Christmann, K., Armitage, R., Whitehead, A., Rogerson, M., 2009. Young People's Involvement in Gangs and Guns in Liverpool. [online] http://eprints.hud.ac.uk/24788/1/acc-guns-and-gangs-report.pdf.

Spicer, J., Moyle, L., Coomber, R., 2019. The variable and evolving nature of 'cuckooing' as a form of criminal exploitation in street level drug markets. Trends Organ. Crime 23, 301–323. https://doi.org/10.1007/s12117-019-09368-5.

Storrod, M., Densley, J., 2017. 'Going viral' and 'going country': The expressive and instrumental activities of street gangs on social media. J. Youth Stud. 20, 677–696.

The Children's Society, 2019. Tackling criminal exploitation. The Children's Society [online]. https://www.childrenssociety.org.uk/what-we-do/our- work/tackling-criminal-exploitation-and-county-lines.

Turner, A., Belcher, L., Pona, I., 2019. Counting Lives. Responding to Children Who Are Criminally Exploited. The Children's Society, London, UK.

Weerman, F., Maxson, C.L., Esbensen, F.A., Aldridge, J., Medina, J., Van Gemert, F., 2009. Eurogang Program Manual: Background, development, and use of the Eurogang instruments in multi-site, multi-method comparative research. https://www.escholar.manchester.ac.uk/uk-ac-man-scw:58536.

Williams, E., Iyere, E., Lindsay, B., Murray, C., Ramadhan, Z., 2020. Therapeutic Intervention for Peace (TIP) Report. Power The Fight [online]. https://www.powerthefight.org.uk/wp-content/uploads/2021/11/tip-report.pdf.

Windle, J., Briggs, D., 2015. "It's like working away for two weeks': The harms associated with young drug dealers commuting from a saturated London drug market. Crime Prev. Community Saf. 17 (2), 105–119.

Young, T., Fitzgibbon, W., Silverstone, D., 2013. The Role of the Family in Facilitating Gang Membership, Criminality and Exit. Catch 22, London.

10d RADICALISATION

LISA CURTIS ■ NIGEL BROMAGE

KEY POINTS

- Understanding radicalisation of children and young people and why it is becoming a growing concern.
- Understanding the role of Prevent.
- Recognising radicalisation and those who are most vulnerable.
- Responding to radicalisation and best practice for practitioners.

INTRODUCTION

Understanding and responding to the emerging nature of radicalisation can present key challenges to practitioners working with children and young people. Practitioners across all agencies need to develop an understanding of the issue and recognise their own roles and responsibility in keeping young people at risk safe from harm. Allowing for the debate about practice issues, this chapter provides guidance that will allow for best practice to be developed and for challenges and barriers to be considered; the importance of recognising opportunities for early intervention will also be discussed.

This chapter provides an outline of the issues all practitioners need to understand in relation to radicalisation. It will start by defining the issue and outlining the Prevent programme. The chapter will then move on to support practitioners in identifying how radicalisation can present, why it can happen, and which young people are vulnerable and why. It will then go on to explore issues around how practitioners can respond to young people at risk, the challenges and best practice.

CLOSER LOOK: RADICALISATION

Definition

'Radicalisation' refers to the process by which a person comes to support terrorism and extremist ideologies associated with terrorist groups – provided in the Prevent Duty Guidance, p.12 3 Section 26 of the Counter-Terrorism and Security Act (CTSA) 2015.

The NSPCC refers to radicalisation as the process through which a person comes to support or be involved in extremist ideologies. It can result in a person becoming drawn into terrorism and is in itself a form of harm (NSPCC, 2021).

Both definitions demonstrate that the child or young person can be drawn into this process This is an important point to note as it potentially means there is time for the process involved in becoming radicalised to be recognised. Key to this is recognising who might be vulnerable and identifying possible contextual indicators.

REFLECTIVE QUESTIONS

- What is your understanding of the term 'extremist ideologies'?
- Does your organisation have a policy for working with children or young people at risk of radicalisation?
- Are you aware of your own professional responsibilities in this area of practice?

RECOGNISING RADICALISATION – WHO MIGHT BE VULNERABLE?

There is no set pattern or route into radicalisation for a child or young person. It often occurs gradually so children and young people who are affected may not realise what it is that they are being drawn into. Radicalisation can be broadly divided into two areas: the first stage is an attitudinal change, where those who are vulnerable are drawn into an ideology, and the second stage is behavioural, where extremist views turn into violence. Both stages are associated with influencing factors or background, environment, friendship groups and unmet psychological needs (Chisholm, Coulter and Public, 2017).

The process used is similar to grooming, and the child or young person can find withdrawing from this process frightening or dangerous. Conversely, the child or young person may be indoctrinated into the belief or ideology as the controlling nature of the relationship evolves, ultimately believing they are right and others, once close to them or known to them, are wrong. Most commonly, the vulnerability of older adolescents to being groomed and exploited is recognised, but the vulnerability of younger children is not, hence the opportunity to protect them is missed.

Children and young people can be drawn into radicalisation for a range of reasons including:

- searching for answers to questions about identity, faith and belonging,
- being driven by the desire for 'adventure' and excitement,
- being driven by a need to raise their self-esteem and promote their 'street cred',
- being drawn to a group or individual who can offer identity, a social network and support,
- being influenced by world events and a sense of grievance resulting in a need to make a difference, and
- feeling they lack purpose, are bored or have been bullied in the past (Educate Against Hate).

Practitioners need to be aware of the range of indicators which suggest a young person may be in the process of being radicalised. These may include:

- acting out of character: changes in dress, behaviour and peer relationships;
- secretive behaviour;

- losing interest in friends and activities;
- isolating themselves from family and friends;
- talking as if from a scripted speech – spending more time online;
- showing sympathy for extremist causes;
- glorifying violence;
- possessing illegal or extremist literature;
- using codes, numbers or graffiti associated with extremist groups;
- new tattoos of numbers or symbols you have never seen before which are codes used to communicate messages to followers;
- advocating messages similar to illegal organisations such as 'Muslims Against Crusades' or other non-proscribed extremist groups such as the English Defence League; and
- new friends that are not known.

Children and young people at risk may display outgoing or risky behaviour, start getting into trouble at school or on the streets and mixing with other children who behave badly, but this is not always the case. Sometimes those at risk may be encouraged by the people they are in contact with not to draw attention to themselves. Children may become quieter and more serious about their studies and may also dress more modestly and mix with a group of people that seems to be better behaved than previous friends. This behaviour can mask the indicators of radicalisation as parents feel their child has settled down. The recruiters/groomers realise that by encouraging this approach, the work needed and those recruited can go undetected.

Small Steps describe how far-right activists have changed the way they operate and recruit members from the upfront vision of the 1980s distributing leaflets to a more sophisticated and harder to detect approach.

Although anyone can be radicalised, there are factors which can increase the possibility of radicalisation. Experienced recruiters/groomers know who to look for and will invest the time required to reach the desired outcome. Some of the factors may include:

- being easily influenced or impressionable,
- having low self-esteem or being isolated,
- feeling that rejection, discrimination or injustice is taking place in society,
- coming from a family who has a sense of grievance,

■ experiencing community tension amongst different groups,

■ being disrespectful or angry towards family and peers,

■ having a strong need for acceptance or belonging,

■ experiencing grief such as loss of a loved one,

■ experiencing a low mood or depression,

■ spending increased time on social media that is not regulated, and

■ having anxiety and uncertainty about their place in the world.

Some children and young people may also be more vulnerable to the impact of digital technology, for example, those with mental health needs such as depression or anxiety, or developmental conditions such as attention-deficit/hyperactivity disorder (Royal College of Psychiatrists, 2020). Trends examined by Malik in her report (Malik, 2019) highlighted that families involved in radicalisation cases had three common denominators, all of which can contribute towards 'pushing' children towards radicalisation. These can be broken down into:

■ isolation (taking children out of school),

■ history (a family that contains a family member who joined Islamic state, or a family who has a history of extremist activity), and

■ home environment, where parents are separated, there is a history of domestic abuse, or a family member has been involved in crime.

Malik (2019) found that 52% of the families examined in this report had backgrounds rooted in extremism, had family members who held convictions related to terrorism or who had been members of extremist groups. Her report demonstrates how family members can play a role in influencing views and values associated with radicalisation.

In the cases examined by Malik, it was noted that boys tended to join Islamic state under the influence of their families whilst girls were more active and independent in seeking out extremist material, which goes against the 'vulnerable bride' narrative. A report from the Henry Jackson Society (2019) think tank agrees, saying that the 'vulnerable bride' narrative, where women are seen as being duped or unduly influenced into joining a terrorist group, does not seem to be the case. This demonstrates the importance of deradicalisation and safeguarding programmes being tailored to gender-specific needs. Similar statistics from the Home Office Key results in the year ending 31 March 2019 (Home Office, 2019) also show a bias towards increased numbers of male participation in extremism.

RECOGNISING RADICALISATION – HOW MIGHT IT HAPPEN?

The NSPCC, 2021 state the process of radicalisation may involve a number of means including:

■ being groomed online or in person,

■ exploitation,

■ psychological manipulation, sometimes referred to as an emotional hook,

■ exposure to violent material and other inappropriate information, (e.g. memes), and

■ the risk of physical harm or death through extremist acts.

Online Grooming and Recruitment

Exit Hate state that while social media platforms can be a useful tool and enjoyed by children and young people, there are powerful programmes and networks in existence that use social media channels to reach out to young people to communicate extremist messages. There are examples of far-right extremists using social media to mobilise young people, organising real-life meetings and demonstrations. Social media is fast becoming the key to the communication infrastructure, operating and recruiting practices of these groups.

Exit Hate give an example: far-right activists understand they can have a greater influence online, and they achieve this by creating multiple fake profiles to recruit a range of different people. Experts in this, they seek to develop and grow their supporter base, encouraging people to get involved, do something, recruit others and, in some cases, take direct action. Because they are trained to groom and can recognise vulnerability in young people and children, recruiters will use any tactic and every opportunity they can. Once they feel connected to the child or young person, things can change swiftly as they are encouraged to troll people, research or create online memes and promote certain items or events.

Exit Hate warn that, although in the past the Facebook and Twitter pages of these groups were easy to identify, this is less possible nowadays because they masquerade as political debating groups where they can recruit new members. Some examples of this include:

- the great British political debate,
- British politics uncut, and
- the real political debate.

As the founder member of Small Steps and Exit Hate, the former extreme right wing activist Nigel Bromage describes that by using chat rooms, forums and gaming platforms, far-right activists can recruit faster by

CASE STUDY 10D.1: JAMES' STORY

James was 15 when his best friend of many years, Mark, showed him a picture on his phone of a soldier who was homeless. The message attached said 'is this right?' The next message stated that Muslims are given priority for housing over British soldiers. James said he just thought this was wrong but could see his friend was very angry. Initially, James felt he was more of a support to his friend, but he became more involved when they were both offered a free lift to a demonstration in London. James thought this was a good offer – he had nothing else to do, it was a free trip and he had never been to London.

James started to research more about this subject online and soon found himself a member of the English Defence League (EDL). (The EDL was a far-right Islamophobic organisation in the United Kingdom. It was a social movement and pressure group that employed street demonstrations as its main tactic.) Once James became a member of the EDL, both he and Mark started to talk openly about their opinions in school. James reflects that up until this point he had always been the class clown and not a trouble-maker. He admits to being openly racist to a teacher and being suspended but nothing else happening. James said at this point he and Mark went their separate ways. He describes that Mark took a path that focussed on white supremacy, wearing white laces in his boots to indicate this, while James, as part of the EDL, used his focus on football to further his support.

James watched hours of far-right propaganda online and took his beliefs to college but still found he was not getting into serious trouble. He describes the Manchester bombing as a turning point for him when, in May 2017, an Islamist extremist suicide bomber detonated a shrapnel-laden homemade bomb as people were leaving the Manchester Arena following a concert. James said he became really angry and stated to promote his opinions more widely, actively promoting the EDL, using college projects to promote hate speech, and finally declaring his true allegiance in a session in college about British values.

At this point James and his mum were asked to come into college and James agreed to be referred to Prevent. He said that having a mentor who understood really helped him to think about alternatives. James said that it took a while for him to turn his back on the far right because he felt he had a role there and a cause; he felt he was not very academic and had been told he would never amount to much. The far right was a way for him to control what was happening but he had also been promised a job within the organisation. James felt loyal to the far right, and he had even been schooled by them in terms of what to say should he be referred to Prevent. He remained interested in the far right for many years before he finally left by ceasing all online contact. It was mentoring that had opened up a different narrative for James and which allowed him to develop different views.

James' family recalled how distressed they were by James' behaviour, but they could not pinpoint what the problem was until a family member witnessed James at a demonstration chanting racist slurs. The family still did not know what to do or who to turn to and are thankful that this was eventually noticed at college.

This example highlights how unchallenged James was and how active he became before he was offered assistance.

Exit Hate outlines how not everyone recruited will be part of a group; some children or young adults will get involved with online activism only, but this will still potentially expose them to threats, making leaving very complex and difficult.

You can view further stories here at https://smallstepsconsultants.com/.

testing out the interest of the young person. The use of social media has also allowed fake news to spread as a way to sensationalise certain news topics, distort the facts and encourage engagement and interest. Children and young people may not be experienced enough to recognise this, even more so when there may be a small element of fact or truth, albeit distorted, within the news story. Exit Hate use their experience as former members of the far right to encourage discussion and are committed to providing first-hand, non-judgemental support and advice, advocating that hate and violence is not the answer.

Case study 10d.1 provides an overview of how James became involved in the far right and how he exited it through the help and support of a Prevent intervention provider (IP). James tells his experience through training to raise awareness.

GOVERNMENT RESPONSES TO RADICALISATION – THE PREVENT STRATEGY

The Prevent programme is part of the Government's counter-terrorism strategy, CONTEST. Its aim is to prevent people from becoming terrorists or supporting terrorism. It is designed to ensure that individuals who are identified as being at risk of being drawn into terrorism are given appropriate advice and support so that they may turn away from radicalisation.

Radicalisation of children and young people is an area of growing concern within the UK. The CTSA (2015) gave local authorities a statutory duty to have 'due regard to the need to prevent people from being drawn into terrorism'. Protecting children from the risk of radicalisation should be seen as part of wider safeguarding duties and responsibilities as described in Working Together to Safeguard Children (2022).

The government's Prevent Duty as written in the CTSA (2015) defines radicalisation as 'the process by which a person comes to support terrorism and extremist ideologies associated with terrorist groups'. The Prevent Duty means that some organisations in England, Scotland and Wales have a duty, as a specified authority under section 26 of the Act, to identify vulnerable children and young people and prevent them from being drawn into terrorism.

These organisations include:

- schools,
- registered childcare providers,
- local authorities,
- the police,
- prisons and probation services, and
- NHS trusts and foundations.

Extremism is defined as a vocal or active opposition to fundamental British values, including democracy, the rule of law, individual liberty and mutual respect and tolerance of different faiths and beliefs. It includes calls for the death of members of the British armed forces (HM Government, 2011). The Department of Education's Prevent Duty: Departmental advice for schools and childcare providers document (Department of Education, 2015) highlights an opportunity to build pupils' resilience to radicalisation by promoting fundamental British values and enabling them to challenge extremist views. It is important to emphasise that the Prevent duty is not intended to stop pupils debating controversial issues. Schools should provide a safe space in which children, young people and staff can understand the risks associated with terrorism and develop the knowledge and skills to be able to challenge extremist arguments.

CLOSER LOOK: BRITISH VALUES

The experience that James shared demonstrates how he quickly moved from listening to his friend and joining his friend on a free trip to actively seeking out information himself. It was a session on British values at college that finally resulted in a referral to Prevent for him. As a result of the discussion on British values, James' feelings were disclosed, highlighting the importance of such discussions.

An Exercise on British Values

As a practitioner think how you could introduce the four British values into a conversation. Each value is presented here with a short explanation for you to expand on. For each value consider the skills that would be helpful for a child/young person to develop and to carry through into adult life.

Democracy:

- where everyone is treated equally and has equal rights.

The Rule of Law:

- understanding that rules matter and that we need to manage our feelings.

Individual Liberty:

- reflect on their differences and understand that we are all free to have different opinions.

Mutual Respect and Tolerance:

- where we learn to treat others as we want to be treated, and
- where we learn how to be part of a community, manage our feelings and behaviour, and form relationships with others.

Both the Prevent Duty (CTSA, 2015) and statutory guidance from the Department for Education for schools and colleges (Department of Education, 2019) recognises radicalisation as a safeguarding issue. These documents should be read in conjunction with Working Together to Safeguard Children (2022) which describes preventative work and the importance of working collaboratively. Specifically, the police, clinical commissioning groups and the local authority are under a duty to make arrangements to work together, and with other partners locally, to help identify and support vulnerable children, young people and families where radicalisation is a potential risk factor.

The Prevent strategy addresses all forms of terrorism, which is prioritised according to the threat posed to national security; the most significant of these threats is currently from terrorist organisations in Syria and Iraq, and Al Qa'ida associated groups. Terrorists associated with the extreme right also pose a continued threat to our safety and security (HM Government, 2015).

The Prevent Strategy, published by the Government in July 2011 (HM Government, 2011a), forms part of the Government's wider counter-terrorism strategy, known as CONTEST. The CONTEST framework comprises Prevent, Pursue, Protect and Prepare. The aim of CONTEST is to reduce the risk to the UK and its interests overseas from terrorism, so that people can go about their lives freely and with confidence (HM Government, 2011b). The strategy recognises the importance of Prevent, Pursue, Protect and Prepare as the key objectives. Coordination between CONTEST and other Government programmes is essential and working closely with other countries a priority in reducing risks. CONTEST reflects our values and human rights, taking proportionate responses to risk.

Prevent aims to safeguard people from becoming terrorists or supporting terrorism. It addresses all forms of terrorism and has three specific strategic objectives:

- respond to the ideological challenge of terrorism and the associated threat faced from those who promote it;
- prevent people from being drawn into terrorism and ensure that they are given appropriate advice and support; and
- work with sectors and institutions where there are risks of radicalisation that we need to address.

The Channel Programme

The Channel programme in England and Wales is an initiative that provides a multiagency approach to support people vulnerable to the risk of radicalisation. Channel forms a key part of the Prevent strategy. The CTSA (2015) placed the Channel programme on a statutory footing and created a duty on each local authority in England and Wales to ensure that there is a panel in place for its area. Statutory guidance for Channel panels was published in March 2015.

Where the police assess there to be a risk of radicalisation, the young person is referred to a Channel panel, where the referral will be discussed. The Channel panel is chaired by the local authority and can include a variety of statutory partners such as the police, children's services, social services, education professionals and mental health care professionals and the Prevent coordinator

The Channel approach protects young people vulnerable to radicalisation by:

- identifying individuals at risk;
- assessing the nature and extent of that risk, e.g. is there engagement with a cause, group or ideology, is there intent to cause harm, is there capability to cause harm?; and

■ developing the most appropriate support plan for the individuals concerned.

Having identified an individual at risk, the Channel panel will assess the nature and extent of the risk, and subsequently develop the most appropriate support plan for the individual concerned.

Currently, only the police can refer an individual identified under Prevent to a Channel panel. New guidance issued in September 2020 (Gov.UK, 2020) would allow local authorities, in addition to the police, to refer an individual to a panel, streamlining the process and removing potential delays.

The way in which Channel is delivered may overlap with the implementation of the wider safeguarding duties of Children's Services. It becomes important therefore that individuals are aware of their roles and responsibilities.

Support Offered Through the Channel Programme

Participation in the Channel programme is confidential, and consent must be obtained from the individual or parent, where this relates to a child, before Channel support is provided. Many types of support are available including addressing educational needs, career advice, vocational, mental health or emotional health issues, substance misuse and other vulnerabilities. Ideological mentoring is common as part of the rehabilitation. If a young person refuses to take part in Prevent via the Channel programme, then there would be continuing engagement with the individual concerned to seek alternative support measures. Exit Hate are an example of this, as James' case study demonstrates. Initially, James agreed to attend sessions with his Prevent mentor believing they would not help him and having already been schooled by the far right in what to say. He saw it as a way to deceive the system. However, James eventually began to adopt a different viewpoint through the support he received from the mentor.

Although anyone can make a referral to Prevent, one of the main challenges is identifying children who may be vulnerable to radicalisation.

The sensitivities involved in determining an appropriate response to radicalisation can make this an uneasy area of practice for some staff. New guidance is called for by Malik (2019) in her report Radicalising our Children:

> to make clear that parents who may be radicalising their children, or who may wish to take them abroad and put them in danger, could also appear to be traditionally good parents and have loving relationships with their children, in a way that other abusive parents do not. A close relationship between the child and parent should not be given undue weighting in deciding whether a child should be made a ward of court or taken into care for safeguarding and protection purposes.

In particular, research also showed widely varying views about the extent to which radicalisation represents a safeguarding or child protection risk (Chisholm, Coulter, Public 2017).

Numbers of Referrals to Prevent

Key results in the year ending 31 March 2019 from experimental statistics from the Home Office show that a total of 5738 individuals were referred to Prevent.

Education

The Education sector made the highest number of referrals (1887; 33%) with most referrals being for males (4991; 87%), which is a continued trend. The majority of referrals were for people aged 20 years or under (3343; 58%) with the mean age of 14 years from the education sector.

Referrals

Of the 561 Channel cases, referrals were most commonly made because of concerns about right-wing radicalisation (254; 45%), followed by Islamist radicalisation (210; 37%). The number of referrals adopted as Channel cases for concerns related to right-wing radicalisation has increased by 50% from the year ending March 2018 to the current year, continuing the upward trend since the 2015 to 2016 financial year. In the same period, the number adopted as Channel cases for concerns related to Islamist radicalisation has increased by 24%.

Types of Radicalisation

- Of the referrals for concerns related to *Islamist radicalisation*, individuals under the age of 15 accounted for the largest proportion referred (402 of 1404; 29%), discussed (166 of 536; 31%) and adopted as a Channel case (69 of 210; 33%).
- For concerns related to *right-wing radicalisation*, individuals aged 15 to 20 accounted for the largest proportion referred (472 of 1389; 34%), discussed (206 of 542; 38%) and adopted as a Channel case (110 of 254; 43%).
- Some individuals are referred with a *mixed, unstable or unclear ideology*, those aged 15 to 20 accounted for the largest proportion referred (695 of 2169; 32%). For all types of radicalisation, the proportion of males referred, discussed at a Channel panel and adopted as a Channel case was higher than females.

Channel Panel Discussions

The number of individuals discussed at a Channel panel (1320) and adopted as a Channel case (561) were the highest recorded compared with previous years, although the previous years had shown a steady increase.

PRACTITIONERS' RESPONSES

A research report on safeguarding and radicalisation commissioned by the Department of Education (Chisholm, Coulter and Public, 2017) demonstrated some themes which impact on practitioner's responses. In particular, there were varying views about the extent to which radicalisation represents a safeguarding or child protection risk. These included staff having an increased confidence in responding to radicalisation in local authorities where safeguarding and child protection teams had made clear decisions about who should take ownership of these cases, and where guidance around assessment and handling of radicalisation cases had been developed and staff had been trained.

The report goes on to discuss three emerging responses from local authorities which impacts on practitioner response:

- Local authorities located in high priority Prevent areas had a strong internal agreement that radicalisation was either a safeguarding or child protection risk to children. There was ownership through early help or statutory social care.
- Local authorities outside of Prevent priority areas, and therefore having fewer cases of radicalisation, had internal agreements that related to universal services, ranging from education to the police.
- Local authorities responded on a reactive or 'needs-driven' basis, largely due to the lack of clarity on risk and lack of understanding of terminology associated with radicalisation.

The report highlights the need for sharing of practice between authorities so staff with less experience in this area can learn from those with more experience. In addition to this, supervision and reflective practice are important for practitioners to explore evidence-based practice and to reflect on their own emotional needs for support (Maclean et al., 2018).

Challenges in Practice

Our learning so far from research and practice highlights the following points:

- Proscribed groups continue to operate under many different aliases, resulting in a continued presence and influence.
- Home schooling, although working for many, can be a way of passing on extremist values.
- There is a need to think about assistance for vulnerable children as they progress into adulthood.
- Practitioners should be working within families on radicalisation issues, while retaining neutrality.
- Focus should be on identifying preventative measures before a child's vulnerabilities can be identified by those who may recruit them and take advantage.
- Preventing terrorism means challenging extremist (and nonviolent) ideas that are also part of a terrorist ideology; the skills to do this require confidence and knowledge not only about the subject matter, but also about safeguarding processes.
- The harm of continuing to expose the child to extremism must be weighed against the harm of separating them from their parents.
- Where the parents are convinced of an extremist ideology or are looking to pledge their allegiance to a group, they are likely to see including their children in a lifestyle that fits an extremist philosophy as good parenting (Malik, 2019).

- When courts act, they must settle upon a course of action which not only protects the child from harm, but also protects them from becoming a person who does harm to themselves or others in the future (Malik, 2019).

The Practitioners Role and Prevention

Practitioners should:

- Help build resilience to radicalisation by promoting British values and enabling children to explore and challenge extremist views.
- Provide a safe space for children and young people to debate and learn about the risks associated with terrorism and develop the knowledge and skills to be able to challenge extremist argument.
- Encourage critical thinking about the news and anything that is seen while using social media.
- Promote safe use of social media. Even if parents are moderating this, there is still a chance the child will come across content you would not want them to see, including religious and extremist propaganda.
- Encourage parental controls and adherence to age limits on Facebook, WhatsApp, YouTube.
- Raise awareness regarding protecting identity online and appropriate sharing of information.
- Raise awareness of the risks associated with using live streaming apps as users can be viewed and contacted by others, including people they do not know.
- Work towards effective engagement with parents/the family as they are in a key position to spot signs of radicalisation.
- Attend Prevent awareness training to equip staff to identify children at risk of being drawn into terrorism and to challenge extremist ideas.

CLOSER LOOK: CREATING POSITIVE CHANGE – IT CAN BE DONE: SMALL STEPS AND EXIT HATE

Small Steps founded Exit Hate to work with children, young adults and adults to help provide a counter narrative. As former members of the Far Right, they know what it is like to feel disillusioned and work to provide first-hand, non-judgemental support and advice to people who have been radicalised. They work from the premise that changing people's minds can be difficult but can be done using a simple process. Initially, the individual must be engaged in a place where they feel comfortable and sessions with young people should be short (no more than an hour). The following section describes the process followed.

The first phase involves getting the young person to relax and talk. Once they are settled, the young person is asked what they think is wrong with the world. Here the aim is twofold: firstly, to find out what they think and secondly to establish if they indicate they are politically active or are being groomed. Without this information, counter narratives to reduce their support for far-right ideology cannot be provided.

Seeking to minimise confrontation and listen to people's concerns, Exit Hate advocates the only way forward is open and honest dialogue. This acceptance approach is based on developing trust-based relationship and can also work to build up relationships with families. Exit Hate was set up by Small Steps to receive self-referrals from people who will not engage with Prevent; it provides a safety valve for people who would otherwise have no-one to talk to. Individuals may choose not to engage with the Prevent agenda because they do not trust this as it feels 'official'.

As described in the real-life story of James, James was schooled by the far right to provide the correct answers to the Prevent mentor. Exit Hate has a unique advantage as former members with experience of leaving this behind, which appears to gain further traction with those who make contact.

The Exit Hate website invites people who may be questioning the far right to talk further with them so they may enter into discussion with mentors at Exit Hate without going via Prevent (if they do not want to) because the main objective is to get people help. Exit groups also exist in Germany, the US, Sweden and Australia, with others forming. Exit combines both deradicalisation and disengagement using the Prevent delivery model (Fig. 10d.1).

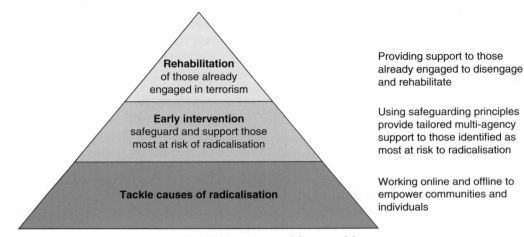

Rehabilitation
of those already
engaged in terrorism

Providing support to those
already engaged to disengage
and rehabilitate

Early intervention
safeguard and support those
most at risk of radicalisation

Using safeguarding principles
provide tailored multi-agency
support to those identified as
most at risk to radicalisation

Tackle causes of radicalisation

Working online and offline to
empower communities and
individuals

Fig. 10d.1 ■ Prevent delivery model.

CONCLUSION

This chapter highlights the process of radicalisation and how this can differ from child to child. Radicalisation is different from other forms of child abuse and harm where actions or harm can perhaps be more clearly defined. Radicalisation has been likened to causing 'moral harm' by Malik (2019) and is increasingly difficult to identify and prove. Practitioners need to be trained and supported by robust procedures to be able to identify and challenge radicalisation and to debate practice issues.

The identification of signs of radicalisation needs to start as early as possible with trained individuals in schools. The quicker the signs are recognised, the easier it is to show young people the reality of life in forms of extremism and how getting involved is harmful and damages the futures both of people who join and those around them. Reducing radicalisation needs long term nationwide investment, with people trained at grassroots level who can respond. Trained to have no outward signs, extremist groups operate like an iceberg, hiding most of their activities and making identification even harder.

KEY POINTS

- Be alert to indicators and have the capacity to challenge and confront radicalisation.
- Local authorities are vital to all aspects of Prevent work. Ensure you are trained to understand the Prevent delivery model.

- Recognise those children and young people who may have existing predisposing indicators and work preventatively.
- Work with children to recognise and manage risk, make safer choices, and recognise when pressure from others threatens their personal safety and well-being.
- Work within existing safeguarding procedures.
- Encourage dialogue with colleagues to raise competence and confidence.
- Understand that success relies on two main areas, co-operation and coordinated activity of partners, and engagement of the child and their families.
- Recognise when the family will not be the connecting factor and use other network connections to reach the individual at risk, e.g. many children attend a range of out of school settings other than childcare which are not regulated. Local authorities should take steps to understand the range of activity and settings in their areas and take appropriate and proportionate steps to ensure that children attending such settings are properly safeguarded.
- Remember that family involvement in extremism can be wider than immediate family.
- Young children can be exposed to violent and terrorist imagery fromw an early age. There is a misconception that very young children would not be radicalised, and there is growing evidence to the contrary (Malik, 2019).

FURTHER READING

https://exithate.org/index.html.

https://smallstepsconsultants.com/the-far-right-threat/spotting-far-right-codes/.

https://educateagainsthate.com/signs-of-radicalisation/.

www.nspcc.org.uk.

https://ParentZone.org.uk.

https://www.childline.org.uk/info-advice/bullying-abuse-safety/online-mobile-safety/staying-safe-online/.

Morrow, E.A., Meadowcroft, J., 2019. The rise and fall of the English defence league: Self-governance, marginal members and the far right. Political Studies 67 (3), 539–556.

REFERENCES

Channel Duty Guidance 2015-Protecting vulnerable people from being drawn into terrorism Statutory guidance for Channel panel members and partners of local panels

Chrisholm, T., Coulter, A., Public, K., 2017. Research Report. Safeguarding and Radicalisation. Department of Education, London.

Department for Education, 2022. Working Together to Safeguard Children. Statutory Guidance on Inter-agency Working to Safeguard and Promote the Welfare of Children.

Department of Education, 2015. The Prevent Duty: Departmental Advice for Schools and Childcare Providers. Department of Education, London. https://assets.publishing.service.gov.uk/government/uploads/system/uploads/attachment_data/file/439598/prevent-duty-departmental-advice-v6.pdf.

Department of Education, 2023. Keeping Children Safe in Education. Statutory Guidance for Schools and Colleges on Safeguarding Children and Safer Recruitment https://www.gov.uk/government/publications/keeping-children-safe-in-education--2.

Educate Against Hate, https://educateagainsthate.com/signs-of-radicalisation/.

Exit Hate, http://exithate.org/index.html.

Gov.UK, 2020. Prevent and Channel Panel Factsheet. https://www.gov.uk/government/publications/counter-terrorism-and-border-security-bill-2018-factsheets/prevent-and-channel-panel-factsheet-accessible-version#what-are-we-going-to-do

Henry Jackson Society (HJS), 2019. https://henryjacksonsociety.org/publications/radicalising-our-children-an-analysis-of-family-court-cases-of-british-children-at-risk-of-radicalisation-2013-2018/

HM Government, 2011. Prevent Strategy. https://www.gov.uk/government/publications/prevent-strategy-2011

HM Government, 2015. Counter Terrorism and Security ACT. https://www.gov.uk/government/publications/counter-terrorism-strategy-contest-2018

HM Government, 2018. Counter-terrorism strategy (CONTEST) https://www.gov.uk/government/publications/counter-terrorism-strategy-contest-2018

Home Office Key Results Individuals referred to and supported through the Prevent programme, England and Wales, April 2018 to March 2019. https://assets.publishing.service.gov.uk/government/uploads/system/uploads/attachment_data/file/853646/individuals-referred-supported-prevent-programme-apr2018-mar2019-hosb3219.pdf

Individuals referred to and supported through the Prevent programme, England and Wales, April 2018 to March 2019 Home Office https://www.gov.uk/government/publications/counter-terrorism-and-border-security-bill-2018-factsheets/prevent-and-channel-panel-factsheet-accessible-version.

Maclean, et al., 2018. Share: A new Model for Social Work. Kirwin Maclean Associates Ltd.

Malik, N., 2019. Radicalising Our Children: an Analysis of Family Court Cases of British Children at Risk of Radicalisation. 2013–2018. Henry Jackson Society, London.

NSPCC, 2021. Recognising and responding to radicalisation. https://learning.nspcc.org.uk/safeguarding-child-protection/radicalisation.

Royal College of Psychiatrists. Technology Use and the Mental Health of Children and Young People January 2020 https://www.rcpsych.ac.uk/improving-care/campaigning-for-better-mental-health-policy/college-reports/2020-college-reports/Technology-use-and-the-mental-health-of-children-and-young-people-cr225.

Small Steps, https://smallstepsconsultants.com/the-far-right-threat/spotting-far-right-codes/.

The Terrorism Act, 2006. https://www.legislation.gov.uk/ukpga/2006/11/contents

FORCED MARRIAGE OF CHILDREN AND YOUNG PEOPLE

RACHAEL CLAWSON

KEY POINTS

- Child marriage and forced marriage happens across the world, including in the UK.
- Girls are most frequently affected, but boys can also become victims.
- Forcing someone to marry is a criminal offence in the UK, punishable by up to 7 years in prison and an unlimited fine.
- Children and young people at risk of forced marriage can be subjected to a range of sexual, emotional and physical abuse both from those forcing them to marry and/or from their spouse.

INTRODUCTION

Forcing someone to marry became a criminal offence in the UK with the implementation of the Anti-social Behaviour, Crime and Policing Act in June 2014. Forced marriage is a child protection issue. It carries risks of sexual, emotional and physical harm as well as potentially impacting upon education and economic independence in adulthood; it is also an abuse of human rights (Clawson and Fyson, 2017). Marriage of children is a complex issue and is tied up in notions of family or community control, gender inequality, patriarchy and perceived traditions. Any discussion of forced marriage needs to be placed within the global context of child marriage, as this helps us to understand why it happens in the UK and helps identify who might be most at risk.

Forced marriage is different to arranged marriage. In arranged marriages, the family of both spouses take a leading role in arranging the marriage, but the decision to accept the arrangement or not remains with the prospective spouses. It is important to remember that in the UK children under 16 cannot consent to marriage because under the Mental Capacity Act 2005 they do not yet have legal capacity. In forced marriage one or both spouses do not, or cannot, consent to the marriage. The giving of consent, however, can be viewed as being on a continuum. Some young people, including those under 18 years, may agree to marry because they believe they have no other option. For some children the consequences of refusing to marry can be life-changing: they may be ostracised by family and community, they might be kidnapped, drugged, poisoned, physically or sexually harmed or even killed. This is sometimes referred to as 'honour-based' violence. These very real consequences need to be held in mind by practitioners whose duty it is to safeguard children and young people.

This chapter will begin by exploring child marriage from a global perspective and will outline the key drivers for the practice. It will then move on to examine the UK context and will include an explanation of the government definition of forced marriage. The chapter will explore who might be most at risk and the harmful impact on health and well-being before moving on to consider the challenges presented to safeguarding practitioners both in recognising the problem and responding to it in an appropriate, safe and sensitive way.

CHILD MARRIAGE AND FORCED MARRIAGE: SOME GLOBAL CONTEXT

Child marriage is defined by UNICEF as 'any formal marriage or informal union between a child under the age of 18 and an adult or another child' (www.unicef.org); forced marriage is defined by the UK Government Forced Marriage Unit as 'where one or both people do not, or cannot, consent to the marriage and duress or abuse is used'. Every year across the world approximately 12 million girls, or 1 in 5, are married before their 18th birthday. That equates to 23 girls every minute or nearly 1 every 2 seconds. Over 650 million women alive today were married as children (www.girlsnotbrides.org). Although girls are most at risk, boys are affected too; the number of boys affected is thought to be around one-sixth that of girls. Globally, approximately 150 million men alive today were married before the age of 18 (www.unicef.org).

Child marriage is a global practice. In some communities, parents believe marriage is the best option for girls, both financially and to protect them from risk of sexual harm. Without marriage, in some countries girls might not survive. Organisations such as UNICEF, Plan and Girls Not Brides are working to empower girls, mobilise communities and families and provide resources to end the practice (there are links to these organisations at the end of the chapter). Marrying early carries a range of consequences, girls (and boys) may be isolated from family and friends and deprived of education, which is their only route to economic security/independence, and health and safety. Many girls who marry young are married to much older men and become victims of domestic abuse. They are physically and emotionally unprepared for marriage and pregnancy carries enormous health risks for both the mother and her baby. There are also great risks associated with refusing to marry as will be discussed later.

Most countries have set the minimum legal age of marriage at 18 years old, but child marriage still happens in countries across the world, including in parts of the UK. Some children who are UK citizens may also marry abroad, and children who are already married may move to live in the UK from other countries.

Across the world forced marriage and child marriage can affect girls and boys of any age, regardless of intellectual or physical disability, ethnic origin, sexual orientation or other characteristic. Data collected by UNICEF shows that girls living in the least developed countries in the world are most at risk with countries in Africa, Latin America and South Asia having the highest rates of child marriage (UNICEF, 2020). Of course, children from all these countries also live within communities in the UK.

Not all child marriages are unlawful, and not all take place in the least developed countries. Notably, child marriage is still lawful in some parts of the UK. In England and Wales, the legal age of marriage was changed in 2022, with the passing into law of the Marriage and Civil Partnership (Minimum Age) Act. This means that child marriage is now unlawful in England and Wales. However, marriage of children aged 16 or 17 remains lawful in Scotland and Northern Ireland. In Northern Ireland, children aged 16 or 17 can marry with the consent of their parents; in Scotland children can freely marry from the age of 16. In some states of the USA, girls as young as 12 or 13 years old can marry in certain circumstances, (e.g. if a girl is pregnant and it is agreed by her parents and the court that she should marry). Unchained at Last, (an organisation affiliated to Girls Not Brides a global partnership of more than 1400 civil society organisations committed to ending child marriage) campaigns against child marriage and has found that these marriages are mostly between girls and adult men, and in some cases the spousal age difference would constitute statutory rape under sexual offences legislation. Many states are now moving to change laws to prevent child marriage from happening. You can find out more information about this at www.unchainedatlast.org.

Countries including Scotland, Northern Ireland and parts of the USA therefore currently sanction marriage below the age at which UNICEF recommends it should take place. Although the majority of those marrying in the UK aged 16 or 17 marry people of the same age or less than 4 years older, in some cases girls are marrying men 20 or more years older than themselves (www.ons.gov.uk). Across all countries of the UK, children under the age of 16 years cannot legally marry, but may nevertheless be forced to marry in religious or cultural ceremonies.

CLOSER LOOK: REASONS FOR CHILD MARRIAGES

The global partnership organisation *Girls Not Brides* outlines the reasons why child marriage happens across the world. They highlight four key driving factors:

1. **Gender inequality.** In many communities where child marriage happens girls are not valued as highly as boys and are seen as an economic burden. They also live within communities driven by patriarchal values which seek to control female sexuality, how girls dress and behave, who they should see, be friends with or marry, etc. In some communities marrying girls early means they are less likely to become pregnant outside of marriage (and therefore less likely to bring shame on the family).
2. **Tradition.** In some communities child marriage happens because it has been this way for generations. Girls are seen as 'of age' when they start menstruation, and marriage is the next step.
3. **Poverty.** More than half the girls from the poorest families in the developing world are married as children. Family members (and sometimes the girls themselves) see marriage as means of addressing poverty. It means one less person to clothe and feed. It also means one less person to educate and enables families to invest in a son's education instead. Sometimes marriage is used as a way to pay off a debt or settle disputes. In communities where a dowry or 'bride price' is paid, marriage of daughters can provide much-needed income for poor families.
4. **Insecurity.** Sometimes parents marry their daughters young because it is thought to be in her best interest. In some communities girls are at high risk of physical and sexual assault – being married is seen as a protective factor. Child marriage can also increase in times of humanitarian crises, such as conflict or natural disaster. Nine out of the ten countries with the highest child marriage rates are considered fragile states (www.girlsnotbrides.org/why-does-it-happen).

REFLECTIVE QUESTIONS

- What are your thoughts about the key drivers highlighted?
- How do they relate to your understanding of forced marriage of children and young people within the UK context?

WHAT ARE THE DRIVERS FOR FORCED MARRIAGE OF CHILDREN IN THE UK AND WHO IS MOST AT RISK?

The reasons why young people in the UK are forced to marry can include: family trying to control behaviour (who a person has a relationship with, how they dress, look and behave, where they go, their sexuality, etc.); perceived tradition relating to age and marriage; protecting family honour (associated with stigma of behaving or looking a certain way); arrangements regarding wealth or property; and long-held family promises.

CLOSER LOOK: REMEMBERING SHAFILEA KHAN

Shafilea Khan, known as Shaf to her friends, was a 17-year-old British Pakistani girl from Warrington, Cheshire. She was in 6th form studying for her A levels and hoped to become a solicitor.

Shafilea was murdered by her parents in front of her siblings (the youngest aged just 7 at the time) at home in September 2003. Her dismembered body was found by the river Kent in Cumbria after a flood in February 2004. In August 2012 both parents were found guilty of her murder and sentenced to 25 years in prison. Her parents were charged after Shafilea's sister staged an armed burglary at the family home in 2010; when interviewed by the police she told them her parents had killed Shafilea in front of her. She said that her parents were trying to force Shafilea into an 'arranged' marriage with an older cousin, and when she refused, her father suffocated her by putting a plastic bag in her mouth. Shafilea was considered 'damaged goods' by her parents; she was murdered for refusing to be married and, in her parents' view, for being too 'westernised'.

Shafilea had been a victim of violence from both parents and had run away from home a number of times, the first time when she was 11 years old. School staff had been concerned about her welfare (she often had bruises) and made a referral to social services who visited her at school. Shafilea played down problems at home, and her case was closed. Six months before her murder she was admitted to hospital in Pakistan after drinking bleach in an attempt to escape her parents. Her father told medical staff it had happened because she mistook the bleach for mouthwash. Shafilea had also written poems outlining her sheer despair at the situation. She had been absent from 6th form for a week before being reported missing to the police by teachers who overheard her siblings talking – they had been told by their parents to say she was missing if asked.

Shafilea's parents were ultra-conservative and did not agree with the way she was choosing to live her life. She was murdered as they believed she had bought shame on the family. The coroner described her as being the subject of 'a very vile murder' and said she had been denied the very basic human right of living her life her own way.

REFLECTIVE QUESTIONS

- What could have been done, and by whom, to better protect Shafilea and her siblings?
- What action would you take now if you were presented with a young person in a similar situation?

Exact figures for forced marriages in the UK are not known – there is a lack of reliable data which makes the full scale of the issue impossible to know (Phillips and Dustin, 2004). In addition, because forced marriage is largely a hidden crime, reported cases are likely to only represent the tip of the iceberg. The UK Government Forced Marriage Unit (FMU) – a unit set up jointly by the Home Office and Foreign and Commonwealth Office in 2005 to tackle the issue – is the only organisation collating and publishing statistics on an annual basis. The FMU data is useful in providing an overview about forced marriage of UK citizens in relation to age and gender of those forced to marry, where they live in the UK and where the marriages took place (i.e. whether the marriage took place in the UK or in another country – the FMU call this the 'focus country').

Since it was established in 2005, the FMU has dealt with cases of forced marriage involving over 90 different focus countries. However, the majority of cases involve young people of Pakistani, Bangladeshi, and Indian origin, and most forced marriages take place overseas. This is partly a reflection of the fact that there is a large, established South Asian population in the UK and partly because of the perceived cultural importance of marriage within some South Asian communities. Forced marriages have also been held in the UK in accordance with the religious laws of Turkish, Middle Eastern and North African cultures, and there is also evidence of forced marriages within Gypsy and Traveller communities. In many cases the perpetrators of the marriage are parents and extended family. Mothers (as seen in the case of Shafilea Khan) as well as fathers and members of the extended family may be involved in forcing a child to marry. It cannot be assumed that any family members will necessarily offer safety and protection to a child at risk.

In 2019 the FMU gave advice and support in 1355 cases of forced marriage, 363 (27%) of these cases involved the forced marriage of children aged 17 years and under, of which 205 were aged under 15 years. Ten cases (8%) of child marriages involved young people with learning disabilities. People with learning disabilities are particularly vulnerable to being forced to marry and have specific needs arising from this, including issues around capacity to consent. It is not possible to adequately cover the issues facing people with learning disabilities in this chapter, but for practice guidance and resources on this aspect of forced marriage see the My 'Marriage My Choice' (Website: http://mymarriagemychoice.co.uk/).

SAFEGUARDING CHILDREN AND YOUNG PEOPLE FROM FORCED MARRIAGE

There are challenges to practitioners in recognising and responding appropriately to forced marriage which must be addressed if children are to be adequately protected. Research shows that there is limited awareness of Government guidelines on forced marriage amongst both statutory and voluntary sector organisations (Clawson, 2016). Sometimes practitioners fail to act on their concerns because they fear being perceived of as racist or culturally insensitive (Clawson et al., 2020; Gangoli et al., 2006). Although guidelines and other supporting materials are available, these are often not incorporated into Local Safeguarding Board and NHS policies and strategic plans, which can lead to inconsistencies in approaches to safeguarding children at risk (Clawson, 2016; Clawson et al., 2020; Wind Cowie et al., 2012).

WARNING SIGNS AND INDICATORS (NOT AN EXHAUSTIVE LIST)

- Absence and persistent absence from school/college/ training or request for extended leave of absence and failure to return from visits to country of origin
- Fear about forthcoming school holidays
- Surveillance by siblings or cousins at school

- Decline in behaviour, engagement, performance or punctuality, poor examination results
- Being withdrawn from school by those with parental responsibility
- Not being allowed to attend extracurricular activities
- Sudden announcement of engagement to a stranger, either to friends or on social media
- Being prevented from going on to further/higher education or employment or having limited choices
- Leaving school/college/work accompanied
- Older siblings forced to marry/early marriage
- Self-harm of self or siblings, suicide of siblings/ substance misuse
- Family disputes/running away from home
- Unreasonable restrictions, e.g. being kept at home by parents/isolation
- Being accompanied to GP surgery, clinics, maternity and/or mental health appointments
- Unwanted or late pregnancy
- Victim or other siblings within the family reported missing
- Reports of domestic abuse, harassment or breaches of the peace at the family home
- Threats to kill and attempts to kill or harm
- Reports of other offences such as rape or kidnap (adapted from HM Govt, 2022)

REFLECTIVE QUESTIONS

- Does your organisation have safeguarding procedures relating to forced marriage?
- What challenges might you or your colleagues have in recognising that a child or young person was at risk of being forced to marry?
- What role might culture or ethnicity play in this if you are working with a child from a different culture or ethnicity to your own?

Forced marriage of children is clearly a child protection issue, and local child safeguarding procedures should be followed when dealing with such cases. However, in addition to knowing about child protection policy and practice, it is crucial that practitioners have a working knowledge of HM Government's (2022) *Multi-agency Statutory Guidance for Dealing with Forced Marriage* and *Multi-agency Practice Guidelines: Handling Cases of Forced Marriage* and understand what their roles and responsibilities are within this. A lack of understanding of the very specific complexities of forced marriage could put victims or potential victims at greater risk of harm. For example, involving families can be dangerous as it may increase the risk of serious harm to the victim. If a child discloses that they are at risk of being forced to marry, practitioners should **never** visit the family to discuss the child's disclosure, as the child may be punished for seeking help. In such cases, families may also bring forward any travel and marriage plans in an attempt to ensure that the marriage takes place before statutory services can intervene to stop it. In any situation involving risk of forced marriage where the victim does not speak English, relatives, friends, community leaders and neighbours should **not** be used as interpreters even if the child thinks this would be acceptable. This is because it cannot be known who can be trusted with such sensitive information. For the same reason, practitioners should also practice safe record keeping and consider who might have access to a child's file. Information should be shared on a strictly 'need to know' basis, and consideration should be given to the 'locking' of electronic files to prevent information being leaked to community or family members.

The FMU provides support to both children and adults at risk of forced marriage, as well as to concerned family or friends and professionals such as police or social workers. It can provide help to any UK national at home or abroad and can arrange repatriation for children and young people who have been removed to another country for the purpose of marriage. A marriage can be deemed forced whether or not it is legally recognised in the UK. So, for example, a religious ceremony taking place in this country or abroad may not be legally recognised but would still count as forced marriage if one or both parties did not freely consent, or did not have capacity to consent, due to age or other factors such as having a learning disability. The Government statutory guidelines and practice guidance for handling cases of forced marriage provides a good overview of all legal measures available to protect a victim. It also provides very clear information on action that should and should not be taken to keep children and young people safe. All practitioners whose role encompasses safeguarding should understand their duties arising from the guidance. One important aspect of the guidance is its emphasis on the 'one chance rule' – that is, that there may only be one chance to intervene to protect a child from forced marriage.

CLOSER LOOK: ONE CHANCE RULE

All practitioners working with children and young people at risk of forced marriage and so-called 'honour-based' abuse need to be aware of the 'one chance rule': in these cases, practitioners may only have one chance or opportunity to speak to the victim (or potential victim) and may therefore only have one chance to take action which could save a life.

All practitioners working within statutory agencies (for example social care, healthcare, education, police, etc.) need to be aware of their responsibilities and duties when presented with a young person at risk of forced marriage. Disclosures of forced marriage should not be dismissed as a 'family matter'. For most young people at risk of forced marriage, seeking help outside the family is a last resort, and all disclosures must therefore be taken seriously. This means that action must be taken to safeguard the child or young person. If the opportunity is allowed to pass without appropriate support being offered and appropriate action being taken, that one chance might be wasted.

This is particularly important in cases where children or young people are taken overseas to be married. Once they leave the UK, the risks to them are greatly increased and it is much more difficult to protect them from being forced to marry.

USING THE LAW TO HELP PREVENT FORCED MARRIAGE

Professionals can use both criminal law and civil law to enable interventions which can prevent forced marriages from taking place. Forcing someone to marry became a criminal offence in England and Wales under the Anti-social Behaviour, Crime and Policing Act 2014. This Act also makes it a criminal offence to use deception with the intention of causing someone to leave the UK (for example, tricking someone into leaving the country by saying that a relative is dying).

The Act stipulates that a person commits an offence if they:

1. Use violence, threats or any other forms of coercion for the purpose of causing another person to enter into marriage, and
2. Believe, or ought to reasonably believe, that the conduct may cause the other person to enter into the marriage without free and full consent

and

In relation to a victim who lacks capacity to consent to marriage, the offence under subsection (1) is capable of being committed by any conduct carried out for the purpose of causing the victim to enter into a marriage (whether or not the conduct amounts to violence, threats or any other form coercion)
Anti-social Behaviour, Crime & Policy Act 2014, s.121

Forced marriage can also be dealt with using civil law. The Forced Marriage (Civil Protection) Act 2007 gives courts across England, Wales and Northern Ireland the power to make forced marriage protection orders (FMPOs). The Forced Marriage (Protection and Jurisdiction) (Scotland) Act 2011 provides this power in Scotland. FMPOs can be used to prevent a forced marriage from taking place, for example, by lodging the individual's passport with the courts to prevent them from being removed from the country. FMPOs can also be used to protect someone who has already been forced to marry and breach of an FMPO is a criminal offence.

CLOSER LOOK: APPLYING FOR A FORCED MARRIAGE PROTECTION ORDER (FMPO)

An FMPO is made by the court and contains conditions that are legally binding. The Anti-social Behaviour, Crime and Policing Act makes breaching an FMPO a criminal offence punishable by up to 5 years in prison.

Applications for an FMPO can be made by the person to be protected by the order (adult or child), a relevant third party (for example, a local authority representative including social workers) or any other person with permission from the court. There is no court fee for making an application to the court and, at the time of writing, legal aid was available for making such applications.

To make an application to the court as a relevant third party, practitioners need to complete a form and provide evidence of the circumstances of the person to be protected and their wishes and feelings (if known). The application process is relatively simple and little evidence (other than information known about the situation) is required. A proforma (which can be obtained from the link below) asks the applicant to provide their own name and that of the person to be protected and then asks for a brief statement outlining the reasons for the application including:

- your connection with the person to be protected;
- what you know of the circumstances of the person to be protected; and
- the wishes and feelings of the person to be protected so far as you know them.

A practitioner should consider applying for an FMPO where they believe a child or adult to be at risk of forced marriage or where a forced marriage has taken place. It is possible to apply for an FMPO without the knowledge or consent of the victim. Further information on applying for an FMPO can be found here: https://www.gov.uk/apply-forced-marriage-protection-order/how-to-apply

CONCLUSION

Forced marriage of children and young people is an abuse of their human rights and is associated with a range of physical, sexual and emotional harms. Although the Government FMU statistics demonstrate that, in the UK, girls from families originating in Pakistan, India and Bangladesh are most at risk of being forced to marry, this can and does happen to children from other cultural backgrounds including children of African heritage and Gypsy and Traveller children. It is also important to note that in Northern Ireland and Scotland children aged 16 and 17 years can lawfully marry and may therefore be at greater risk of being forced to marry. Because of the complex nature of forced marriage, practitioners need to re-think their usual approach to child protection assessments if they are to avoid placing the child at increased risk of harm. Some families will go to great lengths to ensure a marriage takes place and, as a result, protecting children from forced marriage requires careful planning, particularly if there is a risk of the child being removed to another country.

REFLECTIVE QUESTIONS

- What can you do to better inform yourself of the risks of marriage faced by children in your area?
- What can you do within your organisation to ensure statutory guidelines on forced marriage are incorporated into child protection policy?

REFERENCES

Anti-social Behaviour, Crime and Policing Act 2014 (Part 10). https://www.legislation.gov.uk/ukpga/2014/12/part/10/enacted. (Accessed 5 May 2022).

Anti-social Behaviour, Crime & Policy Act, 2014. https://www.legislation.gov.uk/ukpga/2014/12/contents/enacted.

Clawson, R., 2016. Safeguarding people with learning disabilities from forced marriage: The role of Safeguarding Adult Boards. J. Adult Prot. 18 (5), 277–287.

Clawson, R., Fyson, R., 2017. Forced marriage of people with learning disabilities: A human rights issue. Disability & Society 32 (6), 810–830.

Clawson, R., Patterson, A., Fyson, R., McCarthy, M., 2020. The demographics of forced marriage of people with learning disabilities: Findings from a national database. J. Adult Prot. 22 (2), 59–74.

Forced Marriage (Civil Protection) Act 2007. https://www.legislation.gov.uk/ukpga/2007/20/contents. (Accessed 5 May 2022).

Forced Marriage (Protection and Jurisdiction) (Scotland) Act 2011. https://www.legislation.gov.uk/asp/2011/15/contents/enacted. (Accessed 5 May 2022).

Gangoli, G., McCarry, M.J., Razak, A., 2006. Forced Marriage and Domestic Violence Among South Asian Communities in North East England. School for Policy Studies, University of Bristol and Northern Rock Foundation, Bristol, UK.

Girls Not Brides. Why It Happens. www.girlsnotbrides.org/why-does-it-happen. (Accessed 5 May 2022).

HM Government, 2022. The Right to Choose. Multi-agency Statutory Guidance for Dealing With Forced Marriage and Multi-agency Practice Guidelines: Handling Cases of Forced Marriage. https://assets.publishing.service.gov.uk/government/uploads/system/uploads/attachment_data/file/1061641/Forced_marriage_guidance_17.03.22_FINAL.pdf. (Accessed 5 May 2022).

Marriage and Civil Partnership (Minimum Age) Act. https://bills.parliament.uk/bills/2900. (Accessed 5 May 2022).

Mental Capacity Act 2005. https://www.legislation.gov.uk/ukpga/2005/9/contents. (Accessed 5 May 2022).

Phillips, A., Dustin, M., 2004. UK initiatives on forced marriage: Regulation, dialogue and exit. Political studies 52 (3), 531–551.

Unchained At Last. https://www.unchainedatlast.org/. (Accessed 5 May 2022).

UNICEF (2020). Child Marriage. https://www.unicef.org/protection/child-marriage. (Accessed 5 May 2022).

Wind-Cowie, M., Cheetham, P., Gregory, T., 2012. Ending Forced Marriage. Demos, London.

USEFUL WEBSITES

www.girlsnotbrides.org.
https://www.gov.uk/guidance/forced-marriage.
https://karmanirvana.org.uk/.
www.mymarriagemychoice.co.uk.
www.unicef.org.

10f FEMALE GENITAL MUTILATION

LEETHEN BARTHOLOMEW

KEY POINTS

- An overview of female genital mutilation (FGM): what it is, which communities are affected, health complications, who performs it, when and why it is performed.

- FGM and the law – what safeguarding practitioners need to know.

- The factors indicating a girl is at risk of or has undergone FGM and how professionals should respond to concerns.

INTRODUCTION

There is global recognition that female genital mutilation (FGM) is a violation of the human rights of girls and is a harmful practice (OHCHR, 2020; UNICEF, 2016). However, universal acceptance to end it is yet to be attained as girls are still undergoing the practice on every continent except Antarctica (Equality Now, 2019). International movement of populations from FGM affected countries has resulted in women and girls, who have undergone or are at risk of undergoing the practice, living in Europe (European Institute for Gender Equality, 2020; MacFarlane and Dorkenoo, 2015; WHO, 2018). Despite there being only one successful prosecution for FGM in the UK, evidence suggests that girls have undergone the procedure and others are at risk (BBC, 2019; The Guardian, 2018).

This chapter aims to provide professionals with the knowledge and skills to respond appropriately to protect girls where they are at risk of or have undergone FGM. The chapter outlines what FGM is, why it is practiced, possible signs that a girl could be at risk and when it is likely to occur. An overview of the health consequences, both physical and psychological, is provided to illuminate understanding of the extent of the harm girls may experience during their life course and to emphasise the type of support they may require. An outline of the FGM legislation is provided, along with measures available to safeguard girls. To bolster the readers' learning, a case study and key questions to consider are provided. This is followed by further questions aimed at supporting professionals to reflect on their practice.

WHAT IS FEMALE GENITAL MUTILATION?

FGM is an operational term used to refer to a range of practices that involve altering or injury to the external female genitalia for non-therapeutic reasons. More specifically, the World Health Organization (WHO) defines the practice as:

> 'all procedures that involve partial or total removal of the external female genitalia, or other injury to the female genital organs for non-medical reasons.'
> *WHO, UNICEF, UNFPA (1997)*

There are different types of FGM, and the categories have evolved over time (WHO, 2016; 2018). Table 10f.1 outlines the current internationally recognised types of FGM. It is not uncommon for a woman or girl to be unaware of the type of FGM she has suffered or remember the incident.

TABLE 10F.1	
WHO Classification of Female Genital Mutilation (2014)	
Type 1 (clitoridectomy)	Partial or total removal of the clitoris and/or the prepuce
Type II: (excision)	Partial or total removal of the clitoris and the labia minora, with or without excision of the labia majora
Type III: (infibulation)	Narrowing of the vaginal orifice with creation of a covering seal by cutting and appositioning the labia minora and/or the labia majora, with or without excision of the clitoris
Type IV	All other harmful procedures to the female genitalia for non-medical purposes, for example, pricking, piercing, incising, scraping and cauterisation.

WHY IS FMG PRACTICED?

There are a plethora of reasons used for practicing FGM, and these are dependent on the ethnic group and region (WHO, 2018). FGM is seen as a tradition and is practiced as a mark of respect for community elders (WHO, 2018). It is done as a rite of passage from childhood to adulthood, and a girl's entrance into adulthood leads to social acceptance by the community. Therefore, being cut[1] provides a sense of respectability and is intertwined with a sense of identity and personhood (Momoh, 2005).

Understanding the family's motivations for supporting FGM provides insight into which social norms need to be challenged and what educative work is needed to reduce risk.

One of the main reasons for performing it is to control the sexuality of women and girls, as being cut is supposed to 'guarantee' the girl remains a virgin until marriage and is used as a marker to 'confirm' future fidelity. Therefore those undergoing the procedure are seen as the preferred choice for some men, and therefore increases her marriageability

(WHO, 2016). In some communities, a cut girl equates to an announcement of her readiness for marriage (Bjälkander et al., 2013). The completion of the cutting is marked by a community celebration (WHO, 2018).

FGM is also believed to increase a woman's bride wealth, which means her family receives a higher dowry for her hand in marriage compared to a woman who has not undergone the procedure. Those performing the procedure are mainly women who receive an income for their 'duties'. Therefore this commodification of a girl's/woman's body guarantees an income for others and reflects the control and ownership of her body by the prospective husband.

A trenchant analysis of research shows that it is a form of 'honour' based abuse (Gangoli et al., 2018), and there is a correlation between victims/survivors of FGM experiencing other forms of interpersonal violence (Refaat et al., 2001; Salihu et al., 2012). The girl's or woman's experience of FGM is, therefore, one of several forms of violence experienced during her lifetime.

Some groups practice FGM as a form of physical and spiritual cleanliness (WHO, 2018). Physical cleanliness is associated with beliefs that the removal of parts of the external genitalia makes the vagina hygienic, and spiritual purity is linked to beliefs that it is a religious requirement. The practice predates both Christianity and Islam and is not part of the dogma of other religions. There are also links between FGM and beliefs associated with it being done to remove or deliver the family from evil spirits or misfortune (Home Office, 2016).

The practice is also associated with images of femininity and beauty. The clitoris is viewed by some as masculine and if not removed will become penis like, so its removal ensures a woman remains feminine. The removal of the clitoris is also done for aesthetic reasons as its presence makes the vulva appear unsightly. The restriction of the vaginal opening is also believed to heighten sexual pleasure for the male. The presence of the clitoris and beliefs surrounding the threats it poses also extends to the birthing process, as some practicing groups believe death would befall a baby whose head touches the clitoris during childbirth (Roach and Momoh, 2013).

---

[1]The term cut is often used to describe a women/girl who has undergone FGM.

What Are the Signs a Girl Could Be at Risk of FGM?

Between April 2016 and March 2019 children's social care departments in England identified FGM as a reason for completing an assessment in 4040 cases (Department for Education, 2017; 2018; 2019; 2020). Child protection professionals have a responsibility to identify girls at risk and must be aware of the signs. Several factors may indicate a girl may at risk. A family's history (maternal and/or paternal) of practising FGM is considered the most significant risk factor (Home Office, 2016). However, it is important to recognise that whilst some families may have stopped practicing FGM, it is essential to assess the validity of a family's attitudinal change and if it could be sustained over time.

How Do You Assess the Validity of Someone's Claim That They No Longer Support FGM?

In addition to belonging to an FGM-affected community, other potential risk factors may include (a single risk may not indicate there is a risk) (Home Office, 2016):

- a parent disclosing their wish to have their daughter undergo the procedure;
- a girl is born to a woman who has undergone FGM or father comes from an FGM-affected community;
- a girl has a sibling or cousin who has undergone FGM;
- one or both parents or elder family members consider FGM core to their cultural or religious identity;
- a girl from an FGM-affected community is withdrawn from Relationship and Sex Education or its equivalent, may be at risk as a result of her parents wishing to keep her uninformed about her body, FGM and her rights;
- a girl is taken abroad to a country with a high prevalence of FGM;
- a girl may request help from a professional if she is aware or suspects that she is at immediate risk;
- a girl may confide that she is to have a 'special procedure' or to attend a special occasion to 'become a woman'; and

- a woman requesting to be re-infibulated, e.g. following giving birth.

The indicators that a girl has already undergone FGM include (Home Office, 2016):

- a girl discloses to a professional that FGM has taken place (if the professional is a mandated reporter, they must refer this to the police (please see section later on FGM and the law));
- a parent/family member discloses that a female child has had FGM;
- a girl has difficulty walking, sitting or standing or looks uncomfortable;
- a girl has frequent urinary, menstrual or stomach problems;
- prolonged or repeated absences from school or college;
- a girl spends longer than normal in the bathroom or toilet due to difficulties urinating;
- a girl asks for help; and
- increased emotional and psychological needs, e.g. withdrawal or depression, or significant change in behaviour.

WHEN IS FMG PERFORMED?

Evidence on FGM suggests that the age when it occurs depends on the country and ethnic group, as in many countries it is not universally practiced. However, it should be noted that it is an evolving practice, and it can occur between early childhood, adolescence and just before marriage (UNICEF, 2013). Knowing when FGM is most likely to be performed in different affected communities sheds light on the age when a girl is likely to undergo the procedure. However, patterns related to age and when it is performed may change on migration. It is likely that because safeguarding measures are relatively robust in the UK, to evade the authorities, it could be performed at a younger age, as the girl is less likely to remember the incident or make a disclosure. Therefore teachers must be equipped to know how to respond to concerns.

FGM is not necessarily a one-off act that happens in childhood. After giving birth, a women or girl with FGM type III might be re-sutured (Roach and Momoh, 2013). In these cases, professionals should be concerned about a woman and family member's attitude to FGM and the risk to girls in the family.

HOW FMG IS PERFORMED AND HEALTH CONSEQUENCES

There are immediate, short-term and long-term complications associated with FGM. In many FGM-affected communities it is performed by women known as 'cutters', who have no medical training or knowledge of the functions of the different parts of the vulva, using unsanitised equipment, such as knives, razors or fingernails (OHCHR, 1995). 'Cutters' are remunerated for performing FGM, and this acts as a driver for the continuation of the practice (Momoh, 2005). FGM is usually performed without anaesthetic and in unhygienic conditions. The result of this is severe pain and infection which may cause genital swelling. Urine retention may be due to damage to the urethra during infibulation, as a result of pain or fear of urinating, or due to the swelling which may occur. Tissue damage to the clitoris and other genital tissues could also occur. Severe bleeding from cutting may lead to a fall in blood circulation causing haemorrhaging which is life-threatening and could lead to death. 'Cutters' and those assisting in performing FGM are known to pin girls down, holding their limbs tightly or sitting on them to restrict their movement. This act is seen as the first stage of the violence being perpetrated before a girl is cut and could lead to fractures and dislocation of limbs. FGM is mainly a group activity with several girls cut at the same time, sometimes with the same equipment, and this increases the spread of bloodborne viruses.

In some countries, FGM is performed by medical practitioners (Duncan, 2018; WHO, 2018). The medicalisation of FGM is partly based on the erroneous view it will reduce health consequences. Medicalisation is not an accepted alternative to 'cutters' because it violates medical ethics, perpetuates FGM, and it can still lead to death and health complications (WHO, 2018). Some FGM-affected communities where types II and III are practiced have been developing a growing awareness of the health complications associated with the types and are opting to perform types I or IV which are perceived to be less harmful (Hemmings, 2011). For there to be a lasting behavioural change to end the practice, educative work highlighting that all forms of FGM are harmful, illegal and are child abuse must be done with all communities.

The long-term complications of FGM could be experienced throughout a girl's lifespan. Girls may experience one or more complications and may not associate these with the FGM. Psychological impacts are not experienced by all victims/survivors, and they may not interpret what they are experiencing as being such (Coho et al., 2019; WHO, 2018). Table 10f.2 provides an overview of the potential health consequences.

PREVALENCE

It is estimated that over 200 million girls and women alive today in 30 countries are living with the consequences of FGM (UNICEF, 2023). An estimated 22% of those who are cut are under 15 years old (UNICEF, 2016), and some 3 million girls in Africa are at risk of being cut annually (Serour, 2013). The 30 FGM affected countries where the practice is mainly concentrated include 28 in Africa and Yemen and Iraq in the Middle East. A growing body of global research directs attention to FGM also being practiced in South and Central America, India, Indonesia, Israel, Malaysia, Thailand, Oman, Saudi Arabia, United Arab Emirates and Russia (Al-Hinai, 2014; Alsibiani and Rouzi, 2010; Antonova and Siradzhudinova, 2018; Russian Justice Initiative, 2016; UNFPA, 2011; UNICEF, 2016; WHO, 2008; 2018). Professionals must not assume that a woman/girl from an FGM-affected community has had the procedure and must be mindful that FGM is not an 'African' issue, as evidence shows different ethnic groups and communities worldwide are affected by it.

The practice of FGM is not a new phenomenon to the United Kingdom, as the Victorians are known to have performed clitoridectomy (Black, 1997; Sheehan, 1982). The prevalence of FGM in England and Wales is unknown; however, Macfarlane and Dorkenoo (2015) reported that an estimated 137,000 women and girls with FGM, born in FGM-affected countries, were permanently resident in England and Wales. However, caution should be exercised when using this figure (137,000) as some families have changed their attitude to the practice, although, at the same time, there are still concerns about girls being at risk (Macfarlane, 2019).

TABLE 10F.2	
Long-Term Health Consequences of Female Genital Mutilation	
Long-term complications	
Gynaecological & Urogynaecological	Chronic vulvar pain, clitoral neuroma (nerve tumours), reproductive tract infections, urinary tract infections, pelvic infection, vulvar adhesion, vulvar abscesses, painful or difficult urination, epidermal inclusion cysts and keloids in the genital area and menstrual problems (WHO, 2018)
Obstetrics	Increased risk of: caesarean section, postpartum haemorrhage, episiotomy, perineal tears and/or vesicovaginal fistulae or rectovaginal fistulae, prolonged difficult labour, obstetric tears and lacerations and maternal death Babies are at increased risk of: stillbirth and early neonatal death, asphyxia and resuscitation of the baby at birth
Mental health and psychological	The following higher rates of mental disorders have been experienced by girls and women who have experienced FGM: depression, anxiety disorders, posttraumatic stress disorder and somatic (physical) complaints with no organic cause. Psychological: flashbacks during pregnancy, sexual intercourse or childbirth, substance abuse, low self-esteem, shame, nightmares about the genital cutting and self-harm
Psychosexual	Pain during sex, lack of pleasurable sensations, low libido, anorgasmia, fear or anxiety around sexual intercourse, pelvic pain, penetration difficulties, postcoital bleeding, divorce, and marital breakdown

Modified from WHO, 2018

FGM AND THE LAW

In England, Wales and Northern Ireland FGM was criminalised under the Female Genital Mutilation Act 2003 and in Scotland under the Prohibition of Female Genital Mutilation (Scotland) Act 2005. Under the Children Act 1989, girls who have undergone the procedure, regardless of the type, are considered to have suffered 'significant harm'.[2] Girls at risk of FGM are considered likely to suffer 'significant harm.' Where there is reasonable cause to suspect a girl is suffering, or is likely to suffer, significant harm, s.47 of the Children Act 1989 places a duty on children's social care to investigate their concerns. Further information on protective measures available under the Children Act can be obtained from the *Multi-agency statutory guidance on female genital mutilation* (HM Government, 2020).

For the remainder of this section, focus is placed on the 2003 Act. The 2003 Act covers both girls and women and pertains to UK nationals or those habitually resident in the UK. A girl's nationality or residence status is immaterial when considering if an offence has happened.

The WHO definition of FGM (provided earlier) was not incorporated into the 2003 Act, which means it is not necessary to confirm the type of FGM experienced to prove an offence has occurred. Under the 2003 Act, the practice is illegal if excision, infibulation or mutilation of whole or any part of a girl or woman's labia majora, labia minora or clitoris has taken place (CPS, 2019). According to the 2003 Act, there are four FGM offences:

1. It is an offence to perform FGM even if it occurs overseas (section 1)
2. It is an offence to assist a girl to mutilate her genitals (section 2)
3. It is an offence to assist a non-UK resident to mutilate a girl's genital overseas (section 3)
4. It is an offence to fail to protect a girl at risk of FGM (section 3A)

In England and Wales, anyone found guilty on conviction or indictment of an offence under sections 1, 2, and 3 is liable to a fine or a maximum sentence of 14 years imprisonment or both. Any person sentenced on summary conviction will receive imprisonment for a term not exceeding 6 months or a fine or both. For the offence of failing to protect a girl at risk of FGM, under section 3A, the person 'failing to protect' must be 'responsible' for the girl at the time of the offence.

[2][2015] EWFC 3

Those 'responsible' are considered anyone with 'parental responsibility' and having 'frequent contact' with the girl and anyone over 18 years assuming a parenting role. The maximum penalty for this offence is 7 years' imprisonment, or a fine, or both.

Other legal measures under the 2003 Act include:

■ Anonymity for victims of FGM: alleged victims to be given lifelong anonymity which prevents publication of any information leading to their identification.

■ Extended extra-territorial jurisdiction: it is a criminal offence for a UK national or UK resident to perform FGM outside the UK; assist a girl to perform it on herself outside the UK; and/or assist a non-UK national or UK resident to perform FGM outside the UK on a UK national or UK resident.

■ FGM Protection Order: This civil order is designed to protect a girl who may be at risk of FGM or where it has already been perpetrated. An order could be applied for by the person at risk or who has undergone FGM, a relevant third party (e.g. local authority) and any other person with the leave of the court. To obtain an order requires an application, which is free to apply for, to be made at a Family Court in England and Wales. The order allows the court to make restrictions or requirements to protect the subject of the order, (e.g. banning overseas travel). Breaching the order is a criminal offence punishable by a maximum sentence of up to 5 years' imprisonment. A breach of the order could also be dealt with civilly as a contempt of court and punishable by up to 2 years' imprisonment, a fine, or both.

■ Mandatory reporting duty: This requires regulated health and social care professionals and teachers in England and Wales during the course of their work duties to report to the police if (a) they are informed by a girl (under 18 years old) that they have undergone FGM or (b) they observe physical signs that an act of FGM may have been carried out on a girl (under 18 years old). This is a personal responsibility, which means a professional cannot transfer the duty to report to the police to someone else. Failing to comply with this responsibility will lead to the professional being referred to their profession's regulatory body for a review of their fitness to practice. Other professionals still have a responsibility to report cases of FGM by following their organisation's safeguarding guidelines (Home Office, 2015).

RESPONDING TO CONCERNS

Girls at risk of FGM or who have undergone FGM need a multi-agency safeguarding response to protect them. A girl who has undergone FGM will need an individualised, holistic health assessment to determine her health needs and the support required. Responding to concerns must be in line with child protection procedures. Therefore, if a girl is at risk of or has suffered significant harm, a strategy discussion must be held, and professionals should consider if legal measures are needed to protect the girl.

Do you make assumptions about others who are culturally different from you? If yes, what are the consequences of making assumptions, and how do you how do you overcome it?

In all cases professionals should also consider the following when assessing risk:

■ Speak to the girl on her own using an interpreter where needed and observe her behaviour.

■ Assessments should identify other girls in the family and community that could be at risk.

■ FGM is a so-called 'honour' crime and requires an exploration of a family's core beliefs and assumptions about the role and expectations of girls and women along with the role of boys and men within the family.

■ FGM happens within a context of risks being presented at the family and community levels. Using an ecomap to identify family and community networks (including overseas) will identify who presents a risk or provides protection.

■ Identify the generations that have undergone FGM, and the risks they present and protection they provided. Using a genogram[3] will help map family members.

■ Explore the international context as a girl could be taken overseas to have FGM performed, the risk of FGM may have been identified whilst the girl is overseas or 'cutters'

---

[3]A visual representation of the different generations of a family. It is similar to a family tree.

might enter the country with the intention of cutting girls. The likely response to this will be to consider legal measures to protect the girl.

■ FGM may intersect with other safeguarding concerns, e.g. forced marriage or domestic abuse. Therefore assessments must explore other safeguarding concerns.

■ Use an approach based on safety and trust, as talking about FGM might retraumatise a girl.

■ Professionals should consider barriers preventing them from undertaking good assessments. These could be fear of being labelled racists when working with families ethnically different from the professionals or viewing their culture as a gauge for determining what it right or wrong.

CASE STUDY 10F.1: PREVENTING FGM

Michelle and John have been together for 2 years and are the parents of 9-month-old Mary. They are originally from Nigeria and have been residing in the UK for the past 5 years. Michelle overheard a telephone conversation between John and his mother, who lives in Nigeria, where they discussed cutting Mary during a planned trip with her father to Nigeria in 3 days. Michelle is concerned that her daughter may be cut, and she does not feel able to protect her daughter. Michelle shares her concerns with the health visitor, who refers the family to children's social care. Based on the information provided in the referral, within 24 hours children's social care convenes a strategy meeting with the health visitor, general practitioner and police. At this meeting, it was shared that there is a history of domestic abuse and of Michelle having undergone FGM. The professionals devised a plan on how to

investigate their concerns and protect Mary. The social worker and police arranged to meet with Michelle away from the home due to concerns for her safety. Before the meeting, the social worker assessed the risk to Mary using the National FGM Centre's FGM Assessment Tool and used the FGM Toolkit to decide on the best approach to engage the parents.

■ What are your immediate concerns?
■ What are the protective factors present?
■ What further information is needed to in order to assess the level of risk?
■ Does mandatory reporting apply?
■ Would you consider applying for an FGM Protection Order? If yes, what requirements and/or prohibitions are necessary to protect Mary? If no, what are the reasons for this decision?

Following meeting the family, professionals should consider the following reflective questions:

REFLECTIVE QUESTIONS

■ What steps have you taken to minimise the risk to the child(ren)?
■ What steps have you taken to strengthen the protective factors, and how has this affected the child's health or development?
■ Does the parent have insight into your concerns, the impact on their child and the circumstances?
■ What else do you need to do? Have you identified and overcome any barriers?
■ What have you learned, and what would you do differently in future cases and why?

CONCLUSION

FGM is a harmful practice and a form of gender-based violence. It is a complex issue rooted in patriarchal beliefs and driven by cultural, religious and socioeconomic justifications for performing it. The harm caused by the practice can lead to death or short- and long-term health consequences. Professionals must be alert to the risks given the hidden nature of this form of abuse. With all forms of FGM being considered 'significant harm' and girls at risk likely to suffer 'significant harm', a duty is placed on local authorities to make enquires where they are concerned for the safety of a girl. The practice is also a crime, and the 14-year maximum sentence is in recognition of the serious nature of the offence. The legal and civil measures are wide ranging and can be used to protect girls even if they are overseas. Professionals must be aware their personal duties as mandated reporters.

Although professionals may experience discomfort talking about FGM for fear of stigmatising communities or being discriminatory, this should not lead to child protection procedures not being followed. Training should equip professionals to develop competence on how to broach the topic with families and opportunities to share knowledge of what works in practice. Supervision must focus on enabling professionals to reflect on practice. (See Further Reading section for resources available to support professionals on their journey to becoming culturally competent and on how to undertake assessments.)

FURTHER READING

National FGM Centre: http://nationalfgmcentre.org.uk. (Useful resources from this website include: FGM Risk Assessment Tool, direct work tool kit and reflective tool).

National FGM Centre FGM Assessment Tool: https://assessment.nationalfgmcentre.org.uk

Department for Health Guidance and Risk Assessment Tool: https://assets.publishing.service.gov.uk/government/uploads/system/uploads/attachment_data/file/525390/FGM_safeguarding_report_A.pdf.

Home Office FGM Resource Pack: https://www.gov.uk/government/publications/female-genital-mutilation-resource-pack/female-genital-mutilation-resource-pack

NSPCC FGM Helpline: 0800 028 3550 or email: fgmhelp@nspcc.org.uk

28.Too Many – A comprehensive resource library: https://www.28toomany.org/

National FGM Support Clinics: https://www.nhs.uk/conditions/female-genital-mutilation-fgm/national-fgm-support-clinics/

Replace 2: https://www.replacefgm2.org/.

REFERENCES

Al-Hinai, H., 2014. Female Genital Mutilation in the Sultanate of Oman. http://www.stopfgmmideast.org/wp-content/uploads/2014/01/habiba-al-hinai-female-genital-mutilation-in-the-sultanate-of-oman1.pdf. (Accessed 26 January 2020).

Alsibiani, S.A., Rouzi, A.A., 2010. Sexual function in women with female genital mutilation. Fertil. Steril. 93 (3), 722–724.

Antonova, Y.A., Siradzhudinova, S.V., 2018. The Practice of Female Genital Mutilation in Dagestan: Strategies for its Elimination. https://www.srji.org/upload/iblock/957/The_practice_of_ female_genital_mutilation_in_Dagestan_strategies_for_its_ elimination_15.06.pdf. (Accessed 11 January 2020).

Bjälkander, O., Grant, D., Berggren, V., Bathija, H., Almroth, L., 2013. Female genital mutilation in Sierra Leone: Norms, reliability of reported status, and accuracy of related demographic and health survey questions. Obstet. Gynecol. Int. (2), 680926.

Black, J., 1997. Female genital mutilation: A contemporary issue and a Victorian obsession. J. R. Soc. Med. 99, 402–405.

BBC, 2019. Mother Jailed for Female Genital Mutilation on Three-Year-Old. https://www.bbc.co.uk/news/uk-england-london-47502089. (Accessed 14 February 2020).

Children Act 1989. https://www.legislation.gov.uk/ukpga/1989/41/contents (Accessed 25 June 2021).

Coho, C., Sepúlveda, R.P., Hussein, L., Laffy, C., 2019. Female Genital Mutilation: Guidelines for Working Therapeutically with Survivors of Female Genital Mutilation. Dahlia Project, London, UK.

Crown Prosecution Service, 2020. Female Genital Mutilation Prosecution Guidance. https://www.cps.gov.uk/legal-guidance/female-genital-mutilation-prosecution-guidance. (Accessed 14 February 2020).

European Institute for Gender Equality, 2020. Female Genital Mutilation. https://eige.europa.eu/gender-based-violence/female-genital-mutilation. (Accessed 2 February 2020).

Department for Education, 2017. Characteristics of Children in Need: 2016 to 2017. https://www.gov.uk/government/statistics/characteristics-of-children-in-need-2016-to-2017. (Accessed 14 February 2020).

Department for Education, 2018. Characteristics of Children in Need: 2017 to 2018. https://www.gov.uk/government/statistics/characteristics-of-children-in-need-2017-to-2018. (Accessed 14 February 2020).

Department for Education, 2019. Characteristics of Children in Need: 2018 to 2019. https://www.gov.uk/government/statistics/characteristics-of-children-in-need-2018-to-2019. (Accessed 14 February 2020).

Department for Education, 2020. Characteristics of Children in Need: 2019 to 2020. https://www.gov.uk/government/collections/statistics-children-in-need. (Accessed 25 June 2021).

Duncan, B.S., Njue, C., Moore, Z., 2018. Trends in medicalization of female genital mutilation/cutting: what do the data reveal? Evidence to End FGM/C: Research to Help Women Thrive. Population. https://www.popcouncil.org/uploads/pdfs/2018RH_MedicalizationFGMC_update.pdf. (Accessed 13 February 2020).

Equality Now, June 2019. 8 Things You Should Know About FGM. https://knowledgecommons.popcouncil.org/departments_sbsr-rh/571/. (Accessed 14 February 2020).

Female Genital Mutilation Act, 2003. Norwich: The Stationery Office.

Gangoli, G., Gill, A., Mulvihill, N., Hester, M., 2018. Perception and barriers: Reporting female genital mutilation. Journal of Aggression. J. Aggress. Confl. Peace Res. 10 (4), 251–260.

Hemmings, J., 2011. Tackling FGM Special Initiative – Peer Research. Full report. Trust for London, Esmee Fairbarn Foundation, Rosa, Options UK, London.

HM Government (2020) Multi-agency statutory guidance on female genital mutilation. Available at https://assets.publishing. service.gov.uk/government/uploads/system/uploads/ attachment_data/file/1016817/6.7166_HO_FBIS_BN_O__ Leaflet_A4_FINAL_080321_WEB.pdf (Accessed 20 August 2023).

Home Office, 2015. Mandatory Reporting of Female Genital Mutilation – Procedural Information. Home Office, London.

Home Office, 2016. Multi-agency Statutory Guidance on Female Fenital Mutilation. Home Office, London. Available at: FGM_Mandatory_Reporting_-_procedural_information_ nov16_FINAL.pdf (publishing.service.gov.uk) (Accessed 25 June 2021)https://www.gov.uk/government/publications/multi-agency-statutory-guidance-on-female-genital-mutilation

Macfarlane, A., Dorkenoo, E., 2015. Prevalence of Female Genital Mutilation in England and Wales: National and Local Estimates. City University, London, London .

Macfarlane, A., 2019. Tackling female genital mutilation in the UK, The BMJ, 364:l15. https://www.bmj.com/content/364/bmj.l15/ rr-4. (Accessed 25 June 2021).

Momoh, C., 2005. FGM and issues of gender and human rights of women. In: Momoh, C. (Ed.), Female Genital Mutilation. Radcliffe Publishing Limited, Oxford.

Office of the High Commissioner for Human Rights, 2020, Harmful Practice. Available at https://www.ohchr.org/sites/default/files/ INFO_Harm_Pract_WEB.pdf (Accessed 20 August 2023).

Refaat, A., Dandash, F.K., Mohammed, H., Defrawi, E., Eyada, M., 2001. Female genital mutilation and domestic violence among Egyptian women. J. Sex Marital Ther. 27 (5), 593–598.

Roach, M., Momoh, C., 2013. Two steps forward, one step back: The fight against female genital mutilation in the UK. In: Rehman, Y., Kelly, L., Siddiqui, H. (Eds.), Moving in the Shadows: Violence in the Lives of Minority Women and Children. Ashgate Publishing Limited, Surrey.

Russian Justice Initiative, 2016. Female Genital Mutilation of Girls in Dagestan (Russian Federation). Report based on the results of a qualitative study on female genital mutilation performed on girls. https://www.srji.org/upload/iblock/52c/fgm_dagestan_2016_eng_ final_edited_2017.pdf. (Accessed 25 June 2021).

Salihu, H., E. August, J. Salemi, H. Weldeselasse, Y. Sarro, and A. Alio. 2012. "The Association Between Female Genital Mutilation and Intimate Partner Violence. BJOG: An International. J. Obstet. Gynaecol. 119 (13),1597–1605.

Serour, G.I., 2013. Medicalization of female genital mutilation/ cutting. Afr. J. Urol. 19, 145–149.

Sheehan, E., 1982. Victorian clitoridectomy. Med. Anthropol. News 12, 9–15.

The Guardian, 22 March 2018. UK Solicitor Cleared of Forcing Daughter to Undergo FGM. https://www.theguardian.com/ society/2018/mar/22/uk-solicitor-acquited-forcing-daughter-fgm-female-genital-mutilation. (Accessed 13 February 2020).

United Nations Population Fund, December 2011. Project Embera-wera: An Experience of Culture Change to Eradicate Female Genital Mutilation in Colombia – Latin America'. UNFPA, Colombia.

UNICEF, 2013. Female Genital Mutilation/cutting: a Statistical Overview and Exploration of the Dynamics of Change. UNICEF, New York (NY). http:// data.unicef.org/wp-content/ uploads/2015/12/FGMC_Lo_res_Final_26.pdf. (Accessed 23 January 2020).

UNICEF, 2014. Female Genital Mutilation/Cutting: What Might the Future Hold? UNICEF, New York. https://data.unicef.org/ resources/female-genital-mutilationcutting-might-future-hold/. (Accessed 25 January 2020).

UNICEF (2016, February 5). [online] Available at New statistical report on female genital mutilation shows harmful practice is a global concern – UNICEF [Press release]. https://data. unicef.org/resources/female-genital-mutilationcutting-global-concern/. (Accessed 20 August 2023).

UNICEF, 2019. Female genital mutilation. Available at https://data. unicef.org/topic/child-protection/female-genital-mutilation/#_ edn1 (Accessed 20 January 2023).

UNICEF, 2023. Female Genital Mutilation. Available at https://data. unicef.org/topic/child-protection/female-genital-mutilation/#_ edn1. (Accessed 20 January 2023).

UN Office of the High Commissioner for Human Rights (OHCHR), 1995. Fact Sheet No. 23. Harmful traditional practices affecting the health of women and children. August 1995, No. 23 https://www. refworld.org/docid/479477410.html. (Accessed 14 February 2020).

WHO, 1997. Female Genital Mutilation. A Joint WHO/UNICEF/ UNFPA Statement. World Health Organization, Geneva. https:// apps.who.int/iris/bitstream/handle/10665/41903/9241561866. pdf?sequence=1&isAllowed=y. (Accessed 11 January 2020).

WHO, 2008. Eliminating Female Fenital Mutilation: An Interagency Statement UNAIDS, UNDP, UNECA, UNESCO, UNFPA, UNHCHR, UNHCR, UNICEF. UNIFEM, WHO. https://apps.who.int/iris/ bitstream/handle/10665/43839/9789241596442_eng. pdf?sequence=1&isAllowed=y. (Accessed 25 January 2020).

World Health Organization, (2016). WHO guidelines on the management of health complications from female genital mutilation. World Health Organization. Available at https://apps. who.int/iris/bitstream/handle/10665/206437/9789241549646_ eng.pdf (Accessed 20 August 2023).

WHO, 2018. Care of Girls and Women Living With Female Genital Mutilation: A Clinical Workbook. World Health Organization, Geneva.

10g

CHILD ABUSE LINKED TO FAITH OR BELIEF

MOR DIOUM ■ STEPHANIE YORATH

KEY POINTS

- Origins of child abuse linked to faith or belief.
- Definition and prevalence of child abuse linked to faith or belief.
- Law and policy.
- Learning from cases of child abuse linked to faith or belief.
- Protecting children across culture and faith.

INTRODUCTION

This section will consider what social workers and others involved in safeguarding children need to know about child abuse linked to faith or belief (CALFB). Public and professional awareness of this kind of harmful practice first began to emerge in the UK following the death of Victoria Adjo Climbié in 2000. The public inquiry into Victoria's death revealed that she had suffered multiple injuries and had been starved. The injuries were inflicted by Victoria's carers, actions which they claimed were part of their attempts to rid her of the 'evil spirit' they believed was inside her and was causing her to be incontinent; a church pastor had supported them in the belief that 'Victoria's problems were due to her possession by an evil spirit' (Laming, 2003, p. 35). Since Victoria's death, child abuse linked to faith or belief – CALFB – has become the term used to describe this type of child maltreatment.

ORIGINS OF CHILD ABUSE LINKED TO FAITH OR BELIEF

Belief in witchcraft and spirit possession is as old as humanity. Almost every community inherits such a belief system and retains echoes of these beliefs in everyday superstitions, be they cultural or religious. The emergence and expansion of the three Abrahamic religions – Judaism, Christianity and Islam – tended to diminish ancient cultural norms and practices in favour of the belief in one God only, with the worship of animals and natural objects such as the sun, stars and moon being largely abandoned. Nevertheless, the influence of longstanding cultural beliefs in witchcraft, spirit possession and superstition continue to be evident within todays' cultures (Tedam, 2014). For example, in the UK many people consider the number 13 to be 'unlucky' and are superstitious about walking under a ladder, seeing a single magpie, or putting new shoes on the table. Communities across the globe all have their own equally idiosyncratic beliefs and superstitions based on inherited cultural and/or religious (mis)conceptions.

For some communities, belief in witchcraft remains a means of protection and help will be sought from 'traditional healers' in relation to all manner of difficulties, including illnesses. This is a way of life, as ordinary as going to see the GP. For parents or family members who initiate and seek help for a child through a Shaman or a traditional healer, this approach may come from a position of care and compassion. However, a lack of understanding and awareness of how to access public health, social care and educational services for children may also act as an incentive to rely on traditional practices.

In some parts of Africa, the practice of witchcraft has been most often associated with old men and women. Its more recent association with children is a recent development. Some attribute this new phenomenon to poverty and breakdown of family structures which is occurring as a long-term consequence of colonialism. It may also be linked to the consequences of climate change, which results in migration, and hence to intergenerational conflict. Migrant children often pick up language skills and assimilate into their new country faster than their parents, who may seek to maintain social norms and expectations of behaviour from their countries of origin. Conflict may arise as children adopt the attitudes and behaviours of friends at school and of the wider culture in which they are now living. For example, in the UK it is ordinary for children to ask questions and to sometimes 'talk back' to parents and elders, but such behaviours may be less acceptable in other cultures. Or behaviours which a professional might interpret as arising from stress and anxiety, such as Victoria Climbié's bedwetting, may be wrongly ascribed to a supernatural cause.

Whatever its complex causes, a continued belief in witchcraft has resulted in some children being labelled as 'witches' or 'being possessed'. This typically involves the belief that an evil force has entered the child and is controlling them or that the child is able to use an evil force to harm or infect others and to thereby bring bad luck to the family or community (Tedam, 2014). Such accusations may come from family members, from within the community, or from religious and spiritual leaders. In some cases a child may themselves believe that they are possessed, with immeasurable consequences for their emotional and psychological well-being (La Fontaine, 2009; Reis, 2013).

Child abuse linked to faith or belief most often occurs as part of an attempt to exorcise evil spirits or 'deliver' the child from their control. Exorcism is an ancient practice, observed in different forms in most of the major world religions – including Judaism, Christianity, Islam, Hinduism and Taoism. Those who practice exorcism do so in the belief that this will rid a person of evil spirits which are believed to dwell inside them. Attempts at exorcism may be undertaken by family member or may involve religious leaders. Unlike other forms of abuse, CALFB is largely based on *fear* of the unseen or unknown, and people perpetrating such abuse may believe that their actions are necessary to protect the child or wider family and community.

It is important to stress that although the examples used so far have drawn on the case of Victoria Climbié, an African child from the Ivory Coast, child abuse linked to belief or faith can and does occur in families and communities of any religion and any ethnic origin, including White British groups. The 2006 Government-commissioned report *Child Abuse Linked to Accusations of 'Possession' and 'Witchcraft'* found that belief in both witchcraft and in possession by evil spirits is widespread. It concluded that:

- The belief is not confined to particular countries, cultures or religions, nor is it confined to recent migrants.
- The abuse occurs when the carers attempt to 'exorcise' the child.
- There are various social reasons that make a child more vulnerable to an accusation of 'possession' or 'witchcraft'. These include family stress, a change in the family structure, disability, a child with a perceived difference, and a weak bond of affection between the carer and the child.
- The role of places of worship in these cases is unclear.
- The effect on the family and the victim are devastating. The children and their siblings invariably need long-term foster care.
- Police and social workers are not able to change the beliefs of carers (Stobart, 2006, p. 28).

DEFINITION AND PREVALENCE OF CHILD ABUSE LINKED TO FAITH OR BELIEF

No definition of CALFB is provided in the *Working Together* guidance, and there is disagreement about whether this is a specific form of child abuse (Oakley et al., 2017). This is because the harms which children who are subjected to CALFB experience fall within the existing definitions for neglect or for physical, sexual or emotional abuse. However, before further defining what CALFB *is*, it is important to explain what it is *not*.

It is *not* cultural practices that are in themselves a specific form of abuse, for example female genital mutilation or forced marriage (for more on these topics see Chapters 10e and 10f). It is also *not* child abuse in faith settings which are incidental to the abuse – for example, sexual abuse by paedophiles in a religious community as has been widely reported in the *Independent Inquiry into Childhood Sexual Abuse* (2020).

The only Government definition of abuse linked to faith or belief can be found as a reporting category in the annual Children in Need Census. This is the data which all local authorities are required to submit each year to the Government. The guidance on completing this data return (Department for Education, 2021) provides instructions as to when CALFB should be reported as an additional factor, noted at the end of assessment that social workers have identified as being relevant in a case. The guidance states:

> The **abuse linked to faith or belief** *factor should be recorded where a child is at risk of, has been or is being abused because of his or her parents or carers' belief system. This includes, but is not limited to, belief in witchcraft, spirit possession, demons or the devil, the evil eye or djinns, dakini, kindoki, ritual or muti murders and use of fear of the supernatural. The beliefs involved are not confined to one faith, nationality or ethnic community. The abuse concerned may be of any form but can include physical (including excessive physical discipline), sexual, emotional, neglect (including the denial of necessary medical treatment), domestic slavery, sexual exploitation.*
>
> ***Department for Education (2021, p.13)***

The latest available data at the time of writing (Department for Education, 2021) records 1950 cases of CALFB. While this figure is not large in comparison to the 388,490 children reported as children in need, or the 50,010 children who were subject to child protection plans, it is likely that not all cases of CALFB will have been captured within this data. Cases may go unreported because statutory services are never made aware of the abuse, or cases may not be recorded as CALFB because social workers do not link the physical, sexual or other abuses they identify to practices arising from faith or belief.

LAW AND POLICY

In the UK, there is no specific civil or criminal offence of CALFB. Rather, such cases are addressed by tackling whatever fundamental elements of abuse are present (e.g. physical abuse, psychological abuse, etc.) and, where necessary, by the use of related criminal charges (e.g. actual bodily harm, grievous bodily harm, causing or allowing the death of a child, etc.). Specific legislation for CALFB has been opposed in the UK by those who argue that such legislation would be impractical and who consider that applying the existing child protection framework provides for safer practice (Briggs et al., 2011).

In the wake of Lord Laming's report into the death of Victoria Climbié (Laming, 2003) the government published non-statutory guidance on *Safeguarding Children from Abuse Linked to a Belief in Spirit Possession* (HM Government, 2007). This guidance is no longer in force, though remains available online as part of the national archive. *The National Action Plan to Tackle Child Abuse Linked to Faith or Belief* (National Working Group, 2012) provides the only current guidance on how professionals should work to reduce the prevalence of this type of child maltreatment. The key messages from the *National Action Plan* are set out in Box 10G.1 and emphasise that CALFB is a child protection issue.

LEARNING FROM CASES OF CHILD ABUSE LINKED TO FAITH OR BELIEF

Since the death of Victoria Climbié there have been a number of other high-profile child abuse cases in the UK which have involved abuse linked to faith or belief. These cases illustrate how CALFB can arise in families of different faiths and ethnicities:

Samira Ullah: Three-month-old baby Samira Ullah was killed by her father, Sitab Ullah, a British man of South Asian heritage. At the time of the murder, Sitab was a heavy user of heroin and crack cocaine and was exhibiting paranoid and delusional behaviours. His delusional beliefs included thinking that Samira was possessed by jinn, a term used in the Islamic tradition to refer to supernatural beings who occupy a parallel world to mankind (BBC News, 2005).

BOX 10G.1

KEY MESSAGES FROM THE NATIONAL ACTION PLAN TO TACKLE CHILD ABUSE LINKED TO FAITH OR BELIEF (2012)

- **Child abuse is condemned by people of all cultures, communities and faiths, and is never acceptable under any circumstances.** Child abuse related to belief includes inflicting physical violence or emotional harm on a child by stigmatising or labelling them as evil or as a witch. Where this type of abuse occurs, it causes great distress and suffering to the child.
- **Everyone working or in contact with children has a responsibility to recognise and know how to act on evidence, concerns and signs** that a child's health, development and safety is being or may be threatened, especially when they suffer or are likely to suffer significant harm.
- **Standard child safeguarding procedures apply and must always be followed** in all cases where abuse or neglect is suspected including those that may be related to particular belief systems.
- **The number of cases of child abuse linked to a belief in spirits, possession and witchcraft is small**, but where it occurs the impact on the child is great, causing much distress and suffering to the child. It is likely that a proportion of this type of abuse remains unreported.
- **Child abuse linked to faith or belief may occur where a child is treated as a scapegoat for perceived failure.** Whilst specific beliefs, practices, terms or forms of abuse may exist, the underlying reasons for the abuse are often similar to other contexts in which children become at risk. These reasons can include family stress, deprivation, domestic violence, substance abuse and mental health problems. Children who are different in some way, perhaps because they have a disability or learning difficulty, an illness or are exceptionally bright, can also be targeted in this kind of abuse

Foster children of Eunice Spry: Eunice Spry was a White British woman and devout Jehovah's Witness who fostered children for Gloucestershire County Council for almost two decades. Spry punished several of her fostered children for being 'possessed by the devil' and would mete out punishments which including ramming sticks down their throats and making them eat their own vomit and excrement (BBC News, 2007).

Khyra Ishaq: Seven-year-old Khyra Ishaq, a British child of Caribbean heritage died of starvation while living in a house with fridge full of food; her five siblings were also found to be suffering from malnutrition. The Serious Case Review which followed Khyra's death noted her stepfather's strict interpretation of Islam and his 'belief that evil spirits inhabited at least the child [and] led to a tirade of severe physical chastisements, beatings and humiliating punishments for all of the children, including the withdrawal of food' (Radford, 2010, p. 33).

Kristy Bamu: Fifteen-year-old Kristy Bamu, a French child of African heritage, drowned on Christmas Day. Kristy was visiting family in London when his sister's partner accused him of bringing 'kindoki' (witchcraft) into the home, as a consequence of which Kristy was tortured with knives, sticks, metal bars, ceramic floor tiles, bottles, a pair of pliers and a hammer and chisel. He drowned after being put into the bath as part of 'ritual cleansing' (BBC News, 2012).

As well as these high-profile individual cases, work has been undertaken to better understand the dynamics of CALFB in the UK and to help professionals identify when CALFB may be occurring. The Metropolitan Police have recognised the following range of factors as being potential indicators of CALFB:

- physical injuries, such as bruises or burns (including historical injuries/scarring);
- a child reporting that they are or have been accused of being 'evil', and/or that they are having the 'devil beaten out of them';
- the child or family may use words such as 'kindoki', 'djin', 'juju' or 'voodoo' – all of which refer to spiritual beliefs;
- a child becoming noticeably confused, withdrawn, disorientated or isolated and appearing alone amongst other children;
- a child's personal care deteriorating (e.g. rapid loss of weight, being hungry, turning up to school without food or lunch money, being unkempt with dirty clothes);
- it may be evident that the child's parent or carer does not have a close bond with the child;
- a child's attendance at school or college becomes irregular or there is a deterioration in a child's performance;
- a child is taken out of a school altogether without another school place having been arranged; and

■ wearing unusual jewellery/items or in possession of strange ornaments/scripts.

(Metropolitan Police: https://www.met.police.uk/advice/advice-and-information/caa/child-abuse/faith-based-abuse/)

PROTECTING CHILDREN ACROSS CULTURE AND FAITH

Work to raise awareness of abuse linked to faith or belief within UK communities and to encourage reporting is ongoing, largely driven by third sector organisations such as The Victoria Climbié Foundation UK. Nevertheless, because much (though by no means all) CALFB occurs in minority ethnic communities, the fear of being accused of racism continues to make some professionals hesitant to act. There is therefore a danger of cultural relativism within child protection practice related to CALFB, which may leave children from Black and minority ethnic communities at increased risk of abuse.

CLOSER LOOK: WHAT IS CULTURAL RELATIVISM?

Cultural relativism starts with the idea that ethical and social standards reflect the cultural context in which they exist. Because cultures differ around the world, so do the normative attitudes, beliefs and behaviours of people born into those different cultures. Using the perspective of cultural relativism leads to the view that no one culture is superior to any other culture.

An approach to social work which supported cultural relativism would seek to promote understandings of cultural practices that were not typically part of the social worker's own culture and to avoid judging all cultures based on the norms and expectations of White British culture. In many ways cultural relativism is a positive approach to working with diverse communities. It can help us to welcome, value and celebrate difference.

However, when it comes to child protection, too much emphasis on cultural relativism may not always bring about the best outcomes for every child. There remains a tension between cultural relativism and universal rights. Child protection work needs to be culturally sensitive, but also needs to ensure that all children are protected from harm. In relation to CALFB, fully adopting cultural relativism risks ignoring potential harms to children which can arise from faith-based cultural practices.

Culture or religion must never override the right of a child to be protected from abuse. Where there are perceived tensions between culture, faith and rights, the best interest of the child is always of paramount concern. Good practice should aim to be sensitive to the cultural heritage of a child and their family without compromising the protection of the child (Akilapa and Simkiss, 2012).

When working with children who may be subject to CALFB, it is important for practitioners to acknowledge that their own views about religion are likely to influence their practice (Horwarth and Lees, 2010). Research shows that many social workers adopt a 'religion-blind' and 'belief blind' approach to their work and can be reluctant to ask about issues of faith or belief as part of assessments (Gilligan, 2009). This can lead to signs of CALFB being overlooked. Engaging with and reflecting how faith and faith-based practices influence family dynamics is an important aspect of holistic assessment.

Although CALFB may manifest through one or more of the recognised categories of abuse (physical, sexual, psychological, neglect), it cannot be adequately addressed without conversations which directly consider matters of faith and belief. Such conversations should explore belief in relation to the wider social, economic and cultural context of the family. This should include asking about the parents' and caregivers' beliefs about the causes of any difficulties they may face. A key indicator of CALFB is that family misfortune and/or a child's behaviour is explained in terms of witchcraft and spirit possession. This should lead to an exploration of the meaning of misfortune or difficulty in the family and the provision of information about alternative sources of help and support, including therapeutic interventions. Research shows that frontline practitioners who have received faith literacy training are better able to recognise and respond to CALFB (Oakley et al., 2019)

Intervention in individual cases may help individual children but is unlikely to change the beliefs of parents or carers (Stobart, 2006) and so may do little to prevent ongoing abuse within communities where belief in witchcraft is sincerely held. However, community engagement to change perceptions and practices in communities where the belief system is practiced has been found to be a promising approach for reducing the risks of harm (Briggs, 2011). However, as Tedam concludes,

'Any preventive strategy aimed at this form of abuse and violence will require major consideration of cultural and faith-related values and ideas on the part of parents, families and communities' (Tedam, 2014, p.1412).

CASE STUDY 10G.1: CALFB

Akuba is a 10-year-old British child of African heritage living in London with her parents and three younger siblings. Akuba has mild cerebral palsy as a result of complications during birth: she walks with a twisted gait and her speech is slightly slurred, something which the family ascribe to 'bad spirits'. The family are devout Christians and regularly attend an African Spiritualist Church where prayers are sometimes offered in the hope that God will cure Akuba and other disabled members of the congregation.

When Akuba returns to school after the summer break, her teacher notices that she has lost weight and there are several small scars on her arm. When the teacher asks all the children in the class to write about what they did over the summer, Akuba writes about spending time at church and being helped by the new Pastor to be a better person. The teacher is concerned and reports the situation to the local authority child protection team.

1. Was the teacher right to be concerned?
2. What should the social worker do on receiving this referral?
3. How might the social worker begin to introduce questions about faith and belief as part of an assessment of Akuba's needs?
4. What which part of the *Assessment Framework for Children in Need and Their Families* do questions about faith, belief or religion fall?

FURTHER READING

Child abuse linked to faith or belief: national action plan: https://www.gov.uk/government/publications/national-action-plan-to-tackle-child-abuse-linked-to-faith-or-belief.

Metropolitan Police: Child abuse linked to faith or belief: https://www.met.police.uk/advice/advice-and-information/caa/child-abuse/faith-based-abuse/.

NSPCC: learning from Serious Case Reviews where culture or faith were significant elements: https://learning.nspcc.org.uk/research-resources/learning-from-case-reviews/culture-faith.

NSPCC, 2022. Safeguarding in Faith Communities. https://learning.nspcc.org.uk/safeguarding-child-protection/for-faith-communities.

NSPCC, 2014. Culture and Faith: Learning from Case Reviews. https://learning.nspcc.org.uk/media/1332/learning-from-case-reviews_culture-and-faith.pdf.

VCF The Victoria Climbié Foundation UK: https://vcf-uk.org/.

WHRIN The Witchcraft and Human Rights Network: http://www.whrin.org/.

REFERENCES

Akilapa, R., Simkiss, D., 2012. Cultural influences and safeguarding children. PCH 22 (11), 490–495.

BBC News, 2005. Father Murdered 'Possessed' Baby. http://news.bbc.co.uk/1/hi/england/london/4549898.stm.

BBC News, 2007. 'Sadistic' Foster Mother Jailed. http://news.bbc.co.uk/1/hi/england/gloucestershire/6571445.stm.

BBC News, 2012. Witchcraft Murder: Couple Jailed for Kristy Bamu Killing. https://www.bbc.co.uk/news/uk-england-london-17255470.

Briggs, S., Whittaker, A., Linford, H., Bryan, A., Ryan, E., Ludick, D., 2011. Safeguarding Children's Rights: Exploring Issues of Witchcraft and Spirit Possession in London's African Communities. Trust for London, London. https://www.trustforlondon.org.uk/publications/safeguarding-childrens-rights-exploring-issues-witchcraft-and-spirit-possession-londons-african-communities/.

Department for Education, 2021. Children in Need Census: Additional Guide on the Factors Identified at the End of Assessment. Crown Copyright, London. https://assets.publishing.service.gov.uk/government/uploads/system/uploads/attachment_data/file/977581/CIN_Additional_guide_on_the_factors_identified_at_the_end_of_assessment.pdf.

Department for Education/Office for National Statistics, 2021. Reporting Year 2021: Characteristics of Children in Need. https://explore-education-statistics.service.gov.uk/find-statistics/characteristics-of-children-in-need.

Gilligan, PA. (2009). Considering religion and beliefs in child protection and safeguarding work: is any consensus emerging? *Child Abuse Review* 18 (2), 94–110.

HM Government, 2007. Safeguarding Children from Abuse Linked to a Belief in Spirit Possession. Department for Education [Archived on 1 Apr 2013], London. https://webarchive.nationalarchives.gov.uk/ukgwa/20130401151715/http://www.education.gov.uk/publications/eOrderingDownload/DFES-00465-2007.pdf.

Horwath, J., Lees, J., 2010. Assessing the influence of religious beliefs and practices on parenting capacity: The challenges for social work practitioners. Br J Soc Work 40 (1), 82–99.

Independent Inquiry into Childhood Sexual Abuse (IICSA), 2020 https://www.iicsa.org.uk/.

La Fontaine, J., 2009. The Devil's Children: From Spirit Possession to Witchcraft: New Allegations that Affect Children. Routledge, London.

Laming, 2003. The Victoria Climbié Inquiry. CM 5730. Crown Copyright, London.

National Working Group on Child Abuse Linked to Faith or Belief, 2012. National Actionplan to Tackle Child Abuse Linked to Faith or Belief. Department for Education, London. https://assets.publishing.service.gov.uk/government/uploads/system/uploads/attachment_data/file/175437/Action_Plan_-_Abuse_linked_to_Faith_or_Belief.pdf.

Oakley, L., Kinmond, K., Humphreys, J., Dioum, M., 2017. Practitioner and communities' awareness of CALFB: Child abuse linked to faith or belief. Child Abuse & Neglect 72 (10), 276–282.

Oakley, L., Kinmond, K., Humphreys, J., Dioum, M., 2019. Safeguarding children who are exposed to abuse linked to faith or belief. Child Abuse Review 28 (1), 27–38.

Radford, J., 2010. Serious Case Review in Respect of the Death of a Child: Case Number 14. Birmingham Safeguarding Children Board, Birmingham. https://www.basw.co.uk/system/files/resources/basw_94519-10_0.pdf.

Reis, R., 2013. Children enacting idioms of witchcraft and spirit possession as a response to trauma: Therapeutically beneficial, and for whom? Transcultural Psychiatry 50 (5), 622–643. https://doi.org/10.1177%2F1363461513503880.

Stobart, E., 2006. Child Abuse Linked to Accusations of "Possession" and "Witchcraft" [Department for Education & Skills Research Report no. 750]. London: Crown Copyright. https://dera.ioe.ac.uk/6416/1/RR750.pdf.

Tedam, P., 2014. Witchcraft branding and the abuse of African children in the UK: Causes, effects and professional intervention. Early Child Development and Care 184 (9-10), 1403–1414.

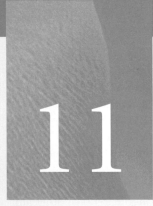

11

CHARACTERISTICS THAT ACCENTUATE VULNERABILITY (EDITORS' INTRODUCTION)

RACHEL FYSON ■ LISA WARWICK ■ RACHAEL CLAWSON

Not all children are equally vulnerable to abuse or equally in need of child protection. This chapter identifies some of the factors which are known to accentuate – or increase – a child's vulnerability to abuse.

In recent years, 'vulnerability' has become an increasingly contested term. It is now recognised that it is unhelpful to think of vulnerability as a characteristic of an individual or group. Vulnerability is better understood as situational: it arises in situations where there is an imbalance of power between two people; or, more often, an imbalance of power between a person or group of people, and an organisation or other social structure. Where imbalances of power exist, the less powerful person is vulnerable to the abusive actions of the more powerful person or social structure. All abuse involves an abuse of power, and all abuse therefore, to a greater or lesser extent, involves powerful individuals or organisations taking advantage of those who have less power. Abusers exploit vulnerabilities created by imbalances of power. Indeed, power is a theme that inevitably runs throughout this handbook.

Power imbalances can often be readily identified when they relate to individuals: a baby is powerless to prevent a parent from neglecting its needs; a toddler is powerless to prevent an older child from hitting them; a 13-year-old is powerless to protect themselves against grooming by a skilled sexual predator. In each of these examples, the abuse is made possible because of physical and/or intellectual power differences between the victim and perpetrator. However, not all babies, toddlers or teenagers are equally likely to be abused, even though most have similar physical and intellectual abilities. Child protection practice therefore needs to be sensitive to how wider power imbalances, created by social structures, can increase the vulnerability of some children.

Returning to the examples given in the previous paragraph will make this clearer. Babies born into families experiencing poverty may be more at risk of neglect because a lack of money creates additional stress in parents' lives and the impacts of stress can make it harder to prioritise the needs of the child. Toddlers regularly left in the care of older siblings, while parents work unsocial hours in poorly paid jobs, may be at greater risk of harm than those left in the care of regulated childminders, but poor families are more likely to rely on siblings and other sources of unregulated care because the costs of a childminder are prohibitive. Any 13-year-old girl may be vulnerable to online grooming, but those from poorer families may be more readily tempted by offers of money or gifts by sexual predators. So poverty undoubtedly creates significant additional vulnerability but, as discussed by Anna Gupta and Brid Featherstone in Chapter 4 (*Poverty and Child Protection*), child protection policy and practice often pays insufficiently attention to this issue.

Additional vulnerabilities may also arise when a child possesses one or more of the 9 'protected characteristics' identified within the Equality Act 2010, namely: age, disability, gender reassignment, marriage and civil partnership, pregnancy and maternity, race, religion or belief, sex and sexual orientation. Some of these protected characteristics will play a greater role than others in relation to increasing the vulnerability of a child. All children are vulnerable due their age. This is because anyone aged under 18 is legally a child and therefore does not have the same legal status or rights as an adult (see Chapter 2: *The Rights of the Child* by Carolyne Willow for more on the legal rights of children). By contrast, only some children will have additional protected characteristics. For example, in Chapter 13: *Culturally Sensitive Child Protection Practice,* Cath Williams discusses how issues related to race can increase the vulnerability of children from minority ethnic communities, and in Chapter 11a Anita Franklin explores the heightened vulnerability to abuse that is known to arise for disabled children.

However, there are also factors which accentuate vulnerability that are associated not with a protected or other characteristic personal to the child, but with the dynamics of the situations in which they find themselves. Three of these situations are explored in this chapter. Robin Sen addresses the impacts of *Being a looked after child* (see Chapter 11b), highlighting how the negative impacts of abuse and neglect - which may lead to a child becoming looked-after - are often compounded by the child's negative experiences within the care system. In this way, child protection processes may sometimes create or exacerbate the vulnerabilities to abuse which they are intended to prevent. Kelly Devenney explores *Being a Refugee or Asylum Seeker* (see Chapter 11c) and considers how global power imbalances which create the impetus for seeking asylum result in individual children being at increased risk of abuse. Finally, Jo Aldridge looks at *Being a Young Carer* (see Chapter 11d) and identifies how family dynamics of care, combined with the inadequacies of adult social care services, may lead some children to provide care for their parents or other family members at the expense of their own education, health and wider welfare.

The factors and situations considered in this chapter are not the only things that may accentuate a child's vulnerability to abuse. However, by highlighting some of these factors and situations, it is hoped that practitioners will be encouraged to think more broadly: about the characteristics of each child, about the situational aspect of each child's life, and about how these might come together in ways that can accentuate their risk of abuse, or limit the extent to which a child is able to protect themselves.

11a

DISABLED CHILD PROTECTION – EVIDENCE FOR IMPROVED PRACTICE IN THE UK

ANITA FRANKLIN

KEY POINTS

- Disabled children and young people face a three- to four-fold increased risk of abuse than their nondisabled peers.

- Practitioners need to see beyond a medicalised notion of disability to understand the structural and attitudinal barriers this group of children face throughout all aspects of child protection.

- Disabled children and young people face specific barriers to disclosing abuse and to having their abuse recognised.

- Disabled children and young people need practitioners to understand, listen, see and embrace all forms of their communication.

- Practitioners need to not lose sight of the child, their impairment or the abuse – disabled children need holistic understanding and responses which address the interplay of all three. Training, time and resources are needed to achieve quality child and family-centred practice.

INTRODUCTION

In England there are approximately 1.5 million children with special educational needs and disabilities (SEND) and .increasing numbers of children with complex needs (Department for Education (DfE), 2022). The term 'disabled children and young people' covers a wide range of impairments that will have differing impacts on a child and their daily lives. The Equality Act (2010) defines a person with a disability if they have a physical or mental impairment, and the impairment has a substantial and long-term adverse effect on a person's ability to carry out normal day-to-day activities.

In this chapter the term children is used for ease of reading to refer to any child or young person under the age of 18 years. The term 'disabled children and young people' is used to reflect the rights-based social model of disability which recognises that children with a wide range of impairments and/or additional needs face social, structural and attitudinal barriers which disable them. These barriers can directly impact on a child's well-being; lead to increased risks of isolation, exclusion, disempowerment and discrimination which can subsequently create vulnerability; and increase the risk of abuse and exploitation. In addition, such barriers also increase the chances that abuse will go unnoticed and not be addressed, and that responses from agencies are not always appropriate to meeting the child's, and their families, needs.

CLOSER LOOK: THE SOCIAL MODEL OF DISABILITY

The Social Model of Disability separates the impairment (the characteristics of a person's body or mind) from disabling barriers (the way society and individuals react to impairment). A disability rights perspective argues that it is not impairment that determines quality of life but attitudes and inequality. Within this perspective the preferred term is disabled children (which describes what society does to children with impairments – it disables them) rather than children with disabilities which defines a child by what their bodies and minds cannot do. Within the social model of disability, the word disability refers to oppression and disabling factors, and not to impairment.

(For further discussion of the social model of disability see work by Thomas, 2004; Connors and Stalker, 2007; Oliver, 2013).

189

Societal attitudes play a role in protection of disabled children from abuse. Historically the focus of child protection services has been nondisabled children. Over the past 20 years or so thinking has shifted; however, in working with disabled children practitioners can easily collude in accepting standards of support that would not be accepted for a nondisabled child. Despite the limited number of studies on disabled child protection in the UK, this chapter sets out what we can learn from research evidence about implementing child protection processes in ways that are accessible and meet the specific needs of this group of children and young people. Evidence on prevention, identification and responses is explored, thus covering all aspects of safeguarding and child protection of this group.

INCREASED RISK OF ABUSE AND EXPLOITATION FOR DISABLED CHILDREN AND YOUNG PEOPLE

She believes anything anyone tells her, if someone offered her a lift she would get in the car, if they had a dog in there, she would be straight in so she is vulnerable that way but I think because she reads loads, she speaks intellectually so people think she's quite old but she's quite young headed really. I do worry. They're not allowed to go anywhere.

Franklin et al. (2019b, p. 11)

Research suggests that disabled children and young people face a three- to fourfold increased risk of abuse compared to their nondisabled peers (Jones et al., 2012; Sullivan and Knutson, 2000). Evidence also indicates that disabled children and young people are overrepresented among children exposed to sexual and criminal exploitation, which may often be associated with 'county lines' (Home Office, 2018). Emerging evidence indicates neurodiverse children and children with learning disabilities are at particular risk from these forms of harm (Berlowitz et al., 2013; DfE, 2018; Franklin et al., 2015; Franklin et al., 2023). Attention has also been drawn to the increased prevalence of online bullying and abuse of disabled children and young people across all social media platforms (Katz and El Asam, 2020) and that disabled children are at a disproportionately higher risk of experiencing significant harm leading to a serious case review, particularly during adolescence (Brandon et al., 2020).

The reasons for these increased risks of abuse and neglect are complex and not well researched or understood (Jones et al., 2012: Leeb et al., 2012). However, increasingly attention is being drawn to the significant and disproportionate impact of austerity and cuts to services, with this having a high impact on this group of children who would be more likely to need and access service provision. In addition, a lack of early help and higher thresholds of support for families with disabled children has been shown to be a contributing factor (Franklin et al., 2022). These families can often face considerable caring responsibilities and without appropriate support can reach a crisis point. Higher levels of poverty (Contact, 2018) and of school exclusion (DfE, 2022) also disproportionately impact disabled children, increasing risk for this group. Some would argue that disablism plays a part throughout all of the discussed (Franklin et al., 2022). Disablism refers to discrimination or prejudice against disabled people.

One specific example of disablism can be seen in the fact that often disabled children and young people are relatively 'invisible' within statistics concerning child protection and children's social care more generally, due to a lack of recording of their disability. Disabled children and young people represent a significant minority of users of children's social care. This is partly due to specific recognition of their increased impairment and family support needs within the Children Act (1989). Evidence indicates, however, that disabled children are also significantly overrepresented within services designed to meet safeguarding needs. Government figures state that 55.9% of children who had been looked after continuously for 12 months (for whom data were available) had a special educational need (SEN) in 2018/19 with the most common type of need being 'Social, Emotional and Mental Health' (SEMH) (DfE, 2019). Disabled children also constitute a high proportion of children placed in residential schools and secure settings (Pinney, 2017), and evidence indicates that 14% of children experiencing incidents leading to Serious Case Reviews are disabled (Brandon et al., 2020). The reasons for these discrepancies remain poorly understood and underresearched (Stalker and MacArthur, 2012).

As mentioned previously, disabled children are significantly more likely to be excluded from school, often due to education provision not being made available to meet their needs, and subsequently become invisible to mainstream services (Martin-Denham, 2020). Or, if the child is known to mainstream services, they can be hidden in plain sight where their impairment-related needs are not recognised. This can often be linked to a lack of diagnosis or assessment of the child's needs, particularly in the case of learning disabilities and neurodiversity (Franklin et al., 2019a), and is exacerbated by the lack of recognition of these needs by practitioners who rarely receive adequate training to support them (Franklin et al., 2022). Such invisibility reduces the chances of signs and indicators of abuse being identified, and limits opportunities for disabled children to tell. Research has indicated that practitioners can often assume that disabled children are being protected by others or that a child will disclose abuse – as will be discussed later, this should not be assumed and can be especially challenging for this group of children (Franklin et al., 2022).

Despite their increased risk of experiencing abuse, disabled children's access to safeguarding and support at all stages of the child protection system has at best been described as patchy, but more often than not, criticised for being inadequate (Ofsted, 2012; Taylor et al., 2016). Research has highlighted that recognising and responding to abuse involving disabled children is often more complex and time consuming, and requires a greater long-term commitment of resources than that concerning nondisabled children (Kelly and Dowling, 2015; Taylor et al., 2016), which is not conducive within the current climate of austerity and service cuts in the UK.

Of course, all disabled children and young people are children with the same equal rights to protection as their nondisabled peers. Therefore all legislative requirements and practice guidelines on the protection of children equally apply to this group. However, the evidence suggests that the application of guidance appears patchy (National Working Group on Safeguarding Disabled Children, 2016) and, given the increased risks, more strategic priority and attention needs to be focused on better prevention, response and recovery (Franklin et al., 2022). In most cases, generic child protection guidance (such as DfE, 2018) highlights the increased risk for this group but rarely offers nuanced insight into how strategic and frontline practitioners can provide improved responses. Previously, specific guidance entitled *Safeguarding disabled children: practice guidance* (Department for Children, Schools and Families, 2009) had offered welcome focused attention for this group of children. However, this guidance was archived by the then Government, and despite sector-wide lobbying for a renewed version, thus far the English government has declined to reissue the guidance. Authors have argued that this needs to be a priority, alongside a much stronger evidence base on which to develop good practice (Franklin et al., 2022).

CLOSER LOOK: RIGHTS BASED APPROACH

As noted, research tells us that disabled children are more vulnerable to abuse than their nondisabled peers and our values, attitudes and assumptions have enormous influence on the way they are (or are not) protected and the way disabled children see themselves. Understanding the reasons why disabled children may be more vulnerable is critical to understanding how they can be better protected. Reasons for increased vulnerability include:

- receiving support services (including intimate care) from a number of different people,
- child becomes used to their body space being 'invaded',
- child receives little or no sex and relationship education,
- child spends a lot of time away from home, e.g. in short breaks or residential schools,
- child spends time in segregated services,
- child is targeted by perpetrators because they appear unlikely to complain successfully to others.

PREVENTION OF ABUSE OF DISABLED CHILDREN

No child is responsible for their own abuse, and a child cannot and should not be assumed to be able to prevent it. However, it is a rights-based issue if disabled children and young people are not taught about abuse, healthy and unhealthy relationships or inappropriate touch and not given accessible information about what to do if they feel unsafe. Such lack of attention in education and support in childhood can lead to lifelong vulnerability.

The case-study example in the text box illustrates the consequences of not talking to disabled young people about the potential dangers of abuse.

CASE STUDY 11A.1: 'TOM' (15)

Tom, a young man with autism aged 15 years, was sexually exploited by an older male who groomed him via Facebook. The older male told Tom that he loved him and wanted to be his boyfriend. He also told him that he was 18, when he was actually 37 years old. Tom explained that, because of his autism, he found it particularly challenging to understand why someone would lie to him and say something they did not mean: 'He said he loved me and wanted to be my boyfriend. Why would he say those things if he didn't mean them? I wanted a boyfriend, so why would I not have someone as my boyfriend who said he wanted to be my boyfriend?'

Tom said he did not tell his social worker, or any other professionals, that he was having a sexual relationship with an older male because no one asked him. When asked whether he would have told his social worker if she had asked him, Tom said he did not know because his older 'boyfriend' had told him that he must not tell anyone about their relationship as Tom would get into trouble: 'He said it was a secret... He said that lots of people thought that people with autism shouldn't have boyfriends, or girlfriends and that they would be angry with me if they knew I had a boyfriend' (Franklin et al., 2015, p. 42).

It is widely known that relationship and sex education (RSE) is poorly delivered to disabled children, either because it is not made accessible or they are denied it as disabled people are wrongly assumed to be asexual (Franklin et al., 2019b). Toft and Franklin (2020) drew attention to the specific needs of LGBTQIA+ disabled young people who had rarely received RSE that was meaningful and accessible to them. In the past social care and youth services may have filled this gap in formal education for disabled young people, whereby informal learning may have taken place through good relational based support. However, many disabled children are isolated and may not be able to have conversations or learn from their peers.

Missing out on important knowledge about safety and life skills leads to an increased level of vulnerability and is a risk factor which all practitioners should be aware of. However, teachers and social care/work practitioners often lack training and the skills and confidence to impart this information. Similarly, research funded by the NSPCC explored what support parents/carers needed to be able to talk about sexual abuse to their disabled children. This indicated that parents often felt unskilled and not adequately prepared to know how to have these conversations with their disabled child in meaningful and accessible ways. Recommendations from the parents/carers were to have the opportunity to work in partnership with practitioners to share knowledge and understanding in order to meet the needs of individual children (Franklin et al., 2019b).

IDENTIFICATION OF ABUSE – DISCLOSING AND DISCOVERY

Although all children face barriers to disclosing abuse, the previous section indicates that for this group of children in particular, additional barriers might exist (Jones et al., 2017). Miller and Brown (2014) highlighted how a disabled child may be isolated, have a limited friendship network or circle of trusted adults, and may feel particularly anxious that they will lose the support of those they depend on for their care and/or communication. Disabled children may not be able to use telephone/internet helplines to report abuse, when they feel in danger or to check information online which might support them. They may also be reliant on their abusers for communication or access to the means to communicate. Taylor et al. (2015) highlighted in their study that a lack of attention and access to suitably qualified British Sign Language (BSL) signers meant that a deaf child's abuser was sometimes called upon to sign for the child. Thus it becomes vitally important for practitioners to notice the child, keep them central and be attuned to their communication and possible expressions of distress (Franklin and Goff, 2018).

Numerous studies have highlighted how professionals may not be proficient in understanding how a child communicates distress, anxiety, pain and fear. Others point to practitioners misunderstanding what might be deemed 'challenging behaviour' or behaviours which have been labelled as 'risk-taking' and wrongly assigning this to an impairment rather than examining possible underlying causes, despite behaviour changes being a potential indicator of abuse/neglect (Franklin et al., 2015; Franklin and Smeaton, 2017; Miller and Brown, 2014). Taylor et al. (2015), who interviewed ten deaf and disabled young people and adults who had experienced abuse as children, illustrated starkly the invisibility of disabled children to services and the tendency for disclosures of abuse to be ignored or discounted. Other studies have shown that when disclosures occur, disabled children are less likely to be believed (Hershkowitz et al., 2007; Kvam, 2004;), such notions being bound up in misconceptions that abuse does not happen to this group of children and/or that disabled children are unreliable and 'make-up stories' (Franklin et al., 2015).

Research has also indicated that practitioners apply higher thresholds to disabled children for safeguarding referrals, which may account for the underrepresentation of disabled children within child protection services (Brandon et al., 2011; Ofsted, 2012; Taylor et al., 2014). Further barriers to making child protection referrals, raised by practitioners, include a lack of confidence and skills communicating with disabled children about abuse and neglect and an associated fear of getting it wrong (Prynallt-Jones et al., 2018; Taylor et al 2014).

Evidence indicates that the protection of disabled children can also lead to polarised responses whereby risks of abuse are either dismissed, leaving children unprotected, or are used to justify disproportionate restrictive measures. These can deny disabled young people autonomy and freedoms that would not be denied to their nondisabled peers, instead of empowering them with knowledge and support (Franklin et al., 2015).

Responses: Working Directly with Disabled Children and Young People

Evidence has shown that there needs to be significant improvements in direct practice with disabled children and young people (Franklin et al., 2022; Jones et al., 2017; Taylor et al., 2015, 2016). For nearly two decades commentators have flagged concerns about the limited training available for social workers who work with disabled children (Morris, 2005). Prynallt-Jones et al. (2018) highlight the lack of attention to disabled child protection in social work degree courses, and others draw attention to the limited access to continued professional development courses due to budgetary constraints for local authorities (Ofsted, 2012). This means that a lack of awareness of disabled children's heightened vulnerability to abuse remains, with many practitioners lacking confidence, knowledge and appropriate skills to meet the specific needs of the group. Of particular concern, noted in a few studies were disablist attitudes permeating within the child protection system which, without training and focus, could remain unchallenged (Franklin et al., 2022).

Specific attention has been drawn to the need for improved communication skills amongst workers so that support can be more effective, targeted and accessible. Statutory legal and policy guidance requires communicating directly with children, including those with learning disabilities and/or complex communication needs. This is an obligation enforced by the Children Acts (1989, 2004), Working Together Guidance (DfE, 2018) and the Children and Families Act (2014). These outline the necessity for children's views to inform assessment alongside the views of their family. Such rights to expression of views and involvement and influence in decision-making in their own lives is enshrined in United Nations Rights Treaties such as on the Rights of the Child (UN, 1989) and of Persons with Disabilities (UN, 2006).

Despite disabled children's rights to be involved in decision making, the Munro review of child protection (Munro, 2011) highlighted that there continues to be a lack of relationship-based practice between social workers and children which can significantly increase risks to children. For children who require additional support concerning their communication and/or understanding of information and processes, relationships built on trust is vital. Prynallt-Jones et al. (2018) highlight the proliferation of desk-based risk-assessment tools and argued that these forms distract from meaningful direct social work activities particularly with children. The result of which means that the needs of children become 'decontextualized, processed and over-simplified whilst good relationships and communication are undermined' (Prynallt-Jones, 2018, p. 96). They also highlight the challenges of safeguarding assessment processes which have a legal timescale. It is of course important to protect children with necessary urgency. However, this can limit quality time for a social worker to appropriately engage with disabled children, a group needing more time to communicate and build trust (Prynallt-Jones et al., 2018), and to process their experiences and the system in which they find themselves.

The lack of relationship-based practice is exacerbated for disabled children who may be isolated, more likely to be living away from home and/or dependent on a small number of care givers and communication facilitators. Practitioners may need to be challenged on overt/covert assumptions that disabled children are not capable of understanding or expressing their views (Franklin and Sloper, 2009). The work of Taylor et al. (2016) highlighted specific issues of discrimination against disabled children. Although disabled children are still children, such practice fails to take account for the impact of impairment and structural and attitudinal barriers which impact disabled childrens' daily lives.

Examples of practitioners undertaking good disabled child-centred work do exist, although there has been little investment in evaluating practice and understanding what interventions work for whom and when (Franklin et al., 2022). With the available resourcing and time, workers can adapt practice to make it accessible. In particular, referring disabled children to advocacy services or ensuring that they have access to British Sign Language signers can make a significant impact on the quality of response a child receives (Franklin and Knight, 2011; Greenaway-Clarke, 2020). While some children may have limited verbal communication, they can successfully communicate using nonverbal and adapted means of communication such as Makaton, symbols, objects of reference, gestures, noises or glances. Working in partnership with others who understand such communication can aid social workers who will often lack training in these methods (Franklin and Sloper, 2009). A lack of investment in communication methods hampers attempts to support children to communicate about abuse or report if they feel in danger.

Evidence indicates that what promotes positive practice is not seeing disabled children as a homogenous group, but instead identifying and meeting the individual needs of the child. Children who communicate nonverbally, or whose behaviour may often be defined as 'challenging', are dependent on professionals spending time with them, understanding their often nuanced, individualised communication methods. Of equal importance is practitioners observing a child in multiple environments and at different times of the day in order to determine any changes in behaviour (Greenaway-Clarke, 2020). Greenaway-Clarke (2020) highlights the important role that advocates can play in seeking the 'voice' of disabled children, and in particularly those with complex communication needs. Independent advocates can often notice and draw attention when there are concerns regarding child protection, although of course advocates perform an entirely different role from that of a child protection practitioner. Child-centred work, which platforms the importance of a child's communication, has been shown to significantly improve assessment processes, build trust, and lead to more holistic assessments and meaningful, effective responses and support.

Responses: Working with Families of Disabled Children and Young People

A number of studies, and serious case reviews have indicated that practitioners can sometimes overempathise with parents/carers of disabled children, assuming they are doing their best in 'difficult circumstances' (Taylor et al., 2016). This is problematic as it can lead to losing sight of the child, marginalising their experiences and an overreliance on parents/carer accounts without seeking the child's views. Conversely, parents/carers of autistic young people in a recent study of child sexual exploitation reported that they often felt blamed by agencies for their child's exploitation, and for not better protecting their child, even though their child have been coerced and control by criminal gangs and highly sophisticated criminal activities (Franklin et al., 2023). Parents in this study spoke at length about their desperation for support from agencies to protect their child, and the wider family, from the criminal targeting of their child (Franklin et al., 2023). Although there is a limited evidence base from which to draw conclusions about what works when working with families of disabled children who have experienced forms of abuse, the importance of communication, involvement in decision-making and a multiagency approach have been highlighted (Franklin et al., 2022).

Responses: Importance of Multiagency Working

Given the often complex needs of this group of children, the importance of multiagency working cannot be underestimated. Liaising with other agencies, particularly those who can facilitate and support direct communication with the child, is vital. Studies have also shown the importance that disabled children place on workers such as advocates, signers, interpreters and specialist IDVAS (independent domestic violence advisors) (Franklin et al., 2015; 2019a).

From the limited research evidence base that exists in the UK, what can be deduced is a vital need for practitioners to not lose sight of the child, their impairment or their abuse. The sharing of information across multiagency services is crucial in creating and holding a holistic understanding of the child's needs regarding their impairment-related needs, risk of abuse and child protection concerns. Disabled children can often fall through the cracks whereby complacency creeps in and assumptions made that these children are being served by other agencies. What is commonly reported in studies, however, is that disability and child protection services can work in silos with both feeling ill-formed and untrained in each other's 'specialism'. Direct communication with disabled children, and their families, is important, but it requires time, a multiagency approach and, importantly, resources.

Once in the care system, disabled children are much more likely to experience placement instability or be placed in residential care than their nondisabled peers, again increasing their potential to become 'invisible' in systems (Kelly et al., 2016). They are also less likely to have access to appropriate therapeutic and mental health support to aid their recovery from abuse (Kelly et al., 2016). Thus the need for ongoing multiagency support for disabled children and young people in the child protection system is evident.

WHAT DISABLED CHILDREN AND YOUNG PEOPLE SEE AS POSITIVE PRACTICE WHICH WILL AID THEIR RECOVERY AND SURVIVORSHIP

A few studies have sought the views of disabled children about the support they have received following abuse. These have found broadly similar findings: disabled children define positive practice in terms of having someone to talk to, someone they can trust, someone who is interested in them as a person not just a victim (Franklin et al., 2019a; Franklin and Smeaton, 2018; Goff and Franklin, 2019).

CONCLUSION

In conclusion, this chapter raises several questions for child protection practice and some reflection points for consideration. These are posed in the context of understanding that for this to be enacted, resources, focus and time must be provided to those on the frontline.

REFLECTIVE QUESTIONS

- Have child protection workers received adequate training in the protection of disabled children and young people? Can they access research evidence to improve their practice?
- Are social workers given the time and resources to directly work with disabled children and, as is required, seek their views, experiences and 'voices' to inform decision-making?
- Do disabled children have access to advocacy or the support of others to enable them to express their views?
- Does your practice seek to empower disabled children and provide them with a professional whom they can trust and communicate with?
- Does your own work/service recognise all forms of communication, see that 'behaviour' is often

a form of communication, and recognise possible signs and indicators of abuse in disabled children?

■ Does your own practice/service recognise the intersectional, individual needs of disabled children and not see disabled children as a homogenous group?

■ Does your practice/service recognise the impact of disablism and other forms of discrimination that affect this group and can increase their vulnerability to abuse?

■ Does your service inadvertently render disabled children invisible?

REFERENCES

Berelowitz, S., Clifton, J., Firimin, C., Gulyurtlu, S., Edwards, G., 2013. "If only someone had listened." Office of the Children's Commissioner's Inquiry into Child Sexual Exploitation in Gangs and Groups. Office of the Children's Commissioner, London.

Brandon, M., Sidebotham, P., Ellis, C., Bailey, S., Belderson, P., 2011. Child and family practitioners understanding of child development: Lessons from a small sample of serious case reviews. Research Report DFE-RR110.

Brandon, M., Sidebotham, P., Belderson, P., Cleaver, H., Dickens, J., Garstang, J., et al., 2020. Complexity and Challenge: A Triennial Analysis of SCRs 2014-2017 Final Report. University of East Anglia & University of Warwick, Department for Education.

Children Act (1989). The Stationery Office, London. https://www.legislation.gov.uk/ukpga/1989/41/contents.

Children Act (2004). The Stationery Office, London.

Children and Families Act (2014). The Stationery Office, London.

Connors, C., Stalker, K., 2007. Children's experiences of disability: pointers to a social model of childhood disability. Disabil Soc. 22 (1), 19–33. https://doi.org/10.1080/09687590601056162.

Contact, 2018. Counting the costs: Research into the Finances of more than 2,700 Families Across the UK in 2018. Contact, London.

Department for Children, Schools and Families, 2009. Safeguarding Disabled Children: Practice Guidance. DCSF, London.

Department for Education, 2018. Working Together to Safeguard Children: A guide to inter-agency working to safeguard and promote the welfare of children. HMSO, London.

Department for Education, 2019. Children Looked After in England Including Adoption: 2018 to 2019. Department for Education, London. https://assets.publishing.service.gov.uk/government/uploads/system/uploads/attachment_data/file/850306/Children_looked_after_in_England_2019_Text.pdf.

Department for Education, 2022. Special Educational Needs and Disability: An Analysis and Summary of Data Sources. Department for Education, London. https://assets.publishing.

service.gov.uk/government/uploads/system/uploads/attachment_data/file/1082518/Special_educational_needs_publication_June_2022.pdf. (Accessed 7 July 2022).

Equality Act (2010). The Stationery Office, London. https://www.legislation.gov.uk/ukpga/2010/15/contents.

Franklin, A., Sloper, P., 2009. Supporting the participation of disabled children and young people in decision-making. Child. Soc. 23 (1), 3–15.

Franklin, A., Knight, A., 2011. Someone on Our Side: Advocacy for Disabled Children and Young People. The Children's Society, London.

Franklin, A., Raws, P., Smeaton, E., 2015. Unprotected, Overprotected: Meeting the Needs of Young People With Learning Disabilities Who Experience, or Are at Risk of, Sexual Exploitation. https://www.pkc.gov.uk/media/39938/Unprotected-Overprotected-Report/pdf/Unprotected__Overprotected_Report.

Franklin, A., Smeaton, E., 2017. 'Recognising and responding to young people with learning disabilities who experience, or are at risk of, child sexual exploitation in the UK'. Child. Youth Serv. Rev. 73, 474–481.

Franklin, A., Goff, S., 2018. Listening and facilitating all forms of communication: disabled children and young people in residential care in England, Child Care in Practice 25. https://doi.org/10.1080/13575279.2018.1521383.

Franklin, A., Smeaton, E., 2018. 'Listening to young people with learning disabilities who have experienced, or are at risk of, child sexual exploitation in the UK.' Child Soc. 32 (2), 98–109.

Franklin, A., Bradley, L., Brady, G., 2019a. Effectiveness of services for sexually abused children and young people. Report 3: Perspectives of service users with learning difficulties or experience of care. https://www.csacentre.org.uk/documents/effectiveness-learning-difficulties-care/. (Accessed 5 October 2023).

Franklin, A., Toft, A., Goff, S., 2019b. Parents' and Carers' Views on How We Can Work Together to Prevent the Sexual Abuse of Disabled Children. NSPCC, London. https://www.csacentre.org.uk/documents/effectiveness-learning-difficulties-care/. (Accessed 5 October 2023).

Franklin, A., Toft, A., Hernon, J., Greenaway-Clarke, J., Goff, S., 2022. UK Social Work Practice in Safeguarding Disabled Children and Young People: From the Perspectives of Disabled Children, Parents/Carers and Practitioners. A Qualitative Systematic Review. What Works in Children's Social Care, London.

Franklin, A., Bradley, L., Greenaway-Clarke, J., Goff, S., 2023. Internal Trafficking and Exploitation of Children and Young People with Special Educational Needs and Disabilities (SEND) within England and Wales: Understanding Identification and Responses to Inform Effective Policy and Practice. Modern Slavery Policy and Evidence Centre, London.

Goff, S., Franklin, A., 2019. We Matter Too: Disabled Young People's Experience of Services and Responses When They Experience Domestic Abuse. Ann Craft Trust, Nottingham. https://www.anncrafttrust.org/wp-content/uploads/2019/12/We-Matter-Too-Final-Report-9-Dec-2019.pdf.

Greenaway-Clarke, J., 2020. Advocacy and 'Non-Instructed' Advocacy with Disabled Children and Young People with Complex Communication Needs. Doctoral Thesis. University of Portsmouth. https://ethos.bl.uk/OrderDetails. do?did=1&uin=uk.bl.ethos.820414.

Hershkowitz, I., Lamb, M.E., Horowitz, D., 2007. Victimization of children with disabilities. Am. J. Orthopsychiatry 77, 629–635. https://doi.org/10.1037/0002-9432.77.4.629.

Home Office, 2018. Criminal Exploitation of Children and Vulnerable Adults: County Lines Guidance. The Home Office, London.

Jones, C., Stalker, K., Franklin, A., Fry, D., Cameron, A., Taylor, J., 2017. "Enablers of help-seeking for deaf and disabled children following abuse and barriers to protection: A qualitative study." Child Fam. Soc. Work 22 (2), 762–771.

Jones, L., Bellis, M.A., Wood, S., Hughes, K., McCoy, E., Eckley, L., et al., 2012. Prevalence and risk of violence against children with disabilities: A systematic review and meta-analysis of observational studies. The Lancet 380, 899–907. https://doi. org/10.1016/S0140-6736(12)60692_8.

Katz, A., El Asam, A., 2020. Vulnerable Children in a Digital World. Internet Matters, London.

Kelly, B., Dowling, S., 2015. Safeguarding Disabled Children and Young People: A Scoping Exercise of Statutory Child Protection Services for Disabled Children and Young People in Northern Ireland. Queens University, Belfast.

Kelly, B., Dowling, S., Winter, K., 2016. Profiling the Population of Disabled Looked After Children and Young People in Northern Ireland. OFMDFM & QUB, Belfast.

Kvam, M.H., 2004. Sexual abuse of deaf children. A retrospective analysis of the prevalence and characteristics of childhood sexual abuse among deaf adults in Norway. Child Abuse Negl. 28, 241–251. https://doi.org/10.1016/j. chiabu.2003.09.017.

Leeb, R., Bitsko, R., Merrick, R., Armour, B., 2012. Does childhood disability increase risk for child abuse and neglect? J. Ment. Health Res. Intellect. Disabil. 5, 4–31.

Martin-Denham, S., 2020. An investigation into the perceived enablers and barriers to mainstream schooling: The voices of children excluded from school, their caregivers and professionals. Project Report. University of Sunderland, Sunderland. http://sure.sunderland.ac.uk/id/eprint/11941.

Miller, D., Brown, J., 2014. "We have the right to be safe": Protecting Disabled Children From Abuse. NSPCC, London.

Morris, J., 2005. Children on the Edge of Care: Human Rights and the Children Act. United Kingdom. Joseph Roundtree Foundation, London.

Munro, E., 2011. Munro Review of Child Protection: A Child-Centred System. Department for Education, London.

National Working Group on Safeguarding Disabled Children, 2016. Safeguarding disabled children in England: How local safeguarding children boards are delivering against Ofsted requirements to protect disabled children: Findings from a national survey. NSPCC, London. https://learning.nspcc.org.uk/ research-resources/2016/safeguarding-disabled-children-england.

Ofsted, 2012. Protecting Disabled Children: Thematic Inspection. https://assets.publishing.service.gov.uk/government/uploads/ system/uploads/attachment_data/file/419062/Protecting_ disabled_children.pdf.

Oliver, M., 2013. The social model of disability: Thirty years on. Disabil Soc. 28 (7), 1024–1026. https://doi.org/10.1080/0968759 9.2013.818773.

Pinney, A., 2017. Understanding the needs of disabled children with complex needs or life-limiting conditions. What can we learn from national data? Exploratory analysis commissioned by the Council for Disabled Children and the True Colours Trust. Council for Disabled Children and the True Colours Trust, London.

Prynallt-Jones, K.A., Carey, M., Doherty, P., 2018. Barriers facing social workers undertaking direct work with children and young people with a learning disability who communicate using non-verbal methods. Br. J. Soc. Work 48 (1), 88–105. https://doi. org/10.1093/bjsw/bcx004.

Stalker, K., McArthur, K., 2012. Child abuse, child protection and disabled children and child protection: A review of recent research. Child Abus. Rev. 21, 24–40 (2012). https://doi. org/10.1002/car.1154.

Sullivan, P.M., Knutson, J.F., 2000. Maltreatment and disabilities: A population-based epidemiological study. Child Abuse Negl. 24, 1257–1273 10.

Taylor, J., Stalker, K., Fry, D., Stewart, A., 2014. Disabled Children and Child Protection in Scotland: An investigation into the relationship between professional practice, child protection and disability. Scottish Government, Edinburgh. https://core.ac.uk/ display/19609940?source=2.

Taylor, J., Cameron, A., Jones, C., Franklin, A., Stalker, K., Fry, D., 2015. Deaf and Disabled Children Talking About Child Protection. NSPCC, London. https://library.nspcc.org.uk/ HeritageScripts/Hapi.dll/filetransfer/2015DeafAndDisabledChil drenTalkingAboutChildProtection.pdf.

Taylor, J., Stalker, K., Stewart, A., 2016. 'Disabled children and the child protection system: A cause for concern.' Child Abus. Rev. 25 (1), 60–73.

Thomas, C., 2004. Disability and impairment. In: Swain, J., French, S., Thomas, C., Barnes, C. (Eds.), Disabling Barriers, Enabling Environments, second ed. Sage, London.

Toft, A., Franklin, A., 2020. Towards expansive and inclusive relationship and sex education: Young disabled LGBT+ people's ideas for change. In: Toft, A. and Franklin, A. (Eds), Young Disabled and LGTB+: Voices, Intersections, Identities. Routledge, London.

United Nations, 1989. United Nations Convention on the Rights of the Child. United Nations, Geneva.

United Nations, 2006. United Nations Convention on the Rights of Persons with Disability. United Nations, New York.

11b

BEING A LOOKED AFTER CHILD

ROBIN SEN

KEY POINTS

- What being a 'Looked after Child', means legally and how this links to issues of child protection and safeguarding.
- A critical overview of the numbers and official reasons due to which children and young people become looked after.
- The vulnerabilities that looked after children may have arising from their enhanced needs, and the implications of these for practitioners who are supporting them.
- An illustration of work that may be undertaken with a Looked after Child to support their well-being.

INTRODUCTION

Looked after children are amongst the most vulnerable groups of children and young people in terms of their needs and consequent support issues. The decisions and practice which professionals take can have significant, sometimes life-long, influence on their well-being. This chapter considers what a Looked after Child means legally and how this status links to issues of child protection and safeguarding. It provides an overview of current care numbers in England and the official reasons as to why children and young people become looked after, inviting readers to reflect critically on these. A case study is used to illustrate particular aspects of work that may be undertaken with a child in care.

LOOKED AFTER CHILDREN – CONTEXT AND OVERVIEW

When children and young people under 18 years become 'looked after', they are formally in the care of the state under English law. They will be cared for in one of three placement types – foster care, formal kinship care or a residential placement. Children and young people become looked after when their parents are unavailable to provide appropriate care or when, in the judgement of professionals and the family court, welfare issues are too considerable for them continue to live in the full-time care of their birth parents. Children and young people become looked after via a so-called 'voluntary' agreement with a parent's consent (s.20, Children Act, 1989), or via a court order which mandates that this should happen. In either case, the state has enhanced legal responsibilities, as corporate parent, to protect and promote their welfare. Legislative provisions also suggest professionals should seek to explore other viable caring arrangements outside the formal care system, as well as formal kinship care, before children are placed in state care with previously unknown carers – there is mixed evidence on whether they do so.

On 31 March 2022, there were officially 82, 170 looked after children in England, (Department for Education (DfE), 2022). In Northern Ireland, Scotland and Wales there were, altogether, another 20,000 children and young people in care. In England, the numbers in care have been increasing in most years since the early 2000s and currently stand at a 30-year high.

It is not clear exactly why this is, but austerity-led cuts to family support services, the ongoing impact of the Peter Connelly case in making child-protection practice more risk adverse, and a more overtly child protectionist direction in Government discourse and policy since 2010 are all likely influences (Sen and Webb, 2019). The numbers and proportions of children in care in Northern Ireland, Scotland and Wales have also generally been rising during the same period.

Each year around 40% of children in care will also leave it – the main routes for them to do so are via 'ageing out' of care on approaching or attaining adulthood, returning to birth family care, or leaving for long-term substitute care outside the care system via adoption, a Child Arrangement Order or Special Guardianship. For those who stay in the care system, there is some stability of placements: around a quarter of all looked after children will be in placements which have lasted 2 years or more (Sinclair et al., 2007). However, a large proportion of care placements intended to be long-term will not last as long as intended: the chances of placement breakdown increase with age, and particularly with the manifestation of marked emotional and behavioural issues in adolescence (Sinclair, et al., 2007).

Table 11b.1 shows the principal recorded reasons, collated by the Department for Education (DfE, 2022), due to which children and young people enter care.

It can be seen that by far, the largest principal official reason is 'abuse or neglect'. This sometimes gets shortened to a statement that most children and young people are in care *due to* or *because of* abuse and neglect. Such statements are worth exploring. Research confirms that 'abuse or neglect' has been a factor in the lives of most children and young people who enter the care system (e.g. Sinclair et al., 2007; Wade et al., 2011). But it is also worth noting that social workers can only record one official 'principal' reason due to which a child or young person is placed in care, and the label of 'abuse or neglect' covers a large range of different circumstances. This fact also helps explain why 'low income' does not feature in the data as a principal reason for entry into care, even though it is well known that poorer children and young people are far more likely to enter care than those in better off households (Morris et al., 2018). Living in poverty is far from synonymous with the absence of good parenting, but it

TABLE 11B.1	
Principal Reasons Why Children and Young People Enter Care	
Principal reason	**%[a]**
Abuse or neglect	66
Family dysfunction	13
Family in acute stress	7
Absent parenting	7
Parent's illness or disability	3
Child's disability	2
Socially unacceptable behaviour	1
Low income	0

[a]Sums to 99% due to rounding effects.
From DfE, 2022

is known that parenting in communities which are less well resourced, in families which have less social support, and in poor quality or insecure housing is a lot harder (Ghate and Hazel, 2002). Therefore, while the Government data appear to provide a clear summary of the key reasons due to which children and young people enter care, they mask a complex interplay of factors.

CLOSER LOOK: JAZ AND ZACH, PART ONE

This chapter will consider Jaz (aged 13 at this point) and Zach (aged 8 at this point). They are full siblings who have recently become looked after following the family court's granting of an Interim Care Order in respect of their care. Their mother, Anita, is of second-generation Bangladeshi ethnicity and has a mild learning disability. Their father, Andrew, is White British. Safeguarding concerns for the children arose from repeated domestic violence between Anita and Andrew, and the impact it was having on the children, as well as concerns about the heavy alcohol misuse of both parents. The violence was sometimes bidirectional and the parents' relationship highly volatile, but professionals believed that Andrew was the primary instigator. The violence gave rise to concerns about their emotional well-being, as well as potentially their physical welfare. The family social worker had made a referral to a domestic violence support group for Anita and to a group work programme for fathers who have been domestically violent for Andrew. However, there were extensive waiting lists for each, and neither parent had started to access them. The social worker had also started to undertake direct work with Jaz and Zach around their wishes and feelings about what was happening in their home. During this time, there was a serious further incident of violence during which Andrew was seriously injured by a knife during a drunken argument involving Andrew, Anita and their next-door neighbour. It is as yet unclear exactly how Andrew was stabbed: the police have interviewed Anita and the neighbour under caution and are continuing their inquiries. Andrew remains stable in hospital. Both children were at home when the incident occurred.

Following this incident, children's services applied for an Interim Care Order to place the children in care. The parents are on low income – Anita and Andrew both work casually and intermittently in poorly paid service sector jobs – and the family home is poor quality social housing in a community known for high levels of social deprivation. Anita had also reported the family were subject to racial harassment from their next door neighbour. Prior to the children's entry to care, Anita had asked for a change of tenancy, but the local authority Housing Officer had refused the request, stating that the family were classed as antisocial tenants themselves due to numerous complaints about the noise and disturbance coming from the family home and rent arrears.

1. Consider the situation of Jaz and Zach – if you were the social worker, what principal reason would you identify due to which they were entered into state care?
2. Which other reasons might you also have chosen, and why would you choose the one you did as the principal one rather than this one?
3. What unmet needs for support might the family have had? If these additional supports had been provided, might the children's entry into state care have been averted ?

LOOKED AFTER CHILDREN – 'VULNERABILITIES' ARISING FROM ENHANCED NEEDS

Certain factors suggest looked after children as having greater vulnerabilities in their lives than their peers. The first is that, by definition, they are not in the care of their birth families and that means that they require additional protections. In the UK this includes legal duties on local authorities to ensure social workers visit children and young people in their placements at set intervals and to periodically review their care at review meetings. The accounts of some prominent care experienced adults, as well as abuse inquiries, illustrate why such additional protections are in place: time in care can be marked by a lack of emotional warmth and denial of a child's cultural heritage (Sissay, 2020), or

destabilised by large numbers of multiple placement moves (Ashcroft, 2013).

Children and young people in care may experience abuse or maltreatment from anyone associated with the placement setting, the wider community, birth family members and from peers in and outside the placement. Each of the different types of maltreatment – neglect, emotional abuse, physical abuse and sexual abuse – may occur when children and young people are in care (Biehal, 2014; Sen et al., 2008). Young people in care, particularly those in residential care, are also at heightened risk of child sexual exploitation (CSE) (Sen, 2017). This is partly because some young people become looked after due to concerns about their sexual exploitation, and being subject to such abuse increases the chance of revictimization. Additionally, some perpetrators may specifically target young people in care, particularly those living in residential homes, due to their perceived vulnerability (Sen, 2017). Greater focus has been given in recent years to children and young people's internet use as a vehicle for abuse, with concerns about the experiences of young people in care prominent within this (Sen, 2016). This abuse can occur directly via the online engagement itself, the online engagement can act as a precursor to offline abuse, or both may co-exist where the online abuse typically underpins and amplifies the offline abuse, including that from peers (Sen, 2016; 2017). Not all maltreatment is the same, and responses to it need to be sensitive to this fact – the impact on a child or young person will be influenced by the type of abuse, its severity and its duration, as well as the support that is available to the child and/or young person afterwards. At the more severe end, however, it is important to recognise that there are life-long impacts from experiencing abuse within the care system (Carr et al., 2019).

In discussing abuse and maltreatment in the care system, it should be noted many carers do provide excellent care, and there is need to balance the desire to keep children and young people in care safe with an acceptance that their engagement in age-appropriate activities is important too. 'Risk' is inherent in life, and it must be managed through judgement. There are, quite correctly, additional systems of protection for children and young people in care due to the fact they are living away from their families. However, overly restrictive practices can be stigmatising and unduly hinder children and young people's engagement in activities that are valued, developmental or simply enjoyable. Where an allegation or any other indication of abuse arises, it is important that it is taken very seriously, but that professionals avoid jumping to conclusions too early, either way. It is known that abuse exists in the care system but also that unfounded allegations against carers and others may sometimes be made (Biehal, 2014). Professional curiosity, sensitivity and judgement is needed while any potential abuse is being explored.

Prevalence data on abuse in care are hard to establish, due to the hidden nature of abuse, the weaknesses in recording systems, and the differences between allegations of abuse and confirmed abuse – an unconfirmed allegation not being the same as an unfounded allegation which is, in turn, potentially different from a knowingly false allegation. While severe abuse does occur in care settings (Sen et al., 2008), issues around poor or inadequate standards of care are more likely occurrences than more serious abuse (Biehal, 2014). Biehal's (2014) evidence review of maltreatment in foster care highlights that there are very varied rates of allegations and confirmed allegations of abuse in foster care by individual research studies, within and between countries. The review does report that foster carers are substantially more likely to be subject to allegations of maltreatment than parents in the general population. Biehal (2014) notes the potential reasons for confirmed abuse by foster carers may include that some carers struggle to respond appropriately to challenging behaviour by children and young people in their care, and that there are also some foster carers in the role who are unsuitable for fostering. Biehal (2014) also noted that allegations against foster carers may be more likely as they are under more scrutiny, and that unfounded allegations may be made against carers by children and young people in their care, as well as birth family members.

Strategies to minimise the chances of abuse in care occurring are focused on carers and the organisational practices surrounding them, whether that be fostering, kinship or residential care. Effective carer assessment and vetting at recruitment stage, and effective training and support for carers in their caring roles are emphasised (Sen et al., 2008). A number of fostering agencies promote 'safer caring' strategies whereby potential risk situations within the foster family are explicitly identified and discussed by the supervising social worker with the family and solutions to managing them articulated. For example, a safer caring plan might outline expected household practices around touch, expression of affection, privacy, health and safety issues, internet use and care arrangements when the main carers are not there.

In terms of identifying abuse where it is occurring, the need for clear whistleblowing procedures for other carers and professionals and complaints procedures for children and young people has been noted (Sen et al., 2008). It must also be acknowledged that the dynamics of child abuse and CSE mean children and young people may struggle to speak out at these times. The most important protective factor, therefore, is professionals who take a caring interest in a child or young person. Establishing trusting, consistent and warm relationships with children and young people is a mechanism for supporting them more broadly, but also means they have trusted people to whom they can speak to about things that are bothering them (Sen, 2018). It is important to recognise, however, that age or communication difficulties mean some children and young people will be unable to communicate about abuse directly and others, who could, may still struggle to do so. Professionals taking the time to notice changes of mood, behaviour or presentation and sensitively exploring these with a child and young person and those who see them regularly is central, therefore. Again, it is important for professionals to avoid jumping to quick assumptions about what may underlie any perceived changes.

MENTAL HEALTH, EDUCATION AND LEAVING CARE

Looked after children also have several other characteristics which give rise to potential enhanced vulnerabilities. It is known that as a group they have consistently higher rates of diagnosable 'mental disorders' (to use psychiatric discourse) as well as poorer mental well-being more broadly. The most comprehensive survey to date suggested these rates were around five times greater for children and young people in care in England than for their peers in the general population (Meltzer et al., 2003). Practitioners should therefore be aware of the potential need for enhanced mental health support for looked after children, while combining this with an awareness of the stigmatising effects that applying a label of 'mental disorder' can sometimes have. Where there is marked mental distress, the provision of appropriate intensive specialist therapeutic support will be required. Where the difficulties are less marked, then efforts to find, or maintain, the supports of a settled, caring placement, and a stable educational setting, will often be the best initial response.

Another area of potential vulnerability is poor educational attainment – this has obvious implications in terms of later employability, earning potential and well-being. Over half of young people in the general population gain 5 GCSEs at grades A to C, but less than 15% of young people in care do so. Around half the general population of young people now go on to higher education, but less than 10% of those who have been in care do so as young people (Sen, 2018). A less pessimistic picture emerges if the comparison is made with those peers who are in 'similar' circumstances. For example, Sebba et al. (2015) found young people in care for more than a year attained better results educationally than those in care for less than a year, or those living at home with social work support. While there is much more progress to be made, this does positively suggest that policy reforms and practice centred on prioritising looked after children's educational needs are having some effect. The key points that emerge for practitioners are of having high, but realistic, expectations of children and young people's educational attainment, and of ensuring that additional educational support is provided in good time where needed.

After leaving the care system it is known that care leavers are statistically considerably more likely than their peers to be involved in the criminal justice system, have mental health difficulties, become homeless and become teenage parents (National Audit Office, 2016). A number of those ageing out of care will also struggle with unemployment, social isolation and substance misuse (Sen, 2018). Broad brush descriptions such as these sound very pessimistic and do mask substantial variation in trajectories and change over time for individual care leavers. A number of care leavers will go on to do very well in their lives, some after initially struggling on leaving care (Stein, 2012). Equally, current data provide a stark reminder of the enduring difficulties a majority of care leavers face on formally leaving state care. Those who struggle the most are more likely to have had multiple placement moves and

to have lacked significant enduring positive relationships (Stein, 2012). Recent policy reform has attempted to address the poor outcomes for care leavers – the Children and Social Work Act (2017) extended local authority duties to provide transitional care to all care leavers until the age of 25, regardless of whether they are in education or training. The 'Staying Put' scheme also gives young people in foster care in England the right to stay in their placements, with the agreement of their carers, until the age of 21. However, there are ongoing gaps. While all local authorities now have a legal duty to provide 'support' until the age of 25 years, the nature of that support is ill-defined in law, meaning there is substantial variation between, and sometimes within, local authorities as to its provision (Field et al., 2021). The Staying Put scheme is also not available to those in residential care in England and is unlikely to be available to those with more difficult relationships with their foster carers.

CLOSER LOOK: THINKING CRITICALLY ABOUT VULNERABILITY

The label of vulnerability is not one that many looked after children apply to themselves – it is instead typically one applied to them by others. This can be illustrated by considering two studies. The first was a study of young women in a secure residential unit (Ellis, 2019). Those placed in the unit due to CSE were often labelled as 'vulnerable' by professionals working with them. Yet the young women themselves rejected that label, finding it to be patronising. They viewed themselves as being in control of their lives and making choices to do the best they could for themselves. The second study considered care-experienced young people's use of mobile phones and social media via the internet (Sen, 2016). Much discourse has highlighted the heightened risks and 'vulnerabilities' which may apply to care-experienced young people's digital media usage. Indeed, young people in this study did recount instances of distressing online engagement, mainly via forms of 'cyber-bullying'. Yet, they also did not see themselves as more vulnerable than other young people in respect of their digital media usage and emphasised that they felt able to manage those distressing situations themselves. As one young person in foster care said in a research interview: 'I feel in control every time. If I ever had any problems I would just tell my foster mum' (Sen, 2016, p. 1071).

While it is important to be aware of the potential vulnerabilities which children and young people in care may have, these examples help illustrate how a label of vulnerability can be rejected by them, because it carries an implication that a person is less able to look after themselves than others. It is therefore important to combine awareness of looked after children's potential additional support needs with a sensitivity to the fact that the label of vulnerability may be unwanted, and sometimes unhelpful. Acknowledging a Looked after Child's strengths, alongside any vulnerabilities, and engaging and respecting their own perspectives of their situation is a balance which practitioners should strive to achieve.

Thinking back to Jaz and Zach, for each of them list
- potential strengths,
- potential vulnerabilities and
- how you might age-appropriately engage their views of their own situations.

WORKING WITH LOOKED AFTER CHILDREN

There are large numbers of different approaches, techniques and therapies which may be used in work with looked after children (e.g. see Sen, 2018, Chapter 3 for an overview; some of these are also referred to in other chapters in this collection). There are, however, some identifiable common characteristics to effective ways of working underlying the different approaches. The importance of a warm, empathic working relationship is emphasised – children and young people need people who are consistent, supportive, trustworthy, interested in their development and willing to seriously engage with what they want for themselves, whether or not that fully accords with what adults think is best for them (Sen, 2018). There is an adage that every child or young person needs at least one trusted adult to fulfil this role, but of course, the more reliable people they can turn to, the better. Building supportive relationships entails spending meaningful time together with a child or young person and doing things that are of interest and importance to them. In social pedagogy the idea of the 'common third' (Ruch et al., 2017) provides a framework for this. It suggests that a child or young person and adult find an activity which is new to each of them and jointly learn it together, without the adult being therefore in a position of expertise and authority in respect of the activity. Through this, joint tasks are accomplished, new skills are learnt and the relationship between both develops.

CLOSER LOOK: JAZ AND ZACH, PART TWO

Jaz and Zach were made subject of a full Care Order after the family court decided there was no realistic prospect of them returning to their parents' care. They are now both in the same foster placement, which is intended to last until adulthood, and perhaps beyond. This case study will focus on Zach. At the age of 10, Zach's behaviour had been very challenging to his carers at home and to teaching staff at school. This behaviour included spitting, hitting and scratching them during frequent outbursts of anger. The school had voiced the view that they would need to exclude him, while his carers questioned if they could continue to provide a placement for him after one highly aggressive outburst: these outbursts gave rise to concerns about Zach's immediate welfare, as well as that of other children and adults around him when an outburst occurred; they also raised concerns about Zach's future emotional well-being, behavioural development and educational progress.

The carers were supported by professionals to work with Zach using a social pedagogic approach focussing on all elements of Zach's development: the head (the reflective and intellectual), heart (the emotional and empathetic) and hands (the practical and concrete). However, it is also possible to see the influence of elements of relationship-based practice, cognitive behavioural therapy (CBT), pro-social modelling and restorative practice within the work undertaken with Zach.

The foster family would sit down as a family unit and discuss matters concerning them all, including ground rules and any breaking of them: they would do so using a restorative model of interaction which allowed Zach, as well as Jaz, to voice their opinions openly, but also take responsibility for communicating openly, and required them to listen to their carers' and each other's views. Zach's carers would encourage Zach to talk through his behaviour in a non-judgemental way that still made clear some of his behaviour was unacceptable. They focussed on rewarding positive behaviour more than sanctioning poor behaviour, with 'time out' sessions framed as an opportunity to help Zach think about his feelings and how his behaviour may be affecting others.

Using the idea of a the 'common third' the family discussed new activities they might do together, outside of school and the home setting. The social worker suggested pairing Zach with his male carer for this activity, thinking it would be easier for them to agree a shared activity of mutual interest and that it would be positive in terms of male role modelling. However, Zach was clearly more willing to open up to Yojitha, his female carer, and when the family discussed it, indicated he wanted to start indoor bouldering/climbing with Yojitha as his activity of choice. Zach's carers accepted his preference, and Zach and Yojitha enlisted on an introductory bouldering course. Zach became more quickly proficient at the activity than Yojitha; he would often try to help and guide Yojitha during the practice sessions, showing both care for her welfare and taking pride in how he was able to help and instruct his carer. They also befriended another carer and child who were taking the same course. Zach and Yojitha's progress was shared and celebrated in family meetings. Zach's birth parents were also included by frequent discussions between Zach, his birth parents and his carers about what he, and Jaz, were doing.

Over and above the work undertaken by Zach's carers, professionals worked closely together regarding his care: an educational psychologist assessment provided tailored support for Zach in school via teaching assistant support within classes and strategies for teachers to help support Zach manage his emotions better. With this, a school exclusion was averted, and he started to make sound academic progress. Zach's carers were actively involved in the educational support plan and reinforced the strategies at home and supported his academic learning by supporting and checking his homework each school night. Zach was also referred to child and adolescent mental health services regarding his aggression: it was decided that longer term mental health input would not be helpful at this point, but with Zach's agreement, he attended a time-limited CBT course to help with anger management. These six sessions included therapeutically integral 'homework' tasks for Zach on implementing self-managed strategies for controlling his emotions and negative though patterns better. Zach's carers were directly involved in some of these sessions and actively supported Zach to work on the tasks given to him by the therapist.

REFLECTIVE QUESTIONS

- If you were a professional working with Zach, would you do anything differently, or in addition to, what is described above? If so what, and why?
- Jaz has also experienced some difficulties in her current placement. These include absconding from her school and, occasionally, her placement with her whereabouts unknown during these times; self-harming by cutting herself; and befriending a group of young people in the community who are reputed to be involved in drinking alcohol and causing criminal damage to local property. What are the key safeguarding risks, based on this short description?
- Map out a plan of work for Jaz to address these risks, and the underlying needs underpinning them?

CONCLUSION

The same child protection concerns which apply to children and young people in the general population apply to looked after children. There are also additional factors which practitioners need to take into account. That there are additional legal safeguards and protections regarding the care of looked after children should not obscure that a good many will have positive experiences within the care system. Such additional safeguards do, however, reflect the fact that a child or young person's separation from their birth family gives rise to the need for additional protections. As an overall group, looked after children also have several characteristics which can give rise to greater vulnerabilities – amongst these are greater levels of mental ill health, greater exposure to CSE, poorer educational attainment and a number of additional challenges they face on leaving state care. It is important that practitioners have an awareness of these broader trends and take action to provide appropriate support where such factors do indeed apply to an individual Looked after Child. Equally, it is important to guard against sweeping and stigmatising assumptions that all of these factors automatically apply to every Looked after Child. Engagement with the detail of a child or young person's individual circumstances is key, and meaningfully gaining a child or young person's views and understanding of their own situation should be seen as a core requirement within this.

REFERENCES

Ashcroft, B., 2013. Fifty-one Moves. Waterside Press, Hook, Hampshire.

Biehal, N., 2014. Maltreatment in foster care: A review of the evidence. Child Abus. Rev., 23(1), pp.48–60.

Carr, A., Nearchou, F., Duff, H., Mhaoileoin, D.N., Cullen, K., O'Dowd, A., et al., 2019. Survivors of institutional abuse in long-term child care in Scotland. Child Abuse Negl. 93, 38–54.

Children Act 1989, c. 41. Available at: https://www.legislation.gov.uk/ukpga/1989/41/contents (Accessed 24 August 2023)

Department of Education (DfE), 2022. Children looked after in England including adoption: 2021 to 2022. DfE, London. https://www.gov.uk/government/statistics/children-looked-after-in-england-including-adoption-2021-to-2022 (Accessed 24 August 2023).

Ellis, K., 2019. Blame and culpability in children's narratives of child sexual abuse. Child Abus. Rev. 28 (6), 405–417.

Field, A., Sen, R., Johnston, C., Ellis, K., 2021. Turning 18 in specialised residential therapeutic care: Independence or a cliff edge? Child. Soc. https://doi.org/10.1111/chso.12450.

Ghate, D., Hazel, N., 2002. Parenting in Poor Environments: Stress, Support and Coping. Jessica Kingsley Publishers, London.

Meltzer, H.,, Gatward, R., Corbin, T., Goodman, R., Ford, T., 2003. The Mental Health of Young People Looked After by Local Authorities in England. The Stationery Office, London.

Morris, K., Mason, W., Bywaters, P., Featherstone, B., Daniel, B., Brady, G., et al., 2018. Social work, poverty, and child welfare interventions. Child Fam. Soc. Work 23 (3), 364–372.

National Audit Office, 2016. Children and Young People in Care. National Audit Office, London. https://www.nao.org.uk/wp-content/uploads/2014/11/Easy-read-Children-and-young-people-in-care-and-leaving-care.A.pdf.

Ruch, G., Winter, K., Cree, V., Hallett, S., Morrison, F., Hadfield, M., 2017. Making meaningful connections: Using insights from social pedagogy in statutory child and family social work practice. Child Fam. Soc. Work 22 (2), 1015–1023. https://doi.org/10.1111/cfs.12321.

Sebba, J., Berridge, D., Luke, N., Fletcher, J., O'Higgins, A., 2015. The Educational Progress of Looked After Children in England: Linking Care and Educational Data. Rees Centre / University of Bristol, Oxford.

Sen, R., 2016. Not all that is solid melts into air? Care-experienced young people, friendship and relationships in the 'digital age.

Br. J. Soc. Work 46 (4), 1059–1075. https://doi.org/10.1093/bjsw/bcu152.

Sen, R., 2017. Child sexual exploitation (CSE): Awareness, Identification, Support and Prevention. South Yorkshire Teaching Partnerships, Sheffield. http://www.southyorkshireteachingpartnership.co.uk/wp-content/uploads/2018/02/CSE-Practice-Resource-Sen-June-2017.pdf. (Accessed 24 August 2023)

Sen, R., 2018. Effective Practice With Looked After Children. Palgrave, London.

Sen, R., Kendrick, A., Milligan, I., Hawthorn, M., 2008. Lessons learnt? Abuse in residential child care in Scotland. Child Fam. Soc. Work 13 (4), 411–422.

Sen, R., Webb, C., 2019. Exploring the declining rates of state social work intervention in an English local authority using Family Group Conferences. Child. Youth Serv. Rev. 106, 104458.

Sinclair, I., Baker, C., Lee, J., Gibbs, I., 2007. The Pursuit of Permanence: A Study of the English Child Care System. Jessica Kingsley, London.

Sissay, L., 2020. My Name Is Why: A Memoir. Cannongate, Edinburgh.

Stein, M., 2012. Young People Leaving Care: Supporting Pathways to Adulthood. Jessica Kingsley Publishers, London.

Wade, J., Biehal, N., Farrelly, N., Sinclair, I., 2011. Caring for Abused and Neglected Children: Making the Right Decisions for Reunification or Long-Term Care. Jessica Kingsley Publishers, London.

11c

BEING A REFUGEE OR ASYLUM SEEKER

KELLY DEVENNEY

KEY POINTS

- Unaccompanied asylum seeking children arrive alone in the UK to seek asylum without a parent or guardian.

- Local Authority children's services have a primary role in supporting unaccompanied children with accommodation, education and well-being.

- Refugee and migrant children should be treated as 'children first and foremost', regardless of their immigration status.

- The immigration status of an unaccompanied child has a significant impact on their well-being and life chances. Many unaccompanied children do not receive 'refugee status' and will be uncertain if they can remain in the UK when they become adults.

- The transition to adulthood and leaving care is a particularly difficult time for unaccompanied young people who have not been granted refugee status.

INTRODUCTION

Increasing numbers of asylum seeking children are arriving in the UK, seeking refuge from war, conflict and persecution (Refugee Council, 2019). Some will arrive with their families, but other children will arrive in the UK alone (Home Office, 2017). Those children (aged under 18 years) who arrive in the UK to seek asylum alone, without a parent or guardian, are referred to as 'Unaccompanied Asylum Seeking Children' (Home Office, 2017). These children are sometimes referred to as 'separated children' or unaccompanied

minors. Figures for 2018 show that 2872 unaccompanied children arrived in the UK that year and over 8000 asylum seeking children arrived with a family or family member (Refugee Council, 2019). Refugee children, whether they arrive alone or with families, are likely to have experienced trauma, either before they left their country of origin or during treacherous and protracted migration journeys (Bronstein et al., 2013). Those refugee children travelling alone are particularly vulnerable to a variety of risks including exploitation and destitution during their migration to the UK (Reed et al., 2012).

Social workers and related professions are most likely to work with unaccompanied children as these children have an automatic entitlement to children's services who will provide them with financial support, accommodation and assess their wider needs (Drammeh, 2019). This chapter will therefore focus primarily on unaccompanied children, although many of the needs and vulnerabilities of 'accompanied' and 'unaccompanied' refugee children are overlapping.

THE LEGAL AND POLICY CONTEXT

The right to seek asylum is embedded in international law (UN, 1951), and the United Nations Convention on the Rights of the Child (UNCRC, 1989) provides a framework for a child-centred approach to children and young people seeking asylum. Similarly, UK immigration law has evolved to emphasise the need to safeguard the welfare of refugee children and for their best interests to be the primary consideration (York and Warren, 2019).

CLOSER LOOK: WHAT IS A REFUGEE?

Under the 1951 Refugee Convention a refugee is 'someone who is unable or unwilling to return to their country of origin owing to a well-founded fear of being persecuted for reasons of race, religion, nationality, membership of a particular social group, or political opinion.'

However, concerns remain about the treatment of children within the context of a 'hostile' immigration policy environment. On arrival in the UK, unaccompanied children seeking asylum will attend an initial 'Welfare' interview, the focus of which should be their welfare needs rather than the basis of their asylum claim. Reports consistently suggest that these initial interviews are incorrectly used to interrogate their asylum claim and are frequently conducted without an appropriate adult or legal professional present (Warren and York, 2014; York and Warren, 2019).

Prior to 2016 the Government was committed to processing children's asylum claims within 25 days, but guidance since 2016 has omitted this requirement and delays of up to 18 months are frequently reported (York and Warren, 2019). Evidence suggests that unaccompanied children find applying for asylum a distressing, confusing and complex process, and they do not always have access to good quality legal advice (Children's Society, 2012). If the asylum claim is successful, the child will receive 'refugee status', which means they will be allowed to stay in the UK on a permanent basis. Many unaccompanied children will be refused refugee status. The trend over the previous few years has been to allow those children who do not receive refugee status a temporary form of leave to remain in the UK known as 'UASC' leave (Refugee Council, 2019). This allows them to remain in the UK until they are seventeen and a half. If, by this stage, they have not successfully appealed the decision or made a fresh claim, they will be expected to return to their country of origin. Concerns have been raised about the impact of such 'enforced temporariness' on unaccompanied young people who may face extreme uncertainty about their future and live with the prospect of detention or deportation when their temporary leave expires (Gupta, 2019). All unaccompanied children are referred to Local Authority children's

services and are treated as looked after children under the Children Act 1989. They have the same legal rights and entitlements as all other looked after children as long as they continue to have the legal right to remain in the UK.

CLOSER LOOK: WELFARE INTERVIEWS

The welfare interview is conducted by the Home Office and is intended to assess if there are any welfare or trafficking concerns about the child; collect fingerprints; and register the child as arriving in the UK, before referring the child to Local Authority children's services.

Age Assessments

When an unaccompanied child arrives in the UK, social care professionals are responsible for assessing their needs and safeguarding their welfare under the relevant domestic legislation. Their rights and entitlements to children's services are the same as 'citizen' children (Drammeh, 2019). Government guidance is clear that migrant and refugee children should be treated as 'children first and foremost and not defined by their immigration status' (Dorling et al., 2017). However, there are ongoing tensions between the protective functions of children's social care policy (e.g. Children Act 1989) and the increasingly punitive function of immigration policy (Drammeh, 2019). The intersection of these conflicting policy agendas is particularly evident in the requirement for social workers to conduct 'age assessments' on unaccompanied children when the Home Office believes there is doubt over the child's claim to be under 18 and no documentary proof of age is available (Busler, 2016). The process of age assessment and the role of social workers within that process has been controversial. Age assessments have been criticised as dehumanising (Matthews, 2014), inaccurate (Busler, 2016) and in conflict with social work values (Cemlyn and Nye, 2012), as well as negatively impacting the well-being of children (Walker, 2011). Whilst medical approaches to assessing age have previously been applied (dental examinations and bone density x-rays were commonly used), recent guidelines following a court case known as 'the Merton judgement' require a more holistic approach. A 'Merton' compliant age assessment takes a psychosocial approach which considers behaviour, social maturity and cultural factors (Dorling et al., 2017).

Significantly, social workers are required to give young people 'the benefit of the doubt', beginning from the presumption that the young person is telling the truth about their age (Association of Directors of Children's Services (ADCS), 2015).

CLOSER LOOK: MERTON COMPLIANT AGE ASSESSMENTS

In the case of B v London Borough of Merton (2003), the high court set out the broad guidelines for conducting age assessments. The elements of a 'Merton Compliant Assessment' are set out below:
Two qualified social workers should conduct the assessment

An assessment cannot be made solely on the basis of appearance.

Any assessment should take into account relevant factors from the child's medical, family and social history. Ethnic and cultural information may also be important.

There is a duty on the decision-makers to give reasons for a decision that an applicant claiming to be a child is not a child.

The young person should be given an opportunity during the assessment to answer any adverse points the decision-maker is minded to hold against him.

If the decision-maker is left in doubt, the claimant should receive the benefit of that doubt.

A young person has a right to be accompanied during the assessment by an appropriate adult.

CASE STUDY 11C.1: CARE AND PROTECTION OF IDRIS

This section will consider the care and protection needs of unaccompanied asylum seeking children using a case study derived from the author's research interviews with unaccompanied children.

Idris arrived in the UK from Eritrea aged 15 years. The first step in working with unaccompanied children is to meet their immediate needs in the present (Kohli, 2007), and finding suitable accommodation may be the first concern. There is a range of evidence to suggest that foster care is the most suitable form of accommodation for unaccompanied children as it can provide a more family-like environment, personalised individual attention and opportunities for integration (Sirriyeh, 2013). Sirriyeh (2013) suggests that the foster placements' ability to meet cultural needs is crucial. Ideally, unaccompanied children should be placed with foster carers who share similar cultural backgrounds, but it will not always be possible to find culturally matched placements, and some unaccompanied children will prefer transcultural foster placements that allow opportunities for integration and the development of language skills (Wade et al., 2012).

Idris was placed with foster carers who had cared for a number of Eritrean young people, and although they were not Eritrean, they had experience of fostering Eritrean children. Idris was initially disappointed that no other Eritrean young people were in the placement at the same time as he was, but he soon became close friends with Gavin, a boy of the same age from the UK who was in the same foster placement. Gavin helped Idris to develop his language skills quickly and introduced Idris to the local area. Unaccompanied children may find comfort and companionship with others who have similar experiences and share cultural similarities but may equally find commonalities in friendships and communities outside of their cultural, national, ethnic and religious identities (Wade et al., 2012). Idris thrived in his foster placement and developed strong connections with his foster family. While Idris benefited from foster care, this option is usually available only to unaccompanied children aged under 16 years (Gupta, 2019). Older children are likely to be placed in semi-independent settings which offer greater freedom and the ability to develop peer support networks but may not be suitable for those who need access to more intensive support (Drammeh, 2019).

Although it took some time to find a school place for Idris, he excelled academically as soon as he settled in. He was particularly interested in science and dreamed of a career in engineering. Education is often a priority for unaccompanied children because it provides a steppingstone to a positive future (Devenney, 2017) and allows them to 'anchor' in the present and establish a routine and regain control over an aspect of their lives (Drammeh, 2019).

Although Idris was doing well in school and had a good relationship with his foster family, he found dealing with the immigration system stressful. Shortly after his arrival and application for asylum, the Home Office decided that Idris did not meet the criteria for 'refugee status' but would be allowed to stay in the UK on a temporary basis until he was 17 1/2. Idris was confused about what the Home Office decision meant and what would happen to him when his temporary leave to remain in the UK expired. Idris was able to appeal the Home Office decision with support from his foster family and social worker, but the uncertainty around his immigration status was having a negative impact on his well-being.

It is well-established that unaccompanied children are at increased risk of suffering from post-traumatic stress disorder symptoms and emotional distress (Bronstein and Montgomery, 2010; Hodes et al., 2008). The roots of such distress may lay in traumatic events prior to and during migration but are also exacerbated by negative experiences after arriving in the UK, including the destabilising effects of the asylum process (Chase and Allsopp, 2013). This is particularly the case for children who do not have the relative security of 'refugee status' and face acute uncertainty about their future (Chase and Allsopp, 2013). Emotional distress and trauma may present in a number of ways including flashbacks, intrusive memories, poor concentration and disturbed sleep (Hughes, 2019). Researchers have identified a variety of coping strategies unaccompanied children use which support resilience including maintaining continuity, seeking distraction, focusing on education and drawing on spiritual faith (Newbigging and Thomas 2011; Ni Raghallaigh and Gilligan, 2010). Idris used a variety of mechanisms to cope and improve his well-being. He was active in his local church community, regularly

played football with friends and developed a wide social network of friends. A number of studies have raised concerns about the social isolation that unaccompanied children may face, due to stigmatised 'refugee identities' (Sirriyeh, 2013); however, recent research has rejected the idea of the 'lonely unaccompanied young person' (Herz and Llander, 2017). Research is emerging with a focus on friendship (Clayton and Willis, 2019) and the important domains of 'every-dayness' (Blazek, 2011, p. 81). As with Idris' experience, sport may provide a key activity through which unaccompanied children and young people can develop informal networks, although it is important to note that this is much more likely to be the case for boys rather than girls (Jeanes et al., 2015). Spiritual faith also provides opportunities to develop networks of support though shared religious practices (Rigby, 2011). Whilst Idris had certainly developed an active social network, he preferred not to tell his friends and church community about his immigration status. This is common amongst unaccompanied children who may use silence and a certain amount of distrust as coping mechanisms which allow them to maintain a sense of control and internal strength (Chase, 2010; Kohli, 2006).

As Idris turned 17 and was transitioning to adulthood, his circumstances were changing. He was transitioning to adulthood and 'leaving care'. He moved out of foster care to live independently, desiring more freedom and independence. Although he had been offered a place at university, he was unable to confirm his place as he was still awaiting the outcome of his latest appeal to the Home Office for refugee status. For unaccompanied children, planning for the transition to adulthood is crucial and should begin as early as possible, especially considering that many unaccompanied children arrive in the UK aged 16 years and over (Wade, 2011). Unaccompanied children face different pathways into adulthood depending on their immigration status. Those who have secured refugee status or are still awaiting a decision on their asylum claim will be entitled to the full range of services for care leavers under the Children (Leaving Care 2000) Act (2002) including a 'pathway plan' which considers support with living independently, accessing work or education and planning for the future (Wade et al., 2012). For those like Idris, who are facing the expiry of their temporary leave to remain or have not yet received a decision, the future is acutely uncertain, and their primary concern is likely to be securing their immigration status, either by extending a period of temporary leave or making fresh claims for asylum and a more permanent status to remain in the UK (Wright, 2014). This is a particularly difficult and anxious time for children and young people who face potential detention and/or deportation when they become adults if their asylum claims are rejected (Kohli, 2011). There is a sharp distinction in the needs and vulnerabilities of unaccompanied children at this stage depending on their immigration status (Devenney, 2017). Those with refugee status may be doing well, planning for the future and moving forward with careers and personal relationships. However, those who face uncertain futures are likely to find it places an extreme burden on their mental well-being and limits their ability to focus on education and develop lasting bonds and relationships (Devenney, 2017).

This was the case for Idris who started to withdraw from his friends as he awaited the outcome of numerous appeals. He was anxious not to talk to people about his situation, but it was hard for him to hide his feelings. He found it easier to isolate himself. Once a busy, sociable, active and proud person, he retreated into his small flat where he mostly watched TV. He no longer attended church or played football in the park and no longer allowed himself to dream of going to university. Immigration status plays a crucial role in isolation, as social connections may begin to shrink the longer asylum seekers continue without any settled and permanent status (Kearns and Whiteley, 2015). As Idris' experience demonstrates, informal social networks can change rapidly for unaccompanied young people, particularly if their immigration status is not confirmed. As friends move into further education and work, they may feel 'left behind' and unable to move forward at the same pace as their friends and peers (Devenney, 2017).

During this period of limbo Idris' primary emotional and financial support was from social services, and Idris began to develop a strong connection with his social workers with whom he shared his fears and anxieties. Whilst the capacity of unaccompanied children to cope and be resilient in certain circumstances is evident across research, consideration should also be given to emotional and therapeutic needs. Kohli (2007) explores the role that social workers can play in 'witnessing' the stories of unaccompanied children and assisting them with 'making meaning' from their experiences. Working with unaccompanied children on this level requires a trusting relationship, delicately developed over time (Devenney, 2019). Not all unaccompanied children and young people will wish to engage with their social worker in this way, valuing the practical support and advocacy of social services while drawing emotional strength from relationships outside of social services (Devenney, 2019). Indeed, the most crucial support that a social worker may be able to offer in these circumstances is to assist the young person to 'navigate the hostile environment of immigration policy in the UK' (Devenney, 2019).

Idris' social worker used the 'pathway planning process' (which all 'care leavers' are entitled to) to explore the future with Idris. However, pathway planning with unaccompanied children who face uncertainty about whether they can remain in the UK can be very challenging. In order to account for the very different pathways unaccompanied children may face depending on their immigration status, a 'triple planning' approach has been suggested. This approach is concerned with ensuring that the pathway plan takes account of the multiple possible outcomes of asylum claims, including refusal, receiving status and a potentially prolonged period of waiting for a decision (Dorling et al., 2017; Wade, 2011). In practice, young people dealing with uncertainty about their future may find it very difficult to discuss the possibility of a negative asylum decision and the potential consequences, which include detention and deportation. Indeed they may struggle to imagine any future at all under the stress of extreme uncertainty (Devenney, 2017). Conversely, where unaccompanied children have some certainty about their immigration status, they are able to plan and take positive steps towards achieving future goals (Devenney, 2017).

Idris found it very difficult to engage with planning for his future with his social worker, even though they had a very good relationship. He found it particularly difficult to discuss his greatest fear, which was receiving a final rejection from the Home Office. When an unaccompanied young person has exhausted all their rights to appeal against a negative asylum decision, they become 'Appeal Rights Exhausted'. At this point they are no longer entitled to any social services and will lose access to their 'leaving care' support (Humphris and Segona, 2017). Unaccompanied young people who become 'Appeal Rights Exhausted' are at risk of detention and deportation. Whilst the government does not use immigration detention for those under the age of eighteen, once unaccompanied children reach legal adulthood, those protections expire. At this point, some young people choose to abscond or 'disappear' out of the system.

For Idris, the final outcome was positive. He was eventually granted refugee status and was able to take up his place at university. Idris threw himself into preparing for university life. When he got there, he once again excelled. He had a big circle of friends and enjoyed meeting other students from different countries and different walks of life. When he completed his degree, his foster parents and his friend Gavin, the first friend he had made in the UK, attended the graduation ceremony.

CONCLUSION

Social workers have a vital role in protecting and promoting the well-being of refugee and unaccompanied children. Migrant children should always be treated as children first and foremost, regardless of their immigration status. However, social workers may have some difficult statutory tasks to undertake with unaccompanied children, which may present difficult ethical dilemmas and values conflicts. The needs and vulnerabilities of unaccompanied children may be exasperated if they do not have certainty about their immigration status. Many unaccompanied children do very well when they are able to plan for the future with the certainty that they can remain in the UK, although they still have a significant range of needs, particularly when they first arrive in the UK. The transition to adulthood may be a particularly difficult time for unaccompanied children as they leave care.

REFLECTIVE QUESTIONS

- Should social workers be required to conduct 'age assessments' on unaccompanied children? Does this conflict with the values of social work?
- Why is it so important to ensure unaccompanied children have access to good quality, supportive education?
- Is the idea of 'triple planning' useful for helping unaccompanied young people who are uncertain about their immigration status plan for the future?

FURTHER READING

ADCS, 2015. Age Assessment Guidance and Information Sharing Guidance for UASC, Publishers are Association of Directors of Children's Services. https://adcs.org.uk/safeguarding/article/age-assessment-information-sharing-for-unaccompanied-asylum-seeking-children.

Department for Education, 2017. Care of Unaccompanied Migrant Children and Child Victims of Modern Slavery: Statutory Guidance for Local Authorities, https://www.gov.uk/government/publications/care-of-unaccompanied-and-trafficked-children.

Coram Children's Legal Centre, https://www.childrenslegalcentre.com/get-legal-advice/immigration-asylum-nationality/.

REFERENCES

Association of Directors of Children's Services (ADCS), 2015. Age Assessment Guidance: Guidance to assist social workers and their managers in undertaking age assessments in England. Association of Directors of Children's Services.

Bronstein, I., Montgomery, P., 2010. 'Psychological distress in refugee children: A systematic review'. Clin. Child Fam. Psychol. Rev. 14 (1), 44–56. https://doi.org/10.1007/s10567-010-0081-0.

Bronstein, I, Montgomery, P., and Ott E., 2013. Emotional and behavioural problems amongst Afghan unaccompanied asylum-seeking children: results from a large-scale cross-sectional study. European child & adolescent psychiatry 22: 285–294.

Blazek, M., 2011. Place, children's friendships, and the formation of gender identities in a Slovak urban neighbourhood,. Child. Geogr. 9(3–4): 285–302.

Busler, D., 2016. Psychosocial age assessment in the UK. Forced Migr. Rev. 52, 86–88.

Cemlyn, S.J., Nye, M., 2012. Asylum seeker young people: Social work value conflicts in negotiating age assessments in the UK. Int. Soc. Work 55 (5), 675–689.

Chase, E., 2010. Agency and silence: young people seeking asylum alone in the UK, British. J. Soc. Work 40, 2050–2068.

Chase, E., Allsopp, J., 2013. 'Future citizens of the world'? The Contested Futures of Independent Young Migrants in Europe. Refugee Studies Centre, Oxford.

Children (Leaving Care) Act 2000. https://www.legislation.gov.uk/ukpga/2000/35

Children Act (1989) https://www.legislation.gov.uk/ukpga/1989/41/contents

Children's Society, 2012. Into the Unknown: Children's Journeys Through the Asylum System. Children's Society, London.

Clayton, S., Willis, K., 2019. Migration regimes and border controls. In: Clayton, S., Gupta, A., Willis, K. (Eds.), Unaccompanied Young Migrants: Identity, Care and Justice. Policy Press, Bristol, pp. 15–38.

Devenney, K., 2017. Pathway planning with unaccompanied young people leaving care: Biographical narratives of past, present, and future. Child Fam. Soc. Work 22 (32), 1313–1321.

Devenney, K., 2019. Social work with unaccompanied asylum-seeking young people: Reframing social care professionals as 'co-navigators'. Br. J. Soc. Work. https://doi.org/10.1093/bjsw/bcz071.

Dorling, K., McLachlan, S., Trevena, F., 2017. Seeking Support: A Guide to the Rights and Entitlements of Separated Children. Coram Children's Legal Centre. www.childrenslegalcentre.com/wp-content/uploads/2017/05/Seeking-Support-2017.pdf.

Drammeh, L., 2019. Spaces of belonging and social care. In: Clayton, S., Gupta, A., Willis, K. (Eds.), Unaccompanied Young Migrants: Identity, Care and Justice. Policy Press, Bristol, pp. 159–186.

Gupta, A., 2019. Caring for and about unaccompanied migrant youth in. In: Clayton, S., Gupta, A., Willis, K. (Eds.), Unaccompanied Young Migrants: Identity, Care and Justice. Policy Press, Bristol, pp. 77–104.

Herz, M., Lalander, P., 2017. Being alone or becoming lonely? The complexity of portraying 'unaccompanied children' as being alone in Sweden. J. Youth Stud. 20 (19), 1–15.

Hodes, M., Jagdev, D., Chandra, N., Cunniff, A., 2008. Risk and resilience for psychological distress amongst unaccompanied asylum seeking adolescents. Child Psychol. Psychiatry 49 (7), 723–732.

Home Office, 2017. National Statistics: Asylum. https://www.gov.uk/government/publications/immigration-statistics-october-to-december-2016/asylum.

Hughes, G., 2019. From individual vulnerability to collective resistance: Responding to the emotional impact of trauma on unaccompanied children seeking asylum. In: Clayton, S., Gupta, A., Willis, K. (Eds.), Unaccompanied Young Migrants: Identity, Care and Justice. Policy Press, Bristol, pp. 135–158.

Humphris, R., Sigona, N., 2017. Outsourcing the 'best interests' of unaccompanied asylum-seeking children in the era of austerity. J. Ethn. Migr. Stud. 45, 312–330.

Jeanes, R., O'Connor, J., Alfrey, L., 2015. Sport and the resettlement of young people from refugee backgrounds in Australia. J. Sport Soc. Issues 9 (6), 480–500.

Kearns, A. & Whitley, E., 2015. Getting there? The effects of functional factors, time and place on the social integration of migrants,. J. Ethn. Migr. Stud. 41(13): 2105–2129.

Kohli, R.K.S., 2006. The sound of silence: Listening to what unaccompanied asylum seeking children say and do not say. Br. J. Soc. Work 36 (5), 701–721.

Kohli, R.K.S., 2007. Social Work with Unaccompanied Asylum–Seeking Children. Palgrave Macmillan, London.

Kohli, R.K.S., 2011. Working to ensure safety, belonging and success for unaccompanied asylum seeking children. Child Abus. Rev. 20 (3), 311–323.

Matthews, A., 2014. What's Going to Happen Tomorrow? Unaccompanied Children Refused Asylum. Office of the Children's Commissioner, London.

Newbigging, K., Thomas, N., 2011. Good practice in social care for refugee and asylum seeking children. Child Abus. Rev. 20, 374–390.

Ni Raghallaigh, M., Gilligan, R., 2010. Active survival in the lives of unaccompanied minors: Coping strategies, resilience and the relevance of religion. Child Fam. Soc. Work 15, 26–237.

Reed, R.V., Fazel, M., Jones, L., Panter-Brick, C., Stein, A., 2012. Mental health of displaced and refugee children resettled in low-income countries: risk and protective factors. Lancet 379, 250–265.

Refugee Council, 2019. Asylum Statistics Annual Trends. https://www.refugeecouncil.org.uk/information/refugee-asylum-facts/.

Rigby, P., 2011. Separated and trafficked children: The challenges for child protection professionals. Child Abus. Rev. 20 (5), 324–340.

Sirriyeh, A., 2013. Inhabiting Borders, Routes Home: Youth, Gender, Asylum. Ashgate Publishing, Ltd, Farnham, UK.

UN General Assembly, Convention Relating to the Status of Refugees, 28 July 1951, United Nations, Treaty Series, vol. 189, p. 137, available at: https://treaties.un.org/pages/ViewDetailsII.aspx?src=TREATY&mtdsg_no=V-2&chapter=5&Temp=mtdsg2&clang=_en. (Accessed 23 August 2023).

Convention on the rights of the child (1989) Treaty no. 27531. United Nations Treaty Series, 1577, pp. 3–178. Available at: https://treaties.un.org/pages/ViewDetails.aspx?src=TREATY&mtdsg_no=IV-11&chapter=4&clang=_en

Wade, J., 2011. Preparation and transition planning for unaccompanied asylum-seeking and refugee young people: a review of evidence in England. Child. Youth Serv. Rev. 33 (12), 2424–2430.

Wade, J., Sirriyeh, A., Kohli, R., Simmonds, J., 2012. Fostering Unaccompanied Asylum Seeking Children: Creating a Family Life Across 'A World of Difference'. British Association of Adoption and Fostering, London.

Walker, S., 2011. Something to Smile About: Promoting Educational and Recreational Needs of Refugee Children. Refugee Council, London.

Warren, R., York, S., 2014. How Children Become Failed Asylum Seekers. University of Kent, Kent, UK.

Wright, F. (2014). Social Work Practice with Unaccompanied Asylum-Seeking Young People Facing Removal,. Br. J. Soc. Work 44(4): 1027–1044.

York, S., Warren, R., 2019. Dilemmas and conflicts in the legal system. In: Clayton, S., Gupta, A., Willis, K. (Eds.), Unaccompanied Young Migrants: Identity, Care and Justice. Policy Press, Bristol, pp. 29–76.

11d BEING A YOUNG CARER

JO ALDRIDGE

KEY POINTS

- Define and describe what it means to be a young carer.
- Present evidence on the prevalence of young caring in the UK and its impact on children's lives.
- Describe and discuss current policy and practice on young carers, including the legal framework and support strategies for young carers and their families.
- Consider the rights and needs of young carers.

INTRODUCTION

Young carers are children and young people under the age of 18 who provide care for a sick or disabled relative, such as a parent, grandparent or sibling, in the home. The focus of policy, practice and research on young carers in the UK is *not* on children's short-term caring responsibilities, when a parent or other relative in the home has temporary illness. Rather the focus is on caring that is long term, unrecognized, unsupported and disproportionate to a child's age and level of maturity. Research demonstrates that level of caring, particularly when this extends for 2 years or more, has the most adverse effects on children's lives, including their transitions into adulthood (Abraham and Aldridge, 2010).

This chapter begins by outlining how many young carers there are in the UK, what young carers do and the effects of caring on children's lives. Following this, the chapter explores the importance of early intervention and outlines how to identify and support young carers, including clarifying relevant legislation. The chapter concludes by advocating for a children's rights approach to supporting young carers. This requires seeing young carers as children first and carers second, advocating for their right to protection and to have a say in decision-making about their lives (United Nations Convention on the Rights of the Child (UNCRC), 1989).

HOW MANY YOUNG CARERS ARE THERE IN THE UK?

Census data from 2011 showed there were just over 166,000 young carers in England and Wales (Office for National Statistics, 2013). In 2010, however, a study conducted by the BBC estimated there were 800,000 young carers in the UK. In 2014, a large scale qualitative and quantitative study was commissioned to understand the prevalence and impact of young caring across England and address the discrepancies in the prevalence data (Aldridge et al., 2016; Cheesbrough et al., 2017). This research included children between the ages of 5 and 17, including those not known to local authorities (often referred to as 'hidden' young carers). In the national omnibus survey of young carers in England (Cheesbrough et al., 2017) – the largest study of its kind to be conducted on young carers across England – 420 young carers were identified out of 79,629 households, giving a figure of 0.5% young carers in the general population.

The notable difference in estimated numbers of young carers in the UK underline three important issues in young carer research and contemporary policy and practice debates. Firstly, methodologies differ across research studies, and in some cases lack rigour; for example the 800,000 young carers finding in the 2010 BBC report was based on extrapolation of data from a small-scale survey of secondary school children (Aldridge, 2019). Secondly, studies use different definitions of young carers and focus on different age ranges of children. Thirdly, and most importantly, focus on the *prevalence* of young caring overlooks the *impact* of caring on children, especially when this is long term and unrecognised or unsupported.

WHAT DO YOUNG CARERS DO, AND WHAT ARE THE EFFECTS OF CARING ON CHILDREN'S LIVES?

Some children carry out caring responsibilities that we would usually associate with adulthood, including nursing type support – administering medications, changing dressings – and intimate care such as toileting and bathing. Others take on a range of tasks that may include domestic chores (cooking and cleaning) and/or emotional care, such as monitoring and supporting the mental and emotional needs of their relative. This is especially the case when parents (or other relatives in the home) have serious or enduring mental health problems (Aldridge and Becker, 2003).

Young carers need help and support, both for themselves and for the person with care needs. They also need opportunities just to be children, to have fun and enjoy being with their families, to care *about* rather than *for* them. In short, children should not have to provide care for their relatives in the home that is long term and/or has a detrimental impact on their lives as children. For some families, in the absence of formal recognition and support, they often have little choice but to rely on children to provide some level of care – in some cases over a prolonged period. Children are also more likely to undertake caring roles in lone parent families, in families living on low income or in poverty, where families are fearful of seeking help and where health and/or social care services are missing or inadequate (Aldridge and Becker, 1993; 2003).

Caring can have adverse impacts on children's and young people's lives, especially when it is not recognised or supported by appropriate and effective services, and

---

CASE STUDY 11D.1: DANI

Dani (14) cares for her mum, Cara, who has multiple sclerosis and depression. Dani does most of the cooking, cleaning, shopping and managing the family finances. She also spends time with her mum trying to keep her spirits up and making sure she takes her medication. This means Dani has little, if any, time for socialising and sometimes does not have time, or energy, to do her homework. Her mother's condition means Dani is sometimes too worried about leaving her mum alone to go out with friends, even though her mum would like her to. School holidays are both good and bad for Dani; it means being home and not having to worry about her mum as much because they are together, but it also means she does a lot more around the house.

REFLECTIVE QUESTIONS

- What are the possible effects of caring on Dani's life?
- Consider some of the likely outcomes if she continues to care like she does now, both in terms of her current circumstances and her future.
- What kind of interventions and support would best help Dani and her mother?

---

without the necessary focus on early intervention and prevention. Caring is more likely to have a profound effect on children's lives when they care unsupported for 2 years or more. In 2010, research on the health and well-being needs of young carers found that:

participants in the 14–17-year age group (who had been caring for longer periods of time – at least two years; more than ten years in two cases) were less optimistic about the future, had a poorer self-view, depleted levels of interest in new things and did not feel as close to other people.

Abraham and Aldridge (2010, p. 4)

Further research has shown that caring can have a negative impact on children's education and their transitions into adulthood. Without any respite from caring or identification of young carers' needs – both as children and as carers (Aldridge, 2019; Children's Society (CS), 2015); and the needs of families through whole family working (see later) – children and young people are more likely to experience poor educational outcomes, as well as opportunity costs. Research findings have shown consistently, for example, that children who have caring responsibilities are more likely to miss school or experience educational difficulties as a result of their caring roles; they often have lower educational attainment at GCSE level, and 16- to 19-year-olds are more likely not to be in education, employment or training (NEET) (CS, 2013; Dearden and Becker, 2004); bullying can also be an issue for children in schools as a consequence of their caring roles (Carers Trust, 2013). When these issues combine, it is more likely that young carers make poor transitions into adulthood.

Gender and ethnicity are significant factors in determining the onset of and outcomes for children and young people who care. Evidence from early studies on young carers showed that girls are more likely to be drawn or elected into caring roles, even when there are other siblings, including older brothers, available to care (see Aldridge and Becker, 1993). Research has also identified a range of barriers and challenges for Black and minority ethnic (BAME) young carers and their families (CS, 2020). Some of these barriers are at a structural (organisational) level that prevent effective community working among professionals who, in some cases (according to CS research), lack the necessary training and skills in diversity and inclusive practice. Additional specific barriers are also identified across health, social care and education, including lack of knowledge among BAME families about what support is available, as well as the lack of and inadequate services to meet the needs of these families.

REFLECTIVE QUESTIONS

- What 'opportunity costs' might young carers experience?
- When does young caring become a child protection concern and what might some of the challenges be in identifying this?

EARLY INTERVENTION AND PREVENTION

Early identification of children's caring responsibilities and wider needs (as children in need) is vital in preventing caring from having an adverse impact on children's lives and transitions into adulthood. Early identification requires professionals to understand:

- the triggers for young caring,
- the contexts in which young caring is likely to occur, and
- Which children might be drawn or elected into caring roles in families affected by chronic illness or disability.

Where early intervention does not occur and caring becomes long term and disproportionate to children's age and level of maturity, they are more likely to experience psychological and emotional problems such as low self-esteem and anxiety-related disorders (Abraham and Aldridge, 2010).

One of the primary triggers for the onset of young caring is the presence of chronic illness, including enduring mental illness, and/or disability among adults who are also parents. Where there are children with illness or disability in families, it is also possible that siblings may be drawn into caring roles. A key first question for any professionals who work with adults who have chronic health problems and/or disability is to establish whether they are also parents (Falkov, 2013) and to consider the impact of the illness/disability on children and the family as a whole. In asking questions not only about the needs of patients/service users with illness/disability, but also the needs of the wider family, including children, it is more likely that professionals will uncover any deficits in care provision that are or could be being made up by children. The focus should then be on identifying what families need to prevent children from being drawn into inappropriate caring roles. Additional early intervention strategies to prevent young caring in families include consideration and assessment of the parenting needs of adults (see Carers Trust, 2020; Falkov, 2013), effective multiagency working (including with schools) and, as is the case in promoting whole family working approaches to young caring more broadly, networking across formal organisations/agencies and informal sources of support.

CASE STUDY 11D.2: JIN

Jin (13) helps to look after his younger brother, An (10), who has autism. Jin's mother died just after An was born, and they were both raised by their father, Lei, who works as a care worker. He works shifts, which means Jin has to care for An while their father is at work, including some late nights. An is becoming increasingly difficult for Jin to look after, especially those times when his behaviour is unpredictable and aggressive – Jin would really like to be able to live with his brother without having to care for him. Their father receives some help and support for An from local children's services and from the National Autistic Society. This support, however, focuses mainly on An's needs, and Lei has been concerned for some time about the needs of his oldest son. Lei relies on Jin to help look after his brother, but he also knows that this is becoming more difficult for him, and especially since he started secondary school. Lei is wary of letting social services and the school know that Jin has to care a lot for An on his own as he is fearful their family might be separated.

One of Jin's teachers recently told Lei about the local young carers project that supports children and families like theirs, and with Lei's consent, she made a referral to the project and a request for support for Jin as well as whole family support. Jin has started attending the project's young carers club and is really enjoying it. The project also provides respite and a homework club. This kind of support has really helped the family, especially Jin who has grown in confidence and whose grades have improved at school. Lei's main concern now, however, is how he will cope with An's needs in the future, especially if Jin goes to university, which is something he would like to do.

REFLECTIVE QUESTIONS

■ How might Lei be encouraged to seek support from social services?

■ Consider some of the barriers to Jin's aspirations to go to university.

■ What is missing from this case study with respect to Jin's needs (think about rights to be heard and to participate)?

As demonstrated in Jin's case study, one of the barriers to successful early intervention and prevention is that some young carers, as well as parents/families, are fearful of disclosing the fact that children are providing care for fear of interventions that might lead to child protection or safeguarding decisions being made. This fear is, in many respects, not misplaced. In 2015, for example, more than 2000 children were placed in care in the UK because of 'parents' illness or disability' (Zayed and Harker, 2015, p. 7). This is more likely in families where parents (or other adult relatives in the home) experience serious mental health problems. For children, caring in these contexts can be especially challenging, as well as stigmatising (Aldridge and Becker, 2003). Some families actively resist children being identified or 'labelled' young carers because of the stigma associated with the term and because it fails to address the real problem, which is that many families lack appropriate and effective family-based interventions that would prevent children from having to provide care in the first place (Aldridge et al., 2016). These are important considerations for professionals (in both adult and children's services) when addressing and preventing young caring in the long term, including children's transitions into young adult caring – young adult carers are categorised variously as aged 16–25; 14–24; and 16–30 (Aldridge, 2019; Learning and Work Institute, 2016).

Identifying and Supporting Young Carers

CLOSER LOOK: LEGAL FRAMEWORK

Prior to 2014, young carers were not recognised or included in legislation; up until this point they were assessed as **children in need** under various Children Act provisions (HM Government, 1989; HM Government, 2004). In 2014, thanks to campaigning by several leading national charities and organisations that support young carers, the needs of young carers were included and addressed in both the **Care Act 2014** (HM Government, 2014a) and the **Children and Families Act, 2014** (HM Government, 2014b) (which amends the Children Act, 1989). The former places a duty on local authorities to identify young carers in their area, while the latter addresses specifically young carers' assessment, transitional (from children's to adult services) and wider needs.

The welcome change in young carer legislation aimed to ensure the needs of young carers and their families were identified and assessed. Evidence has shown, however, that such assessments vary in quality and consistency (see Aldridge et al., 2016; Children's Commissioner for England, 2016). In part this has occurred due to poor screening practices and a lack of resources and tools to identify young carers. To some extent, this has been addressed by the introduction, in 2016, of the YC-QST-20 screening tool, a questionnaire developed from the national study of young carers (Aldridge et al., 2016; Cheesbrough et al., 2017). This enables professionals working with children and families to identify young carers and then route them to appropriate services.

When conducting effective young carer needs assessments, two issues are important: young carers are *children* first; and the needs of families should be addressed (and assessed) through whole family working. With respect to the first of these, the provisions set out in the Children and Families Act (CFA) 2014 (HM Government 2014b) are important in recognising young carers' additional needs and in requiring professionals to ascertain children's views and wishes about caring, their needs outside of their caring roles, and to consider preventive strategies. Following the introduction of both the CFA and the Care Act (CA) 2014 (HM Government 2014a), the guidance states that young carers' needs assessments should 'recognize that each child is a unique person on their own journey to adulthood and maturity,' and that local authorities should 'offer services to promote their welfare as a *child in need*' (CS, 2015; emphasis added). With respect to the need for whole family working, this is vital in ensuring that the needs of families are identified and met rather than only those of the child (young carer), or the person with care needs.

This requires an approach to assessment that starts with understanding why children are providing care in families, what their needs are (as carers and as children), as well as those of the person with care needs and other members of the family. The kind of support that should then be offered would vary, although much depends on the availability of appropriate services, including, for example, parenting support, practical and emotional support, and promoting positive activities for all family members. These provisions should also be underpinned by identifying and developing wider support networks for families that may include other family members, friends, neighbours and more formal interventions such as family group conferences (Carers Trust, 2020).

THE RIGHTS OF YOUNG CARERS AND PROTECTING CHILDHOODS

One of the main challenges young caring presents – and one that has been consistently overlooked in policy and practice discourses on, and in outcomes for, young carers – is that when children provide care, they are often undertaking the kinds of roles and responsibilities that are inappropriate for children, and that we usually associate with adulthood. When these roles are also disproportionate to children's age and level of maturity, it is more likely that their childhoods and transitions into adulthood will be disrupted and compromised; in these contexts, their rights as children become equally precarious. From a critical rights-based perspective, however, the rights of young carers must be balanced with their needs both as children (first) and as carers (including the right and desire/wish not to provide care) but set against the reality of a political context in which unpaid care provision by family members (of all ages) is condoned, regardless of whether people want to care or not (for many this is simply not a choice). Evidence shows, for example, that unpaid caring saves the UK government substantial sums of money each year – estimates suggest between £57 billion and over £100 billion, the latter more than four times the amount spent by local authorities (Parliamentary Office of Science and Technology, 2018).

With respect to the UK government's strategy on carers, one of the central aims was to give children greater recognition for their caring roles both in policy and in practice. In some respects, this has been helpful, especially to those families who are not able to access the kinds of services they need, or where children want to provide help and support that is not onerous and does not have a negative impact on their lives as children. In other ways, however, some of the strategies to support young carers fail to consider their rights as children. In 2020, for example, the government tested the viability of a national young carers recognition scheme that would enable children to identify themselves as young carers in order to benefit from discounts in a range of different settings and outlets (transport, the cinema and so on), thus confirming their roles as carers as an extant (and immutable?) fact (in the end the scheme was not introduced following the results of a feasibility study). In the Carers Action Plan (CAP) 2018–2020, the government also made a commitment to 'making sure young carers are not left behind' (Department of Health and Social Care, 2018, p. 22), with, once again, the emphasis on support for children as (established) *carers* rather than as *children* (mention of children in need is made only with reference to children and young people's mental health; Department of Health and Social Care, 2018, p.23). In the dedicated chapter on young carers in the CAP, no mention is made of prevention or of young carers' rights as *children*, and reference to safeguarding is made mainly with respect to improved strategies for the identification of young carers in families. Suggestions for supporting (identified and established) young carers in the CAP include 'groups to share experiences, mental health support or counselling, information provision through schools and educational establishments, and flexible educational support and careers planning' (Department of Health and Social Care, 2018, p. 22).

When considering young carers' rights as children, including their right to protection (which is enshrined in international children's rights under the UNCRC, 1989), the point at which caring becomes a dominant and negative aspect of children's lives is when needs assessments must take into consideration the risks and harms of caring. This is also where an approach that considers young carers as *children first* is crucial. Understanding and assessing young carers as children from a children's rights perspective (including their right to protection and to have a say in decision-making – UNCRC, 1989), rather than simply as carers, also inevitably and necessarily shifts the focus to early intervention and prevention considerations. Without this and without the kinds of interventions that recognize and address the needs of children and parents using both children's rights and whole family

approaches, then it is likely that children will continue to take on inappropriate caring roles.

REFLECTIVE QUESTIONS

- What would be an appropriate rights-based approach to addressing the needs of young carers?
- How can the needs of young carers *and their families* be addressed most effectively?
- What kinds of interventions are necessary to prevent children taking on inappropriate caring roles?

CONCLUSION

It is recognized that, for children, providing care that is *long-term, unrecognised and unsupported* in families affected by chronic illness and/or disability has a detrimental impact on their lives. Young carers and their families need interventions that prioritise whole family working and that recognize the rights and needs of children to ensure their caring responsibilities do not adversely affect their childhoods or their futures. Early interventions are critical in this process.

REFERENCES

Abraham, K., Aldridge, J., 2010. The Mental Well-being of Young Carers in Manchester. Young Carers Research Group with Manchester Carers Forum and Child and Adolescent Mental Health Services (CAMHS), Manchester.

Aldridge, J., 2019. Where are we now? Twenty-five years of research, policy and practice on young carers. Crit. Soc. Policy 38 (1), 155–165.

Aldridge, J., Becker, S., 2003. Children Who Care for Parents With Mental Illness: Perspectives of Young Carers, Parents and Professionals. The Policy Press, Bristol.

Aldridge, J., Becker, S., 1993. Children who Care: Inside the World of Young Carers. Young Carers Research Group, Loughborough University, Loughborough, UK.

Aldridge, J., Clay, D., Connors, C., Day, N., Gkiza, M., 2016. The Lives of Young Carers in England: Qualitative Report to Department for Education. https://www.gov.uk/government/uploads/system/uploads/attachment_data/file/498115/DFE-RR499_The_lives_of_young_carers_in_England.pdf.

Carers Trust, 2020. Whole Family Approaches. https://professionals.carers.org/whole-family-approaches.

Carers Trust, 2013. Protecting Young Carers From Bullying: A Guide for Schools, Community Groups and Policy Makers. https://professionals.carers.org/sites/default/files/protecting_young_carers_from_bullying_a_guide_for_schools_community_groups_and_policy_makers.pdf.

Cheesbrough, S., Harding, C., Webster, H., Taylor, L., Aldridge, J., 2017. The Lives of Young Carers in England: Omnibus Survey Report, January, 2017. Department for Education. https://www.gov.uk/government/uploads/system/uploads/attachment_data/file/582575/Lives_of_young_carers_in_England_Omnibus_research_report.pdf.

The Children's Commissioner for England, 2016. Young Carers: The Support Provided to Young Carers in England, Office of the Children's Commissioner. http://www.childrenscommissioner.gov.uk/sites/default/files/publications/Young%20Carers%20report%20December%202016.pdf.

The Children's Society, 2020. Barriers and Experiences (BAME and young carers). https://www.childrenssociety.org.uk/youngcarer/engage-toolkit/barriers-and-experiences.

The Children's Society, 2015. No Wrong Doors: Working Together to Support Young Carers and Their Families. https://www.local.gov.uk/sites/default/files/documents/no-wrong-doors-working-to-27d.pdf.

The Children's Society, 2013. Hidden from View: The Experiences of Young Carers in England. The Children's Society, Winchester.

Dearden, C., Becker, S., 2004. Young Carers in the UK: The 2004 Report. Carers UK and The Children's Society, London.

Department of Health and Social Care, 2018. Carers Action Plan 2018-2020: Supporting Carers Today. https://assets.publishing.service.gov.uk/government/uploads/system/uploads/attachment_data/file/713781/carers-action-plan-2018-2020.pdf.

Falkov, A., 2013. The Family Model Handbook: An Integrated Approach to Supporting Mentally Ill Parents and Their Children. Pavilion, London.

HM Government, 2014a. The Care Act, 2014. http://www.legislation.gov.uk/ukpga/2014/23/contents/enacted.

HM Government, 2014b. Children and Families Act, 2014. http://www.legislation.gov.uk/ukpga/2014/6/contents/enacted.

HM Government, 2004. Children Act, 2004. http://www.legislation.gov.uk/ukpga/2004/31/contents.

HM Government, 1989. Children Act, 1989. http://www.legislation.gov.uk/ukpga/1989/41/contents.

Learning and Work Institute, 2016. Young Adult Carers. https://learningandwork.org.uk/what-we-do/social-justice-inclusion/young-adult-carers/.

Office for National Statistics, 2013. 2011 Census Analysis: Unpaid Care in England and Wales. https://www.ons.gov.uk/peoplepopulationandcommunity/healthandsocialcare/healthcaresystem/articles/2011censusanalysisunpaidcareinenglandandwales2011andcomparisonwith2001/2013-02-15.

Parliamentary Office of Science and Technology, 2018. Unpaid Care, no 582, July 2018. Houses of Parliament, London.

United Nations Convention on the Rights of the Child (1989). https://www.ohchr.org/en/professionalinterest/pages/crc.aspx

Zayed, Y., Harker, R., 2015. Children in Care in England: Statistics. Briefing paper 04470. House of Commons Library, London.

12

FROM 10S TO TEENS: WORKING WITH YOUNG PEOPLE (EDITORS INTRODUCTION)

LISA WARWICK ▪ RACHEL FYSON ▪ RACHAEL CLAWSON

Public attention and sympathy lie largely with young children and babies, in contrast with young people (or teenagers) who are more often conceptualised as problematic. Mainstream media representation of child protection, for example, often focus on the 'failures' of professionals to protect young children and babies, who are presented as innocent victims of unimaginable adult aggression. In contrast, stories involving young people typically present them as aggressors or blame them for 'life choices' even when these so-called choices might more reasonably be regarded as the consequences of prior abuse or neglect. Any links between the now 'problematic' teenagers and the 'innocent' young children they were until recently are removed from the narrative.

This portrayal of child protection is unhelpful. Over half of all children who require child protection services are between the ages of 10 and 17 (Department for Education (DfE), 2021a; 2021b), and practitioners need to be equipped to support children of all ages. Media portrayals therefore not only perpetuate unhelpful narratives, but also generate unrealistic representations of what child protection actually entails. This chapter seeks to address this imbalance by focussing on child protection with young people aged 10 to 17 years.

Work with young people is perhaps best understood as supporting the transition from childhood to adulthood. This period can present challenges for young people, as they navigate their own increasing freedom, with all the opportunity and risk this incorporates. It can also present challenges for parents, carers and other adults involved in young people's lives, including professionals. Much of the tension that exists between adults and young people during this period is based on conflicting perspectives on experience, choice and trust. Just as young people may struggle to accept adult's 'wisdom', so may adults struggle to accept that young people need increasing autonomy. This is despite the fact that the Mental Capacity Act 2005 enshrines in law the right to make decisions for oneself from the age of 16, and that legal concepts such as 'Gillick Competence' support independent decision-making from mid-teens. These issues are central to child protection practice with young people and are addressed by Leslie Hicks and Mike Stein in Chapter 12a: *Child Protection in Adolescence*.

It is also important to recognise that experiences of children and young people may change radically between the generations. The children and young adults of today have, in many senses, grown up in a different world than that of their parents. Whilst all young people experience puberty and the accompanying sexual and bodily changes, how puberty is experienced will be shaped by the intersection of wider socioeconomic factors such as gender, ethnicity, sexuality, culture, poverty, social class, disability and more. Legal changes have both made young people more responsible (e.g. the lowering of the age of criminal responsibility in England from 12 to 10) and reduced the range of decisions they are judged old enough to make (under the age of 18 it is unlawful to buy cigarettes or alcohol or to get married; compulsory education is now extended to age 18 years). The advancement of communications technology – mobile phones, the internet, social media – shape young people's experiences of the world.

Political, economic and social changes have affected the expectations of young people in relations to education, employment and housing. More young people go on to university, but there are also more young people on minimum-wage zero-hour contracts and young people typically live with their parents for longer. Transitions from school to work or higher education and from parental home to independence are negotiated by (almost) everyone, but not everyone has the same experience. Young people with care experience may face particular challenges, as discussed by Jo Dixon in Chapter 12b: *Leaving Care*.

Child protection concerns are raised for a variety of reasons, and for some young people the concerns may be due to their own behaviours, because they are a risk to themselves or others. In these areas of practice the complexities of care and control are acute, as professionals seek to balance the harms young people may have experienced and the harm they now present towards others. Some examples of these more complex areas of practice are addressed within the latter half of this chapter. In Chapter 12c, Joe Yates and Steph Yates explore practice with young people involved with the criminal justice system, in *Safeguarding and Children in Conflict with the Law*. In Chapter 12d, *Children and Young People Who Sexually Harm Others,* Stuart Allardyce and Peter Yates explore how to intervene, understand and manage young people who display harmful sexual behaviours towards others. And finally, in Chapter 12e, Helen Bonnick explores an emerging area of professional practice in *Child to Parent Violence and Abuse*. Each of these chapters explore behaviours that put other people and the young people themselves at risk. They also each acknowledge and explore how complex this work is when seeing and understanding the young person as a legal child who needs protecting in the here and now, protecting those who may be being harmed by the young person and hoping to prevent the recurrence of these behaviours in the young person's future.

REFERENCES

Department for Education, 2021a. Characteristics of Children in Need (2020-2021). https://explore-education-statistics.service.gov.uk/find-statistics/characteristics-of-children-in-need/2021#dataBlock-87ec9f7f-69e0-434b-64cc-08d987e087b8-charts. (Accessed 8 August 2022).

Department for Education, 2021b. Children Looked After in England Including Adoptions (2020-2021). https://explore-education-statistics.service.gov.uk/find-statistics/children-looked-after-in-england-including-adoptions/2021. (Accessed 8 August 2022).

12a

CHILD PROTECTION IN ADOLESCENCE

LESLIE HICKS ■ MIKE STEIN

KEY POINTS

- Setting the scene in relation to trends in adolescence.
- Discussing young people's emergent needs.
- Identifying complexities in addressing adolescent needs.
- Examining the implications for developing child protection practice.

INTRODUCTION

All aspects of child protection involve extensive complexities for consideration. When working with young people, practice frequently has to move beyond the home and family nexus to incorporate wider environments, in line with the broadening experiences that are associated with psychological, social and physical development in adolescence. Widening horizons bring potential for an increase in risks and thereby a very broad range of factors to consider when aiming to keep young people safe from harm.

For the purposes of considering issues faced in the period stretching between childhood and adulthood and considering the preferences expressed by young people themselves, wherever possible, we use the term 'young people' when referring to those within an age range of 10 to 18, unless in special circumstances, such as young people with special educational needs or those involved with Youth Offending Teams. This period aligns with that acknowledged as adolescence by legal systems in the UK (HM Government, 2018) and the United Nations Convention on the Rights of the Child (United Nations, 1989).

TRENDS IN ADOLESCENCE

Young people aged between 10 and 19 years and 10 and 24 years constitute approximately 11% and 18% of the total UK population, respectively (Hagel and Shah, 2019). Although age-specific data are reported a little differently across nations and data sets and legislative frameworks and categorisations differ, 'data on age distribution of children on the child protection register are broadly similar in all four [UK] countries' (Rees, 2016, p. 278).

In England, 53% of young people categorised as children in need in 2019 were aged 10 years or over (Department for Education, 2019a). The figure for those aged 10 to 15 who were the subject of a child protection plan in 2019 was quite similar to those aged 5 to 9 years (15,580 and 15,180, respectively) and lower than the figure for 0 to 4 years (17,950). Adding those who were 10 to 16 years and over brings the 10 to 16+ figure to 17,920 (NSPCC, 2019). Excluding unborn babies, this represents approximately 35% of those subject to a plan. In Wales, those between 10 and 18 years on the child protection register in 2018–19 numbered 940 (50%) in comparison with 1880 aged between 0 and 9 years (Statistics for Wales, 2019). Correspondingly, the figures for 2018 in Scotland for 11 to 16+ years were 450 (21%) and 2111 for 0 to 10 years, and for Northern Ireland in 2019, for 0 to 11 years there were 1739 children registered, with 12 to 16+ year olds numbering 481 (28%) (Scottish Government, 2019; Information Analysis Directorate, 2019). There is an overall taper with age; however, it is evident that young people represent a considerable proportion of overall vulnerable populations.

Added to this clear, widespread need for protection is an extensive portrait of the state of well-being amongst young people. This is measured in various ways, including via 'objective' quantitative measures that focus on aspects such as health, education and deprivation (for example, data collected by the Office for National Statistics (ONS, 2018)), as well as 'subjective' measures, drawn from young people's own views about factors such as their happiness, satisfaction with their lives and general psychological well-being (see for example, *The Good Childhood Report 2019* from The Children's Society (TCS, 2019)). The different sources of data portray multifaceted experiences that increase in complexity as children age. Chief findings from the TCS report indicate that 'an estimated quarter of a million 10-15 year olds in the UK may be unhappy with their lives; boys are becoming less happy with their appearance; happiness in friendships is in decline, any experience of financial strain or poverty in childhood is linked to lower well-being by age 14 (TCS, 2019) and financial disadvantage in childhood relates to 'lower well-being by age 14 years'. Similarly, a report from the Department for Education (2019b), focusing primarily on England, integrates data on children and young people's well-being and indicates that well-being declines as children and young people age, with a particular decrease during adolescence through to early adulthood.

In England, messages drawn from analysis of serious case reviews (SCRs; known as 'safeguarding practice reviews' (SPRs) at the time of writing) highlighted that issues experienced prior to suicide and risks relating to child sexual exploitation for those aged 11 to 18 years were 'growing areas of concern' (Sidebotham et al., 2016, p. 98). These trends have continued, and in the sixth triennial review of SCRs, Brandon et al. (2020, p.113) record that almost one-third of the 368 reviews related to children of 11 years old and above, with the most common causes being '(i) risk-taking or violent behaviour by the young person, and (ii) child sexual exploitation'.

Added to these indicators of need and distress is a broader portrait relating to those who increasingly find themselves transitioning between education and employment without opportunities for either, who are thereby categorised as 'not in education, employment, or training' (NEET). In the UK in February 2020, 11.1% of young people aged 16 to 24 years were identified in this way, of whom 39.6% were unemployed, with the remainder being classified as 'economically inactive' (Office for National Statistics, 2020). This is a slightly downward trend; however, the scale of the situation becomes clearer if the total *number* of young people represented in the 11.1% grouped as NEET is stated: 763,000 young people were in this position in the UK at the time of data collection.

Although this represents a troubling picture overall, it is encouraging to see that these and related issues are recognised nationally and internationally and are now receiving extensive attention from major organisations. For example, both the World Health Organisation (WHO) and UNICEF now focus on the key challenges in this life stage and their implications for positive development (UNICEF, 2012; WHO, 2017).

From this brief consideration of categorisations, classifications and the situations of young people, it is evident that patterns of need in adolescence are quite different from those of younger children. Where young people experience multiple disadvantages, the potential for agency, achievement, enjoyment and safety may become very limited, pointing to the continuing need to invest in protecting and supporting young people from within children's services, in order to lay positive foundations for future lives.

EMERGENT NEEDS IN ADOLESCENCE

It is clear from the breadth of training courses, practitioner insight, theoretical models and research findings that a wealth of knowledge has been established about the way that development in adolescence brings with it a broad range of convergent, changing characteristics (Coleman, 2010). These include extensive physiological, psychological and social factors (Aldgate et al., 2006).

Longstanding knowledge about brain growth has indicated its influence on 'thinking and reasoning' aspects, such as cognitive and moral development, and the ways in which these stimulate a range of behaviours, such as impulsivity, swift decision-making and heightened risk-taking (Coleman, 2010). Attention more recently has been paid to neurological development and the ways in which the brain continues to grow into the early to mid-twenties (Research in Practice, 2014). Brain plasticity influences greater receptivity to environmental stressors and 'adolescents demonstrate heightened effects of peer influence on risk taking, risk perception and reasoning, hypersensitivity to social exclusion, and reduced use of other people's perspective in decision making' (Foulkes and Blakemore, 2018, p. 316).

This extended period clearly represents a phase ripe with opportunities for social reinforcement (Jones et al., 2014). Set alongside broader and evolving ecological interrelationships, such as those within families and with friends, schools, neighbourhoods and wider influences, this is often a tumultuous time. All of these fluctuating factors are prominent in shaping youthful aspirations towards independence, adult expectations of young people and their capacity to 'stand on their own two feet', plus a burgeoning sense of identity and corresponding agency in relation to the social world. The extent to which young people have a sense of agency in their lives varies according to individual circumstances and histories (Morrison et al., 2019). Choices made by young people need to be assessed in context – there may be powerful factors influencing choice, serving to either push or pull, thereby compromising a young person's ability to perceive risk.

Risk and Resilience in Adolescence

Alongside these changes, an increase in threats to the well-being of adolescents arising from external environments means that risks to safety have increased greatly in 21st century life. A clear example of this lies in the relatively easy access to online and potentially harmful communication at local and global levels. Learning to perceive, assess and contend satisfactorily with risk are vital aspects of human growth. As adolescents' horizons broaden beyond their families, exposure to risky situations increases, along with opportunities to actually take risks by trying new experiences, and to learn

from doing this. Amidst an array of individual, family and societal factors (Fitzsimons et al., 2018), the influence of past experiences may determine the extent to which behaviour manifests as increasingly risky, possibly emanating from earlier experiences of abuse and/or neglect (Hanson and Holmes, 2015).

Contemporary awareness of the exposure of young people to a range of risk-laden situations includes a bleak catalogue of potential harms, within the dynamics of families and increasingly, beyond into much broader contexts. These wider domains frequently sit beyond the view or control of parents and carers, and importantly, may not be straightforwardly addressed by use of child protection categories, as shown effectively in Table 12a.1.

As Table 12a.1 illustrates, both intra- and extra-familial risks are important. Concerningly, as vulnerability increases in this widening world, there is potential for several risk factors to align concurrently and in turn, the potential for external, predatory influences to escalate. Combined with an emerging sense of agency, addressing such risks and their effects becomes a complex business (Rees and Stein, 1999).

The influence of peers is often immense at this life stage, both directly and in virtual worlds. Peer encouragement to experiment and to conform to norms may result in anxieties and extreme pressures being experienced by young people, and social influence of peers is frequently stronger than that of families, including parents (Knoll et al., 2015). There are many relatively new fields for research focusing on this period, including the effects of social media use on young people, and prevalence of the onset of mental health issues, such as anxiety and self-harm (Lockwood et al., 2017; Marino et al., 2020). Increases in risk and social influences on behaviours combine to make this a perplexing time for young people.

Professionals may assume that adolescents are more resilient than younger children, more able to contend with maltreatment and more equipped to seek help (Horwath, 2007; Rees et al., 2010). However, such perceptions may result in a failure to intervene (Rees et al., 2011). There is evidence that promoting resilience can be positive if this incorporates factors that serve to potentially strengthen young people's lives, including those within environmental contexts, such

TABLE 12A.1

Serious Risks Facing Adolescents in the UK Today (by Closest Child Protection Categories)

Child protection category within which risks fit, or are closest to	Some of the risks adolescents face in the UK (often distinctive within adolescence, either in prevalence or impact)
Sexual abuse	Sexual exploitation by gangs or groups Sexual abuse by peers Duress/coercion to sexually exploit/abuse others Online sexual abuse Intrafamilial sexual abuse Sexual abuse by those in positions of trust or authority
Physical abuse	Family violence – adult(s) to adolescent Mutual family violence between adult(s) and adolescent(s) Gang-related and community violence Violence from relationship partner
Neglect	Neglect from family members including rejection and abandonment, and parental mental health or substance misuse problems that disrupt parenting capacity and incur caring responsibilities on part of the young person Overly restrictive parenting Neglect in custody[a]
Emotional abuse	Emotional abuse from family members towards adolescents Emotional abuse between family members and adolescent Extensive bullying by peers and/or online Exposure to other risks listed above and below Living with domestic abuse between parents Emotional abuse from relationship partner
None of the above	Homelessness Self-harm including deliberate self-harm, suicide attempts, eating disorders Gang involvement Substance misuse

[a]Neglect is the persistent failure to meet a child's basic physical and/or psychological needs. In young offender institutions, arguably children are not looked after by a parent or parental agent who aims to meet the child's basic psychological needs (The Howard League for Penal Reform, 2010). This is in stark contrast to homes with authoritative parenting and also to residential care homes underpinned by a caring ethos. (See Implications for Developing Child Protection Practice in Relation to Adolescence for further discussion of the extent and impact of this.)
Source: Hanson and Holmes, 2015.

as social and economic factors, family situations and community resources (Hicks and Stein, 2010). In this way, developing resilience entails a consideration of protective factors, which in turn, requires a strengths-based approach to practice with young people, based on a commitment to participation and children's rights (Stein, 2009).

COMPLEXITIES IN ADDRESSING ADOLESCENT NEEDS

A Time of Change and Transition

Adolescence represents a period of biological change and social transition that is unlike other developmental stages. For some young people, encouragement to contend with these transformations requires no external intervention, whilst for others, a level of help and support may be needed or required. Much depends on individual circumstances and the extent to which supportive networks exist. Where maltreatment is involved, either episodic or experienced over time, increased support may be necessary to address vulnerabilities and importantly, to protect young people from further harm.

Adolescents as a group lack homogeneity, and needs will vary according to individual circumstances, such as gender, sexuality, faith, ethnicity, disability, poverty and potentially the intersection of a considerable range of these and related factors (Sankar et al., 2019). In order to attain well-being, needs in adolescence cluster around feeling safe and secure, being loved and cared for, having freedom, independence and scope for self-expression, developing a sense of achievement, alongside feeling listened to and respected. Attaining an acceptable balance between offering 'safety and security' and sufficient 'freedom to grow' often presents challenges for all concerned. Although self-evident, it is perhaps worth drawing attention to the formative nature of this part of the life course, insofar as the quality of experiences here have been shown to bring implications throughout life and forwards into subsequent generations (Azzopardi et al., 2019).

Adding to the rapidly changing nature of young people's development and their environmental contexts, research focusing on adolescent neglect (Rees et al., 2011) indicates that practitioners are keenly aware of age-related variations in experience and achievements. The legal context for determining what is permissible at particular ages is not particularly helpful in situating young people. Just a few examples of variation in England illustrate a potential for uncertainty. There are clear differences in the ages at which a child is seen to be equipped to take criminal responsibility, join the army without parental consent, leave education or training, vote in parliamentary elections, donate blood or consent to have sex. This variation contributes to an unclear status for adolescents. Similarly, norms surrounding the behaviour of young people vary according to perspective. What is expected of adolescents and thereby considered to be usual and acceptable will differ considerably between different contexts and parties. In this way, norms, legal prescriptions and social expectations combine to offer a rocky springboard into adult responsibilities.

While assessing needs is rarely a straightforward matter, the fluid nature of influences external to families brings added complexities to the largely family-focused concerns associated with assessment of younger children's needs. For the first time, the 2018 revision of government guidance for England, *Working Together to Safeguard Children*, draws attention to the inclusion of factors beyond relationships within families:

Interventions should focus on addressing these wider environmental factors, which are likely to be a threat to the safety and welfare of a number of different children who may or may not be known to local authority children's social care.

HM Government (2018, 33, p. 22)

This quotation refers to potential invisibility, which is a further factor for concern when identifying needs. In adolescence, engagement with adults can be problematic, particularly when grappling with the transitions characteristic of this life-stage. Frequently, feelings of insecurity may make it difficult to develop communicative, trusting relationships with adults, including with professionals (Jobe and Gorin, 2013). Reports of feeling intimidated and stressed by encounters with professionals indicate that forging relationships that enable young people to participate in child protection decision-making is not easy to attain (Buckley et al., 2011). Correspondingly, young people may be regarded by practitioners as putting themselves at risk and exacerbating the situation through their own behaviour (Rees et al., 2010; Rees and Stein, 2012). These factors may be compounded by practitioners' experiences of the related challenge of engagement with parents and carers (Hicks, 2014). It is particularly important to recognise the complexities resulting from changing family relationships and structures, and the corresponding fluctuations in attachment and a sense of security. Since effective assessments require consideration of different viewpoints – those of young people, families and carers, and practitioners – the combination of these perspectives may in itself become difficult to establish as congruent, making an holistic assessment of circumstances hard to accomplish. Whilst addressing these factors is complex, it is worth emphasising that, taken together, the transitions and shifts experienced during adolescence represent important opportunities for interventions. Such turning points can lead to lasting, positive change for young people.

Assessing Adolescent Needs

The long established domains and dimensions of the *Framework for the Assessment of Children in Need and their Families* used in England and Wales (HM Government, 2018) include developmental needs, parenting capacity and family and environmental factors (Fig. 12a.1). Similar assessment areas are utilised in Scotland and Northern Ireland (Calder et al., 2012;

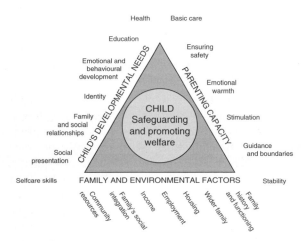

Fig. 12a.1 ■ Framework for the assessment of children in need and their families. (Working Together to Safeguard Children, HM Government, 2018, p. 27)

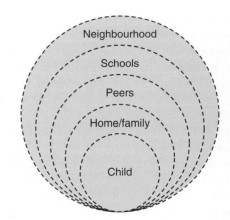

Fig. 12a.2 ■ Context of adolescent safety and vulnerability. (Firmin, 2013, p. 47.)

Northern Ireland Department of Health, Social Services and Public Safety, 2011). These lay firm foundations for the development of assessment tools generally and are reflected in detail in 'Early Help Assessments'. Importantly, the base of the triangle (see Fig. 12a.1), focuses on aspects in the wider environment and provides useful indicators for identifying the emerging needs of young people.

A heartening appreciation of the importance of safety and well-being in adolescence, coupled with growing recognition that the current child protection system is predicated on a vital need to protect young children from neglect and abuse, argues for reconsidering approaches to protecting older children. Many local authorities in England are seeking to develop ways to aid practitioners in the complex identification of risks. Building on these factors, a conceptualisation of adolescent safety and vulnerability (Firmin, 2013) highlights the need for contextual safeguarding, where an understanding is developed of both risk and the dynamics within wider contexts, together with recognition of 'push and pull factors' that young people experience when making choices (Fig. 12a.2). Firmin et al. (2019) distinguish between three potentially overlapping terms when considering ways to protect the safety and well-being of young people. 'Complex safeguarding' relates to 'criminality and exploitation', such as child criminal and/or sexual exploitation,

county lines and trafficking. 'Contextual safeguarding', as above, requires assessing and intervening in contexts outside families. 'Transitional safeguarding' recognises the developmental needs of older young people, on the basis that a 'more fluid and transitional approach is needed for young people entering adulthood' (Firmin et al., 2019, p. 6) (Case Study 12a.1).

Again, the breadth of these factors argues for the need to work across agencies, and perhaps most importantly, for 'extrafamilial risk' to be incorporated into all assessment tools for young people (Peace and Atkinson, 2019). To determine which agency/ies may be most appropriate to support a young person, it is essential to consider the various contexts in which interaction takes place.

IMPLICATIONS FOR DEVELOPING CHILD PROTECTION PRACTICE IN RELATION TO ADOLESCENCE

Here and elsewhere (Hicks and Stein, 2010; Rees et al., 2011) we highlight the value of utilising the concepts of primary prevention (addressed via universal services), secondary interventions (addressed via early intervention and assessment) and tertiary interventions (designed to prevent recurrence of difficulties) to guide practice with young people. More broadly, in this section we offer 'factors for practitioners to consider' (Table 12a.2), discuss implications in terms of

CASE STUDY 12A.1: COMPLEX SAFEGUARDING CASE EXAMPLE

Take the example of a teenage boy who is struggling to fit into his new school – and his behaviour at school and at home is becoming challenging. In an attempt to fit in, he frequently meets his peers at the local bus station. But at the bus station he is threatened and coerced into passing packages of money between drug dealers and storing weapons at his house. Traditional interventions may have focused solely on his behaviour and what he and his parents can do to change it – including stopping him from going to the bus station. He may also have been treated as a criminal.

A complex or contextual safeguarding approach would instead focus on a spectrum of his needs. This may include helping him access positive activities and hobbies to nurture his overall well-being and increase opportunities to make healthier friendships. They may also include ensuring the bus station is well lit and that its CCTV system is working. They could also include working with his parents to help educate them about child exploitation.

Source: Marsh, N. (2019)

young people's needs, and consider multiagency working and empowerment.

Changing Notions of Needs in Adolescence

A major point for consideration relates to redefining the period of 'adolescence' to accommodate changing biological and social patterns. Arnett's theory of 'emerging adulthood' (Arnett, 2000), and more recently, the work of Sawyer and colleagues (2018), recognises the fluidity of boundaries between adolescence and early adulthood. To some extent, these changes are starting to be acknowledged, for example by legislation in England and Wales that addresses the duty to support young people deemed particularly vulnerable, such as those with special educational needs and disabilities (SEND) and those who are leaving care (Stein, 2012). Further to this, the assumption that young people should be capable of 'standing on their own two feet' at the age of 16 years merits challenge, not least in light of heightened vulnerabilities and the prominent risk of exploitation in a network connected world.

Multiagency Working

Owing to the broadening interrelationships that are characteristic of adolescence, the capacity to protect young people may be stretched for practitioners who work from within a single agency. Furthermore, young people's needs may be identified initially from within a wide range of systems, including education, health, youth justice and social care. Those working with young people need to engage across agencies in order to attain a full picture of experiences and changes, and when/where/with whom these occur. This indicates a compelling and ongoing need to strengthen multiagency working, particularly in light of broadening opportunities to enhance resilience (Case Study 12a.2).

Frameworks and processes to aid collaboration and information-sharing between professionals from different disciplines are essential. These need to be founded on close working relationships between practitioners, robust communication mechanisms and the agreement of clear, common goals that practitioners feel free to own. Assumptions made about young people's behaviour, their development and notions of expectations and responsibilities need to be overtly clarified so that common standards of practice can be achieved.

Shared understanding of young people's risks and difficulties are vital to establish, underpinned by confidence in systems such as information sharing processes. These demand an understanding of agency thresholds to guarantee that young people's needs are identified and addressed by services.

Young people themselves need to be placed at the centre of multiagency working, where positive relationships are established over time. Duplication of effort between services and unnecessary repetition of histories and needs are likely to be counterproductive to enabling trust and importantly, to result in despondency and disengagement.

TABLE 12A.2		
Understanding Adolescent Needs: Factors for Practitioners to Consider		
Key factors associated with adolescence	**What this involves for young people:**	**Practitioners need to be alert to:**
Complex developmental life stage	Intensive period of growth: ■ Physical ■ Psychological ■ Social	■ Young people may be experiencing strain in adjusting to convergent changes ■ What is happening for young people may not be recognisable by young people themselves ■ Communicating feelings and anxieties and/or developing trusting relationships may not be easy for young people ■ Being able to spend time in developing trusting relationships with young people is essential
Period of transition	■ Ambiguities associated with co-terminus childhood vulnerabilities and developing a sense of independence ■ A period where identity develops, fluctuates and changes ■ Increased sense of agency, self-determination ■ Potential for turning points, both negative and positive	■ What is seen as 'normal' and/or acceptable behaviour varies according to surrounding expectations ■ Each young person's experience is individual, varies according to circumstances (e.g. special needs ■ Importance of being alert to both intra- and extra-family issues, and the dynamics between the two
Widening horizons	Broadening social worlds potentially leads to increases in: ■ Vulnerability and uncertainty ■ Risk of being harmed ■ Risk-taking behaviours – 'testing' ways of being ■ Opportunities to maximise positive experiences	■ Factors outside the family are influential ■ Peer influence is often more important than that of parents/carers/families ■ Potential for practitioners to assume active choice in relation to risk-taking, rather than looking holistically at influences beyond the individual young person and/or their family situation ■ Need for professional proactivity/curiosity about young people's lives, challenging responses to exploitation that locate blame within young people themselves ■ Risk reduction is an insufficient response ■ Longer term approaches are essential ■ Developing resilience requires working to strengthen wider contextual relationships and supports, including family, friends, mentors, school/college/employers, communities
Heightened vulnerabilities	Specific situations may lead to greater potential for protection needed in adolescence, for example: ■ Disabilities ■ Special Educational Needs and Disability (SEND) ■ Young carers ■ Unaccompanied asylum-seeking children ■ Sexual orientation ■ Gender identities ■ Contexts where female genital mutilation is practised ■ Diminished parenting capacity	■ Changes in family structures/situations/dependencies ■ Intersecting situations/needs ■ Potential for isolation/alienation/bullying/withdrawal ■ Emerging mental health issues ■ Ensure cultural competence, e.g. cultural sensibilities and roles, need for interpreters

CASE STUDY 12A.2: MULTIAGENCY WORKING CASE EXAMPLE

Surrey youth support service

In 2012, Surrey disbanded its youth offending team and incorporated the YOT's functions into a wider youth support service (YSS). The Surrey YSS comprises 11 local teams, and utilises a proactive keyworker approach to help and support young people experiencing one or more of a range of risks. Those risks include homelessness, disengagement from education, employment or training, mental health difficulties (where the young person is open to but not engaged with CAMHS) and offending. The team also work with adolescents categorised as 'children in need'.

A young person's caseworker will work with the young person to understand their view of the situation and to develop a holistic package of support. Support is mostly delivered by the caseworker, who brings in suitably qualified specialists for advice and co-work when required. In this way, the relationship between the young person and their keyworker is developed and harnessed as the central driver of change. Keyworkers focus on young people's strengths and work with the young person to find opportunities to develop these.

The YSS works closely with other council-led teams, such as housing, and also has developed partnerships with public, voluntary and private sector employers and local economic partnerships to provide a route to training and employment opportunities for young people.

This 'one-stop shop' approach and having one individual keyworker means young people don't have to navigate complex pathways (with the associated risks of rejection and delay) and can instead have multiple needs met through one holistic package. Labelling is also minimised when young people are supported by the generic YSS rather than a YOT. The YSS approach also has the potential for cost-savings.

Source: Hanson and Holmes (2015)

All of these factors rely on meaningful discussions. Mutual understanding needs to be established between multiagency professionals, young people, their families and communities of support.

Empowering Young People

Coming to understand young people requires relationship-based practice. In turn, this can enable robust assessment of needs, as informed by both present and past experiences. Young people frequently may hold views that differ from those of adults, meaning that practitioners' communication skills are essential to developing an understanding of young people's lives. It is important to recognise the potential negative influence that vocabulary can have, for example, if implying that young people are making lifestyle choices when risk-taking behaviours may be resulting from bullying or grooming. Using strengths-based approaches to enable young people to make choices can help to build a positive sense of self and overall agency.

Listening to and understanding young people's views, particularly on issues such as risk and maltreatment, form a vital part in developing trusting relationships. Identifying a reliable key worker who provides consistency in support can serve to build young people's confidence and is central to facilitating well-coordinated multiagency working. Locating positive peer support networks can help to reduce isolation and to offer empathic reassurance and inspiration.

In terms of information, lengthy documents can be counterproductive to good communication. Material provided in concise formats that are accessible to young people, for example audio or video clips, online resources and pocket-sized infographics can be useful aids to supporting needs as these arise.

In conclusion, the changes characteristic of adolescence include widening social worlds that potentially lead to an increase in risks being encountered outside the home. In turn, this requires practitioners to 'stretch' their assessment of needs to beyond the family nexus. Responses need to be predicated on young person-centred approaches, where children's rights and empowerment are prioritised.

For some young people, their immediate context involves multiple disadvantages and potential to 'slip through the net' of protection. For many young people, this period represents a time of optimism about the future, where opportunities are welcomed and aspirations are high. The challenge for those involved in protecting children is to enable the latter set of ambitions to become a shared concern for all.

REFLECTIVE QUESTIONS

- How do the needs of adolescents differ from those of younger children, and what concepts and theories have informed your understanding of these?
- What are the implications for the 'assessment process', arising from your understanding of the needs of specific groups of vulnerable young people?
- What principles should underpin multiagency working, and how would these translate into policy and practice?
- What is your understanding of 'relationship-based practice', 'resilience', 'vulnerability' and 'empowerment', and how may these concepts inform your work with young people?

FURTHER READING

Hanson, E., Holmes, D., 2015. That Difficult Age: Developing a More Effective Response to Risks in Adolescence: Evidence Scope. Research in Practice, Dartington.

Hicks, L., Stein, M., 2010. Neglect Matters: A Multi-agency Guide for Professionals Working Together on Behalf of Teenagers. Department for Children Schools and Families, London. Available at http://eprints.lincoln.ac.uk/id/eprint/4859/1/Hicks_and_Stein_Neglect_Matters.pdf. (Accessed 28 June 2020).

Rees, G., Stein, M., Hicks, L., Gorin, S., 2011. Adolescent Neglect: Research Policy and Practice. Jessica Kingsley Publishing, London.

Useful websites

Action for Children: https://www.actionforchildren.org.uk/
National Youth Agency: https://nya.org.uk/
NSPCC (National Society for the Prevention of Cruelty to Children): https://www.nspcc.org.uk/
The Children's Society: https://www.childrenssociety.org.uk/

REFERENCES

Aldgate, J., Jones, D., Rose, W., Jeffery, C. (Eds.), 2006. The Developing World of the Child. Jessica Kingsley Publishing, London.

Arnett, J., 2000. Emerging adulthood. A theory of development from the late teens through the twenties. Am. Psychol. 55 (5), 469–480.

Azzopardi, P., Hearps, S., Francis, K., et al., 2019. Progress in adolescent health and wellbeing: Tracking 12 headline indicators for 195 countries and territories, 1990–2016. The Lancet 393, 1101–1118.

Brandon, M., Sidebotham, P., Belderson, P., et al., 2020. Complexity and Challenge: A Triennial Analysis of SCRs 2014-2017 Final Report. Department for Education, London.

Buckley, H., Carr, N., Whelan, S., 2011. 'Like walking on eggshells': Service user views and expectations of the child protection. Child Fam. Soc. Work 16 (1), 101–110.

Calder, M., McKinnon, M., Sneddon, R., 2012. National Risk Framework to Support the Assessment of Children and Young People. Scottish Government, Edinburgh.

Coleman, J., 2010. The Nature of Adolescence, 4th edn. Routledge, Hove.

Department for Education, 2019a. Characteristics of Children in Need: 2018 to 2019 England. Department for Education, London.

Department for Education, 2019b. State of the Nation 2019: Children and Young People's Wellbeing. Department for Education, London.

Firmin, C., 2013. Something old or something new: Do pre-existing conceptualisations of abuse enable a sufficient response to abuse in young people's relationships and peer groups? In: Melrose, M., Pearce, J. (Eds.), Critical Perspectives on Child Sexual Exploitation and Related Trafficking. Palgrave Macmillan, Hampshire, pp. 38–51.

Firmin, C., Horan, J., Holmes, D., Hopper, G., 2019. Safeguarding During Adolescence– the Relationship Between Contextual Safeguarding, Complex Safeguarding and Transitional Safeguarding. Research in Practice, Dartington.

Fitzsimons, E., Jackman, J., Kyprianides, A., Villadsen, A., 2018. Determinants of Risky Behaviour in Adolescence: Evidence from the UK. Centre for Longitudinal Studies, UCL Institute of Education, London.

Foulkes, L., Blakemore, S., 2018. 'Studying individual differences in human adolescent brain development'. Nat. Neurosci. 21, 315–323.

Hanson, E., Holmes, D., 2015. That Difficult Age: Developing A More Effective Response to Risks in Adolescence: Evidence Scope. Research in Practice, Dartington.

Hagel, A., Shah, R., 2019. Key Data on Young People's Health. Association for Young People's Health, London.

Hicks, L., 2014. Responding to adolescent risk: Continuing challenges. In: Blyth, M. (Ed.), Moving on From Munro: Improving Children's Services. Policy Press, Bristol.

Hicks, L., Stein, M., 2010. Neglect Matters, a Multi-Agency Guide for Professionals Working Together on Behalf of Teenagers. Department for Children Schools and Families, London. http://eprints.lincoln.ac.uk/id/eprint/4859/1/Hicks_and_Stein_Neglect_Matters.pdf. (Accessed 28 June 2020).

HM Government, 2018. Working Together to Safeguard Children. A Guide to Inter-Agency Working to Safeguard And Promote the Welfare of Children. Department for Education, London. https://assets.publishing.service.gov.uk/government/uploads/system/uploads/attachment_data/file/729914/Working_Together_to_Safeguard_Children-2018.pdf. (Accessed 28 June 2020).

Horwath, J., 2007. Child neglect: Identification and Assessment. Palgrave Macmillan, Basingstoke, Hampshire.

Information Analysis Directorate, 2019. Children's Social Care Statistics Tables 2018/19. Northern Ireland Department of Health, Belfast.

Jobe, A., Gorin, S., 2013. 'If kids don't feel safe they don't do anything': Young people's views on seeking and receiving help from Children's Social Care Services in England. Child Fam. Soc. Work 18 (4), 429–439.

Jones, R., Somerville, L., Li, J., et al., 2014. 'Adolescent-specific patterns of behavior and neural activity during social reinforcement learning'. Cogn. Affect Behav. Neurosci. 14 (2), 683–697.

Knoll, L., Magis-Weinberg, L., Speekenbrink, M., Blakemore, S., 2015. Social influence on risk perception during adolescence. Psychol. Sci. 26 (5), 583–592.

Lockwood, J., Daley, D., Townsend, E., Sayal, K., 2017. Impulsivity and self-harm in adolescence: A systematic review. Eur. Child Adolesc. Psychiatry 26, 387–402.

Marino, C., Gini, G., Angelinia, F., Vienoa, A., Spada, M., 2020. Social norms and e-motions in problematic social media use among adolescents. Addictive Behaviors Reports. https://doi.org/10.1016/j.abrep.2020.100250. (Accessed 28 June 2020).

Marsh, N., 2019. Teenagers are vulnerable too – how social workers are trying new ways to keep them safe. Blog, 13 September. https://world.edu/teenagers-are-vulnerable-too-how-social-workers-are-trying-new-ways-to-keep-them-safe/. (Accessed 28 June 2020).

Morrison, F., Cree, V., Ruch, G., Winter, K., Hadfield, M., Hallett, S., 2019. Containment - exploring the concept of agency in children's statutory encounters with social workers. Childhood 26 (1), 98–112.

Northern Ireland Department of Health, Social Services and Public Safety, 2011. Understanding the Needs of Children in Northern Ireland. Northern Ireland. Department of Health, Social Services and Public Safety, Belfast.

NSPCC, 2019. Child Protection Plan Statistics: England 2015-2019. NSPCC, London.

Office for National Statistics, 2018. Children's Well-being Measures. ONS, London.

Office for National Statistics, 2020. Young People not in Education, Employment or Training (NEET), UK: February 2020. https://www.ons.gov.uk/employmentandlabourmarket/peoplenotinwork/unemployment/bulletins/youngpeoplenotineducationemploymentortrainingneet/february2020. (Accessed 28 June 2020).

Peace, D., Atkinson, R., 2019. Learning project 3: Holistic Approaches to Safeguarding Adolescents. University of Bedfordshire: The International Centre Researching Child Sexual Exploitation, Violence and Trafficking.

Rees, G., 2016. 'Child maltreatment' in J. Bradshaw. The Well-being of Children in the UK. Policy Press, Bristol.

Rees, G., Gorin, S., Jobe, A., Stein, M., Medforth, R., Goswami, H., 2010. Safeguarding Young People: Responding to Young People Aged 11 to 17 who Are Maltreated. The Children's Society, London.

Rees, G., Stein, M., 1999. NSPCC Policy Practice Research Series. The abuse of adolescents within the family. NSPCC, London.

Rees, G., Stein, M., 2012. Older children and the child protection system. In: Blyth, M., Solomon, E. (Eds.), Effective Safeguarding for Children and Young People: What Next After Munro? Policy Press, Bristol.

Rees, G., Stein, M., Hicks, L., Gorin, S., 2011. Adolescent Neglect: Research Policy and Practice. Jessica Kingsley Publishing, London.

Research in Practice, 2014. Risk-taking Adolescents and Child Protection. Research in Practice, Dartington.

Sankar, S., McCauley, H.L., Johnson, D.J., Thelamour, B., 2019. Gender and sexual prejudice and subsequent development of dating violence: Intersectionality among youth. In: Fitzgerald, H., Johnson, D., Qin, D., Villarruel, F., Norder, J. (Eds.), Handbook of Children and Prejudice, Integrating Research, Practice, and Policy. Springer Nature, Switzerland, pp. 289–302.

Sawyer, S., Azzopardi, P., Wickremarathne, D., Patton, G., 2018. 'The age of adolescence'. Lancet Child Adolesc. Health 2 (3), 223–228 Viewpoint.

Scottish Government, 2019. Children's Social Work Statistics Scotland, 2017-2018: Publication Tables. Scottish Government, Edinburgh.

Sidebotham, P., Brandon, M., Bailey, S., et al., 2016. Pathways To Harm, Pathways to Protection: A Triennial Review of Serious Case Reviews 2011-2014. Department for Education, London.

Statistics for Wales, 2019. Children on Child Protection Register By Local Authority, Category of Abuse and Age Group. https://gov.wales/social-services-activity-april-2018-march-2019. (Accessed 28 June 2020).

Stein, M., 2009. Resilience and young people leaving care. Child Care Pract. 14 (1), 35–44.

Stein, M., 2012. Young People Leaving Care: Supporting Pathways to Adulthood. Jessica Kingsley Publishers, London.

The Children's Society, 2019. The Good Childhood Report 2019. The Children's Society, London.

The Howard League for Penal Reform, 2010. Life Inside 2010: A unique insight into the day to day experiences of 15-17 year old males in prison. London: Howard League.

United Nations, 1989. Convention on the Rights of the Child. United Nations, New York.

UNICEF., 2012. Report Card on Adolescence. UNICEF, New York. https://www.unicef.org/publications/index_62280.html. (Accessed 28 June 2020).

World Health Organisation, 2017. Global Accelerated Action for the Health of Adolescents (AA-HA!): Guidance to Support Country Implementation. World Health Organization, Geneva. https://data.unicef.org/resources/progress-children-report-card-adolescents-number-10-april-2012/. (Accessed 28 June 2020).

12b LEAVING CARE

JO DIXON

KEY POINTS

- An introduction to leaving care and care leavers.
- Statistics, research and young people's views.
- The UK leaving care policy context.
- Leaving care journeys – experiences, risk and protective factors affecting post-care outcomes.
- Examples of what helps.

INTRODUCTION

Moving to independent adulthood is a time of opportunity but also one of risk and vulnerability for many young people who have been looked after in state care. Childhood trauma, placement instability and separation from support networks can result in many care leavers struggling during the transition from care. For some, difficulties and disadvantage continue throughout adult life. It is the responsibility of the state and related services, as corporate parents, to protect and support these young people in and after care.

This chapter discusses the characteristics and experiences of care leavers, what can help or hinder their post-care outcomes, and the UK policy and practice context for protecting them. Definitions, legislation and data-reporting vary across the four countries of the UK, so directly comparable information is unavailable; however, official statistics from each country suggest a broadly similar picture (Rees and Stein, 2016).

LEAVING CARE AND CARE LEAVERS

Leaving care refers to moving out of care towards independent adult living. It refers to a process rather than a single event. UK legal definitions (Children (Leaving Care) Act 2000) of a care leaver encompass being in care as a child and for some time after their 16th birthday. This includes being in care in foster, kinship or residential placements and, in Scotland, the parental home. The term usually refers to young people aged 16 years and over who:

- are leaving or have left their care placement for semi-independent or independent accommodation aged 16–17, or
- legally cease to be in care on turning 18 and move from their care-placement or remain with foster carers either on a formal basis up to age 21 (known as staying put) or informally as a member of their foster family for as long as both parties wish.

In both scenarios, and providing they meet the eligibility criteria (see Child Law Advice website [see under Resources at the end of this chapter] for eligibility criteria for England), they will be considered care leavers and have access to leaving care or aftercare services up to age 25 (and 26 in Scotland). The term care-experienced is increasingly used to refer to any child or adult who has been in care.

EXPLANATORY BOX

- *Eligible:* aged 16–17 years who have been looked after by the local authority for 13 weeks since age 14 and are still in care.

■ *Relevant:* aged 16–17 years who meet the criteria for eligible children, but who left care after reaching their 16th birthday.

■ *Former relevant:* young people aged 18–21 years and were eligible and/or relevant prior to becoming 18. The Children and Social Work Act (2017) enables care leavers to request support up to 25.

Care leavers are not a homogenous group. They vary in characteristics, needs and pathways through care, including different pre-care, in-care and post-care experiences. Some have additional needs, such as asylum-seeking children (Chapter 11c; Devenney, 2017; Mitchel, 2003), young parents (Chapter 11d; Craine et al., 2014, Fallen and Broadhurst, 2015), those with disabilities (Chapter 11a; Kelly et al., 2016; Rabiee and Priestly, 2001) and those involved in offending (Prison Reform Trust, 2016). Some care leavers will have spent all or most of their childhood in care, others will have alternated between care and home, and some who enter care as older adolescents will have spent very little time in care. Each of these journeys will affect young people's experiences and outcomes after care.

Research highlights the vulnerability of care leavers and their experiences of post-care difficulties and poor outcomes in employment, accommodation and well-being. This raises awareness of the need for improved service support. It is also important to consider care leavers who do well, in order to understand the protective and facilitative factors that enable positive outcomes after care.

POLICY CONTEXT

Policies particular to care leavers emerged around four decades ago. The Children Act 1989, one of the first pieces of legislation to recognise the state's role in supporting care leavers, introduced duties and powers for local authorities and other services to provide advice and assistance for care leavers in England and Wales. The 1989 Act also presented the notion of what is now known as corporate parenting (see Closer Look: Corporate Parenting), stating that responsibilities for supporting children in care and care leavers did not solely lie with children's services, but that they should call upon other services to help fulfil these responsibilities.

CLOSER LOOK: CORPORATE PARENTING

Corporate parenting (CP) remains one of the underpinning tenets of good, effective services for children in care and care leavers across the UK. It refers to the collective responsibility to ensure that policies, services and support are good enough to enable care-experienced young people to have the same aspirations and opportunities as any other child. The principle of CP was established in 1998 by Frank Dobson MP, who succinctly and powerfully articulated the State's legal and moral duty towards children in and leaving care; that is to act as any good and reasonable parent would towards their child. As a benchmark for performance and provision, he suggested that services ask, 'would this be good enough for my child?'

Corporate parents include public agencies and providers such as health services, education, employment and training providers, housing providers, leisure services and benefits agencies, amongst others. CP is embedded across the UK. The Children and Young People (Scotland) Act 2014 was the first to install duties for public bodies defined as Corporate Parents in legislation, followed by England via the Children and Social Work Act 2017 (see also Social Services and Well-being (Wales) Act 2014 and Children's Services Co-operation Act (Northern Ireland) 2015 (CSCA)).

As an example, CP is central to England's Care Leaver Strategy (DfE, 2016b) and government guidance to local authorities (DfE, 2018a), which articulates its approach to care leavers and the expectations for the services that support them. At local level, CP boards provide cross-departmental and multiagency stakeholder forums for debating policies and developments to improve services and outcomes for care-experienced young people. CP sits at the heart of the care leaver covenant, which task local authorities and other organisations to publish their offer of support for care leavers. (See Children and Social Work Act 2017 and Spectra first-care leaver covenant.)

CP provides a tool to advocate for care-experienced young people. Examples include providing ring-fenced jobs or work experience within the council and local businesses, council tax exemption for care leavers, free access to sport and leisure opportunities and support to access university.

REFLECTIVE QUESTIONS

■ What examples of CP are you aware of in your area?
■ How can you use CP in your practice?
■ Think of ways that CP can be used to enhance and challenge wider policy, practice and services affecting care-experienced young people.

While the 1989 Act contributed to the growth of dedicated services for care leavers, the discretionary nature of its application meant that leaving care support varied from patchy to nonexistent across local authorities (see Biehal et al., 1995 and the consultation document *Me Survive Out There?* (DoH, 1999)).

In response, subsequent UK legislation has aimed to improve consistency and continuity of provision as well as outcomes for care leavers (see Children (Leaving Care) Act 2000, Children (Leaving Care) Act (Northern Ireland) 2002, Children and Young Person's Act 2008, Social Services and Well-being (Wales) Act 2014, Children and Young People (Scotland) Act 2014, Children and Families Act 2014 and Children and Social Work Act (2017)).

The first specific leaving care legislation was the landmark Children (Leaving Care) Act 2000. Some sections of the 2000 Act covered Wales and Scotland; the equivalent in Northern Ireland was introduced in 2002. Designed to create a major shift in leaving care policy and practice, the 2000 Act sought to increase the quality and consistency of leaving care services, delay leaving care until young people were ready, and improve post-care outcomes. To reduce service variation, it required that all local authorities provide a specialist leaving care service and adopt a consistent framework for leaving care planning and support. This included:

- creating the role of personal adviser (PA) – a worker specialising in support for teenagers transitioning from care to adulthood;
- requiring a multiagency needs assessment for all care leavers;
- local authorities having responsibility for supporting young people financially up to age 18 years; and
- introducing the pathway plan, completed jointly by young people and their PA and reviewed at least 6-monthly, setting out goals across life areas and the support needed to attain them (see Closer Look: Pathway Plans).

All underpin leaving care services today, with subsequent amendments extending access to services to age 25 in England and 26 in Scotland, introducing education-focused support, including for those attending university, and increasing policies to delay the move from care at 18 (see UK legislation

> ## CLOSER LOOK: PATHWAY PLANS
>
> - Begin as soon as possible after Needs Assessment
> - Young person centred – it is their document
> - Not just a paper exercise
> - 'Living document' kept under regular review – at least 6 months
> - Include name of personal adviser and other relevant staff
> - Help young people to identify their goals
> - Provide nature and level of contact and support to help them achieve their stated goals
> - Reflect high and realistic expectations and aspirations
> - Allow more than one chance to succeed
> - Empower young people as they mature, to make decisions and hold services to account
> - Identify adult community-based support
>
> Support areas:
> - Relationships (family, friends and social support networks)
> - Practical & other life skills
> - Financial needs and arrangements
> - Emotional & behavioural needs and skills
> - Physical and mental health care needs
> - Accommodation
> - Plans for education, training and employment
> - Identity and understanding their past
> - Contingency plans
> - Knowing where to access support and Services

2011–2017). Further policies have increased the criteria for receiving care and leaving care services such as the 2009 Southwark Judgement, which provided that 16–17-year-olds generally who were at risk of homelessness should be treated as looked after children with access to leaving care support.

CARE LEAVERS IN THE UK: CHARACTERISTICS

Annual leaving care statistics are gathered separately across the UK. In 2022, leaving care services supported around 45,940 care leavers aged 17 to 21 years in England, 700 aged 16+ in Wales and 8,132 16 to 25-year-olds were eligible for aftercare support in Scotland. Northern Ireland reported 320 care leavers aged between 16 and 18 (see resources for access to statistics).

The characteristics of care leavers are, by definition, the same as the care population (see Chapter 11a).

Some characteristics and experiences apparent within the care population are particularly pertinent to understanding leaving care experiences. Specifically, age at entry and at leaving care, placement stability, education participation and reasons for entering care. These have been identified throughout research literature as predictors of post-care outcomes, as discussed in the following section.

Characteristics of the care population are similar throughout the UK (Rees and Stein, 2016). Data gathered annually from English local authorities are used here as an illustration. During 2021–2022, 82,170 children were in care, the highest number since 1985. The number leaving care is also increasing, rising from 10,600 in 2017 to 11,220 in 2020. The most common age-band for entering care in 2022 was 10 to 15 years, accounting for 27%, while 25% were aged 16 to 17 (DfE, 2020; DfE, 2022). This has implications for services in terms of the different support needs of older children and the timescales for supporting them. Past research suggests that those who enter care later (aged 14+) tend to leave care before their 18th birthday, meaning that the length of time they spend in foster or residential care is relatively short. Furthermore, they tend to have poorer post-care outcomes in housing, employment and well-being than those who enter care younger and remain with foster carers beyond 18 (Dixon et al., 2006; Dixon and Lee, 2015).

The most common reason for entering care has remained consistent over many years, with abuse or neglect being the most cited category of primary need. In England, this accounts for 65% (DfE, 2020) indicating that most looked after children, and thereby care leavers, have a history of maltreatment and adverse childhood experiences. As discussed later, this can carry a long-lasting impact for young people's well-being.

The most common placement type in the UK is foster care. Most care leavers, therefore, leave from foster placements, though some may have experienced several placement types. There is some evidence that those leaving residential care are more likely to do so before their 18th birthday, experience difficult transitions and poorer post-care outcomes. This reflects findings that those in residential care are often older entrants who have been unable to settle and who exhibit more complex difficulties (Action for Children, 2014),

highlighting the need for a tailored service response to meet their specific needs.

Placement instability continues to affect the UK care population. Statistics for England report over a third move placements and 11% experience three or more placements per year (DfE, 2020). Research indicates that some care leavers experience in excess of 10 placements. Placement instability is associated with poor attachment and educational attainment, and a predictor of post-care instability and difficulties (Sinclair et al., 2007). Young people describe feelings of rejection and confusion arising from placement movement:

Every time you move, you feel rejected and this affects your self-esteem and confidence.

Care leaver, Barnardo's (2006)

I have been moved several times without being told why, so I am used to being moved with no apparent reason.

Care leaver, Dixon and Lee (2015)

REFLECTIVE QUESTIONS

- How might some of these features of the care experience impact on young people's lives in and after care?
- What can carers, social/leaving care workers and other corporate parents do to mitigate that impact?

EXPERIENCES OF LEAVING CARE

Although some care-experienced young people do well after care, a considerable number struggle with poor outcomes, particularly during the early years post-care. Experiences of childhood trauma, estrangement from family and community, placement instability, education disengagement and higher rates of risk behaviour can undermine the possibility of a settled childhood and positive transition to adulthood. Without support, these can compromise long-term personal, social and economic well-being (Baker, 2017; Dixon and Stein, 2005; Dixon and Lee, 2015; Stein, 2012). A lack of longitudinal research on care leavers means that much of what is known about longer-term outcomes derives from studies of marginalised adult groups. These show that care leavers are overrepresented in adult unemployed, homeless and prison populations (Gill and Daw, 2017; Ministry of Justice, 2012).

TRANSITIONING FROM CARE

Many care leavers move to semi-independent or independent living before their 18th birthday, with studies reporting between 33% (National Audit Office (NAO), 2015) and 48% (Dixon and Lee, 2015) leaving aged 16 to 17. Statistics suggest some reduction in the percentage of 16 year olds leaving care (17% in 2012 to 14% in 2016) (DfE, 2016a). Nevertheless, this is in stark contrast to trends within the general population, where the average age at which young adults leave the family home varies between 25 and 28 across the UK (Office for National Statistics, 2016).

In addition to moving to independent living earlier, care leavers take on the responsibilities of adulthood in a shorter space of time than other young people, which Stein (2006) describes as accelerated and compressed transitions. Care leavers are expected to set up home, finance their independent status and sustain education, employment or training (EET) soon after leaving care. For some, this includes reconnecting with family or embarking upon a family of their own, with care leavers being significantly more likely to become young parents than young people generally (Craine et al., 2014). Furthermore, young care-experienced parents are themselves more likely to have social care involvement in their child's lives, perpetuating the legacy and impact of care and leaving care, as described by care leavers quoted in Baker's 2017 review; *my kids are going through the same thing, history is repeating itself*. Most care leavers undertake these instant adult responsibilities without the emotional, practical and financial support that most young adults receive from their families. Some, therefore, report feeling poorly prepared, afraid and lacking the practical and emotional skills and support networks for such a challenge.

The age that care leavers embark upon independent adulthood is an important factor in post-care outcomes. Of equal importance, however, is that they experience a well-planned and supported transition from care and can exercise choice and agency in when and how they leave and where they go. Studies show that care leavers can feel disempowered during the transition from care. Dixon and Lee's study (Dixon and Lee, 2015) found that 32% had 'no choice' and 42% had 'insufficient information' when leaving care. Care leavers also report feeling '*rushed out of care*' and '*cast adrift*', experiencing a '*crash course*' in preparation (Dixon and Baker, 2016).

Reasons for leaving care early, as demonstrated by young people interviewed in Dixon et al., 2006 and Dixon and Ward, 2017 can be categorised as:

- Young person-led (choice/planned) 'The time felt right, we negotiated the timing'
- Placement breakdown/difficulties (they opted to or had to leave) 'My foster carer gave notice on me so now I am a sofa surfer'
- Resource pressures (insufficient placement options for older young people and care leavers or having to free-up places to meet the demand of increased numbers entering care). 'I didn't really want to move but I had no choice. I would rather have stayed at the foster parents ... I miss being there' (Dixon et al., 2006; Dixon and Ward, 2017)

Strategies have been developed to improve preparation and increase choice and decision-making for young people leaving care. These include pathway planning, children in care councils, care leaver forums and care leaver advocacy organisations, which offer opportunities for young people to have their say in decisions about their own lives as well as in shaping services that support them. Nevertheless, the requirement for services to act as a good parent continues to place emphasis on enabling young people to remain with carers until they feel well prepared and ready to leave.

REFLECTIVE QUESTION

What can corporate parents do to ensure care leavers' views are heard and acted upon, and to ensure they are able to make informed choices about their leaving care journeys?

ACCOMMODATION

For most care leavers, finding a home takes priority over other needs and adult milestones, such as embarking on career pathways, addressing personal difficulties and forming support networks. The importance of good accommodation (a safe, suitable home that meets the young person's needs and where they feel happy) is evident in the level of practice focus and by its impact on other outcomes. Research identifies a positive accommodation outcome as a protective factor that mediates the impact of pre-and in-care difficulties, is associated with increased levels of post-care well-being, and can provide a firm foundation from which to sustain EET participation. Care leavers who achieve positive accommodation outcomes tend to have left care later (18+), exhibited fewer difficulties and received ongoing and individualised support with practical and emotional needs (Dixon and Ward, 2017; Wade and Dixon, 2006).

Some care leavers, however, experience multiple post-care moves, housing breakdown, temporary or unregulated housing and around one-third become homeless in the early years after care. This can result from a lack of preparation and independent living skills and the presence of wider personal difficulties, as well as from the type, location, poor state or high cost of accommodation, all of which can conspire to reduce young people's ability to find a settled home (Dixon and Stein, 2005; Gill and Daw, 2017; Stein and Morris, 2010).

Local authorities have a duty to support care leavers to find suitable accommodation, and to provide a range of options, including transitional, semi-independent accommodation with support (e.g. hostels, supported lodgings) and independent options (e.g. house/flat). This requires working alongside housing providers to source and allocate appropriate accommodation.

Since 2014, care leavers have the option to remain with former carers beyond 18. This includes Staying Put with foster carers to age 21 years in England, Continuing Care post-18 in Scotland, Going the Extra Mile in Northern Ireland and When I am Ready provision in Wales. A similar approach for residential care leavers (Staying Close) is being tested (Allen et al., 2020; Neagu and Dixon, 2020). Such options can offer longer-term stability and continuity, often alongside tailored support. By delaying the move to transitional or independent accommodation, such options offer care leavers security, time and space at a crucial age, to focus on EET and to develop the practical and emotional skills for independent adulthood. Data show

increasing numbers staying put with carers beyond their 18th birthdays (DfE, 2020).

Independent, single-occupancy tenancies, however, remain the most common accommodation type for care leavers aged 19 to 21 (DfE, 2019). Research with care leavers suggests that some prefer to move directly from care into a long-term home of their own, rather than experiencing the stepping-stones of short-term, semi-independent options. Initiatives such as Centrepoint's Housing First for care leavers and The House Project in England and Scotland aim to meet that need by helping care leavers to find and remain in their own tenancy, using a programme of tailored support designed to develop tenancy related skills as well as address emotional and other needs (Dixon and Ward, 2017). For example, care leavers in the House Project were encouraged to create a peer community to support each other to leave care together, as one described;

> *'this project means that I can still be part of a group of people and I won't always be on my own'*
> **(Dixon and Ward, 2017).**

Such support can reduce the loneliness that many care leavers, as quoted here, report as the worst aspect of independent living:

> *'I feel very isolated and lonely. I don't like living by myself'* and *'it's the fear of having to face things alone, suddenly all the support you were familiar with has gone'*
> **(Baker, 2017; Dixon and Baker, 2016).**

REFLECTIVE QUESTION

What can corporate parents do to support care leavers to overcome the individual and structural challenges facing them as they move to independent living?

EDUCATION, EMPLOYMENT AND TRAINING

A significant, longstanding gap exists between the educational achievement of care-experienced young people and their non-care peers. Data in England for Attainment 8 score (a measure of pupils' average GCSE grades across eight subjects) show an average of 18.8 for care-experienced children compared with

44.4 for all children (DfE, 2018b). Family disadvantage, trauma, placement instability and risk behaviour (running away or truancy) have been identified as risk factors for education disruption and poor attainment. Additionally, children in care are three times more likely to have special education needs (DfE, 2018b) and five times more likely to have a fixed period exclusion than all school pupils (DfE, 2017), which can impact education experiences.

Research by Sebba et al., (2015) identified a settled care experience as a protective factor for education success. This resonates with earlier studies that found girls who enter care early and remain in stable foster care tend to do better in education (Dixon et al., 2006). Furthermore, international research identifies educational success as a protective factor for other positive outcomes (Berlin et al., 2011), indicating that positive care and education experiences are mutually and cumulatively beneficial.

Education disruption and poor attainment, however, can have a lasting impact on post-care EET participation. Care leavers aged 19 to 21 years have lower participation in employment and training (25%), further education (21%) and higher education, which despite an increase from 1% to 6% over the past decade, compares to 47% of the general population who go to university (Centre for Social Justice (CSJ) 2016). Although research suggests that for some care leavers, education journeys are delayed rather than derailed (e.g. over half of care-experienced students entering university are over 21), Ellis et al., (2019) emphasise the importance of continued support to reduce dropout rates.

Consequently, the risk of being NEET (not in education, employment or training) is higher for care leavers. In England, 39% were reported NEET compared to 12% of 19- to 24-year-olds generally (DfE, 2019). In Scotland, 30% were unemployed 9 months after leaving school compared to 5% of young people generally (Scottish Government, 2019). Reasons for being NEET include disrupted education and care experiences. Furthermore, the timing of education milestones can often negatively coincide with milestones within the care experience. For example, choosing subjects and sitting end of school exams coincide with the age that many young people enter care (14–16 years) and when many are in the process of leaving care (16–18 years). In such circumstances, EET is likely to be disrupted or delayed until care leavers have secured a settled home life.

Being NEET carries a cost to society (see NAO, 2015) as well as to the individual (e.g. lack of social integration and emotional and financial well-being). Research by The Children's Society (2017) identified care leavers on benefits as three times more likely than other claimants to be sanctioned, placing them at increased risk of debt and homelessness. Strategies for improving EET outcomes for care leavers is a key challenge for policy and practice. Research indicates

CASE STUDY 12B1: SUPPORTING SUCCESSFUL OUTCOMES

Gemma is amongst 6% of care leavers at university. She entered care aged 7 and settled well with foster carers until moving to university aged 19 years. During a settled school career, Gemma achieved three A levels.

When asked what had helped her achieve her goals, she described support and encouragement from her foster carers throughout her childhood and after care, which had helped raise her aspirations and motivation.

'I still have contact with my foster carer, she helps me a lot, getting involved ...to sort of guide you; "Look there's this going on, get involved" and stuff like that. You need positive reinforcement to be proud of your achievements, but it's also needed when you are at your lowest ebb'.

Her foster carer had high expectations for Gemma and instilled a sense of confidence that enabled her to overcome stereotypes attached to care leavers.

'For me 1 wanted to do that, 1 didn't want to be different and everyone else going to university... 1 didn't want to be the Leaving Care girl who didn't do it. 1 wanted to be the girl who did do it.'

Her personal adviser explained what had helped,

'It takes [her] own motivation and encouragement from staff and family. This determination has helped a lot and the issue of education is always discussed during [pathway plans]'.

REFLECTIVE QUESTION

What are the learning points from Gemma's experience, for carers, social workers, PAs and education professionals in how they can support care-experienced young people in their education journeys?

the need for earlier support to broaden young people's EET opportunities. Factors that can foster EET success, identified by care leavers in research (see Case Study), include personal aspirations and motivation, high expectations of carers, supportive networks that can signpost EET opportunities (Dixon and Lee, 2015) and resilience (South et al., 2016).

Participation also relies on access to opportunities, including training and employment options that can financially support independent living, alternative access routes into further and higher education and the availability of pre-employment support and training to help young people overcome the impact of disrupted education or other difficulties.

REFLECTIVE QUESTION

The introduction of designated teachers and virtual school heads in 2008 brought a focus to the education of children in care, while corporate parenting and the local offer provide scope to engage with post-18 EET providers. How can services work with education, training and employment professionals to support care-experienced young people to reach their goals and potential?

HEALTH

Research highlights the impact of adverse experiences (e.g. maltreatment, separation from family, posttraumatic stress, drug-use and self-harm) and the psychological effects of entering care and leaving care, on young people's health (Braden et al., 2017; Dixon, 2008; Luke et al., 2014; Smith, 2017).

Statistics on health needs and the extent that they are met is not readily available; however, research shows problems associated with poor eating and sleeping, chronic health conditions, emotional difficulties and unhealthy lifestyles (Dixon and Lee, 2015; Sempik et al., 2008). A Scottish study reported that care leavers had one of the highest rates of youth smoking (ScotPHO, 2009), whilst others report higher substance misuse compared to non-care peers (Alderson et al., 2019).

Mental health needs are particularly evident. Care-experienced children are five times more likely to experience mental distress, even when compared to children from the most deprived areas (Ford et al.,

2007; Meltzer et al., 2003). Additionally, some groups within the care population have greater vulnerability. McCann et al. (1996) found that 96% of children in residential care, compared to 57% in foster care, had a psychiatric disorder, again reflecting the complex needs of the residential group.

Research with the general population shows that mental health problems often emerge in late adolescence/early adulthood (McCrory et al., 2010) and studies of care leavers confirm higher rates of mental health needs. Saunders and Broad (1997) reported that 48% of care leavers in their study had mental health difficulties, and Dixon and Lee (2015) reported that care leavers were twice as likely to have mental health problems compared to children in care.

Some research indicates that the leaving care process itself can initiate or exacerbate health problems (Dixon and Lee, 2015; Matthews and Sykes, 2012). Care leavers participating in the Scottish Health Survey (2001) reported that leaving care had a negative impact on their overall health, while research with care leavers in England reported deterioration in mental well-being and a twofold increase in health problems one year post-care, with care leavers commenting on the stress associated with leaving care (Dixon, 2008).

The prevalence of mental health problems within the care population is also linked to the high numbers that come into care due to maltreatment. Studies of the impact of maltreatment identify associations with conduct disorder, emotional problems, bipolar disorder, depression, suicide attempts and poor physical health and development (Agnew-Blais and Danese, 2016; Arseneault et al., 2011; Banduccia et al., 2013). Despite this, there is a lack of mental health support for care leavers. Practice and research evidence highlights difficulties in obtaining child and adolescent mental health services for all young people and suggests that care-experienced young people have lower levels of engagement in such interventions and are likely to fall into the gap between child and adult services (Alderson et al., 2019; Kelly et al., 2016). This has implications for how services can best respond. For example, the use of therapeutic approaches and mental health specialists within leaving care teams and using trauma informed practice are becoming more common within support for care-experienced young people in the UK (Buckley et al., 2016; Furnivall and Grant, 2014).

REFLECTIVE QUESTIONS

- What factors, evident in reasons for entering care and experiences of being in and leaving care, might impact on care-experienced young people's health?
- What can help reduce the impact?

CONCLUSION

Accumulated evidence demonstrates the vulnerability of some care leavers post-care. It also shows that a positive leaving care journey depends on:

- a positive and settled care experience;
- identifying needs early and putting in place multiagency support to address them;
- having support networks and positive relationships;
- consistent and holistic adult support to accompany care leavers throughout the journey to independent living alongside timely preparation and opportunities for skills-development, choice and agency;
- access to a range of safe, affordable post-care accommodation to meet the diverse needs and wishes of care leavers at difference stages of the transition to independent living, including the option to remain with carers;
- encouragement and assistance to engage with, or return to, education;
- early and long-term access to specialist help and opportunities to improve employment readiness;
- access to timely and effective health support from practitioners who understand the impact of childhood trauma; and
- investment and improvement in services that support care leavers, underpinned by bold policies, effective corporate parenting, evidence of what works, and the voices of care-experienced young people.

FURTHER READING

Legislation, Policy and Guidance

- Children Act 1989: http://www.legislation.gov.uk/ukpga/1989/41/contents
- Children (Northern Ireland) Order 1995: http://www.legislation.gov.uk/nisi/1995/755/contents/made
- Children (Leaving Care) Act 2000: http://www.legislation.gov.uk/ukpga/2000/35/contents
- Children (Leaving Care) Act (Northern Ireland) 2002: http://www.legislation.gov.uk/nia/2002/11/contents
- Governments promise to young people leaving care (2012). Care Leavers Charter.
- Children and Young People (Scotland) Act 2014: http://www.legislation.gov.uk/asp/2014/8/contents/enacted
- Social Services and Well-being (Wales) Act 2014: http://www.legislation.gov.uk/anaw/2014/4/contents
- Staying Put – Arrangements for care leavers aged 18 and above to stay on with their former foster carers, 2013: https://assets.publishing.service.gov.uk/government/uploads/system/uploads/attachment_data/file/201015/Staying_Put_Guidance.pdf
- Young People's Guide to Staying Put, 2014. Staying Put: What Does it Mean for You? Catch 22 National Care Advisory Service: https://www.basw.co.uk/system/files/resources/basw_113930-2_0.pdf
- Children's Services Co-operation Act (Northern Ireland) 2015 (CSCA): https://www.legislation.gov.uk/2015?title=children%27s%20services%20co-operation%20act
- Revised guidance for young people leaving care – Children Act 1989 Guidance and Regulations Volume 3: Planning Transition to Adulthood for Care Leavers (Revised January 2015), 2015.
- Government strategy to improve services and support for care leavers – Keep on Caring: Supporting Young People from Care to Independence, 2016.
- The Children and Social Work Act 2017: http://www.legislation.gov.uk/ukpga/2017/16/contents/enacted
- Extending Personal Adviser (PA) Support to Age 25: Guidance for local authorities, 2018: https://www.gov.uk/government/publications/extending-personal-adviser-support-to-age-25
- Applying Corporate Parenting Principles to Looked-after Children and Care Leavers, 2018. https://www.gov.uk/government/publications/applying-corporate-parenting-principles-to-looked-after-children-and-care-leavers.
- The care leaver covenant – Local Offer Guidance: Guidance for local authorities, 2018: https://www.gov.uk/government/publications/local-offer-guidance

Resources

- Become – The Charity for Children in Care and Young Care Leavers – The facts about being a care leaver. https://www.becomecharity.org.uk/care-the-facts/being-a-care-leaver/
- Care Inspectorate Wales, 2019. National Overview Report: In Relation to Care Experienced Children and Young People. Care Inspectorate Wales, Llandudno. https://careinspectorate.wales/sites/default/files/2019-06/190619-national-overview-report-en_2.pdf
- Care leaver covenant website. https://mycovenant.org.uk/
- Child Law Advice – local authority support and services for young people leaving care (Eligibility for service). https://childlawadvice.org.uk/information-pages/services-for-children-leaving-care/
- Children's Commissioner – Leaving Care information: https://www.childrenscommissioner.gov.uk/help-at-hand/leaving-care-your-rights/

- Coram Voice – Information for young people leaving care on rights and entitlements: https://coramvoice.org.uk/myrights/all-you-need-to-know-about-leaving-care/
- Drive Forward – Closing the gap for care leavers in London: https://www.globalgiving.org/pfil/24106/projdoc.pdf
- GOV.UK – Information for young people leaving care: https://www.gov.uk/leaving-foster-or-local-authority-care
- LawStuff – Information on leaving care support: https://lawstuff.org.uk/childrens-services/leaving-care-support/
- Leverhulme Trust – Pathways to University from Care: Findings Report One
- National Homelessness Advice Service – duties to support care leavers find housing: https://www.nhas.org.uk/improving-outcomes/advising-young-people/when-young-people-have-to-move-out/care-leavers/local-authority-duties-to-care-leavers
- The care leaver covenant: https://mycovenant.org.uk/
- Statistics – For UK leaving care statistics see:
  Who Cares Scotland, 2019. Statistics. Who Cares Scotland, Glasgow. Available from https://www.whocaresscotland.org/who-we-are/media-centre/statistics/ (Accessed 12 September 2023).
England
https://www.gov.uk/government/statistics/children-looked-after-in-england-including-adoption-2018-to-2019
https://explore-education-statistics.service.gov.uk/find-statistics/children-looked-after-in-england-including-adoptions/2022
N. Ireland
https://www.health-ni.gov.uk/sites/default/files/publications/health/nicl-21-22.pdf
Scotland
https://www.gov.scot/publications/childrens-social-work-statistics-scotland-2021-22/documents/
Wales
https://statswales.gov.wales/Catalogue/Health-and-Social-Care/Social-Services/Childrens-Services/Children-Looked-After/Care-Leavers-Aged-16-and-Over/episodesfinishingforchildrenlookedafteraged16andoverduringyearto31march-by-localauthority-reasonforfinishing

REFERENCES

Action for Children, 2014. Too Much Too Young: Helping the Most Vulnerable Young People to Build Stable Homes after Leaving Care. Action for Children, Watford. https://www.actionforchildren.org.uk/our-work-and-impact/policy-work-campaigns-and-research/policy-reports/too-much-too-young-report/#:~:text=What%20did%20we%20discover%3F,the%20most%20vulnerable%20young%20people. (Accessed 10 September 2023).

Agnew-Blais, J., Danese, A., 2016. Childhood maltreatment and unfavourable clinical outcomes in bipolar disorder: a systematic review and meta-analysis. Lancet Psychiatr. 3, 342–349.

Alderson, H., Brown, R., Copello, A., Kaner, E., Tober, G., Lingam, R., et al., 2019. The key therapeutic factors needed to deliver behavioural change interventions to decrease risky substance use (drug and alcohol) for looked after children and care leavers: A qualitative exploration with young people, carers and front line workers. BMC Med. Res. Methodol. 19 (2019), 38. https://doi.org/10.1186/s12874-019-0674-3.

Allen, D., Heyes, K., Hothersall, G., O'Leary, C., Ozan, J., 2020. Bristol City Council Staying Close Pilot. Department for Education, London.

Arseneault, L., Cannon, M., Fisher, H.L., Polanczyk, G., Moffitt, T.E., Caspi, A., 2011. Childhood trauma and children's emerging psychotic symptoms: a genetically sensitive longitudinal cohort study. Am. J. Psychiatr. 168 (1), 65–72. https://doi.org/10.1176/appi.ajp.2010.10040567.

Baker, C., 2017. Care Leavers' Views on Their Transitions to Adulthood: A Rapid Review of the Evidence. Coram Voice, London.

Banduccia, A., Hoffmana, E., Lejueza, C.W., Koenenb, K., 2013. The impact of childhood abuse on inpatient substance users: Specific links with risky sex, aggression, and emotion dysregulation. Child Abuse and Neglect 38 (5), 928–938.

Barnardo's, 2006. Failed by the System: The Views of Young Care Leavers on Their Educational Experiences. Barnardo's, London.

Berlin, M., Vinnerljung, B., Hjern, A., 2011. School performance in primary school and psychosocial problems in young adulthood among care leavers from foster care. Child. Youth Serv. Rev. 33 (12), 2489–2497.

Biehal, N., Clayden, J., Stein, M., Wade, J., 1995. Moving on: Young People and Leaving Care Schemes. HMSO, London.

Braden, J., Goddard, J., Graham, D., 2017. Caring for Better Health: An Investigation into the Health Needs of Care Leavers. The Care Leavers Association, London.

Buckley, A.M., Lotty, M., Meldon, S., 2016. "What Happened to Me? Responding to the Impact of Trauma on Children in Care: Trauma Informed Practice in Foster Care". The Irish Social Worker Spring 2016, pp. 35–40.

Craine, N., Midgley, C., Zou, L., Evans, H., Whitaker, B., Lyons, M., 2014. Elevated teenage conception risk amongst looked after children; A national audit. Publ. Health 128, 668–670.

Centre for Social Justice (CSJ), 2016. Delivering a Care Leavers' Strategy for Traineeships and Apprenticeships. Centre for Social Justice, London.

Department for Education (DfE), 2016a. London. Children Looked after in England Including Adoption: 2015 to 2016. Office for National Statistics SFR 41/2016. (Accessed 12 September 2023).

Department for Education (DfE), 2020. Children Looked after in England Including Adoptions: Statistical Release for the Year Ending March 2020. DfE, London. https://explore-education-statistics.service.gov.uk/find-statistics/children-looked-after-in-england-including-adoptions/2020. (Accessed 19 December 2020).

Department for Education (DfE), 2022. *Children looked after in England including adoptions: Statistical release for the year ending March 2022.* London: DfE. https://explore-education-statistics.service.gov.uk/find-statistics/children-looked-after-in-england-including-adoptions/2022. (Accessed 12 September 2023).

Department of Health (DoH), 1999. Me survive out there? New Arrangements for Young People in and Leaving Care. Department of Health, London.

Devenney, K., 2017. Pathway planning with unaccompanied young people leaving care: Biographical narratives of past, present, and future. Child Fam. Soc. Work 22 (3), 1313–1321.

DfE, 2016b. Care Leaver Strategy: A Cross Departmental Strategy for Young People Leaving Care. https://assets.publishing.service.gov.uk/government/uploads/system/uploads/attachment_data/file/535899/Care-Leaver-Strategy.pdf. (Accessed 12 September 2023).

DfE, 2017. Outcomes for Children Looked after by Local Authorities in England 31 March 2017. National Statistics, DfE, London.

DfE, 2018a. Applying Corporate Parenting Principles to Looked-After Children and Care Leavers: Statutory Guidance for Local Authorities. Office for National Statistics, London. https://assets.publishing.service.gov.uk/government/uploads/system/uploads/attachment_data/file/683698/Applying_corporate_parenting_principles_to_looked-after_children_and_care_leavers.pdf. (Accessed 12 December 2019).

DfE, 2018b. Outcomes for Children Looked after by Local Authorities in England 31 March 2018. Office for National Statistics, London.

DfE, 2019. Children Looked after in England Including Adoption: 2018 to 2019. Office for National Statistics, London.

Dixon, J., 2008. Young people leaving care: Health, well-being and outcomes. Child Fam. Soc. Work 13 (2), 207–217. https://doi.org/10.1111/j.1365-2206.2007.00538.x.

Dixon, J., Baker, C., 2016. New Belongings: An Evaluation. Department for Education, London.

Dixon, J., Lee, J., 2015. Corporate Parenting for Young People in Care – Making the Difference? Summary report of key findings. Catch 22, London.

Dixon, J., Stein, M., 2005. Leaving Care: Throughcare and Aftercare in Scotland. Jessica Kingsley Publishers, London.

Dixon, J., Ward, J., 2017. Making a House a home: The House Project Evaluation. (Children's Social Care Innovation Programme). Department for Education, London.

Dixon, J., Wade, J., Byford, S., Weatherly, H., Lee, J., 2006. Young People Leaving Care: A Study of Costs and Outcomes: Final Report to the Department for Education & Skills. Social Work Research and Development Unit, University of York, York.

Ellis, K., Johnston, C., 2019. Pathways to University from Care: Findings Report One. https://doi.org/10.15131/shef.data.9578930.

Fallon, D., Broadhurst, K., 2015. Preventing Unplanned Pregnancy and Improving Preparation for Parenthood for Care-Experienced Young People: A Comprehensive Review of the Literature and Critical Appraisal of Intervention Studies. Coram, London.

Ford, T., Vostanis, P., Meltzer, H., Goodman, R., 2007. Psychiatric disorder among British children looked after by local authorities: Comparison with children living in private households. Br. J. Psychiatry, 190(4), 319–325. doi:10.1192/bjp.bp.106.025023

Furnivall, J., Grant, E., 2014. Trauma Sensitive Practices with Children in Care. Insights 27 Evidence Summaries to Support Social Services in Scotland. IRISS, Institute for Research and Innovation in Social services.

Gill, A. and Daw, E., 2017. From Care to Where? Care Leavers' Access to Accommodation. Centrepoint, London.

Kelly, B., McShane, T., Davidson, G., Pinkerton, J., Gilligan, E., Webb, P., 2016. Transitions and Outcomes for Care Leavers with Mental Health And/or Intellectual Disabilities: Short Report. QUB, Belfast.

Luke, N., Sinclair, I., Woolgar, M., Sebba, J., 2014. What works in preventing and treating poor mental health in looked after children NSPCC.

Matthews, S., Sykes, S., 2012. Exploring health priorities for young people leaving care. Child Care in Practice 18 (4), 393–407.

McCann, J.B., James, A., Wilson, S. and Dunn, G., 1996. Prevalence of psychiatric disorders in young people in the care system. BMJ, 313(7071), pp.1529–1530.

McCrory, E., De Brito, S., Viding, E., 2010. Research review: The neurobiology and genetics of maltreatment and adversity. J. Child Psychol. Psychiatry 15, 1079–1095 110 95.

Meltzer, H., Gatward, R., Corbin, T., Goodman, R. and Ford, T., 2003. The mental health of young people looked after by local authorities in England. London, England: Office for National Statistics. https://doi.org/10.1037/e616412007-001

Ministry of Justice (MoJ), 2012. Prisoners' Childhood and Family Backgrounds. Results from Surveying Prisoner Crime Reduction (SPCR) Longitudinal Cohort Study of Prisoners. Ministry of Justice, London.

Mitchell, F., 2003. The social services response to unaccompanied children in England. Child Fam. Soc. Work 8 (3), 179–189.

National Audit Office (NAO), 2015. Care Leavers' Transitions to Adulthood. National Audit Office, London. https://www.nao.org.uk/wp-content/uploads/2015/07/Care-leavers-transition-to-adulthood.pdf.

Neagu, M., Dixon, J., 2020. The Portsmouth Aspiration Staying Close Project: Evaluation Report. Department for Education, London. https://assets.publishing.service.gov.uk/government/uploads/system/uploads/attachment_data/file/932012/Staying_Close_Portsmouth.pdf.

ONS, 2016. Young Adults Living with Their Parents: November 2016. ONS data online. https://www.ons.gov.uk/peoplepopulationandcommunity/birthsdeathsandmarriages/families/articles/whyaremoreyoungpeoplelivingwiththeirparents/2016-02-22. (Accessed 12 September 2023).

Prison Reform Trust, 2016. In Care, Out of Trouble: How the Life Chances of Children in Care Can Be Transformed by Protecting Them from Unnecessary Involvement in the Criminal justice System. Prison Reform Trust, London.

Rabiee, P., Knowles, J., Priestley, M., 2001. Whatever Next? Young Disabled People Leaving Care. First Key Limited.

Rees, G., Stein, M., 2016. Children and Young People in Care and Leaving Care. In: Bradshaw, J. (Ed.), The Well-Being of Children in the UK, fourth ed. Policy Press, Bristol.

Saunders, L. and Broad, B., 1997. The Health Needs of Young People Leaving Care. De Montfort University, Leicester.

ScotPHO, 2009. Knowledge, Attitudes and Motivations to Health, 2008-2009. The Scottish Public Health Observatory, Edinburgh. https://www.scotpho.org.uk/media/1200/scotpho101214_kam200809.pdf. (Accessed 12 September 2023).

Scottish Health Feedback, 2001. A Study of the Health Needs of Young People with Experience of Being in Care in Glasgow. Scottish Health Feedback, Edinburgh.

Scottish Government, 2019. Children's social work statistics 2017-2018. Scottish Government, Edinburgh.

Sebba, J., Berridge, D., Luke, N., Fletcher, J., Bell, K., Strand, S., et al., 2015. The Educational Progress of Looked after Children in England: Linking Care and Educational Data. Nuffield Foundation. https://research-information.bris.ac.uk/en/publications/the-educational-progress-of-looked-after-children-in-england(f58855fe-cc01-4908-a497-74ccecb528d5).html. (Accessed 12 September 2023).

Sempik, J., Ward, H., Darker, I., 2008. 'Emotional and behavioural difficulties of children and young people at entry into care'. Clin. Child Psychol. Psychiatr. 13 (2), 221–233. https://doi.org/10.1177/1359104507088344.

Sinclair, I., Baker, C., Lee, J., Gibbs, I., 2007. The Pursuit of Permanence: A Study of the English Care System. (Quality Matters in Children's Services Series). Jessica Kingsley, London.

Smith, N., 2017. Neglected Minds: A Report on Mental Health Support for Young People Leaving Care. Essex: Barnardo's, Barkingside.

South, R., Jones, W.,F., Creith, E., Simmonds, M.,L., 2016. Understanding the concept of resilience in relation to looked after children: A Delphi survey of perceptions from education,

social care and foster care. Child Psychol. Psychiatry 21 (2), 178–192.

Stein, M., 2006. Research review: Young people leaving care. Child Fam. Soc. Work 11 (3), 273–279. https://doi.org/10.1111/j.1365-2206.2006.00439.x.

Stein, M., 2012. Young People Leaving Care: Supporting Pathways to Adulthood. Jessica Kingsley, London.

Stein, M., Pinkerton, J., Kelleher, P., 2000. Young people leaving care in England, Northern Ireland and Ireland: A comparative research perspective. Eur. J. Soc. Work 3 (3), 235–246.

The Children's Society, 2017. Claiming after Care: Care Leavers and the Benefits System. https://www.basw.co.uk/system/files/resources/basw_35341-9_0.pdf (Accessed 12 September 2023).

The Children's Society, 2017. Good Childhood Report 2017. The Children's Society: London.

Wade, J., Dixon, J., 2006. Making a home, finding a job: Investigating early housing and employment outcomes for young people leaving care. Child Fam. Soc. Work 11 (3), 199–208. https://doi.org/10.1111/j.1365-2206.2006.00428.x.

12c SAFEGUARDING AND CHILDREN IN CONFLICT WITH THE LAW

JOE YATES ■ STEPH YATES

KEY POINTS

- Children in conflict with the law can pose a risk but are often in need of safeguarding themselves.

- Children who come into conflict with the law are often drawn from the most marginalised and disadvantaged sections of society.

- Children's involvement in crime can be the result of criminal exploitation.

- Children are vulnerable and 'at risk' in a range of ways, and these vulnerabilities and risks interlock. Understanding the intersectional manner in which these factors interlock helps us better understand and respond to these children.

- The safeguarding issues evident in the lives of these young people are often overshadowed by their criminal actions. As a society we often respond to these children through criminal justice rather than safeguarding processes.

- Practitioners who come into contact with these children need to be aware of the risks that these children could be victims of criminal exploitation even when they themselves resist this label.

INTRODUCTION

Children and young people who come into contact with the criminal justice system pose a risk, sometimes significant, in terms of their law breaking and are often at risk and vulnerable themselves. In this chapter we will outline the intersectional nature of vulnerability and risk in the lives of children and young people in

trouble with the law. The chapter will argue that these children and young people are largely drawn from the most vulnerable sections our society and that their offending behaviour needs to be understood in the context of the multiple, complex vulnerabilities which typify their lived experiences. The chapter will briefly outline, by way of example, some of the vulnerabilities and structural disadvantages which are evident in the lives of children and young people who come into contact with the criminal justice system. The chapter will then move on to critically appraise the interplay of vulnerability, risk and safeguarding in the case of child criminal exploitation through the 'county lines' model – critically appraising recent policy developments in this area.

CHILD VULNERABILITY, INTERSECTIONALITY AND THE YOUTH JUSTICE SYSTEM

Children and young people in conflict with the law are largely drawn from poor families living in some of the most marginalised sections of our community (Yates, 2009). It is well established that children growing up in poverty (which is a growing number – see Social Metrics Commission, 2019) are more likely than their middle-class counterparts to become caught up in the criminal justice system (Yates, 2009). They are also more likely to experience social and economic conditions associated with a higher likelihood of coming into conflict with the law, and they are more likely to have encountered a range of other challenges during their adolescent transitions (Pitts, 2008). The evidence is also clear that they are also often victims of crime as well as perpetrators (Pitts, 2008).

CLOSER LOOK: INTERSECTIONALITY

Intersectionality is a sociological concept which explains how a person or a group of people can experience, and be affected by, a variety of discriminations and disadvantages. It shows how these can overlap in people's lives and how people's identities can overlap. Understanding these overlapping identities and experiences can help us better understand the complexity of their lived experience of discrimination and oppression at a micro and macro level.

Many of the children and young people who come into conflict with the law often also have troubled life experiences which have brought them into contact with social services and the care system. The Youth Justice Trust, which surveyed the case files of 1027 children and young people under the supervision of Youth Offending Teams, identified that more than 90% had 'significant experience of loss or rejection, usually losing contact with a parent because of family breakdown, bereavement, or the onset of mental illness or physical disability for a parent' (Youth Justice Trust, 2003, p. 28). The Prison Reform Trust also reported that 'around half of the children currently in custody in England and Wales have been in care at some point' with 'children who had been in care being six times more likely to be cautioned or convicted of an offence than other children' (Prison Reform Trust, 2016, p. 48). It is clear that factors which can result in children being taken into care are also factors which are linked to their offending behaviour. Indeed, the Taylor report observed that it was likely that the way care homes and the police respond to minor offending by this group, by criminalising their behaviours, contributed to their overrepresentation (Taylor, 2016, p. 24). The Howard League (2018) identified that living in a care home made children at least 15 times more likely to be criminalised compared to other children of a similar age.

There is also evidence that children and young people from Black and minority ethnic (BAME) communities disproportionately come into conflict with the law. Youth Justice Statistics (2017/18) (Youth Justice Board,

2019) indicate that the proportion of cautions or sentences given to Black children and young people has been increasing and is now three times that of the general 10- to 17-year-old population. In 2016 the Lammy review, set up to review racial bias in the criminal justice system, illustrated how people from BAME backgrounds experience differential treatment and outcomes from the criminal justice system. The report provided a detailed overview of why people from ethnic minorities, including children, are overrepresented. Outlining the process from early decisions about exclusion from education, responses to behaviour in care, application of stop and search powers by the Police, right through to decisions around whether to arrest, prosecution and diversion decisions, about advocacy, plea and, ultimately, sentencing (Lammy, 2016).

It is also apparent that young people with diagnosable mental health problems and specific learning disabilities are disproportionately caught up in the criminal justice system (Fyson and Yates 2011; Yates, 2009). The Seen and Heard report by Talbot, published by the Prison Reform Trust report in 2010 identified that Youth Justice workers were reporting that 'children who offend with learning disabilities, communication difficulties, mental health problems, ADHD, and low levels of literacy were more likely than children without such impairments to receive a custodial sentence' (Talbot, 2010, p.6). In addition many children who offend have mental health, behavioural or learning difficulties which have gone undiagnosed (Chitsabesan et al., 2006). More recently The Youth Justice Board statistics (2017/18) indicated that more than one-third of children and young people in custody had a diagnosed mental health disorder with children who end up in custody being three times more likely to have mental health problems than those who do not. We also know they are very likely to have more than one mental health problem, to have a learning disability, to be dependent on drugs and alcohol and to have experienced a range of other challenges. Research evidence also indicates that many of these needs go unrecognised and unmet. The work of Singleton et al. (1998) illustrated that young people caught up in the criminal justice system have a higher level of mental health problems than other sections of the youth population.

In terms of general health, there are similar concerns. The survey by the Youth Justice Trust (2003)

identified that the health of children and young people under supervision by the Youth Offending Teams surveyed was not 'generally good'. They identified characteristics including 'poor nutrition; low levels of immunisations; poor take-up of appointments to see GPs; particularly low levels of health education awareness and examples of prematurely restricted growth or chronic health conditions where the children involved have never sought assistance' (Youth Justice Trust, 2003, p.26). These findings are reflected in a range of other studies (see Griggs and Walker, 2008). More recently, the Taylor review in 2016 noted that the health of children in the criminal justice system was of frequent concern and that this was particularly acute among those entering the secure estate (Secure Care and Young Offender Institutes). Griggs and Walker (2008) identified that children in custody often display poor physical health and many have not visited a doctor or dentist for years, with a number entering custody with undiagnosed sight or hearing problems.

Many of these children and young people are also educationally challenged. They have poor records of school attendance and educational achievement; learning and communication difficulties are common which can, in turn, compound the challenges they are facing educationally (see Fyson and Yates, 2009 and Prison Reform Trust, 2016). We have also, in recent years, become more aware of the high number of children on the autistic spectrum and with learning disabilities who are caught up in the criminal justice system – often with un-diagnosed needs (Fyson and Yates, 2009).

There is a significant body of evidence which indicates that children and young people who come into conflict with the law have complex, multiple and interlocking patterns of risk, disadvantage and vulnerability, which, if seen through the lens of the Children Act 2004 or through the Working Together Guidance (2018), could lead them to being identified as children at risk, and in need of a safeguarding, rather than criminal and in need of criminalisation (Goldson, 2005; Jamieson and Yates, 2009; Yates, 2009). The case of child criminal exploitation is an area which starkly illustrates the complex intersectional nature of vulnerability, risk, safeguarding and public protection in the lives of children who come into conflict with the criminal justice system.

REFLECTIVE QUESTIONS

- Consider your own case load. Can you identify these factors in the lives of the young people you work with?
- Consider how the different challenges they face could be seen as intersectional.
- Also consider how this might impact how you approach your work with them.

SAFEGUARDING: CHILD CRIMINAL EXPLOITATION

The Serious Violence Strategy (2018) defines child criminal exploitation as where:

> *an individual or group takes advantage of an imbalance of power to coerce, control, manipulate or deceive a child or young person under the age of 18 into any criminal activity (a) in exchange for something the victim needs or wants, and/or (b) for the financial or other advantage of the perpetrator or facilitator and/or (c) through violence or the threat of violence.*
>
> *Home Office (2018, p. 8)*

While child criminal exploitation can take many forms, dealing drugs – across county lines – has become a particularly pernicious and widespread problem.

CLOSER LOOK: 'COUNTY LINES'

The National Crime Agency (NCA) has been reporting on the 'county lines' phenomena since 2016 (NCA, 2016) and identifies the 'county lines' model as a significant national threat. A common feature of this model of supply is the recruitment of children and young people by 'elders' (Spicer, 2019) to carry out low level criminal activity (NCA, 2019). The business model is predicated on exploitative labour undertaken by vulnerable populations (Moyle, 2019) driven by organised criminal gangs. It is aggressive, thrives on exploitation and relies on the offenders' ability to target vulnerable individuals and to traffic them to distribute drugs at a local level in areas the gang is seeking to 'colonise' (Coomber and Moyle, 2018). Victims are targeted and trafficked across county lines to act as runners and to deal drugs from addresses in different locations where the homes of vulnerable individuals are occupied. Here, the occupants can also be the victims of abuse (see Robinson et al., 2019). It is acknowledged that children have always been exploited within the drug trade. However, widespread availability of mobile phones and encrypted applications has seen this exploitation evolve and expand.

The National Crime Agency (NCA) identifies that any 'vulnerability is a potential target, resulting in a broad profile of victims of exploitation in county lines offending' (NCA, 2019) with vulnerable children and young people targeted. Prosecutions of offenders can occur under the Modern Slavery Act 2015, this legislation was introduced to protect those being trafficked into this country and is not straight forward when being applied to county lines (see Stone, 2018 for a detailed overview).

Turner et al. (2019), in research conducted for the Children's Society, identify the 10- to 17-year age range as the most at risk of this form of criminal exploitation. These children are targeted by the criminal groups due to their vulnerability and are groomed with promises of money, drugs, status and affection, and also controlled through violence, fear, threats to their families and sexual abuse (see NCA, 2019; Moyle, 2019; Turner et al., 2019). In 2018 the NCA identified the majority of referrals (through the National Referral Mechanism under Modern Slavery Act 2015) for involvement in county lines as being between the ages of 15 and 17 because they are easier to 'control, exploit and reward than adults' (NCA, 2019). The NCA cite behaviour by offenders similar to the strategies employed by paedophiles to groom sex abuse victims and that this grooming takes place before the criminal exploitation takes place – with children being approached as young as 11 years. Turner et al. (2019) cite examples of children and young as 7 years being groomed and highlights a lack of recognition of the potential for young children to be exploited, leading to missed opportunities to protect them.

The NCA intelligence reports identify that 'children displaying vulnerabilities such as poverty, family breakdown and intervention by social services, looked after status, frequent missing episodes, behavioural and developmental disorders and exclusion from mainstream schooling are frequently targeted by county lines offenders' (NCA, 2019, p. 22). The NCA also note that offenders target children and young people with limited economic opportunities and those who have already been in conflict with the law along with those whose parents are drug users or are already, as adults, themselves being exploited by county lines offenders. In their research Turner et al. (2019) also identify children living in poverty, children with learning difficulties, those excluded from school and those being looked after by the local authority as being particularly vulnerable to being targeted by offenders for criminal exploitation. They highlight that children and young people with special education needs and learning disabilities are easier still to exploit and exert power over, and therefore easier to influence and control, due to their additional vulnerabilities, mirroring the strategies paedophiles employ to exploit the vulnerabilities of individual victims.

Both the NCA and Turner et al. (2019) identify recruitment through social media, pupil referral units, special educational needs schools, foster homes and homeless centres (also see NCA, 2019, p. 30). The NCA also highlight that, as with the sexual exploitation of children, the children and young people will often not identify themselves as victims or realise they have been groomed. The Children's Society research also identified that children were not likely to recognise their victimisation. This can add a further level of vulnerability if apprehended as the child might be considered to be more of a willing accomplice than a victim of exploitation. Vulnerable female children, who Turner et al. identify as often lost in narratives around child criminal exploitation (Turner et al., 2019, p.32), are also targeted and can often also be the victims of sexual violence and sexual exploitation within the county lines model. County lines offenders have been identified as being involved in the direct sexual exploitation of vulnerable young people (NCA, 2019). Victims also have difficulty leaving the county lines, with threats of violence towards victims and their families should they attempt to leave.

SAFEGUARDING AGAINST CHILD CRIMINAL EXPLOITATION

At present, despite the NCA identifying the county lines model as representing a significant national threat (NCA, 2019), and the vulnerability of children being exploited criminally being recognised in the Serious Violence Strategy and by the NCA Intelligence Reports, Her Majesty's Inspection of Constabulary and Fire and Rescue Services (HMICFRS) identify that there is no statutory definition of child criminal exploitation. The legal framework and definitions which relate to these children as children in need and at risk and in need of safeguarding, as well as children who are in conflict with the law, are complex. With no statutory definition, different services can take different positions on the levels of risk (HMICFRS, 2020). HMICFRS note that this can lead to one agency being more committed to working with an exploited child, on the basis of perceived risk, than another. This compounds the challenges around how intersectionality of risk and need interact – cutting across legal frameworks – vacillating between constructions of the child as a victim (being exploited and in need of safeguarding) and as a risky child offender. Furthermore, Tuner et al. (2019) observe a tendency to respond to these children through criminalisation rather than safeguarding and also identify a lack of consistent safeguarding strategies, at a national and local level, for children who are being criminally exploited and that the responses from statutory agencies are reactive, too variable and often come too late. A concerning lack of data and reporting about children at risk of criminal exploitation has also been identified, with the National Referral Mechanism using the Modern Slavery Act 2015 to record incidences of child criminal exploitation. The majority of police forces and local authorities are also not able to share figures on the number of children affected by criminal exploitation, and there are no consistent markers being used by agencies to flag children at risk of this type of activity (Turner, 2019; HMICFRS, 2020), thus highlighting how statutory agencies are struggling to respond effectively to organised criminal groups exploiting children. It is also clear that responses are most likely after the exploitation has occurred and as such a reaction to the criminal activity the child is involved in as a result of their exploitation,

rather than a systematised practice response to prevent harm, safeguard and protect those vulnerable to this form of exploitation.

Moreover even when the children and young people are apprehended for their involvement in drug supply as part of the county lines model, the Youth Justice Legal Advice Centre identify that 'there is currently poor awareness and understanding of CCE (child criminal exploitation) and it is often the case that victims are mistakenly viewed as having made a 'choice' to engage in criminal behaviour. This is often exacerbated by the child's refusal to recognise themselves as a victim' (Sands, 2018, p. 3). As a result the children who are the victims of exploitation are more likely to be labelled as criminal and criminalised rather than receive a safeguarding response. Indeed, where children are being criminally exploited '[p]rofessionals reported that many children come to attention of statutory agencies when exploitation is already present in their lives and criminal groups are controlling them to deliver drugs. Typically, in these instances professionals report that law enforcement takes precedence over safeguarding responses' (Turner et al., 2019, p. 9). They also noted how gender, age and ethnicity can impact on how professionals respond to the child or young person as an offender or as a victim who needs safeguarding – raising further questions regarding how discrimination, stereotyping and bias can impact on the decisions made.

Therefore children and young people who are being exploited through the county lines model often come to light because they are arrested for controlled drug possession and/or supply. If arrested for possession of controlled drugs, in order to be recognise as a victim, they need to be considered as victims of trafficking under the Modern Slavery Act 2015. The Crown Prosecution Service (CPS) current guidance states 'Where it is found that the child committed an offence as a direct result of their situation, prosecutors should follow the CPS guidance on suspects in a criminal case who might be victims of trafficking or slavery and consider the statutory defence for slavery or trafficking victims' (CPS, 2020). The NRM refers to the National Referral Mechanism which refers for a decision on whether a suspected victim is the victim of human trafficking or modern-day slavery. As the Children Society research indicates, this can often mean that children are simultaneously being prosecuted whilst also waiting on an NRM decision on whether they are a victim of trafficking or modern slavery.

CONCLUSION

The Children Acts of 1989 and 2004 identifies duties around safeguarding. Section 17 of the Children Act 1989 puts a duty on the local authority to provide services to children in need in their area, regardless of where they are found, and requires local authorities to undertake enquiries if they believe a child has suffered or is likely to suffer significant harm (Section 47). Under Section 10 of the Children Act 2004, the local authority is also under a duty to make arrangements to promote cooperation between itself and organisations and agencies to improve the well-being of local children. According to the Working Together guidance (2018) this cooperation should be effective at all levels of an organisation, from strategic level through to operational delivery.

The Working Together guidance promotes a child-centred approach and defines safeguarding and promoting the well-being of children as 'protecting children from maltreatment, preventing impairment of children's health or development, ensuring that children grow up in circumstances consistent with the provision of safe and effective care, taking action to enable all children to have the best outcomes' (Working Together, 2018, p. 5). The guidance recognises that children may be vulnerable to neglect and abuse or exploitation not only from within their family and from individuals they come across in their day-to-day lives, but also from exploitation by criminal gangs and organised crime groups. This is a welcome move to a more contextual understanding of safeguarding away from a narrow focus on familial risks (see Firmin, 2015 for a discussion of contextual safeguarding). The guidance is clear that 'whatever the form of abuse or neglect, practitioners should put the needs of children first when determining what action to take' (Working Together, 2018, p. 8) recognising the extrafamilial threats to safeguarding children and young people from criminal gangs – specifically citing criminal child exploitation and the county lines model. It also specifically references that 'children who are encountered as offenders, or alleged offenders, are entitled to the same safeguards and protection as any other child and due regard should be given to their safety and welfare at all times' (Working Together, 2018, p. 62).

However, as this chapter has illustrated, it remains clear that many of the risk factors which could place a child at risk in safeguarding terms can also be factors which increase the risk of them becoming involved in the county lines model (Coliandris, 2015) and coming into conflict with the criminal justice system. Indeed within the county lines model of child criminal exploitation, children and young people are purposively targeted by criminal groups due to their vulnerability and are systematically exploited. They are also, due to the very nature of the model, committing criminal acts themselves and, due to their positioning in the hierarchy, carry a greater risk of apprehension. They are also, through their criminal exploitation, exposed to further contextual risks and a 'spectrum of harm' (Moyle, 2019) due to the harmful and risky environments they encounter (see Windle and Briggs, 2015). They therefore occupy victim and perpetrator status simultaneously, and this is illustrative of how safeguarding and vulnerability interact in the context of children and young people's exploitation in the county lines model. In the absence of robust early intervention to develop protective factors and resilience, they are first and foremost reactively drawn into contact with the criminal justice system, a system which itself can be damaging and can pose safeguarding risks to the vulnerable children and young people who encounter it (Goldson and Yates, 2008).

REFERENCES

Chitsabesan, P., Kroll, L., Bailey, S., Kenning, C., 2006. Mental health needs of young offenders in custody and in the community. Br. J. Psychiatry 1 (6), 534–540.

Children Acts of 1989. https://www.legislation.gov.uk/ukpga/1989/41/contents.

Children Act 2004. https://www.legislation.gov.uk/ukpga/2004/31/contents.

Coliandris, G., 2015. County lines and wicked problems: Exploring the need for improved policing approaches to vulnerability and early intervention. Australasian Policing: A Journal of Professional Practice and Research 7 (2), 25–36.

Coomber, R., Moyle, L., 2018. 'The changing shape of street-level heroin and crack supply in England: Commuting, holidaying and cuckooing drug dealers across 'county lines''. Brit. J. Criminol. 58, 1323–1342.

Crown Prosecution Service (CPS), 2020. Human Trafficking, Smuggling and Slavery. https://www.cps.gov.uk/legal-guidance/human-trafficking-smuggling-and-slavery. (Accessed 26 April 2021).

Firmin, C., 2015. Contextual Safeguarding: An Overview of the Operational, Strategic and Conceptual Framework. University of Bedfordshire: Contextual Safeguarding Network.

Fyson, R., Yates, J., 2011. 'Anti-social behaviour orders and young people with learning disability'. Crit. Soc. Policy 31 (1).

Goldson, B., 2005. 'Taking liberties: Policy and the punitive turn'. In: Hendrick, H. (Ed.), Children and Social Policy: An Essential Reader. The Policy Press, Bristol.

Goldson, B., Yates, J., 2008. 'Youth justice policy and practice: Reclaiming applied criminology as critical intervention'. In: Yates, J., with, Stout, B., Williams, B. (Eds.), Applied Criminology. Sage, London.

Griggs, J., Walker, R., 2008. The Costs of Child Poverty for Individuals and Society. Joseph Rowntree Foundation, York.

Her Majesty's Inspection of Constabulary and Fire and Rescue Services, 2020. Both Sides of the Coin: The Police and National Crime Agency's Response to Vulnerable People in 'County Lines' Drug Offending. www.justiceinspectorates.gov.uk/hmicfrs. (Accessed 30 April 2021).

Home Office, 2018. Serious Violence Strategy. HM Government, London. https://assets.publishing.service.gov.uk/government/uploads/system/uploads/attachment_data/file/698009/serious-violence-strategy.pdf.

Howard Leagues, 2018. Ending the Criminalisation of Children in Residential Care. Briefing one. https://howardleague.org/wp-content/uploads/2017/07/Ending-the-criminalisation-of-children-in-residential-care-Briefing-one.pdf.

Jamieson, J., Yates, J., 2009. 'Young people, youth justice and the state'. In: Coleman, R., Sim, J., Tombs, S., Whyte, D. (Eds.), State, Power, Crime. Sage, London.

Lammy, D., 2016. The Lammy Review: An Independent Review into the Treatment of, and Outcomes for, Black, Asian and Minority Ethnic Individuals in the Criminal Justice System. https://assets.publishing.service.gov.uk/government/uploads/system/uploads/attachment_data/file/643001/lammy-review-final-report.pdf.

Modern Slavery Act 2015. https://www.legislation.gov.uk/ukpga/2015/30/contents/enacted.

Moyle, L., 2019. 'Situating vulnerability and exploitation in street-level drug markets: Cuckooing, commuting, and the "county lines" drug supply model'. J. Drug Issues 49 (4), 739–755.

National Crime Agency, 2016. County Lines: Gang Violence Exploitation and Drug Supply 2016. https://www.nationalcrimeagency.gov.uk/who-we-are/publications/15-county-lines-gang-violence-exploitation-and-drug-supply-2016/file.

National Crime Agency, 2019. Initial Intelligence: County Lines Drug Supply, Vulnerability and Harm 2018. https://www.nationalcrimeagency.gov.uk/who-we-are/publications/257-county-lines-drug-supply-vulnerability-and-harm-2018/file.

Pitts, J., 2008. Reluctant Gangsters: The Changing Face of Youth Crime. Willan, Cullompton.

Prison Reform Trust, 2016. In Care, Out of Trouble: Full report, https://prisonreformtrust.org.uk/publication/in-care-out-of-trouble-full-report/

Robinson, G., McLean, R., Densley, J., 2019. 'Working county lines: Child criminal exploitation and illicit drug dealing in Glasgow and Merseyside'. Int. J. Offender Ther. Comp. Criminol. 63 (5), 694–711.

Sands, C., 2018. Child Criminal Exploitation: County Lines Gangs, Child Trafficking and Modern Day Slavery Defences for Children. Youth Justice Legal Centre, London. https://yjlc.uk/wp-content/uploads/2018/02/Modern-Slavery-Guide-2018.pdf.

Serious Violence Strategy (2018). https://www.gov.uk/government/publications/serious-violence-strategy.

Singleton, N., Meltzer, H., Gatwood, R., 1998. Psychiatric Morbidity Among Prisoners in England and Wales. Office for National Statistics. Stationery Office, London.

Social Metrics Commission, 2019. Measuring Poverty. A report of the Social Metrics Commission Chaired by Philippa Stroud, CEO of the Legatum Institute. https://socialmetricscommission.org.uk/wp-content/uploads/2019/07/SMC_measuring-poverty-201908_full-report.pdf

Spicer, J., 2019. 'That's their brand, their business': How police officers are interpreting county lines. Policing and Society 29 (8), 873–886.

Stone, N., 2018. Child criminal exploitation: 'county lines', trafficking and cuckooing. Youth Justice 18, 285–293.

Talbot, J., 2010. Seen and Heard: Supporting Vulnerable Children in the Youth Justice System. Prison Reform Trust, London https://www.prisonreformtrust.org.uk/wp-content/uploads/old_files/Documents/SeenandHeardFinal%20.pdf.

Taylor, C., 2016. Review of the Youth Justice System in England and Wales. Ministry of Justice, London. https://assets.publishing.service.gov.uk/government/uploads/system/uploads/attachment_data/file/577103/youth-justice-review-final-report.pdf.

Turner, A., Belcher, L., Pona, I., 2019. Counting Lives: Responding to Children Who Are Criminally Exploited. Children's Society, London.

Yates, J., 2009. 'Youth justice: Moving in an anti-social direction. In: Wood, J., Hine, J. (Eds.), Work with Young People: Theory and Policy for Practice. Sage, London.

Youth Justice Board, 2019. Youth Justice Statistics 2017/18. Youth Justice Board, London. https://assets.publishing.service.gov.uk/government/uploads/system/uploads/attachment_data/file/774866/youth_justice_statistics_bulletin_2017_2018.pdf.

Youth Justice Trust, 2003. On the Case: A Survey of Over 1,000 Children and Young People Under Supervision. Youth Justice Trust, Manchester.

Windle, J., Briggs, D., 2015. 'It's like working away for two weeks': The harms associated with young drug dealers commuting from a saturated London drug market. Crime Prevention and Community Safety 17, 105–119.

Working Together to Safeguard Children, 2018. A Guide to Inter-Agency Working to Safeguard and Promote the Welfare of Children. Https://assets.publishing.service.gov.uk/government/uploads/system/uploads/attachment_data/file/779401/Working_Together_to_Safeguard-Children.pdf.

12d CHILDREN AND YOUNG PEOPLE WHO SEXUALLY HARM OTHERS

STUART ALLARDYCE ■ PETER YATES

KEY POINTS

- The term 'harmful sexual behaviour' describes a continuum of sexual behaviours displayed by children and young people, from inappropriate through to abusive behaviours.

- The majority of children and young people who have displayed harmful sexual behaviour do not become sex offenders as adults.

- Children and young people who sexually harm others are more likely than other young people to have a history of maltreatment and family difficulties.

- Assessment should be proportionate to the behaviours displayed.

- Interventions need to be holistic, addressing both the behaviours the child has displayed and their wider welfare needs, and involve families as well as other relevant agencies, such as schools.

- Services should maintain a perspective that these are children first and foremost, not mini adult-sex offenders.

INTRODUCTION

Between 2012 and 2016, 32,452 reports were made to police in England and Wales involving alleged sexual offences where both perpetrator and victim were under the age of 18 years. This represents an average of over 22 initial concerns raised every day (Barnardo's, 2017). Most child protection professionals will therefore work with cases involving children and young people who sexually harm others at some point during their career, and many will do so on a regular basis.

However, a UK survey of 597 childcare professionals found that many practitioners and carers felt that they did not have the knowledge and skills for working directly with these young people (Clements et al., 2017). Over half (56%) of the practitioners and carers who responded to the survey said that they had worked with between one and five children or young people displaying harmful sexual behaviour in the previous year, but many said they lacked confidence in working with this client group. The 190 service managers, strategic managers and commissioners who participated in the study said that they found leading multiagency partnerships and the design and commissioning of services particularly challenging and an area in which most lacked confidence.

Nonetheless, in recent years, research has outlined clear principles for effective work with children and young people who have sexually harmed others. This chapter focuses on effective child protection responses to this issue.

CASE STUDY 12D.1: EVA

Mary is a mother of Harry (14) and Sophie (6). Mary contacted social services in a state of some distress. Her neighbour, Jane, had angrily accused Harry of sexually abusing Eva, Jane's 5-year-old daughter. Jane had said that yesterday afternoon, Eva had been playing with Sophie in their back garden after school and

Harry had joined them. Harry took Eva behind a bush and told her that he wanted to 'show her what grown-ups do when they love each other'. He put his hand between her legs, under her clothes, and then put his finger 'right inside her flower'. She told him this hurt and asked him to stop. She ran home and was very upset but was only able to tell her mother what had happened the following morning when she refused to go to school. Mary says that she thinks the allegation is malicious because she recently fell out with Jane. She cannot believe that Harry would have acted in this way. She asked Harry about what happened, and he denied he was there at the time before becoming very distressed.

REFLECTIVE QUESTIONS

- What feelings and thoughts are raised for you by this case example? How do you feel towards Harry, to Eva, and to Mary? What relevance do these thoughts and feelings have for your practice?
- How serious do you consider this situation to be?
- What immediate actions need to take place in terms of child protection?
- What further information would you need to develop a robust child protection plan that responds to the needs of all children involved and manages and reduces risks over time? What would be the key components of this plan?

ATTITUDES AND VALUES

Child sexual abuse is a demanding and highly complex issue for child protection practitioners. Child sexual abuse by children and young people themselves adds extra complexities to the tasks of identifying risks, assessing strengths and vulnerabilities within families, acting to prevent further immediate harm, and intervening effectively to reduce risks.

This is in part because practitioners tend to conceptualise sexual abuse as a form of harm carried out by adults on children: it is not a form of behaviour expected of children themselves. Accordingly, approaches to assessment and intervention are mostly framed to address adults who abuse. The lack of anchoring of this practice issue within a traditional childcare policy and practice context means that encountering harmful sexual behaviour by children and young people can leave practitioners feeling overwhelmed and underskilled. On the one hand, some practitioners find it difficult to accept that children can act in abusive ways and may dismiss sexual behaviours that harm as experimentation, or by normalising them (e.g. 'boys will be boys'). Practitioners may appreciate the vulnerability and welfare needs of these children but fail to respond effectively to the genuine risks that they may present or the harm they have caused. On the other hand, practitioners may be inclined to treat the young person as a 'mini adult sex offender'. Anxiety about risk may lead to professional practices and decisions that are defensive, even punitive, and that fail to appreciate the child or young person's welfare needs and their rights as a child. This can lead to responses that are inappropriate for the child's age and do not support the child and their family to move on from harm (Hackett et al., 2015).

A disclosure of this nature will typically lead to an investigation involving police and social work, necessitating interviews with Eva as the alleged victim and Harry as the alleged perpetrator of a serious crime. Eva and her family will need sensitive support and practical assistance. Professionals will need to engage with Mary, giving her an opportunity to process and make sense of the allegations, offering practical advice and support whilst assessing her capacity to protect. There are many things professionals will then need to establish. Was the behaviour experimental and opportunistic, or more ingrained and planned, and perhaps an indicator of a more deep-seated problem? Does Harry present a continuing risk to Eva and/or to other children, including Sophie, his sister? Is it safe for Harry to remain living at home? Can he continue to attend his school? How safe will Harry be within his own community further to this allegation? How can these families continue to live together safely as neighbours? And why has Harry acted in this way? Does this mean that he has been sexually or otherwise abused himself, and if so, by whom, and is he still at risk? All of these questions need to be addressed, recognising that as child protection professionals we must draw on our reflective capacity to address the interplay of feelings, values, thoughts and actions raised for ourselves and other practitioners when working with the families and children in this kind of practice situation.

DEFINITIONS AND KEY CHARACTERISTICS

Although the term is consistently used by practitioners and in policy and practice guidance in the UK, there is no universally agreed meaning of the term 'harmful sexual behaviour'. The following definition is, however, commonly used:

> *Sexual behaviours expressed by children and young people under the age of 18 years old that are developmentally inappropriate, may be harmful towards self or others and / or be abusive towards another child, young person or adult.*
>
> *Hackett et al. (2019, p. 13)*

Practitioners' ability to determine if a child's sexual behaviour is harmful will therefore be based on an understanding of what constitutes developmentally appropriate, healthy sexual behaviour in childhood as well as an awareness of informed consent, power imbalances and exploitation.

Children and young people may display normative or expected sexual behaviours from early childhood onwards. For prepubescent children this means:

> *Natural and healthy sexual exploration… an information-gathering process wherein children explore each other's and their own bodies by looking and touching (e.g. playing doctor), as well as exploring gender roles and behaviours (e.g. playing*

> *house)….The child's interest in sex and sexuality is balanced by curiosity about other aspects of his or her life…The feelings of the children regarding the sexual behaviour are generally light-hearted and spontaneous.*
>
> *Johnson (2016, pp. 1–2)*

For adolescents this means behaviours that may include 'kissing, flirting and foreplay (touching, fondling), [that] are more goal orientated towards intimacy, sexual arousal and orgasm' (Araji, 1997, pp. 20–22).

Assessing what constitutes 'normal' sexual behaviour at each developmental stage is not straightforward and needs to take into account the social, emotional and cognitive development of the individual child or young person. Some behaviours that are normal in young children are concerning if they continue into adolescence; other behaviours, normal in adolescence, would be worrying in younger children (Friedrich et al., 1998).

Detailed assessment of children's sexual behaviour is indicated if the behaviour meets any or all of the following criteria:

- it occurs at a frequency greater than would be developmentally expected;
- it interferes with the child's development;
- it occurs with coercion, intimidation, or force;
- it is associated with emotional distress;
- it occurs between children of divergent ages or developmental abilities;
- it repeatedly recurs in secrecy after intervention by caregivers (Chaffin et al., 2002).

Sexual behaviour outside the normative range may be called 'harmful' as it may cause physical or emotional harm to others and/or to the child or young person themselves. It may range from activities that are simply inappropriate in a particular context through to serious sexual assault. Children's sexual behaviour may therefore best be described as lying on a continuum from normal through inappropriate, problematic, abusive and violent behaviours (Fig. 12d.1; Hackett, 2010).

Critically, they can occur in four different contexts:

Family settings: The vast majority of sexual abuse by children and young people takes place within domestic spaces such as the family home or the homes of relatives or friends (Finkelhor, 2009). Close family relatives, including siblings, or neighbours' children typically feature as victims in these settings, although abuse in substitute care settings can also occur.

Organisational settings: This would include harmful sexual behaviour in primary and secondary schools as well as residential group living environments. Such sexual abuse generally involves peers. There is growing awareness of abuse in school settings, and data collected by the BBC in 2015 found that 5500 sexual offences, including 600 rapes, were recorded in UK schools over a 3-year period (BBC, 2015).

Community settings: Sexual abuse in public spaces is less prevalent than in domestic and organisational settings (Smallbone and Wortley, 2000). Stranger rape offences by adolescents is rare. Acts of public indecency or peer sexual abuse, such as girls being pressured and coerced into sexual acts by boys, often in gang or group settings, are more common. This may occur in community spaces where young people congregate (e.g. parks, playgrounds, shopping centres, fast food outlets, disused houses and stairwells).

Online: This involves harmful sexual behaviour taking place exclusively online or taking place in-person but facilitated by new technologies. In an analysis of online sexual offences in Scotland between 2013 and 2016, in a quarter of cases both the victim and perpetrator were under 18 (Justice Analytics Service, 2017). The term 'technology assisted harmful sexual behaviour' is

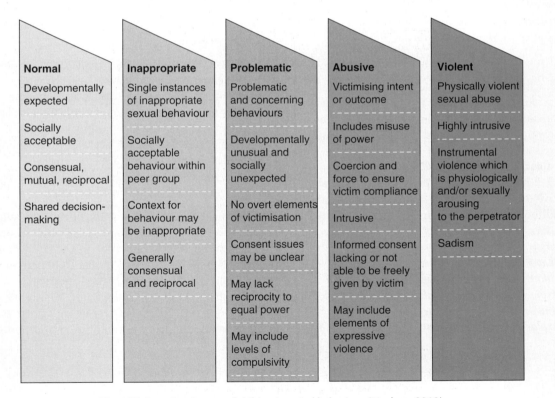

Fig. 12D.1 ■ Continuum of children's sexual behaviour (Hackett, 2010).

increasingly used to describe these scenarios, defined as 'One or more children engaging in sexual discussions or acts – using the internet and/or any image-creating/sharing or communication device – which is considered inappropriate and/or harmful given their age or stage of development. This behaviour falls on a continuum of severity from the use of pornography to online child sexual abuse' (Hollis et al., 2017, p. 11).

There is considerable variation in the level of seriousness of the incidents that come to the attention of child protection agencies. Many of the sexual crimes committed by children and young people in the UK are of the utmost severity: 15% of rapes in England and Wales in 2016 involved a perpetrator under the age of 18 years (Criminal Justice Statistics, 2017). Some, however, are lesser infractions: 35% of juvenile sexual offences in 2016 attracted a caution, suggesting that they may have been below the level of seriousness requiring prosecution (Bateman, 2017). Just as there is a continuum of behaviours, there also needs to be a continuum of responses to harmful sexual behaviour, ranging from broad educational inputs on consent and relationships for inappropriate and some problematic behaviours, through to multiagency public protection arrangements for the most serious sexual offences.

CLOSER LOOK

Sexual abuse is regulated in law by a number of statutes, chiefly the Sexual Offences Act 2003 in England and Wales and the Sexual Offences (Northern Ireland) Order 2008 and Sexual Offences (Scotland) Act 2009 in other parts of the UK. In particular, young people under the age of 13 years are considered in law to be unable to give consent to sexual activity. The law places a strict interpretation on the responsibility of those who engage in sexual activity, which means that young people over the age of 10 years (12 in Scotland) who sexually abuse others are expected to take responsibility for their actions.

PREVALENCE IN UK

The Office for the Children's Commissioner for England and Wales (Office of the Children's Commissioner, 2015) estimates that only around one in eight children who have been sexually abused are ever known to police and social services. Establishing the prevalence of any form of sexual abuse is methodologically challenged by the hidden nature of this form of harm.

Hackett et al. (2019) estimate that at least one-third of all child sexual abuse in the UK is carried out by other children and young people. Information gathered from the police on the perpetrators of sexual offences against children in England and Wales by the Office of the Children's Commissioner (2015) identified 34,241 perpetrators over a 2-year period (April 2012–March 2014). One-third of the perpetrators – where age was known – were under the age of 18. Of the 58,900 proven offences committed by children and young people under the age of 18 in the year to March 2019, 2% were sexual offences. Some 8% of those in youth custody were remanded or sentenced in relation to a sexual offence (Youth Justice Board, 2020).

THE NEEDS OF YOUNG PEOPLE WHO HAVE DISPLAYED HARMFUL SEXUAL BEHAVIOUR

It may appear obvious to state that children are different from adults, with distinct needs and vulnerabilities arising from their developmental status. Nonetheless, children and young people who have displayed harmful sexual behaviour are often responded to in ways that are shaped fundamentally by assessment and risk management strategies designed for adult who have committed sexual offences. Research has conclusively shown that children and young people represent a distinct population from adults who commit sexual offences, and pathways into – and out of – these behaviours are very different for children when compared to adults (Lussier and Blokland, 2014). There is now a large body of scientific evidence to support the view that children and young people who have displayed harmful sexual behaviour are not 'mini adult sex offenders'.

They are also a highly heterogeneous population, although some general characteristics emerge from relevant research:

- **Gender**: Most children and young people who abuse are boys: only between 3% and 7% of those who come to the attention of services are girls (Finkelhor et al., 2009; Fox, 2017; Hackett et al., 2013).

- **Ethnicity:** Where it is reported, the ethnic background of the young people in studies are broadly in line with that of the UK population (Hackett et al., 2013).

- **Age at onset of behaviour**: Most research has shown a significant rise in harmful sexual behaviour from the age of 12 and peaking at age 14 (Finkelhor, 2009; Fox, 2017; Hackett et al, 2013).

- **Cognitive abilities**: Learning disability is consistently overrepresented in studies describing children and young people who have displayed harmful sexual behaviour, representing about one-third of young people referred to specialist services (Hackett et al., 2013).

- **Experiences of abuse and maltreatment**: Hackett et al. (2013) found that 66% of a UK sample of young people who had displayed harmful sexual behaviour were known to have experienced some form of maltreatment. Such maltreatment may include physical abuse, witnessing physical and domestic abuse, sexual abuse and exploitation, emotional abuse and neglect, with many children having experienced multiple forms of trauma. A meta-analysis by Seto and Lalumiere (2010) found that young people who had committed sexual offences were five times more likely to be sexually abused than young people known to statutory services for nonsexual offending.

- **Families of young people who have displayed harmful sexual behaviour**: Many studies report that a significant minority of the parents of children who have displayed harmful sexual behaviour may have problems with mental health and substance misuse, and a significant proportion may themselves have experienced poor parenting and childhood maltreatment (Cherry and O'Shea, 2006; Duane and Morrison, 2004).

- **Victim characteristics**: While the majority of children and young people who have displayed harmful sexual behaviour are boys, the majority of victims are girls, with only around 20% being boys (Finkelhor et al, 2009; Kjellgren et al., 2006). Other studies have recorded higher levels of victim crossover, with Hackett et al. (2013) finding that 30% of their sample abused both males and females, while 51% abused females only and 19% males only. The victims of adolescents tend to be either peers or prepubescent children, with sexual assaults of adults being statistically uncommon. In Finkelhor et al.'s 2009 study of 13,471 US cases involving recorded sexual crime perpetrated by a child or young person, 59% of victims were under the age of 12. Aside from these age and gender characteristics, the majority of victims are known to the young people who have harmed them. Somewhere between one-third and one-half of child sexual abuse perpetrated by children and young people is intrafamilial in nature (Allardyce and Yates, 2013).

- **Nature and causes of behaviour**: A wide range of sexually abusive behaviours are described in various studies, although there is considerable diversity in how behaviours are defined and classified. In Finkelhor et al.'s (2009) sample, 24% of cases involved rape, 13% sodomy and 49% fondling. Current research suggests that key aetiological factors include unmet emotional needs and attachment difficulties; use of coercion and aggression as coping strategies; poor emotional regulation skills; social isolation; experiences of preadolescent sexualisation and/or unresolved trauma. Atypical sexual interests may be present for a proportion of young people, including a sexual interest in prepubescent children (Seto and Lalumiere, 2010).

- **Reoffending**: Reitzel and Carbonell's meta-analysis (Reitzel and Carbonell, 2006) of relevant studies found sexual recidivism rates of 19% for young people who had not participated in interventions and 7% for those who had, while UK data suggests that the overall sexual reoffending rate for young people charged with sexual offences in the UK is 15% (Youth Justice Board, 2020). Rates of nonsexual reoffending can be considerably higher (Caldwell, 2002). Welfare outcomes in relation to employment, physical and mental health and family and intimate partner relationships are also often poor for a significant minority of young people who come to the attention of services because of harmful sexual behaviours (Hackett et al., 2011). Assessment and intervention must therefore address risks beyond those of sexual harm as well as the wider welfare outcomes for these young people.

- Research tells us that many children and young people who sexually harm others have experienced maltreatment and/or have other vulnerabilities (e.g. intellectual impairments). How should this inform initial child protection responses when sexual abuse perpetrated by a child or young person has been identified?
- Research also tells us that many parents of children who sexually harm others have also experienced adversity in childhood and/or adulthood. Parents often report feelings of shock, denial, confusion, guilt, shame, anger, isolation and powerlessness when they find out their child has acted in a sexually abusive way. What might a trauma-informed response look like when working with a family where this issue has emerged?

RESPONDING TO HARMFUL SEXUAL BEHAVIOURS

The level of assessment should be proportionate to the behaviours displayed, requiring only brief assessment when the behaviour is judged to be inappropriate, but more comprehensive assessment if initial indications are that the behaviour is abusive.

Immediate responses to harmful sexual behaviour depend on interacting considerations relating to the level of risk to and from the child/young person, their age and the contexts in which they live and in which the harmful sexual behaviour has taken place. The primary professional consideration must be to safeguard and promote the well-being of all the children involved, which will include deciding whether action should be taken under child protection procedures, both to protect the victim and to address concerns about what may underpin the child's harmful sexual behaviour. Where concerns are below the threshold of significant harm towards or caused by a child, there may still be a need for coordinated assessment and support to address underlying needs.

Parents have a critical role to play in promoting safety and helping their child to move on from

their harmful behaviour. The parents' strengths and protective capacities need to be identified and harnessed, as well as offering sensitive support to help parents to understand the likely causes of the harmful behaviour and the recommended collaborative responses to it.

A risk assessment should be carried out to determine whether the child or young person should remain within the family home and, if necessary, to inform the decision as to what might be an appropriate alternative placement. Such assessments should draw on a recognised and validated tool where possible, and this would also need to be bolstered by an analysis of family dynamics, including sibling dynamics where relevant. The assessment should formulate:

- the predisposing factors underlying the behaviour;
- the precipitating factors that help us to understand the dynamic nature of risk;
- the perpetuating factors that may serve to maintain the behaviour; and
- the protective factors that can help to mitigate risks and reduce risks in the longer term to explain the underlying mechanism of the presenting behaviour and direct intervention (Logan, 2014).

In simple terms, the assessment needs to answer the following questions:

- Why has the young person behaved in this way?
- How likely are they to do it again? To whom? And in what circumstances?
- What do we need to do now to manage the risks that are presented?
- What do we need to do in the longer term to reduce the levels of risk presented and to help the child to move on from their harmful behaviour?

It is likely to be helpful to consult with practitioners experienced in the area of children and young people's harmful sexual behaviour when attempting such a risk formulation.

Situations involving adolescent harmful sexual behaviour should both be referred to children's services for multiagency assessment and response. Risk assessment tools commonly used by childcare practitioners in the UK include AIM-3, J-SOAP II or PROFESOR

(Leonard and Hackett, 2019; Prentky and Righthand, 2003; Worling, 2017). Further advice can be found in relevant practice guidance.

In the event that an alternative placement is needed, residential staff or foster carers need to be fully informed about the harmful sexual behaviour and a risk management plan drawn up to support the placement. Teamwork between all involved is the key to safety.

Every child's plan must be holistic and tailored to the needs of the particular child, the risks they may present and the context in which they live. Proportionate risk management measures are essential but must be balanced with nurture, encouragement and opportunities for the child to develop healthier social and relationship skills. Disproportionate risk management plans which stifle children's opportunities to develop social skills are likely to increase the risks of harmful behaviour in the future. Such skills need to be developed within the community, so it is essential to involve the family, the school and other community agencies. Plans should build on those skills and relationships that promote resilience. In general, each child requires individual attention within a systemic approach so they become more able to:

- overcome any problems with emotional and sexual regulation;
- understand their own feelings and behaviours as well as the feelings and behaviours of others;
- work towards resolution of any past trauma;
- develop social and relationship skills in the context of home, school and community;
- meet their own needs in a socially acceptable way; and
- encourage and sustain longer-term change, anticipating future stresses the child may encounter.

CONCLUSION

Children who have displayed harmful sexual behaviour are children first and foremost, and whilst we must take seriously any risks they may present, this needs to be balanced by a supportive approach to help children to meet their wider welfare needs. Children may display harmful sexual behaviours in different contexts: family; organisational; community and online. Risk and needs assessments and safety planning must be responsive to these different contexts. The risks of engaging in further harmful behaviour for most – although not all – children are low, and great care must be taken neither to over- or under-respond to the risks and needs of these children. Practitioners need to maintain a level of reflexivity around their attitudes and values so as not to respond to these children as mini adult sex offenders.

FURTHER READING

NSPCC's Harmful Sexual Behaviour Framework. https://learning. nspcc.org.uk/research-resources/2019/harmful-sexual-behaviour-framework/

This 2019 framework helps local areas develop and improve multiagency responses to children displaying harmful sexual behaviour (HSB). It provides a coordinated, systematic and evidence-based approach to recognising and responding to the risks and needs of this vulnerable group.

National Institute of Clinical Excellence Guidelines on Harmful Sexual Behaviour Among Children and Young People. https://www.nice.org.uk/guidance/ng55

This 2016 guideline covers children and young people who display harmful sexual behaviour, including those on remand or serving community or custodial sentences. It aims to ensure these problems don't escalate and possibly lead to them being charged with a sexual offence. It also aims to ensure no-one is unnecessarily referred to specialist services.

Prevention of and Responses to Harmful Sexual Behaviour by Children and Young People. https://www.gov.scot/publications/expert-group-preventing-sexual-offending-involving-children-young-people-prevention-responses-harmful-sexual-behaviour-children-young-people/

Commissioned by Scottish Government, this 2020 report sets out proposals from an expert group on tackling sexual offending involving children and young people to improve prevention and early intervention.

Working With Children and Young People Who Have Displayed Harmful Sexual Behaviour (Allardyce and Yates, 2018, Dunedin Press). https://www.dunedinacademicpress.co.uk/page/detail/?K=9781780460680

This 2018 single volume provides a comprehensive overview of the subject for practitioners, including approaches to assessment and intervention as well as work with special populations (prepubescent children who display HSB, working with girls, working with those who abuse in intrafamilial contexts etc.).

REFERENCES

Allardyce, S., Yates, P.M., 2013. Assessing risk of victim crossover with children and young people who display harmful sexual behaviours. Child Abus. Rev. 22, 255–267.

Araji, S.K., 2004. Preadolescents and adolescents: Evaluating normative and non-normative sexual behaviours and development. In *The handbook of clinical intervention with young people who sexually abuse* (pp. 19–51). Psychology Press.

12e

CHILD TO PARENT VIOLENCE AND ABUSE

HELEN BONNICK

KEY POINTS

- Child to parent violence is often hidden and emerges as part of other issues and crises within the family.
- Child to parent violence causes harm to all members of the family.
- Levels of risk are often misunderstood by safeguarding practitioners and a lack of joined up thinking leads to inadequate support for child and parent.
- Parents and young people can find it difficult to access help.
- Parents want to work in partnership with practitioners and often remain committed to supporting their child and achieving the best for them.

INTRODUCTION

The abuse of parents by their own children is something many people would find hard to imagine or accept. It challenges traditional understandings of power within families and requires a re-think about family functioning and child protection. Despite references in the literature to 'battered parents' as far back as the 1970s (Harbin and Madden, 1979), understanding of child to parent abuse and violence is still developing. Attention to the issue has grown as parents, academics and campaigners have created wider public and media awareness. However, there is still limited research on the topic, despite suggestions that child to parent violence and abuse affects as many as 1 in 10 families (Gallagher, 2008).

Child to parent violence and abuse can involve children of any age and does not only involve physical abuse. This form of abuse can also include siblings and extended family members. This chapter seeks to explore why child to parent violence occurs, what the risks are and how families can be best supported by professionals working within child protection. In this chapter, 'parent' is used to include all those in a parenting relationship and 'child' denotes anyone from birth to the age of 18.

DEFINING CHILD TO PARENT VIOLENCE AND ABUSE

There is no one agreed definition for the violence towards, and abuse of, parents by their children, though the terms 'Child to Parent Violence and Abuse' (CPVA) and 'Adolescent to Parent Violence and Abuse' (APVA) are most commonly used. This chapter will use the term Child to Parent Violence and Abuse (CPVA) to reflect that the issue can occur across all ages and not just in the teenage years. The wider terminology encapsulates the relationship, direction and type of behaviour exhibited. Holt (2016, p.1) offers a helpful definition of CPVA:

> A pattern of behaviour, instigated by a child or young person, which involves using verbal, financial, physical and /or emotional means to practice power and exert control over a parent [...] The power that is practised is, to some extent, intentional, and the control that is exerted over a parent is achieved

through fear, such that a parent unhealthily adapts his/her own behaviour to accommodate the child.

The issue can also be viewed through the broader lens of domestic abuse, for example, as 'a form of family violence that falls under the cross-government definition of domestic violence and abuse, most often (although not exclusively) directed towards mothers' (Condry et al., 2020, p. 4). New legislation is beginning to acknowledge the issue in legal terms, and for children over the age of 16 'CPVA is considered domestic abuse in accordance with the statutory definition under the 2021 Act' (Domestic Abuse Act, 2021, p. 21). However, a formal, legal definition of CPVA remains absent.

PREVALENCE AND EMERGING TRENDS

Accurate figures relating to incidences of CPVA are currently unknown. Abuse often remains unreported and hidden within families; therefore CPVA incidents reported to the police are likely to represent only a small proportion of all cases (Holt and Retford, 2013). As indicated in the introduction, limited research on the topic has suggested that CPVA may affect up to 1 in 10 families (Gallagher, 2008). In 2008, the organisation *Parentline Plus* reported that 8% of 30,000 calls to their helpline were from parents worried about their child's physical aggression towards them (Condry and Miles, 2013). Between 2009 and 2010, data from the Metropolitan Police indicated there were 1892 incidents of violence/threats of violence by 13- to 19-year-olds towards a parent in the home. During the COVID-19 pandemic, perhaps unsurprisingly, practitioners noted an increase in both the number and severity of referrals (Condry et al., 2020). Certainly, the period of restrictions during the pandemic demonstrated the impact of increased stress and loss of support for many experiencing CPVA; as one parent put it *'We're trapped with a caged lion and there is no rest'* (Condry et al., 2020, p. 11). In this respect, although there is limited data available, it is clear CPVA warrants urgent further research to develop knowledge in the area.

CPVA can affect any family and involve children of any age; however, there are some key trends within emerging data. Within this data, it is clear that gender is a significant factor when accounting for prevalence. The vast majority of CPVA (around 75%) is directed towards women, particularly mothers (Gallagher, 2008). Young men are the most common perpetrators (around 75%), and the most common occurrence overall (around 50%) is between sons and mothers (Gallagher, 2008). Further research echoes this conclusion, finding 87% of instigators were sons and 77% of victims were woman, usually mothers (Condry and Miles, 2013). Current definitions therefore do not necessarily wholly account for the gendered dynamics of the issue, which predominantly exists between young men and their mothers.

Additional learning needs and/or previous experiences of trauma are also amongst factors which can increase prevalence. There is a higher incidence of autism diagnosis and other learning disabilities among families where CPVA is reported (Routt and Anderson, 2014). However, it is also important to note that, in general, children with a diagnosis will not use violence. Previous experiences of trauma have also been linked to CPVA through research. For example, CPVA was a notable issue for adoptive families wherein children have experienced multiple losses (Selwyn et al., 2014). One research project found that around 50% of families who have experienced domestic abuse in the past report CPVA (Gallagher, 2008). Importantly, however, only 25% of young people who have experienced domestic abuse in their childhoods will go on to demonstrate abusive behaviour (Coordinated Action Against Domestic Abuse (CAADA), 2014). Thinking carefully about language will be an important aspect of this topic's development in research, policy and practice. Current definitions classify the child as an 'abuser', which may not be appropriate or helpful in terms of understanding and responding to the problem (Sanders, 2020).

The limited data presented here makes it clear that there remain serious gaps in research data about CPVA overall, although there are some important trends emerging. Therefore, despite developments in wider recognition, the issue remains underresearched, which impacts upon understandings of why problems occur and how best to address them. Further research is urgently required to explore the scope of this topic in more depth. This would be particularly beneficial in relation to less represented groups, for example knowledge around the LGBTQIA+ community, the experience in particular of fathers, and diverse ethnic groups.

REFLECTIVE QUESTIONS

- Have you encountered CPVA in any of your cases?
- Were you aware of any surrounding literature/support available when you encountered this in your practice?
- How does this limited knowledge base impact upon your ability to protect and support families effectively?

WHY DOES CPVA OCCUR, AND WHAT DOES IT LOOK LIKE?

The current political, policy and professional narratives often hold parents responsible for the behaviour of their children, shaping the assumption that CPVA is at heart an issue of 'poor parenting' (Bonnick, 2019, p. 117). However, emerging research contradicts this and suggests the issue is underpinned by a variety of factors (Holt and Retford, 2013). These can include children and young people with multiple diagnoses struggling to regulate their emotions; children whose own experience of violence has caused deep harm or modelled harmful ways of behaving; children dealing with traumatic loss, whether through adoption, bereavement or parental imprisonment; disrupted family relationships; poor physical or mental health; bullying at school; substance use; or involvement in gangs (Bonnick, 2019). Ultimately, there are a range of factors underpinning CPVA and no single cause (Holt and Retford, 2013). These children and young people are increasingly understood as using their behaviour to communicate needs which they may not be able to articulate in other ways, whether fear, anxiety, pain – or indeed a need for control over their environment.

Research on the behaviours demonstrated within CPVA are still emerging; however, the limited research available suggests there are a range of behaviours exhibited by young people and that some families are living with high levels of fear. CPVA can include physical and/or emotional violence and can

include patterns of coercive control (Stark, 2007). SafeLives data shows physical violence (57%) is the most frequent form of abuse utilised with CPVA, with jealous or controlling behaviour (24%) also featuring regularly Safe Lives (2017). Sometimes, behaviour develops slowly over time and becomes normalised within the family or it is tolerated because the child has a learning or physical disability or experiences mental distress.

> **CLOSER LOOK**
>
> CPVA is likely to be a pattern of behaviours which can include:
> - extended rages,
> - physical threats,
> - physical harm,
> - theft of sentimental items,
> - being 'nocturnal' (especially during lockdown),
> - damage to property,
> - shaming language, threats, swearing and shouting,
> - fraud and forgery, and
> - threatening and/or causing harm to themselves as a form of control.

Impact on Family Members

We are very different people to what we used to be, now we are less sunny and optimistic. Two of us are on antidepressants. Seeing others in the household be shouted at, called names and get hurt has made us all at times feel shocked and angry and we don't know what to do with that feeling. Two of us have expressed the feeling that if he is going to kill us we wish he would just get on with it and give us some release.

Parent reporting to Condry et al. (2020, p. 15)

Abusive and violent behaviour can be very frightening, and the impact of CPVA on parents and other family members should not be underestimated. Parents may respond by changing their own parenting practices to 'keep the peace' within increasingly tense environments and have reported a range of coping strategies including locking doors, hiding knives away, carefully navigating the family home and 'tiptoeing round' the child to avoid escalation (Bonnick, 2019). The organisation Who's in Charge?, set up to support families experiencing the issue, describes parents as feeling a range of emotions including hopelessness, feeling powerless, guilty, isolated and ashamed when their child exhibits this behaviour.

Parents' mental and physical health can be affected as they face uncertainty of what will happen next, when it will happen and what the consequences will be. This is very different to 'normal' patterns of difficult teenage behaviour (Bonnick, 2019). Consequences of experiencing child to parent violence can also extend beyond the family home: parents may be forced to leave work to supervise a child excluded from school, face eviction because of damage to property or complaints from neighbours, and experience financial implications due to loss of employment. Parents report feeling socially isolated as a result of their child's behaviour and judgements of both the child and their own parenting from friends, family and professionals.

CLOSER LOOK

The organisation Who's in Charge? provides advice for parents who sometimes find it difficult to recognise whether the behaviour of their child is violent or abusive. The following indicators may help identify the problem:

Parents:

- Changing behaviour to avoid confrontation with child
- Fearful for their own safety or that of wider family
- 'Walking on eggshells' to keep the peace

Children:

- Verbally or physically causing fear or distress to wider family
- Stealing or damaging possessions of wider family
- Threatens parent or wider family
- Threatens to harm themselves[a] or engage in risky behaviour
- Critical and dismissive of parent and parents' interests
- Blames parent or others for their behaviour
- Cruel to pets
- Threatens to run away from home, call others (i.e. ChildLine/other professionals) if demands are not met

[a] *Always take threats of self-harm seriously and seek support if required.*

LEGISLATION, POLICY AND PRACTICE RESPONSES

Despite some increased recognition of CPVA in policy and practice, the absence of a rigorous research base has arguably hindered the development of an appropriate and coordinated policy response (Condry et al., 2020). CPVA lies at the periphery of domestic abuse policy; therefore responses to the issue by agencies are often uncoordinated. The Domestic Abuse Act (2021) places new duties on authorities to support victims of abuse and their children, and at the time of writing this chapter, the outcome of the consultation on the Draft Statutory Guidance (England and Wales) is awaited. The draft guidance does include a specific reference to CPVA, acknowledging although there is still no legal definition:

> *If the child is 16 years of age or over, the abuse falls under the statutory definition of domestic abuse in the 2021 Act.*
>
> **Statutory guidance (2022, p. 25)**

However, some practitioners believe the guidance fails to adequately encapsulate the complexities of the problem and the experiences of families (Sanders, 2020). There are also crucial differences to be considered between abuse perpetrated by and towards ex/partners and that perpetrated by a child towards a parent. In this situation the young person themselves is frequently vulnerable and parents are often, understandably, unwilling to criminalise their child (Condry et al., 2020). Other relevant policy includes the *Information Guide to Adolescent to Parent Violence and Abuse* (Home Office, 2015), which sets out how various agencies and departments should fulfil their responsibilities to families. However, the underpinning research informing this was largely from the criminal justice field, and CPVA was widely contextualized as a 'teen' issue, linked to the challenges of adolescence. As such, professionals are largely left to tread ambiguous terrain, and families with younger children exhibiting CPVA are left without much support at all.

Agency responses to CPVA vary, with domestic abuse, youth justice and children's social care services all adopting varying approaches to framing the issue and offering support (Hunter et al., 2010). Austerity, cuts to wider public services, rising thresholds for support and a lack of wider policy commitment and training have further intensified this issue. Social workers are (perhaps unknowingly) already engaged in CPVA work. Biehal (2012) found that CPVA was a key feature for many families where children were 'on the edge of care'. Similar findings are echoed in Bonnick (2019, p. 9) by 'Sandi', a social worker:

> At one point I was the social worker who'd get those cases where teenagers were being relinquished into local authority care [...] part of it was the violence, I think probably with our cases with adolescents, it's a feature with nearly every case.

However, in children's services, with a legal duty to protect children rather than parents and an absence of a clear support route, social workers often approach families seeking support for CPVA in one of three ways. First, families are referred onto other services due to a reluctance to become involved (Hunter et al., 2010). Second, parents are offered responses to a 'parenting problem', through a failure of practitioners to fully explore the issues, or to reflect on their own assumptions (Bonnick, 2019; Cook and Gregory, 2019). For example, some families arriving at assessments prepared with their own information have been perceived as demanding and threatening (Bonnick, 2019). A combination of these two approaches can often lead families to experience more harm (direct and indirect). When the harm experienced by CPVA becomes unmanageable for families, they may choose to ask the local authority to voluntarily accommodate their child under Section 20 of the Children Act (1989). This is a difficult decision for families to make and can be an elongated process when trying to obtain support from local authorities managing the financial impact of 10 years of austerity.

The third approach, and arguably most unhelpful, is that some families are themselves subject to (or threatened with) child protection investigations due to social workers concerns about their parenting (Selwyn et al., 2014). The use of the term 'threatened' is itself of interest, in a field of work where both parents and social workers may behave defensively, each fearing the response of the other (Ferguson et al., 2020). This can be incredibly demoralizing for parents who approach services for support, and it

is worth exploring whether assumed *disengagement* may actually be the result, rather than the cause, of abuse (Cottrell, 2004). In some cases the local authority may pursue a care order under Section 31 of the Children Act (1989), in which care or supervision orders are granted if the child is suffering or is likely to suffer significant harm, which is attributed to being 'beyond parental control' (Children Act, 1989, p. 31 2.ii). It is noteworthy that courts have determined the 'beyond parental control' clause carries no implication of blame (British and Irish Legal Information Institute (BAILII), 2016).

REFLECTIVE QUESTIONS

- What assumptions are held about those who seek help with difficulties in the family, and how might these affect understandings of CPVA?
- Families experiencing CPVA experience a loss of power in the family and sometimes report feeling revictimized by their experiences with professionals. Why might this happen, and how might it be avoided in future?

SUPPORTING FAMILIES EFFECTIVELY

Supporting families experiencing CPVA effectively begins with building respectful relationships with families that seek to understand and explore issues, rather than invoke shame or turn families away until circumstances worsen. Practitioners should approach situations from a position that recognises that most parents actively seek to protect their children from harm, and those who do not often have their trauma histories that inform their ability to do so. Even where young people are reluctant themselves to engage in work to address their behaviour and underpinning causes, the value of working with parents alone cannot be overstated in bringing about and maintaining change. Practitioners need to ask, 'Is this family safe?' in addition to 'What is this young person trying to communicate?' Apportioning individual blame should be avoided, and instead each person should be encouraged to take responsibility for their own actions, for improving communication, for learning to avoid escalation and for identifying the priorities for change.

These are fundamental building blocks and need to be used within a context of addressing the specific needs of the individual child and other family members. Safeguarding practitioners should also seek to discover any other contributing factors such as ongoing abuse, mental health challenges and/or harm from external factors. Children can, and do, use allegations as a method of abuse and control; however, they may be using harmful behaviour as a result of the harm they have themselves received. Importantly, this harm may have taken place beyond their family. Investigations need to take place within a context that understands the issue of CPVA and the background of the specific family. Practitioners need to fulfil the requirements of the agency, while maintaining a respectful, compassionate – and knowledgeable – approach in which attention should be on the needs of each family member (Firmin, 2020).

Finally, recognising and naming CPVA can very helpful when working with families who often find it very difficult to talk about their experiences. Professionals will need to explore information and, at times, probe further, as shame can lead families to describe their experiences in abstract terms (such as 'out of control', 'throwing tantrums', or 'in with a bad crowd') rather than explicitly naming the abuse. When the possibility of CPVA is acknowledged by all parties, practitioners can go on to more accurately explore the experience and name the issue as abuse and violence – perhaps for the first time for that family. This can reduce the stigma and shame families can feel surrounding CPVA.

The experience of Craig's family mirrors that found within multiple reports (Albiston, 2016; Yexley, 2014). A lack of curiosity and poor communication between agencies meant there was no larger picture of the harm being caused within this family. The defining of the difficulties as a 'behaviour problem' and the emphasis on the parents asking for help meant statutory agencies failed to understand the difficulties and potential dangers, now widely recognised within domestic abuse practice. As noted earlier, a domestic abuse lens can be useful for understanding CPVA, but Craig's age precludes him from falling within the

---

CASE STUDY 12E.1: CRAIG

Craig was removed from his birth parents' care due to severe neglect and physical abuse and was adopted by Rachel and Tony aged 3 years. His birth parents both used illegal drugs, and his father was violent and abusive to his mother. Craig's behaviour as a child was difficult to manage, but with support from Children's Services and Craig's primary school, Rachel and Tony managed. With transfer to secondary school, a new and more frightening family life began. Craig struggled with the larger environment; he often arrived home angry and was physically and verbally aggressive towards Rachel. He then began self-harming. Meetings in school focussed on his behaviour, with an expectation that Rachel and Tony would enforce strict boundaries. Craig began to be sent home regularly and was eventually excluded permanently aged 14. Rachel was forced into a position where she had to give up work and home school Craig. Craig's behaviour at home was becoming more and more difficult; he smashed Rachel and Tony's possessions and physically assaulted Rachel numerous times. Tony wanted to call the police, but Rachel resisted as she was worried what would happen to Craig. The couple sought support from Children's Services and were given advice on de-escalating behaviour and parenting strategies around boundary setting. Things deteriorated to a point where Craig held a knife to Rachel and threatened to stab her, Tony called the police and Craig, now aged 15, was arrested. Both Rachel and Tony refused to have him home.

REFLECTIVE QUESTIONS

- Could more effective help have been offered earlier? If so, what would this be?
- What might Craig have been thinking and feeling and why?
- What are the risks to Craig? To his parents? To the wider public?

---

legislation, and the remedies available for adults are arguably not appropriate for younger people. Nevertheless, without intervention and support he may go on to become an adult perpetrator. Many of the programmes designed for young people have taken on board insights from the domestic abuse field, often within multiagency teams, adapting them to the different circumstances.

CONCLUSION

Early identification and appropriate assessment of CPVA offers the possibility of therapeutic intervention and transformative change. It enables professional and peer support for families, modelling new ways of relating for parent and child. Some families may reach a point where abuse is not eliminated but remains at a tolerable level. Sometimes it is necessary for a child to leave the home – for example they may have psychiatric needs requiring inpatient treatment; may be more safely placed in secure accommodation; or have attachment issues which make family life too difficult. Sometimes parents will ask for respite, knowing they can carry on with a short break, but, even with permanent removal, parents often remain closely attached to their children 'parenting at a distance'.

CLOSER LOOK

Good practice when working with families experiencing CPVA includes:

- working in partnership with the whole family;
- relational working, built on trust and non-judgementalism;
- adopting the shared language of CPVA for clarity;
- earlier diagnosis and support for children's mental health and learning needs;
- early intervention for children and survivors of domestic abuse;
- automatic postadoption support;
- close cooperation between agencies and appropriate sharing of information;
- thorough risk assessments that identify escalating levels of danger; and
- training and awareness for all agencies, so responsibility is transparent and clear.

Supporting families experiencing CPVA requires a move away from thinking of parents as part of the problem, to understanding them as part of the solution. Putting aside all assumptions, in an atmosphere of enquiry and learning, it remains possible to complete a thorough assessment of risk and, through timely, comprehensive, evidence-based interventions, to enable families to return to a safe and healthy life, the violence and abuse a thing of the past. The key must be to intervene early, armed with developing knowledge and understanding, to prevent harm, and to safeguard individuals as well as the integrity of the family as a whole. Such an approach upholds an evolving humane model of child protection work.

FURTHER READING

1. The Home Office, 2015. Information Guide: Adolescent to Parent Violence and Abuse, https://safelives.org.uk/sites/default/files/resources/HO%20Information%20APVA.pdf.
2. Holes in the Wall, https://holesinthewall.co.uk.
3. Bonnick, H., 2019. Child to Parent Violence and Abuse, A Practitioner's Guide to Working With Families. Pavilion Publishing and Media, West Sussex.
4. The Youth Justice Board Effective Practice Library includes programmes such as Break4Change, RYPP and Who's in Charge? https://yjresourcehub.uk/effective-practice.html.
5. Guidance for Health Services. This document gives advice on routine questioning about the experience of domestic abuse. https://assets.publishing.service.gov.uk/government/uploads/system/uploads/attachment_data/file/597435/DometicAbuseGuidance.pdf.

Other Books Include

Routt, G., Anderson, L., 2014. Adolescent Violence in the Home, Restorative Approaches to Building Healthy, Respectful Family Relationships. Routledge, New York.

Holt, A. (Ed.), 2015. Working with Adolescent Violence and Abuse Towards Parents, first ed. Routledge, London.

Coogan, D., 2017. Child to Parent Violence and Abuse, Family Interventions with Non Violent Resistance. Jessica Kingsley Publishers, London.

Yvonne Newbold Offers Support for Families Experiencing Violent Challenging Behaviour. https://yvonnenewbold.com.

REFERENCES

Albiston, K., 2016. Domestic Homicide Review into the Death of 'Sarah'/2016, Executive Summary. https://www.northumberland.gov.uk/NorthumberlandCountyCouncil/media/Safer-Northumberland-docs/DHR-Executive-Summary-Sarah.pdf.

BAILII, 2016. WBC v A. http://www.bailii.org/ew/cases/EWFC/OJ/2016/B70.html.

Bonnick, H., 2016. 'Beyond Parental Control: No Attribution of Blame', Holes in the Wall. 7 November. https://holesinthewall.co.uk/2016/11/07/beyond-parental-control-no-attribution-of-blame/.

Biehal, N., 2012. 'Parent Abuse by Young People, on the Edge of Care: A Child Welfare Perspective'. Soc. Policy Soc. 11 (2), 251–263.

CAADA, 2014. In Plain Sight: Effective Help for Children Exposed to Domestic Abuse, 2nd National Policy Report. https://safelives.org.uk/sites/default/files/resources/Final%20policy%20report%20In%20plain%20sight%20-%20effective%20help%20for%20children%20exposed%20to%20domestic%20abuse.pdf.

Children Act, 1989. c. 41. https://www.legislation.gov.uk/ukpga/1989/41/contents.

Condry, R., Miles, C., 2013. Adolescent to Parent Violence Project Briefing Paper 1. https://www.law.ox.ac.uk/sites/files/oxlaw/briefing-paper-1-general.pdf.

Condry, R., et al., 2020. Experiences of Child and Adolescent to Parent Violence in the COVID-19 Pandemic. University of Oxford. https://www.law.ox.ac.uk/sites/files/oxlaw/final_report_capv_in_covid-19_aug20.pdf.

Cook, L., Gregory, M., 2019. 'Making Sense of Sensemaking: Conceptualising How Child and Family Social Workers Process Assessment Information'. Child Care in Pract. 26 (2), 182–195. https://doi.org/10.1080/13575279.2019.1685458.

Cottrell, B., 2004. When Teens Abuse their Parents. Fernwood Publishing, Halifax.

The Domestic Abuse Act, 2021 chapter 17 https://www.legislation.gov.uk/ukpga/2021/17/pdfs/ukpga_20210017_en.pdf

Ferguson, H., et al., 2020. 'Hostile relationships in social work practice: Anxiety, hate and conflict in long-term work with involuntary service users'. J. Soc. Work Pract. https://doi.org/10.1080/02650533.2020.1834371.

Firmin, C., 2020. Contextual Safeguarding and Child Protection, Rewriting the Rules. Routledge, London.

Gallagher, E., 2008. Children's Violence to Parents: A Critical Literature Review. Master's Dissertation. Monash University. http://www.eddiegallagher.com.au/Child%20Parent%20Violence%20Masters%20Thesis%20Gallagher%202008.pdf.

Harbin, H.T., Madden, D.J., 1979. 'Battered parents – a new syndrome'. Am. J. Psychiatry 136 (10), 1288–1291.

Holt, A., 2009. 'Parent abuse: Some reflections on the adequacy of a youth justice response'. Internet J. Crim. 1–9. Available at: https://docs.wixstatic.com/ugd/b93dd4_5720f359696f4324bdc27b08f8e38803.pdf.

Holt, A., Retford, S., 2013. 'Practitioner accounts of responding to parent abuse – a case study in ad hoc delivery, perverse outcomes and a policy silence'. Child Fam. Soc. Work. https://onlinelibrary.wiley.com/doi/10.1111/j.1365-2206.2012.00860.x.

Holt, A. (Ed.), 2016. Working with Adolescent Violence and Abuse Towards Parents, first ed. Routledge, London.

Home Office, 2015. Information Guide: Adolescent to Parent Violence and Abuse. https://safelives.org.uk/sites/default/files/resources/HO%20Information%20APVA.pdf.

Hunter, C., Nixon, J., Parr, S., 2010. 'Mother abuse: A matter of youth justice, child welfare or domestic violence'. J Law Soc. 37 (2), 264–284.

Routt, G., Anderson, L., 2014. Adolescent Violence in the Home, Restorative Approaches to Building Healthy, Respectful Family Relationships. Routledge, New York.

Safe Lives, 2017. Safe Young Lives: Young People and Domestic Abuse. https://safelives.org.uk/sites/default/files/resources/Safe%20Young%20Lives%20web.pdf

Sanders, R., 2020. 'Adolescent to Parent Violence and Abuse'. https://www.iriss.org.uk/resources/esss-outlines/adolescent-parent-violence.

Selwyn, J., Wijedasa, D., Meakings, S., 2014. Beyond the Adoption Order: Challenges, Interventions and Adoption Disruption. Department for Education. https://assets.publishing.service.gov.uk/government/uploads/system/uploads/attachment_data/file/301889/Final_Report_-_3rd_April_2014v2.pdf.

Stark, E., 2007. Coercive Control: The Entrapment of Women in Personal Life. Oxford University Press, Oxford.

Statutory guidance, 2022. https://assets.publishing.service.gov.uk/government/uploads/system/uploads/attachment_data/file/1089015/Domestic_Abuse_Act_2021_Statutory_Guidance.pdf

Yexley, M., 2014. Overview Report into the Homicide of CJ, Tower Hamlets Community Safety Partnership. https://www.towerhamlets.gov.uk/Documents/Community-safety-and-emergencies/Domestic-violence/DHR_4_Final_Executive_Summary.pdf.

PART 3 Child Protection Practices

13

CULTURALLY SENSITIVE CHILD PROTECTION PRACTICE

CATH WILLIAMS

KEY POINTS

- How culture, race and ethnicity impact on children's well-being.
- How far issues of race, ethnicity and culture should be considered in safeguarding children.
- What cultural competence is and how can it be used in safeguarding children.
- How social workers and other practitioners can respond competently to the needs of children and young people from diverse cultures and backgrounds.

INTRODUCTION

The boundaries between culture, race and ethnicity are unclear, overlapping and sometimes contradictory. This can cause problems working with Black and ethnic minority children and families, in part due to how these concepts are defined and understood. The chapter begins with an explanation of some key terms and descriptions, followed by a short history of multiculturalism in British society. Following this, the chapter explores how culture, race and ethnicity interact in the lives of Black and ethnic minority children and young people. By drawing upon Cross et al.'s (1989) Cultural Competence Continuum model, the chapter undertakes a critical discussion on assessment, decision-making and intervention practices, exploring the extent to which practitioners need to both understand and consider matters of culture, race and ethnicity in relation to safeguarding. The chapter concludes by considering best practice in culturally competent social work and calls for urgent on-going work in this vital area of child protection work.

UNDERSTANDING CULTURE, RACE AND ETHNICITY

Terms Used Throughout the Chapter

BAME – Black and Asian Minority Ethnic

'Black' – children and families of African, African–Caribbean descent. It is also sometimes used to reference the shared experiences of racism and discrimination amongst some visible BAME groups and communities

Ethnicity – common values and cultural practices of a particular ethnic group defined by geography, politics, history, religion and culture

Race – the social categorisation of people defined by skin colour

Identity – individual and group characteristics that interact to form a personal sense of self and a collective sense of belonging

Eurocentrism – favouring European (usually dominant) cultural beliefs and practices

Cultural Absolutism – the idea that there is only one right standard or rule (all abuse and neglect is wrong, regardless of culture)

Cultural Relativism – the idea that every culture practice is equally valid (neglect and abuse must be understood within its cultural context)

Cultural Competence – accumulation of knowledge, skills and understanding about the norms, behaviours, values and practices that exist within a particular cultural group in order to practice effectively

Note: Some of these terms are contested descriptions adopted for the purpose of this chapter. The use of the term **ethnic minority children** is a synonym for Black ethnicities and can render invisible those of White minority ethnicities such as Irish, Jewish and travelling communities (Goldstein, 2005).

The starting point to understanding the importance of culturally competent practice in safeguarding Black and ethnic minority children is the historical context, in which Britain became a significant multicultural society. British multiculturalism really began following the end of World War 2. Thousands of citizens from across the Commonwealth (for example, in the Caribbean and Asia) left their families and travelled to the UK to fulfil the need for labour (Wilkinson and Craig, 2011). These diverse ethnic groups brought their varied languages, styles of dress, cultural beliefs and practices. They settled in the UK with their families, working and bringing up their children. Scholars have described their encounters with racism and discrimination in myriad areas, including (but not exclusive to) housing, employment, health and welfare (Fryer, 1984; Knowles, 2009; Panayi, 1999; Phillips, 1999). Important other aspects of their experience, for example the impact of child and family separation and family reunification, have been less documented (Arnold, 2006; Chamberlin, 1995; Williams, 2019). This lack of exploration and understanding is an important feature for those working in child protection.

British multiculturalism has been based on the key policy notion of cultural diversity and has involved the promotion of religious tolerance and cultural interaction between different ethnic communities (Bleich, 2001). Multiculturalism has also sought to increase awareness of – and respect for – ethnic minorities' cultural backgrounds, identities and experiences (Blunkett, 2003; Chiarenza, 2012). There has been a wide range of legislation and policy on issues affecting ethnic minority communities including immigration, mental health and criminal justice, which have all *shaped discourses about race, culture and ethnicity in the wider society*' (Bloch and Solomos, 2010, p. 2).

One problem for practitioners working with diverse cultural groups is the terminology used to classify and identify ethnic minority people. **Race, ethnicity and culture** are often used interchangeably in research, policy and practice, but their meanings are complex and not always effectively defined. **Culture** comprises psychological, physical and social aspects; its meaning is not a simplistic notion, but one that recognises a *variety of meanings* (Virkama, 2010). Culture broadly

refers to the shared values and way of life that exist amongst a group of people and includes the rules that guide and give meaning to how people live and behave in society (Kohli et al., 2010). Language, dress codes and child rearing customs are all examples of the diverse practices through which people function and create shared meaning and belonging. For many people such cultural diversity is inherently positive; for others, however, cultural diversity, based on distinctions of skin colour and differences of language, beliefs and customs, can become a major cause of conflict (Parekh, 2008).

The notion of **race** is both problematic and controversial. Historically, it has been used to attempt to differentiate and discriminate between human populations, including skin colour, physical features and other visible or cultural characteristics (Blank et al., 2004). The perception of racial differences affects personal and social relationships. In Western countries that privilege whiteness, Black people and other visible racial minorities are positioned as 'outsiders' and are subject to marginalisation and discriminatory practices (Bopal, 2018). Whilst race often has a negative and exclusionary meaning, ethnicity, according to Eriksen (2002) usually implies a positive group status. **Ethnicity** refers to distinct groups of people who share a similar heritage, encompassing language, culture and nationality, that together shape relationship, values and behaviour (Connolly et al., 2006).

Race, ethnicity and culture are therefore entirely interconnected and together play a major part in how individuals are identified and responded to by others (Kanyeredzi, 2018). Another characteristic related to race, ethnicity and culture is **identity**. What makes a person who they are is made up of personal (individual) and social identity (Parekh, 2008). Our **individual identity** contains our unique experiences that define us as well as distinguish us from others. Our **social identity** is embedded in membership of different ethnic, religious, cultural and other groups and relationships. It helps to create a sense of belonging and affects the roles we take on, how we live and conduct our lives (Parekh, 2008). Fearon (1999) notes that identity is not fixed and unchanging but is changed and constructed over time.

In summary, ethnic minority children and young people living in the UK have wide-ranging cultural and racial backgrounds, '*multi-faceted and shifting*' social identities and influences that can be difficult to disentangle (Mullen et al., 2014, cited in Robertson and Wainwright, 2020, p. 5).

ASSESSING BLACK, ASIAN AND MINORITY ETHNIC CHILDREN AND THEIR FAMILIES

All assessment and investigation in child protection occurs within a cultural context.
Welbourne (2002, p. 347)

Child protection is a contentious area of practice, partly due to how race, ethnicity and culture are defined, but also due to the range of differing cultural values and interpretations of risk, vulnerability and need within and between families and safeguarding professionals. Social work is a profession underpinned by principles of human rights, equality and social justice (Hare, 2004), and the importance of anti-oppressive perspectives has been explored in depth (Dominelli, 1996; Dalrymple and Burke, 1995; Laird, 2008; Maxime, 1989). Anti-oppressive practice requires professionals to explore their own personal power, to ensure they are not oppressing, or further oppressing and discriminating against, minority groups. It also requires critical analysis of broader structural issues, such as the use of language, cultural systems and political institutions.

To assess the needs of Black and ethnic minority children, practitioners need appropriate knowledge and understanding. However, learning about cultural or ethnic differences or following guidance on cultural diversity does not necessarily lead to culturally competent practice: education and training can only provide a limited level of knowledge of cultural diversity. Practitioners often still lack sufficient knowledge and understanding, and fear of being seen as racist can result in reluctance to explore other people's cultures, or sensitively challenge their childcare practices and beliefs (Kalra, 2003; Rodger et al., 2020).

Child abuse occurs in all cultures, ethnicities and across all socioeconomic groups. Irrespective of race, culture or ethnicity, the starting point for social work assessment and intervention is that the child's welfare is paramount (Children Act, 1989). The official guidance *Working Together to Safeguard Children* underpins safeguarding practice with all children and young people and clearly emphasises the need to undertake sensitive assessment of children with particular needs and vulnerabilities (HM Government, 2018). *The Framework for Assessing Children in Need and their Families* remains the formal guidance for social worker's assessment of vulnerable children and their families (DoH, 2001). The *Assessment Triangle'* is still a helpful framework for holistic assessment of strengths and vulnerability factors, and its practice guidance provides a full chapter on assessing the specific needs of Black children and their families. It stresses that race, ethnicity and culture are often significant in a Black child's life experiences and should be integral to social work assessment (DoH, 2001). This however can be challenging when practitioners '*apply subjective assumptions based on skin colour or cultural stereotypes*' (Jivraj and Simpson, 2015, p. 2).

Culturally competent and anti-oppressive practice requires an on-going commitment from practitioners to proactively keep up to date with emerging areas of practice guidance, including (but not exclusive of) transracial adoption (Kirton, 2000), female genital mutilation (Barrett et al., 2020), modern slavery (Edwards and Mika, 2016), child sexual exploitation (Hallett, 2016), forced marriage (Clawson, 2013), migration and citizenship (Valtonen, 2008), family separation (Arnold, 2006; Chamberlin, 1995), Islamophobia and asylum-seeking children (Lathan, 2016). This work will continue throughout practitioners' careers in their own continuing professional development.

Lack of effective professional knowledge of the child and family's language, ethnicity and cultural background is a repeated concern within serious case reviews. Young Black men specifically have been identified as being frequently misunderstood and underassessed (Bernard and Harris, 2019). The public and media racialised perception of young Black men (often represented as physical threats, gangsters and antisocial) has been persistently critiqued (Knight, 2015; Laird, 2008; Guerrero, 1995). Practitioners need to consider the ways Black young men are perceived and in turn safeguarded, developing a better understanding of how norms and beliefs about culture and race can prevent effective safeguarding (Rodger et al., 2020). Child Y, a 15-year-old African Caribbean boy, was the victim of a fatal stabbing in his local area (Croydon Safeguarding Children Board, 2019). The Serious Case Review highlighted that:

- Child Y was labelled by some professionals as a gang member, which was not validated via any formal assessment and the perception never challenged. Yet, this classification did not change the approach to working with him. Child Y and his father Mr F were not visited by any Police, YOT or gangs' team to warn them of any potential danger despite being aware of a violent feud between two local rival gangs.
- The decision was to exclude Child Y from school with no consultation and no assessment of the impact of his move to a PRU.
- Mr F's methods of parental discipline were deemed to cause Child Y harm, although the courts endorsed the view that Child Y's needs were met by being in the care of his father. Despite this, Child Y was made the subject of a child protection plan and an Interim Supervision Order.
- There were differences within the professional network in how physical chastisement was viewed and defined.
- Mr F felt criticised and unsupported in his parenting and care of Child Y.
- The role of family members/kind (Child Y's sister Ms S) was not acknowledged or supported.
- Child Y was the victim of a stabbing and admitted to hospital. Yet, there was no alternative planning put in place such as a discharge planning meeting and no coordinated multi-agency plan to respond to Child Y's needs to ensure consistency of approach.

REFLECTIVE QUESTIONS

- Why do you think there was a lack of an integrated multiagency approach?
- How might professionals' responses have been shaped by assumptions about Child Y's race and ethnic identity?
- What other assessments might have better safeguarded Child Y?

In summary, evidence from serious case reviews, education, research and training suggests a lack of cultural proficiency amongst practitioners and a failure to incorporate sensitive cultural competence in assessment and care planning with vulnerable BAME children and their families (Bernard and Harris, 2019).

BAME CHILDREN AND FAMILIES WITHIN THE CHILD WELFARE SYSTEM

The ethnic diversity of the UK is increasing and can be seen in the UK Office for National Statistics (ONS) census records:

Ethnicity	Census (ONS, 1991)	Census (ONS, 2012)
White	94%	86%
Other ethnic groups	6%	14%

There is wide diversity between ethnic groups, which inform children and families' opportunities, experiences, attainment and challenges (Mason, 2003). Black and ethnic minority children and their families are more likely to live in areas of high deprivation, experiencing multiple disadvantages including poverty, unemployment and racism (Nazroo and Williams, 2005; ONS, 2018). Ethnicity disproportionately plays a part in patterns of representation in the child welfare system, and whilst poverty and deprivation are significant predictors of entering care, this is disproportionality related to socioeconomic factors rather than ethnicity itself (Bywaters et al., 2014; Barn et al., 2005). Children from Black and ethnic minority communities are more likely to be 'in need' than White children (Owen and Statham, 2009; Webb et al., 2002); however, formal support available to ethnic minority children is lower than for White children (Welbourne, 2002). When ethnic minority families do receive services, they are often viewed by professionals as 'harder to work with', can experience *'excessive scrutiny'* (Bywaters et al., 2015, p. 99) and families themselves often perceive the child protection process as discriminatory (Bell, 2007; Farmer and Owen, 1995). Black and mixed race children are overrepresented amongst looked after children, who together make up around 13,000 (27%) of the looked after population, whilst Asian children are underrepresented (3500 or 4%). Asian children on the child protection register are one-third of those of White children (Owen and Statham, 2009).

Within adoption services, ethnically mixed and Black children wait longer to be adopted (Ali, 2014; Barn, 1999). Policy and practice has varied swinging between opposition to, and support for, interracial and intercultural adoption (Barn and Kirton, 2012). Legislation has supported the need for permanence and the impact of placement delay on children's well-being, generating support for interracial adoption and repealing the former duty for social workers to prioritise the adopted child's ethnic and cultural background (Ali, 2014; DfE, 2012). In contrast, same-race advocates have argued that the child's racial, cultural and ethnic identity matters – therefore Black children should be placed with Black families (Barn and Kirton, 2012; De Souza, 2017; Maxime, 1993). There are many cultural practices and requirements that are necessary for Black and ethnic minority children to acquire for them to gain a positive sense of their ethnic and cultural identity. Adoption practice has reflected these polarised positions and has been slow to offer nuanced responses to permanence for mixed heritage children in care (Bhatti-Sinclair and Price, 2016). In consequence, *the best interests of the child are often lost in struggles over racialized and racializing difference'* (Ali, 2014, p. 96).

In the broader welfare system, ethnic minority children also experience further challenges. Some children and young people from ethnic minority groups are casualties of military conflict or war and are at high risk of physical violence and abuse as displaced and/ or unaccompanied minors (Quiroga, 2009). They have complex personal histories and experiences of trauma, loss and separation – which are often neglected in current practice (Newbigging and Thomas, 2011). Black and ethnic minority children, particularly young Black and mixed-race boys, are also far more likely to become part of the criminal justice system than the mental health system (Cross et al., 1989; Phillips and Bowling, 2017), demonstrating further how broader welfare services are not provided in culturally sensitive ways. A main message for practice should be that Black and mixed-race boys are amongst the most vulnerable groups who become involved with children's social

care. Overall, there are multiple and frequent negative impacts and outcomes for Black and ethnic minority children involved not only with children's services, but the wider social welfare network. At the heart of these issues lies cultural competence.

REFLECTIVE QUESTIONS

■ Why are children from Black and mixed ethnicity families more vulnerable to formal contact with children's services?

■ Reflecting on your own practice, how can you help to safeguard Black and mixed ethnicity children?

THE CULTURAL COMPETENCE CONTINUUM

Cultural competence is a key principle that underpins culturally sensitive and anti-oppressive practice with diverse communities (Carpenter, 2016). It advocates professional knowledge, skills and self-development and its features incorporate cultural awareness, cultural sensitivity, cultural knowledge and cultural skill (Duan-Ying, 2016). Cultural competence involves a set of values and competencies that work at three levels: the practitioner level, the service delivery and the policy level. According to Cross et al. (1989) culturally competent behaviours and practices exist along a continuum:

Cultural Destructiveness ⇒ Cultural Incapacity ⇒ Cultural Blindness ⇒ Cultural Pre – Competence ⇒ Cultural Competence ⇒ Cultural Proficiency

At one end of the continuum is **cultural destructiveness**, which are extremely devastating actions, processes and policies that actively seek to destroy other ethnic cultures, for example ethnic cleansing. A related form of cultural destructiveness is **cultural incapacity** or **incapability** (Cross et al., 1989), which is the overt exclusion of any different cultural practices from the norm. Policies of assimilation are perpetuated based on beliefs in racial, ethnic and cultural superiority; they often require ethnic minority groups to abandon their cultural identity and assume the dominant culture's practices and beliefs to receive rights from the host country (Hanley, 1999). The consequence of this Eurocentrism is that people with cultural behaviours or beliefs that differ from the dominant culture become viewed as problematic and deficient (Gambe et al., 1992; Goldstein, 2005). Safeguarding Black and ethnic minority children in this context would be interpreted as 'correcting the deficit' or 'rescuing' the child from the problematic culture (Egonsdotter et al., 2020, p. 363). In addition, accent, dress and skin colour can all play a part in reinforcing the practitioner's biased assumptions about ethnic and cultural differences.

Through the mid-point of the continuum is **'cultural colour-blindness'** (Cross et al., 1989). This approach subscribes to the idea that race, ethnicity and culture do not matter. It adopts an equal opportunity and treatment for all and an 'unbiased', universal approach to service delivery (Cross et al., 1989). The emphasis is on fitting Black and ethnic minority service users into existing mainstream services, ignoring the uniqueness and strengths of different cultures and overlooking their needs. Assumptions that 'we are all the same' can lead childcare practitioners to impose Eurocentric standards of practice onto Black and ethnic minority families, in the belief they are providing appropriate interventions and services (Korbin, 2007). It can also lead to misdiagnosis of cultural practices of some ethnic minority groups as physical abuse (Vitale and Prashad, 2017), for example, 'coining' (rubbing the skin with metal coins or ceramic implements to stimulate blood flow and restore balance), 'cupping' (applying suction cups to the skin to treat pain or remove toxins) and the misdiagnosis of Mongolian blue spot, the visible birthmarks on Black and ethnic minority babies (Chin, 2005).

Further along the continuum is the **cultural pre-competency** stage. As successive Governments recognised the need for strengthening cultural awareness and cultural competence (UNESCO, 2009), policies have explicitly required health and social care agencies to deliver culturally appropriate services. For example, the Department of Health (1991), Department of Health (2008) and Department of Health and Social Care (2004) all highlighted the importance of considering culture in assessment and service delivery (Laird, 2008). At a basic level, such practice includes, for example, offering services such as interpreters and translators to facilitate communication for non-English language speakers. For childcare practitioners, cultural pre-competency recognises that different beliefs and practices exist about parenting and child rearing, as well as understanding that what is defined as neglect or abuse can vary greatly across cultures (Korbin, 2007). Pre-competency involves learning about ethnic minorities, valuing and respecting diversity and deepening understanding of forms of child abuse that may have been labelled as '*cultural practices*', such as female genital mutilation (FGM) or forced marriage (Tedam, 2013, p. 61).

The cultural continuum model culminates in **cultural proficiency**, an advanced cultural competence where practitioners pay '*careful attention to the dynamics of difference*' and '*continual self-assessment regarding culture*' (Cross et al., 1989, p. 17). According to Duan-Ying (2016) cultural competence is an ongoing process of developing knowledge and skills, critical reflection of the practitioner's own prejudgements and assumptions and sensitive and respectful communication alongside a developed awareness of culture. Cultural proficiency is the highest level of cultural competence, whereby staff and agency perspectives, policies and practices on culture and diversity are fully aligned. The cultural competence of practitioners is integrated within a service that is itself embedded within a wider, learning institution. At these service and organisational levels, the recruitment and retention of multicultural staff, service user involvement, and the building of meaningful policies and strategies are all prioritised.

Social workers have an ethical responsibility to be culturally competent, to have knowledge of and respect for diverse cultures and be able to demonstrate competence in the provision of services that are sensitive to others' cultures. They must be self-aware and able to examine their own cultural identity, beliefs, assumptions and privileges, recognising how these affect and influence relationships with service users. Congress and Kung (2012) assert that culturally competent practitioners need knowledge of a wide range of factors when assessing children and families from diverse backgrounds. This also involves social workers demonstrating appropriate communication skills, models and methods of assessment and care planning that are attuned to the cultural experiences of the service users they work with.

CASE STUDY 13.1: THE KHAN FAMILY

Mia (14), Nila (11) and Hassad (9) have been living with their grandparents, Hamza and Khalida Khan since 2016. Their mother, Jula, lives and works in London as a live-in domestic, only coming home once every few months due to the cost and restrictions of her employment. Hamza works as a taxi driver; he often sleeps during the day and works late at night. Hamza and Khalida are of Muslim faith, although Khalida is more liberal. Since moving to England, she has not been to the mosque and mainly cooks English food for the children. Hamza speaks Arabic to the children who also mainly speak English at home.

Nila and Hassad attend the same school. Nila has some learning difficulties and requires an assessment of her learning needs, but the school has been struggling to gain the family's cooperation. She is quiet and withdrawn at school. Nila is very thin, and there have been some worries from school about her eating behaviour. She was recently seen with bruising on her arms, and when questioned about this by her teacher, she said she had fallen over. Children's social care were not informed because the teacher was not sure it was actually bruising and did not want to report the family unnecessarily. Nila is very close to her mother and misses her. She would like to attend mosque more often but needs Khalida to help with this.

School staff describe Hassad as difficult and aggressive towards other children, especially younger males. He is at risk of exclusion following an incident where he was found with a knife in class. At home, he tends to ignore his grandmother, and she tolerates this behaviour. The girls are expected to help with chores, while Hassan sits playing on his Nintendo. Mia shares a small bedroom with her sister, while Hassan has the larger bedroom to himself, causing friction between Mia and Hassad. Mia disclosed to a teacher she has an older boyfriend named Josh, who is not a Muslim. Mia is terrified of her family finding out. Mia told her teacher Josh wants to sleep with her.

The younger children have been reported as being regularly late for school, and family members are often late collecting them. Mia is supposed to pick them up but often does not. Instead, she spends time with her friends, who are older girls with boyfriends. This has caused conflict between Jula and Khalida. Kalida does not think it is an issue and that Hassad and Nila can walk home alone. However, Hassad often leaves Nila to make her way home alone while he goes off with his friends. He sometimes comes back late, smelling of cannabis and sometimes alcohol. As this is against Islam, Hamza has threatened to physically punish Hassad. Hassad also seems to have access to money as he claims he bought the Nintendo himself; however, Hassad does not do any kind of paid work.

There is financial stress in the house, but Jula cannot afford to send more money. This has led to arguments and threats of physical violence between Khalida and Hamza. The family have no car, and the mosque is two miles away. The local community has little ethnic diversity, leaving the couple rather socially isolated.

Case Discussion

Within this case, alongside concerns around domestic violence and mental health, there are also clear risks of physical and/or sexual harm towards Mia and neglect towards Nila and Hassad. Some practitioners may choose to undertake all their assessments from a *fixed cultural perspective*, meaning their assessment and intervention would subject the family to the *'same rules as everyone else'*. This kind of **cultural absolutism** would assess that the neglect and abuse issues within the family are a result of their culture (Howard, 1993). However, a rigid focus on culture and risk can hamper social work practice in several ways. First, by (mis)interpreting the Khan family's arrangements as malfunctioning, attributing these as weaknesses. Second, by emphasising Hamza, Jula and Khalida's *problems* rather than their *strengths* – attributing these to their ethnicity or culture. Third, by ignoring cultural practices that can serve as protective factors (such as faith), this overemphasises the children's vulnerabilities rather than their resiliencies (Bernard and Thomas, 2016). Finally, this approach also overlooks research that highlights poorer outcomes for children of different ethnic and cultural backgrounds (Lu, 2018).

In many ethnic minority families, the family incorporates a wide kinship network, in which the child's views and wishes are considered in the context of wider obligations to the family group. Yet too often, social workers still assume **Eurocentric** cultural practices and contexts that:

> *do not take into account the network of bonding obligations found in groups of highly structured kinship systems.*
>
> **Lau (1988) cited in Gambe et al. (1992, p. 33)**

Eurocentric models of practice include those where children are informed or advised on ways to be increasingly autonomous and independent from their parents and families, without reference to their family system (Bernard and Gupta, 2006; Karasz et al., 2016). Consequently, the Khan family's resistance to this model of assessment and practice may be viewed as further evidence of problematic or defective parenting or dysfunctional family life (Karasz et al., 2016).

In the Khan case, a **culturally relative** approach would recognise the family have had to adapt to living in a new cultural environment, where their faith, language, culture and history differ significantly from that of the majority culture. This approach would ensure the family's culture and strengths were taken account of, rather than imposing biased Western parenting expectations. Raud (2016) supports the use of strength-based and systems perspectives as methods for engaging with the complex dynamics of culture, identity and ethnicity. While this level of cultural competence is helpful, one tool that can enhance understanding of the social and cultural context of ethnic minority children and families is the culturagram. A culturagram is a family assessment tool that is used to assist practitioners in exploring the cultural experiences, beliefs and practices of BAME children (Congress and Kung, 2012). Placing the child and family in the centre, the tool examines multiple areas of cultural influence and experience (Fig. 13.1).

In the Khan case, the culturagram can assist practitioners to explore their experiences and gain deeper understanding of their cultural influences and beliefs. Congress and Kung (2012) suggest an individualised assessment and plan can then be created that can also guide appropriate interventions.

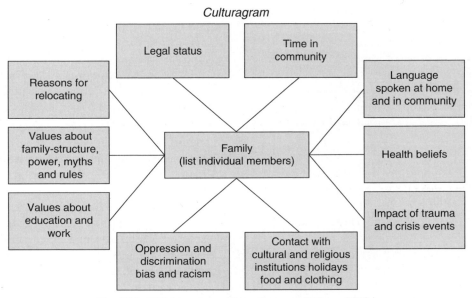

Fig. 13.1 ■ **Culturagram.** (From Congress & Kung, 2012.)

REFLECTIVE QUESTIONS

- Draw your own culturagram of the Khan family.
- Outline a list of protective and risk factors in relation to this family.
- Reflect on your own practice experience with a BAME family: did you adopt a **cultural absolutist** or **cultural relativist** approach? How could you have worked in a more culturally relativist way with the family?

CONCLUSION

This chapter has outlined how (mis)definitions of race, ethnicity and culture can contribute to biased assumptions and stereotypes about Black and ethnic minority children. It has demonstrated the need for cultural competent practice in the context of the persistent inequities experienced by many BAME children who come to the attention of child welfare services. The chapter outlined how a lack of culturally sensitive knowledge, skills and practice negatively influences outcomes for ethnically and culturally diverse children across many areas. For example, a lack of cultural awareness has been the principal driver in many serious case reviews when accounting for how such children and their families are perceived by safeguarding professionals. The chapter therefore urgently calls for culturally competent practice to be further embedded into social work education, training and practice as a fundamental requirement of effective safeguarding practice with culturally diverse children and their families.

Culturally sensitive safeguarding practice is still developing, and there is no easy recipe for working competently with culturally diverse children and their families. It involves the practitioner in an active, dynamic process that takes place throughout the career of the social worker (Jani et al., 2016). Alongside individual practitioners' self-reflection and learning, equally necessary is a diverse workforce and positive organisational culture, which shift polices and practice towards safeguarding solutions and interventions that work in partnership with diverse communities. It demands a holistic, systemic approach and the role of childcare managers and supervisors is critical. Supervision is an important source in supporting practitioners to manage complex cases and unpick cultural issues.

Peer and group supervision can provide further spaces for shared learning experiences, exploring new ways of working and building supportive environments and alliances where changes to accepted policies and practices may be fostered.

FURTHER READING

Carballeira's (1997) **LIVE and LEARN model** supports practitioners to engage in reflective thinking and capture the nuances of culture more effectively for ethnic minority children and families.

Newcastle Safeguarding Children Board (2019) developed useful practice guidance that identified six competences for effective safeguarding of ethnic minority children and families. The guide highlights many factors that affect cross–cultural interactions (including self-reflection, adapting existing tools and interventions and integrating cultural knowledge into the whole service).

Tedam (2013) has developed a useful tool for trainee social workers that connects the domains of the professional capabilities framework (PCF) to culturally competent knowledge, behaviour and values.

REFERENCES

Ali, S., 2014. Governing multicultural populations and family life. The British Journal of Sociology 65 (1), 82–106.

Arnold, E., 2006. Separation and loss through immigration of African Caribbean women to the UK. Attachment & Human Development 8 (2), 159–174.

Barn, R., 1999. 'White mothers, mixed-parentage children and child welfare'. The British Journal of Social Work 29 (2), 269–284 April 1999.

Barn, R., Andrew, L., Mantovani, N., 2005. Life after Care – the Experiences of Young People from Different Ethnic Groups. Joseph Rowntree Foundation, York. policycommons.net. (Accessed 25 August 2023).

Barn, R., Kirton, D., 2012. Transracial adoption in Britain: Politics, ideology and reality. Adoption & Fostering 36 (3–4), 25–37.

Barrett, H.R., Brown, K., Alhassan, Y., Leye, E., 2020. 'Transforming social norms to end FGM in the EU: an evaluation of the REPLACE Approach'. Reprod. Health 17, 40.

Bell, M., 2007. Safeguarding children and case conferences. In: Wilson, K., James, A. (Eds.), The Child Protection Handbook, third ed. Elsevier Health Sciences, London.

Bernard, C., Gupta, A., 2008. 'Black African children and the child protection system'. The British Journal of Social Work 38, 476–492 (2008).

Bernard, C., Harris, P., 2019. Serious case reviews: The lived experience of Black children. Child & Family Social Work 24, 256–263.

Bernard, C., Thomas, C., 2016. 'Risk and safety: a strengths-based perspective in working with black families when there are safeguarding concerns'. In: Williams, C., Graham, M. (Eds.), Social Work in a Diverse Society: Transformative Practice with Ethnic Minority Communities. Policy Press, Bristol.

Bhatti-Sinclair, K., Price, D., 2016. 'Evaluation of serious case reviews and anti-racist practice'. Chapter 13. In: Williams, C., Graham, M.J. (Eds.), Social Work in a Diverse Society: Transformatory Practice with Black and Minority Ethnic Individuals and Communities.

Blank, R.M., Dadady, M., Citro, C.F., 2004. Measuring Racial Discrimination: Panel on Methods for Assessing Discrimination. The National Academies Press, Washington DC.

Bleich, E., 2001. The French model: color-blind integration. In: Skrentny, J.D. (Ed.), Color Lines: Affirmative Action, Immigration and Civil Rights Options for America. University of Chicago Press, Chicago.

Bloch, A., Solomos, J., 2010. 'Key questions in the sociology of race and ethnicity'. Chapter 1. In: Bloch, A., Solomos, J. (Eds.), Race and Ethnicity in the 21st Century. Palgrave Macmillan, Hampshire.

Blunkett, D., 2003. Speech on Multi-Faith Britain. https://www.ukpol.co.uk/david-blunkett-2003-speech-on-multi-faith-britain/ UK (Accessed 25 August 2023).

Bopal, K., 2018. White Privilege: The Myth of a Post-Racial Society. Policy Press, Bristol.

Bywaters, P., Brady, G., Sparks, T., Bos, E., 2014. Inequalities in child welfare intervention rates: the intersection of deprivation and identity. Child & Family Social Work 21 (4), 452–463.

Bywaters, P., Brady, G., Sparks, T., Bos, E., Bunting, L., Daniel, B., et al., 2015. Exploring inequities in child welfare and child protection services: Explaining the 'inverse intervention law'. Children and Youth Services 57, 98–105.

Carballeira, N., 1997. The Live & Learn Model for culturally competent family services. Continuum 17 (1), 7–12 PMID: 10165619.

Carpenter, L. 'The Development of Cultural Competence in Social Work Practice and Education'. Master of Social Work Clinical Research Paper. Retrieved from Sophia, the St. Catherine University repository website: https://sophia.stkate.edu/msw_papers/568. (Accessed 25 August 2023).

Chamberlin, M., 1995. Family narratives and migration dynamics: Barbadians to Britain. New West Indian Guide 69 (3&4), 253–275.

Chiarenza, A., 2012. 'Developments in the concept of cultural competence'. Chapter 3. In: Ingleby, D., Chiarenza, A., Devillé, W., Kotsioni, I. (Eds.), COST Series on Health and Diversity. Inequalities in Health Care for Migrants and Ethnic Minorities - Vol. 2. Garant, Antwerp.

Children Act, 1989. The National Archives. https://www.legislation.gov.uk/ukpga/1989/41/contents (Accessed 25 August 2023).

Chin, W.Y., 2005. Blue spots, coining and cupping: How ethnic minority parents can be misreported as child abusers. The Journal of Law and Society 7 (1), 88–115.

Clawson, R., 2013. Safeguarding people with learning disabilities at risk of forced marriage: Issues for inter-agency practice. Social Work and Social Sciences Review 16 (3), 20–36.

Congress, E.P., Kung, W.W., 2012. Using the culturagram to assess and empower culturally diverse families. In: Congress, E.P., Gonzalez, M.J. (Eds.), Multicultural Perspectives in Social Work Practice with Families, third ed. Springer Publishing, New York.

Connolly, M., Crichton-Hill, Y., Ward, T., 2006. Culture and Child protection: Reflexive Responses. Jessica Kingsley Pubs, London.

Cross, T.L., Bazron, B.J., Dennis, K.W., Isaacs, M.R., 1989. Towards a Culturally Competent System of Care: A Monograph on Effective Services for Minority Children Who Are Severely Emotionally Disturbed. CASSP Technical Assistance Center, Georgetown University Child Development Center, Washington DC.

Croydon Safeguarding Children Board, 2019. Serious Case Review Summary: Child Y. https://library.nspcc.org.uk/ (Accessed 25 August 2023).

Dalrymple, J., Burke, B., 1995. Anti Oppressive Practice and the Law. Open University Press, Buckingham.

Department for Education, 2012. An Action Plan for Adoption: Tackling Delay. DfE, London.

Department of Education/Department of Health and Social Care. Children and Families Act 2014. London: The Stationery Office. legislation.gov.uk. (Accessed 25 August 2023).

Department of Health, 1991. Care Management and Assessment Guide. The Stationery Office, London.

Department of Health, 2001. Framework for the Assessment of Children in Need and Their Families. The Stationery Office, London.

Department of Health and Social Care, 2004. National Service Framework for Children, Young People and Maternity Services. The Stationery Office, London. https://www.gov.uk/government/publications/national-service-framework-children-young-people-and-maternity-services.

Department of Health, 2008. National Carer's Strategy: Carers at the Heart of 21st-century Families and Communities. The Stationery Office, London.

De Souza, S., 2017. Black, Asian and Mixed Ethnicities in Adoption and Fostering: An Interview with Coram BAAF Consultant Savita de Sousa. Corum Academy Ltd, London. https://corambaaf.org.uk/-interview-corambaaf-consultant-savita-de-sousa.

Dominelli, L., 1996. Deprofessionalizing social work: anti-oppressive practice, competencies and postmodernism. The British Journal of Social Work 26, 153–175.

Duan-Ying, C., 2016. A concept analysis of cultural competence. Int. J. Nurs. Sci 3 (3), 268–273.

Edwards, L., Mika, K.M., 2017. Advancing the efforts of the macro-level social work response against sex trafficking. International Social Work 60 (3), 695–706.

Egonsdotter, G., Bengtsson, S., Israelsson, M., Borell, K., 2020. Child protection and cultural awareness: Simulation-based learning. Journal of Ethnic & Cultural Diversity in Social Work 29 (5), 362–376.

Eriksen, T.H., 2002. Ethnicity and Nationalism: Anthropological Perspectives. Pluto Press, Bristol.

Farmer, E., Owen, M., 1995. Child Protection Practice: Private Risk and Public Remedies—Decision Making, Intervention and Outcomes. Protection Work HMSO, London.

Fearon, J.D., 1999. 'What Is Identity (As We Now Use the Word)'? Unpublished Manuscript. Stanford University, Stanford.

Fryer, P., 1984. Staying Power: The History of Black People in Britain. Pluto Press, London.

Gambe, D., 1992. Improving Practice with Children and Families: A Training Manual (Vol. 2). Central Council for Education and Training in Social Work. CCETSW, London.

Goldstein, B., 2005. Introduction. In: Thoburn, J., Chand, A., Procter, J. (Eds.), Child Welfare Services for Minority Ethnic Families: The Research Reviewed. Jessica Kingsley Pubs, London.

Guerrero, E. The black man on our screens and the empty space in representation. Callaloo, Vol.. 18, No. 2 (Spring, 1995), pp. 395–400.

Hallett, S., 2016. An uncomfortable comfortableness: Care, child protection and child sexual exploitation. The British Journal of Social Work 46, 2137–2152.

Hanley, J., 1999. Beyond the tip of the iceberg: five stages toward cultural competence. Reaching. Today's. Youth 3 (2), 9–12.

Hare, I., 2004. Defining social work for the 21st century: the international federation of social workers' revised definition of social work. International Social Work 47 (3), 407–424.

HM Government, 2018. Working Together to Safeguard Children, 2018. https://assets.publishing.service.gov.uk/media/5fd0a8e78fa8f54d5d6555f9/Working_together_to_safeguard_children_inter_agency_guidance.pdf

Howard, R.E., May, 1993. Cultural absolutism and the nostalgia for community. Human rights 15 (2), 315–338.

Jani, J.S., Osteen, P., Shipe, S., 2016. Cultural competence and social work education: Moving toward assessment of practice behaviors. Journal of Social Work Education 52 (3), 311–324.

Jivraj, S., Simpson, L., 2015. How has ethnic diversity grown? In: Jivraj, S., Simpson, L. (Eds.), Ethnic Identity and Inequalities in Britain: The Dynamics of Diversity. Policy Press, Bristol.

Kalra, V., 2003. Police lore and community disorder: Diversity in the criminal justice system. In: Mason, D. (Ed.), Explaining Ethnic Differences: Changing Patterns of Disadvantage in Britain. Policy Press, Bristol.

Kanyeredzi, A., 2018. Race, Culture, and Gender: Black Female Experiences of Violence and Abuse. Palgrave Macmillan, London.

Karasz, A., Gany, F., Javier, E., Flores, C., Prasad, L., Inman, A., Kalasapudi, V., Kosi, R., Murthy, M., Leng, L., Diwan, S., 2016. Mental Health and Stress Among South Asians. Immigrant Minor Health, pp. 1–12.

Karasz, A., Gany, F., Escobar, J., Flores, C., Prasad, L., Inman, A., et al., 2019. Mental health and stress among South Asians. The Journal of Immigrant and Minority Health 21, 7–14.

Kirton, D., 2000. 'Race', Ethnicity and Adoption. Open University Press, Buckingham.

Knight, D.J., 2015. Beyond the stereotypical image of young men of color. The Altantichttps://www.theatlantic.com/education/archive/2015/01/beyond-the-stereotypical-image-of-young-men-of-color/384194/ (Accessed 23 February 2021).

Knowles, C., 1999. Race, identities and lives. Chemical Society Reviews 47 (1), 110–135.

Kohli, H.K., Huber, R., Faul, A.C., 2010. Historical and theoretical development of culturally competent social work practice. Journal of Teaching in Social Work 30 (3), 252–271.

Korbin, J.E., 2007. Issue of culture. In: Wilson, K., James, A. (Eds.), The Child Protection Handbook, third ed. Elsevier Health Sciences, London.

Laird, S.E., 2008. Anti-oppressive Social Work: A Guide for Developing Cultural Competence. Sage Publications, London.

Lathan, S. The global rise of Islamophobia: whose side is social work on? J. Soc. Altern. Vol.35, Issue 4, pp.80-84.

Lu, M.C., Halfon, N., 2003. Racial and ethnic disparities in birth outcomes: a life-course perspective. Matern Child Health J. 7 (1), 13–30.

Mason, D., 2003. Explaining Ethnic Differences: Changing Patterns of Disadvantage in Britain. Policy press, Bristol.

Maxime, J., 1989. The Effects of Positive Self Reference Material on Seven to Twelve Year Old Children of the African Diaspora. Doctoral thesis, Institute of Education, University of London.

Maxime, J., 1993. The therapeutic importance of racial identity in working with black children who hate. Chapter 6. In: Varma, V. (Ed.), How and Why Children Hate. Jessica Kingsley, London.

Nazroo, J.Y., Williams, D.R., 2005. The social determination of ethnic/racial inequalities in health. In: Marmot, M., Wilkinson, R.G. (Eds.), Social Determinants of Health, second ed. OUP, Oxford.

Newbigging, K., Thomas, N., 2011. Good Practice in social care for refugee and asylum–seeking children. Child abuse review 20, 374–390.

Newcastle Safeguarding Children Board and Newcastle Safeguarding Adults Board, 2019. Cultural Competence: Practice guidance, awareness and advice in the context of safeguarding. https://www.newcastlesafeguarding.org.uk/?s=cultural+competence.

Office for National Statistics (1991). https://www.ons.gov.uk/census/historiccensusdata/1991andearliercensusdata

Office for National Statistics, 2012. Ethnicity and National Identity in England and Wales 2011. https://webarchive.nationalarchives.gov.uk/20160107112033/http://www.ons.gov.uk/ons/dcp171776_290558.pdf.

Office for National Statistics, 2018. People Living in Deprived Neighbourhoods. Department for Communities and Local Government. https://www.ethnicity-facts-figures.service.gov.uk/uk-population-by-ethnicity/demographics/people-living-in-deprived-neighbourhoods/latest#people-living-in-the-most-deprived-10-of-neighbourhoods-by-ethnicity.

Office for National Statistics, 2019. Children Looked after in England (Including Adoption). Year Ending 31 March 2019. https://webarchive.nationalarchives.gov.uk/20200303005132/https://www.gov.uk/government/statistics/children-looked-after-in-england-including-adoption-2018-to-2019.

Owen, C., Statham, J., 2009. Disproportionality in Child Welfare. The Prevalence of Black and Minority Ethnic Children within the 'Looked After' and 'Children in Need' Populations and on Child Protection Registers in England. Institute of Education, University of London, London.

Panayi, P., 1999. The Impact of Immigration: A Documentary History of the Effects and Experiences of Immigrants in Britain since 1945. Manchester University Press, Manchester.

Parekh, B., 2008. A New Politics of Identity: Political Principles for an Interdependent World. Red Globe Press, London.

Phillips, C., 1999. A dream deferred: Fifty years of Caribbean migration to Britain. Kunapipi. 21 (2). https://ro.uow.edu.au/kunapipi/vol21/iss2/17.

Phillips, C., Bowling, B., 2017. 'Ethnicities, racism, crime and criminal justice'. Chapter 8. In: Liebling, A., Maruna, S., McAra, L. (Eds.), The Oxford Handbook of Criminology. Oxford University Press, Oxford.

Pon, G., 2009. Cultural Competency as New Racism: An Ontology of Forgetting. J. Progress. Hum. Serv. 20, 59–71. https://www.kcl.ac.uk/cultural-competency.

Quiroga, J., 2009. Torture in children. Torture 19 (2), 2009.

Raud, R., 2016. Meaning in Action: Outline of an Integrated Theory of Culture. Polity Press, Cambridge.

Robertson, L., Wainwright, J.P., 2020. 'Black boys' and young men's experiences with criminal justice and desistance in england and wales: a literature review'. Genealogy 4 (2), 50.

Rodger, H., Hurcombe, R., Redmond, T., George, R., 2020. "People Don't Talk about it": Child Sexual Abuse in Ethnic Minority Communities. Independent Inquiry Child Sexual Abuse. https://www.iicsa.org.uk/publications/research/child-sexual-abuse-ethnic-minority-communities (Accessed 23 February 2021).

Sawrikar, P., 2017. Working with Ethnic Minorities and across Cultures in Western Child protection Systems. Routledge, London.

Tedam, P., 2013. Developing cultural competence. In: Bartoli, A. (Ed.), Antiracism in Social Work Practice. Critical Publishing, St Albans.

UNESCO Framework for Cultural Statistics (FCS) (2009). Quebec, Canada. http://www.uls.unesco.org. (Accessed 25 August 2023).

Valtonen, K., 2008. Social Work and Migration: Immigrant and Refugee Settlement and Integration. Ashgate, Farnham.

Vitale, S.A., Prashad, T., 2017. Cultural awareness: coining and cupping. International Archives of Nursing and Health Care 3 (3), 1–3.

Virkama, A., 2010. From othering to understanding: Perceiving 'culture' in intercultural communication education and training. In: Kohornen, V. (Ed.), Cross-cultural Lifelong Learning. University of Tampere.

Webb, E., Maddocks, A., Bongilli, J., November/December 2002. Effectively protecting black and minority ethnic children from harm: Overcoming barriers to the child protection process. Child Abuse Review 11 (6), 394–410.

Welbourne, P., 2002. Culture, children's rights and child protection. Child Abus. Rev. 11, 345–358.

Wilkinson, M., Craig, G., 2011. Wilful negligence: migration policy, migrants' work and the absence of social protection in the UK. In: Carmel, E., Cerami, A., Papadopoulos, T. (Eds.), Migration and Welfare in the New Europe: Social Protection and the Challenges of Integration. Policy Press, Bristol.

Williams, C., 2019. 'Windrush is not History: The Past in the Present'. Research Seminar. School of Sociology and Social Policy, 23 October 2019, University of Nottingham.

Yadav, R., 2019. Decolonised and Developmental Social Work: A Model from Nepal. Routledge, Abingdon.

14 MODELS OF CHILD PROTECTION PRACTICE

SIOBHAN MACLEAN

KEY POINTS

- The inter-relationship between approaches, theories, models and methods.
- The Hackney model (reclaiming social work).
- Signs of Safety.
- Family Group Conferencing.

INTRODUCTION: THE RELATIONSHIP BETWEEN THEORIES, MODELS AND METHODS

Very often, in social work, the word theory is used as a 'catch all' word to cover not just theory, but also approaches, models and methods. This means that there is often a confusion about the difference between theories, models, methods and approaches (Maclean et al., 2018). In fact, each is a separate concept, although they are closely related and influence each other (Fig. 14.1).

Throughout my social work career, I have used a What? Why? How? framework (Maclean 2019). This might mean exploring:

- What is happening for this child and their family? What risks are there?
- Why is this happening? Why does this pose risks?
- How do I work with the family to bring about change? How do I ensure this child is protected?

This basic, but powerful, framework can help to clarify the difference between a theory and a model.

A theory provides a way of understanding a situation. It helps us to understand the 'what?' and 'why?' but not the 'how?' of a situation. So, a theory can help a social worker to understand what is happening to a child or young person and why this poses risks, but it does not provide a social worker with a plan for intervention. A theory can inform intervention, but it does not structure intervention.

A model, on the other hand, does not help us to understand what is happening, or why it is happening, but it provides a clear structure for intervention, so it helps to answer the question, 'What do we need to do to protect this child or young person?'

A method is a specific technique or tool which is used as part of a model. So, a model should have a range of methods which a practitioner can draw on in practice.

An approach describes an overall way of working. The way that a practitioner approaches their work will effectively flavour everything that they do, such that two social workers could use the same model to intervene in a situation, but it would look different because they take a different approach to their work and that has flavoured the model in a different way. Indeed, different organisations can take different approaches to practice so that the same model used in two different local authorities might look very different. I use the analogy of a model being a curry. A Thai curry tastes very different from an Indian curry, and a Jamaican curry is different again. You can get a curry sauce in a fish and chip shop. McDonald's provide a pot of curry sauce to dip your chips in. They are all curries, but they look, smell and taste totally different. The flavouring of the curry (approach) really matters.

The main contemporary approaches in social work with children and young people which have significantly influenced the development of models of child protection practice, and which continue to 'flavour' their use, are outlined in the following explanatory box:

APPROACHES IN CONTEMPORARY SOCIAL WORK WITH CHILDREN AND FAMILIES

Strengths-based approach: A strengths-based approach focuses on the strengths rather than the deficits of a family. It challenges traditional notions that the professional 'knows best' and works from the basis that families are the experts on their own situations.

Systemic approach: Building on the ideas outlined in systems theory, this approach recognises that there are a range of systems involved in anyone's life ('no-one is an island'). A systemic approach looks at how systems are impacting on the life experiences of a child or young person and seeks to harness all the systems that surround the child in reaching solutions to difficulties.

Relationship-based/relational approach: This builds on the basis that relationships are the most important aspect of bringing about change. Professionals need to work on the development of an effective relationship with the child and family.

Restorative approach: This comes from the criminal justice field and provides a way to work in situations where there is conflict. Working restoratively stresses the importance of working in partnership with people to heal any harm which has occurred (to restore relationships).

Managerialist/bureaucratic approach: This approach focuses on the organisational agenda, rather than that of the child or family. It involves the use of tick box criteria to identify concerns and calculates outcomes in terms of standard measurements.

Protectionist approach: This sees the professional as the expert. The focus is on deficits and risks within a family, and the response is risk averse. A protectionist approach often pushes towards early state intervention in families.

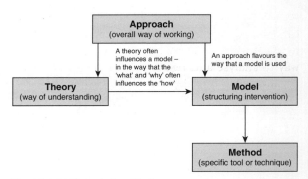

Fig. 14.1 ■ The relationship between a theory, model, method and approach.

Many of the contemporary models used in child protection come from a strengths-based, systemic or restorative approach. However, practitioners continue to report being pushed towards a managerialist or bureaucratic approach through organisational pressure which includes a high workload, tight timescales and a focus on risk management (Ferguson, 2014; Rogowski, 2015). Trying to implement a model which comes from one approach into an environment which promotes another approach is potentially very problematic – effectively the flavours don't work together. Pawson (2006, p. 35) perhaps explained this best describing intervention models as 'complex systems thrust into complex systems'.

THE HACKNEY MODEL

Originally named 'Reclaiming Social Work', the Hackney model was developed in 2008 by Steve Goodman and Isabelle Trowler, who were then assistant directors in Hackney's children's services. Trowler and Goodman (2012) describe the way that they sought to profoundly change everything in Hackney model, effectively 'reclaiming' social work. This 'reclaiming' came from a fundamentally systemic approach, which considered the systems surrounding social work professionals, leading to whole system change in the way that services were delivered to children and their families.

Trowler and Goodman (2012) describe the way that they used the 7S Framework to assist in conceptualising and delivering the whole system change, and the 7S framework has been used by others to summarise the model (Munro, 2011). Developed in the 1980s by

Waterman et al. (1980) working in the McKinsey Consulting firm, the 7S framework (or McKinsey model) has been very influential in the business world as a way to analyse and restructure organisations based around seven interdependent factors. Fig. 14.2 outlines the 7S framework and design of the Hackney model:

One of the most significant aspects of the model is the restructuring of traditional social work teams, from Figs 14.3 to 14.4.

In this structure, children and their families are known by one social worker, who, along with their line manager, is responsible for risk assessment and management. There are limited links between different workers. This can lead to a risk-averse culture based on the fear of blame should something happen to a child or young person.

In the Hackney model, social workers work in small groups known as a social work unit, illustrated in Fig. 14.4.

In this structure, the consultant social worker has overall responsibility, but everyone in the team knows the children and their families, and at different stages, different people may work with the family. This leads to a culture where risk is more shared and reflective discussions which focus more on the management,

The S component	What this means	The Hackney model
Shared values	The central 'cog' of the 7S framework, in that organisational values will impact on each of the other S factors, and these must therefore be agreed by all involved.	The shared values outlined in the hackney model include: • An understanding of the importance of keeping children safely in their families, limiting the role of state involvement • Where intervention is required, this should be done with speed and depth working in partnership with parents and other professionals • Building on collaborative, respectful working where families are supported to gain confidence in themselves and rely on their own strengths • Judgements and decisions must always be made within a context of emotional intelligence and empathy
Structure	The way an organisation structures its component parts.	The structure used within the hackney model is perhaps what it has become most known for. The model involves small specifically designed, multi-professional, socialwork units made up of a consultant social worker, a children's practitioner, a social worker, a clinician (often family therapist) and a unit co-ordinator. Each family is known to everyone in the unit and direct work can be undertaken by any team member with the lead undertaken by the person who is seen as best placed, although overall responsibility always remains with the consultant social worker.
Systems	The policies, procedures and routines which are set up to support the work of the organisation.	Systems are significantly redesigned to move social workers away from bureaucracy, freeing them up to spend more time with families. Procedures are limited so that social workers are encouraged to think about the why and how of their work rather than simply the what (what should I do now?) Decision making is located as close to the social worker as possible.
Skills	The capabilities and skills of staff members, and the way the best use of skills is made across the organisation.	The model requires specific skills in social workers which revolve around a systemic style of working, the use of social learning theory and behavioural based interventions, such as motivational interviewing. Reflective practice skills are essential in ensuring that social workers are able to analyse information to develop a range of hypotheses in relation to the circumstances of the children they are working with. The involvement of a unit co-ordinator who is responsible for tasks such as minute taking, administration and diary management recognises the skills of different professionals and considers the way that these can be best used to improve the experiences of families and the delivery of services.
Staff	The recruitment and treatment of staff.	The recruitment and retention of staff with the right skill base and supporting staff through training and effective appraisal systems is seen as essential in the model. Investment in training and development is seen as particularly cost effective in the longer term.
Style	The culture of organisation and the way the leadership style of managers promotes the organisation's culture and vision.	Everyone is required to work collaboratively and respectfully, ensuring that everyone involved in the child's life systems (for example, family, school and wider services) works together to locate solutions to the presenting issues. Everyone in the organisation works on the basis that decision-drivers are the interests of children not service specifications. Children and young people are at the very heart of everything the organisation does.
Strategy	The organisation's plan to reach their identified goals, in many ways this is the sum of the other 6 S components.	Trowler and Goodman (2012:17) are clear that implementation of the hackney model takes a significant length of time (three to five years) because of the significance of the fundamental widespread changes required within an organisation – addressing every aspect of the system. The model involves creating a strategy where social workers can be proud of what they do, with a frontloading of resources towards early intervention and spending on staff, which is offset in the longer term by fewer children going into long term care.

Fig. 14.2 ■ The 7S components and their influence on the design of the Hackney model.

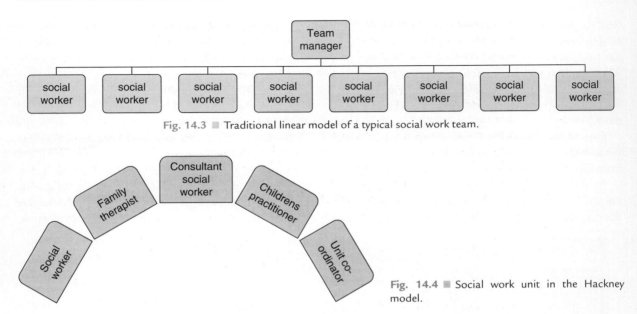

Fig. 14.3 ■ Traditional linear model of a typical social work team.

Fig. 14.4 ■ Social work unit in the Hackney model.

rather than the elimination, of risk. In an evaluation of the model, Cross et al. (2010) reported that social work units were 'consistently better' than traditional teams.

> *The multi-skilled nature of the social work units aims to enable good assessment of whether the child is suffering harm or is likely to suffer harm in the future and to manage the risk by identifying and possibly providing interventions that reduce the risk and improve the child's well-being.*
>
> **Cross et al. (2010, p. 11)**

The Munro review (2011) identified that social workers working in social work units were much more likely than those working in traditional teams to agree that they had the autonomy they needed to carry out their job. The social work unit meets regularly to discuss their work with families in a reflective way, and practitioners overwhelmingly regard unit meetings as positive forum promoting reflective practice (Bostock et al., 2017).

A key aspect of the Hackney model is the use of systems-based thinking in the assessment process. Social workers gather information about the relationships that children and young people have and the way that the systems that surround them are operating. Social workers should develop a range of hypotheses

about what they think is happening in a situation, testing these and ruling them in or out as they gather further information. Professional curiosity is central to the model.

Four key aspects have been identified as impacting on the quality of social work practice in the Hackney model:

- Training in systemic practice
- Consultant social workers involvement in a specific development programme
- The quality of group systemic case discussion
- Presence of clinicians in group case discussion (Bostock et al., 2017)

The Hackney model became very popular in a very short space of time, with the Munro review referring to the model as 'promising' (Munro, 2011) and government departments and think tanks evaluating the model very positively (Bostock et al., 2017). Indeed, the Policy Exchange 2013 report 'Reforming Social Work' suggested that the model 'ought to inform the thinking of local authorities when considering their social work departments' (Holmes et al., 2013, p. 53). Although an evaluation of extending the use of the model into a small number of differing local authorities recognised that there were significant challenges in creating the fundamental change required to fully implement the model, identifying particular barriers in reducing bureaucracy (Bostock et al., 2017).

There has been significant criticism of the way that the Hackney model has been 'commoditised'. Effectively, a model which was developed using public sector finances has been used to make money in the private sector. Goodman and Trowler set up Morning Lane Associates to promote the model, selling consultancy services to local authorities. Jones (2015) claims that between December 2010 and January 2013, Cambridgeshire County Council paid Morning Lane Associates £474,750, citing this as an example of the marketisation and privatisation of child protection practice.

THE HACKNEY MODEL: THE EVIDENCE BASE

Initial evaluation of the use of the model in Hackney was almost entirely positive. For example, Cross et al. (2010) evaluated the model in relation to three areas: context (particularly organisational culture), processes (mechanisms of care) and outcomes. It reported significant positives in every area.

However, when the model began to be used in other localities, more negative findings emerged in the evidence base.

- There can be a tendency for practitioners to be over-optimistic about change (Cross et al., 2010).
- When one person in the social work unit is away for a period of time, there is a significant impact on the rest of the unit, which can result in heavy workloads and staff feeling stressed (Cross et al., 2010).
- There have been significant difficulties in recruiting to the consultant social worker role (Bostock et al., 2017).

SIGNS OF SAFETY

Signs of Safety is a trademarked model, created in Western Australia by Andrew Turnell and Steve Edwards, working in partnership with child protection caseworkers in the late 1990s. Designed as a child protection casework model, it is now used across the UK, Europe, Asia, North America and Canada.

The What Works Centre for Children's Social Care (2018) explain that the founders of the Signs of Safety model caution against simplistic applications of the model, and indeed it can be difficult to provide a clear overview of the model in a limited word count. However, there are three core principles of Signs of Safety model:

1. Establishing constructive working relationships and partnerships between professionals and family members, and between professionals: Relationships must enable honest, respectful discussions about concerns and worries, drawing on positives, considering multiple perspectives, and incorporating a skilful use of authority. Social workers should work with families towards a shared understanding of what needs to change, agreeing on purpose and goals. The relationship needs to be based on more transparent processes and decision-making.

2. Thinking critically and maintaining a stance of critical inquiry: In order to minimise error, a culture of shared reflective practice and a professional willingness to admit that you may have got something wrong are vital. Risk assessment is a core task and requires constant balancing of strengths and dangers to avoid the common errors of drifting into an overly negative (risk focused) or overly positive view of the situation.

3. Grounded in everyday experience: Signs of Safety values both professional and family knowledge. Work with families within Signs of Safety is about ensuring a family's full involvement in assessing risk and developing solutions. The child/young person's experience is central to this, and children, young people and their families are fully engaged in developing and delivering their plans.

SIGNS OF SAFETY: ASSESSMENT AND ANALYSIS

Traditionally assessment is viewed as gathering information, analysing this information and using this information to create plans (Milner and O'Byrne, 2009). Signs of Safety places a significant focus on how information is analysed, proposing that this enables faster and more accurate assessment practice.

Child protection assessment always tends to become bogged down in information gathering with professionals feeling too anxious to analyse and judge. The Signs of Safety assessment and analysis cycle aims for agility, asking practitioners to move quickly through all three stages. Completion is expected in around fourteen days.

Munro et al. (2016, p. 15)

The Signs of Safety assessment and analysis cycle 'maps' the strengths, worries and required safety in a family, in plain language. The areas of enquiry and exploration for the mapping process are:

■ *What is working well?*
■ *What are we worried about?*
■ *What needs to happen?*

The question 'what are we worried about?' is also broken down further into: what do we know has happened in the past that has caused harm to the child? and what are we worried might happen to cause harm in the future? The purpose of this is both about understanding and naming the actual risk more clearly and seeing risk firmly in the context of the impact on each child's well-being, health and development.

These questions are utilised to explore and understand both the strengths and protective factors within the family, and the concerns and risks, making it clear what the family and professionals are working to achieve, and what needs to happen to get there. Scaling questions (drawn from Solution Focused Brief Therapy, de Shazer, 1985) are used to show how all parties judge the risk to the child or young person supporting people to see the situation from the perspective of others and enabling a shared understanding about the level of concerns.

Initial 'danger statements' and 'safety goals' are created to support the development of a safety planning trajectory (Munro et al., 2016).

Danger statements: essentially outline the concerns about a child or young person. They provide 'clearly understandable, simple language descriptions of danger' (Turnell et al., 2017, p. 7) Signs of Safety works on the basis that danger statements which are clearly laid out in a language that professionals and families can understand should be used as the basis for safety planning. Danger statements should identify who is worried, what they are worried about and what specifically they are concerned could happen if nothing changes.

Safety goals: are shared goals agreed between professionals and families. They clarify what needs to happen for children to be safe. Safety and well-being statements should be generated for each danger statement and need to show what the parent will be doing that is different, what the child's experience will be, and what professionals will see that proves something has changed.

Effectively, the mapping stage is about discovering (through the combination of danger statement and a consideration of what is working) **where are we now?**

The safety goals identify **where do we want to be?**

Safety planning can then be developed to look at how to get from where we are to where we want to be. There is a need for precise and understandable language as part of the plan, with the avoidance of words such as 'monitoring'. Responsibility for demonstrating progress needs to sit with families, who must be clear about what needs to be done to ensure their children are safe. An essential aspect of the Signs of Safety model is that safety planning should be viewed as a journey and not a one-off event or a document. Every aspect of progress, even small steps, needs to be acknowledged.

SOME SIGNS OF SAFETY METHODS

'Three houses' is a direct work tool which enables a professional to work with a child or young person to explore what is working, what the child or young person's worries might be and what they would like to happen. This has been an incredibly popular direct work tool with many social workers drawing on the method in their practice, even where they are not using the Signs of Safety model. Anecdotally, many children and young people are beginning to report that they have done this activity many times with social workers and they are bored of it.

'Words and Pictures' is a method to communicate concerns and actions to children and families. A story board of words and pictures is created (usually in conjunction with a child) to use with children, young people and parents to explain what is happening for them, in a way which is easy to understand, and child focussed. This results in children and young people understanding why services are involved, who is doing what to make things better, and what the short-/long-term plans are.

'Fairies and Wizards' is another direct work tool which enables children to talk to a practitioner about what is working well for them, their worries, what helps them to escape their worries and what they wish for. There are criticisms of the gendered nature of this tool which is described in specific terms as 'using a drawing of a fairy with a magic wand (for girls) or a wizard figure (for boys)' (Turnell et al., 2017, p. 48).

Essentially each of these methods is about promoting the voice of children and young people and making the child protection process itself more meaningful and accessible for those at the heart of it.

SIGNS OF SAFETY: THE EVIDENCE BASE

Since the model was first developed, there have been a number of small studies in areas using the approach, including Western Australia, the Netherlands, various Minnesota counties, Gateshead, England, Copenhagen boroughs and New Zealand. These studies have concluded that Signs of Safety model:

■ increases worker morale,
■ increases practitioner clarity and decision-making,
■ improves and focuses relationships between practitioners and families,
■ improves collaboration between child protection and other professionals,
■ reduces rates of child removal, and
■ reduces the length of time cases are open to child protection services (Bunn, 2013; Caslor, 2011; Holmgård Sørensen, 2013; Idzelis Rothe et al., 2013; Keddell, 2014; Salveron et al., 2015; Skrypek et al., 2012).

However, in a comprehensive mixed-method review of Signs of Safety, Sheehan et al. (2018, p. 6) concluded that 'The evidence base for Signs of Safety urgently needs developing. The approach is currently widely used with little evidence of positive impact'.

CASE STUDY 14.1: SIGNS OF SAFETY

Jaxxon (18 months) and Marley (3) are the children of Mel, who has recently moved out of a refuge to resume a relationship with the children's father, Paul. Social care complete an assessment of the children's needs, and they decide to convene a child protection conference using the Signs of Safety model. A danger statement is agreed which states:

Children's Social Care, the health visitor, Mel and her parents are concerned because there have been fights between Mel and Paul in the past, which have resulted in Mel being in hospital with a broken arm and bruises to her face. Jaxxon and Marley have seen this, and they and Mel moved to a refuge for 2 months. If there are more fights, this may mean that Jaxxon and Marley are worried about Mel, they could be unable to sleep, and they and Mel could get hurt.

The family's goal is:

For us all to live together and not argue and fight, so the children are happy, and so that we do not have to be on a child protection plan.

The agency's goal is:

For the children to be safe and happy, and not to get hurt or upset because of fights and arguments.

A child protection plan is agreed which includes these goals, and the following indicators which would show services that there were changes to the children's safety:

For Paul to complete a course around his anger with the local domestic abuse charity, to attend all sessions, and for there to be no police call outs to the family home.

For Jaxxon and Marley to attend nursery three times a week, and for staff to see them playing with other children and happy when they see both Paul and Mel come to collect them.

For Mel's parents to see Mel, Jaxxon and Marley regularly and for them to feel that Mel and the children seem safe, well and happy.

For Mel to attend all appointments offered by Women's Aid, and for there to be no hospital attendances or concerns about her safety reported by professionals or Mel.

For the family to see social workers and family support staff once a week (announced and unannounced) over the 6 months, and to be honest with all professionals about these Signs of Safety.

FAMILY GROUP CONFERENCING

Family Group Conferencing, often referred to as FGC, originates from the cultural traditions which frame New Zealand's child welfare legislation. Family Group Conferences were introduced to the UK by the Family Rights Group in 1992 (Edwards, 2018). Essentially Family Group Conferencing is a model for decision-making and planning, which should not be an isolated intervention, but should be placed in a wider approach which sees families as partners in the child protection process. A Family Group Conference is different to traditional decision-making arenas in five key ways (Maclean and Harrison, 2015):

1. **Involvement of extended and wider family and kin:** Central to Family Group Conferences is the involvement of extended family members and the broader kinship network. In the context of Family Group Conferencing, 'family' can mean close friends, neighbours, community leaders and peer supporters as well as aunts, uncles, cousins and grandparents. This definition of family recognises the importance of informal networks in strengthening people's relationships and addressing risk factors for the child.
2. **Values and power base:** Family Group Conferencing starts from the premise that families can make good plans for the care of their children, no matter how complex the nature of the difficulties they are facing. There is wide agreement that, for this reason, a Family Group Conference is not usually appropriate in cases of intergenerational sexual abuse, but it may be used in many other complex situations. Family Group Conferences aim to shift power away from people who represent organisations, so that the family are enabled to plan for themselves.
3. **Neutrality:** The Family Group Conference coordinator is neutral which means they do not attend other meetings, do not complete assessments and are not responsible for case management or care planning. This is critical as the coordinator's independence is what means that the family have a true opportunity to develop their own plan and make their own decisions about their own child/ren's future. Family Group Conferences are usually held in community venues (a church hall or community centre), and often food and drink are provided. This is crucial as a physical manifestation of the transfer of power in decision-making. Services offer support, but it is up to the family to decide which support they will access, as long as their plan keeps the child safe.
4. **Cultural competence:** Family Group Conferencing is a culturally competent model as each family's conference will differ according to their preferences, needs and wishes. These differences could relate to the family choosing the venue, or might be around the provision of food, or through allowing children and families to agree and own the ground rules for the meeting. Family Group Conferences celebrate diversity (e.g. by enabling religious preference to be incorporated into the introduction of the meeting, or by looking at the status of some family members in terms of who speaks first and who sits where, etc.).
5. **Presence and voice of the child:** The model works to provide children and young people with a voice via a trained advocate. This could either be someone who the child already knows and trusts who is supported to take on that role, or a practitioner or volunteer who is brought in just to perform that function. Family Group Conferences work on the premise that young people should be present for all discussions concerning them, and that younger children or those who are not able to participate for the whole meeting should be supported so their views are fully considered and represented.

The Family Group Conference process can be broken down into five key stages, as illustrated in Fig. 14.5.

Good preparation with all participants is what leads to good outcomes, so at the referral stage, the referrer will outline the concerns, the decisions which the family need to make and the 'bottom line' – for example, anything which the family could not include in their plan, and what could happen if the family do not participate or do not stick to their plan. The coordinator spends time with everyone in the network in the preparation stage, considering what each individual is prepared to offer. This planning stage time ensures that everyone has space to consider how anything they

Stage 1 (Referral): There needs to be an identified need and consequently a plan to address the presenting needs. At this stage a co-ordinator is appointed who is independent of the family and the social care agency. It is important to consider the cultural needs of the family.

Stage 2: The co-ordinator, in consultation with the child and family, issues invitations, agrees the venue, date and timing of the family meeting. The co-ordinator also prepares the participants.

Stage 3: At the start of the meeting the co-ordinator chairs the information sharing. Professionals explain their roles, responsibilities, any concerns and available resources.

Stage 4: Private planning time for the family. The co-ordinator and professionals withdraw whilst the family agree a plan, which should include a contingency plan and review arrangements.

Stage 5: The co-ordinator and professionals re-join the family / kinship and hear the plan. Resources are negotiated and the plan is agreed.

Fig. 14.5 ■ The Family Group Conference process. Maclean and Harrison (2015) p 203

offer could be sustained alongside their own lives, work, children or commitments. The coordinator will explore the network, engage the child to ascertain their views and wishes, consider access issues (disability, venue accessibility, literacy, language, childcare, transport, etc.), and think with each person about what they could offer, but crucially without telling them what they have to put into a plan. Preparation work also covers conflict, recognising that not all conflict is negative, and some issues may need to be aired in order for the family to plan. However, adults do need to attend, ready to focus on the future and put conflict to one side to focus on the needs of the child.

The information sharing stage of the Family Group Conference should be reasonably brief, so that it is experienced as different from other meetings which families have attended. Family Group Conferences should feel as comfortable as possible for families, more neutral in terms of the environment and lack of 'blame', and more focused on the future than the reasons for services becoming involved. Social workers may feel unsettled by the experience of being invited into the family's meeting, as well as leaving the family for private time, and it is important that the coordinator

prepares professionals, so that their experience of the meeting is not disempowering, as professionals retain case management responsibility.

Private family time can take a while, and no time limits should be set, so that the family feel enabled to make the plan which they have been asked to consider. This can be difficult for practitioners to manage in terms of diary planning. However, only when the family have had as much time as they need to create a plan should professionals (including the coordinator) be invited back into the meeting to look at the plan. Professionals should be on hand during this private time in case the family wish to ask for clarification on specific points or on services which might be available.

It is relevant to note that the family plan should not place the child or young person at any risk. The plan should address concerns and lead to an improved outcome and family plan to ensure the well-being and development of the child or young person. When the family plan is being heard by the social worker, it may be that more detail is requested, and it may be that the family are asked to take further private time to add detail and specifics into their plan. This is so that the plan is the family's own and in their own words as much as possible (Cashmore and Kiely, 2017).

Family plans should be agreed, providing they address the concerns and do not put children at risk. Everyone needs to leave the meeting feeling clear about:

- How the plan will be monitored and implemented by the family
- How and when the plan will be reviewed
- If the plan will be considered within the court arena, how and when this will take place

FAMILY GROUP CONFERENCES: THE EVIDENCE BASE

Up until recently the evidence base (going back some time) has been very positive in relation to Family Group Conferencing, such that it was perhaps seen as the most evidence-based model used in child protection:

- Family Group Conferences increase the number of children in kinship care placements (Pakura, 2004). The Who Cares Trust (2015) report that children in kinship care in the UK experience higher degrees of self-worth and a reduction in emotional and behavioural difficulties.
- Family Group Conferencing supports effective anti-discriminatory practice with families from black or minority ethnic communities as it validates families' own social and cultural values (Love, 2017; Tapsfield, 2003).
- Social workers believe that risks to children are addressed and reduced as a result of the plan (Cashmore and Kiely, 2017).
- In Leeds, the adoption of Family Group Conferences across the city as the way to work with all families pre-child protection has led to a reduction of 40% in the number of children who are subject to a child protection plan (Mason et al., 2017). Leeds have also shown a reduction in the number of children coming into care, and they report that Family Group Conferences prevented 90 children coming into care in 1 year, as well as an increase in the number in kinship care.

- In a Children's Innovation Fund project, Southwark and Wiltshire children's services offered a Family Group Conference to all families where there was an intention to initiate care proceedings. Where families had a Family Group Conference, there were proceedings in 29% of cases compared to 50% of cases where there was no Family Group Conference (Munro et al., 2017). All key stakeholders reported a high level of satisfaction, and all family members agreed or strongly agreed that they knew what was going to happen (Munro et al., 2017).

However, a recent randomised control trial (Dijkstra et al., 2019) has shaken this evidence base, identifying through an extensive study, that Family Group Conferencing resulted in a longer period of involvement with child welfare services and more out of home placements. Sanders (2019) suggests that while this study is important, aspects of it should be taken 'with a pinch of salt'. Certainly, further research and exploration is required.

> ### CASE STUDY 14.2: FAMILY GROUP CONFERENCING EXAMPLE
>
> Shakira, aged 5, is subject to a child protection plan because her parents continue to use substances in a way which impacts on her health and development. The local authority has taken legal advice and held a pre-proceedings meeting, at which it was agreed a Family Group Conference was needed to explore what support the wider family could offer, especially in terms of making sure Shakira's parents attend appointments with drug services. The Family Group Conference was also asked to ascertain if any family members would put themselves forward to care for Shakira if this was required in the future.
>
> The independent coordinator engaged two aunts and three uncles, three of Shakira's grandparents and a close family friend in the Family Group Conference. Shakira's wishes and feelings were explored and shared at her conference, and she drew a picture of her family and who she feels is close to her. Family members agreed to

increase the level of drop ins with Shakira's parents, to have her overnight once a week at maternal grandparents, and for one aunt to take responsibility for taking parents to their drug service appointments. This aunt also considered what it may entail if she put herself forward for a viability assessment, and this was actioned following inclusion of this in the family plan by Shakira's social worker. Other family members considered putting themselves forward but did not commit to this in the plan, meaning that if Shakira were to be removed from parents, all options had then been considered in advance of any court proceedings.

CONTEMPORARY COMMONALITIES

This chapter has explored three of the main contemporary models used in child protection. Several common principles and practices can be drawn out of these. Working within these may be an aspect of what defines a contemporary child protection worker in the UK:

- Families are seen as experts in their own situation and are supported to find their own solutions to the difficulties they face.
- Professionals need to work in partnership with families and the wider systems that surround children and young people.
- The voice of the child or young person must be central to decision-making.
- Analysis and reflective practice are vital aspects of risk assessment and management.
- Decision-making should be shared.
- There is a need to move away from a culture of blame.

CONCLUSION

Social workers take a 'person in environment perspective', which is becoming even more embedded in light of the move towards contextual safeguarding (Firmin et al., 2019). It follows, therefore, that it is important to adopt a 'social worker in organisation' perspective when considering models of child protection. What works well in one context may not work as effectively

in another organisation. There is a growing understanding that services, models and interventions can retraumatise children and their families (Shelley et al., 2016). It is therefore vital that social workers remain fully conversant with models of intervention, that they take a critical stance to the use of these and that they consider how they might adopt a trauma-informed position and work relationally with parents regardless of the model adopted.

REFLECTIVE QUESTIONS

- How do you understand the difference between a theory, model, method and approach?
- Which of the models covered in this chapter interest you the most? Why?
- Is there a case for a nationwide model of child protection? What should that look like?

REFERENCES

Bostock, L., Forrester, D., Patrizo, L., Godfrey, T., Zonouzi, M., Antonopoulou, V., et al., 2017. Scaling and deepening the Reclaiming Social Work model: Childrens Social Care Innovation Programme Evaluation Report 45. Department for Education, London.

Bunn, A., 2013. Signs of Safety in England: An NSPCC Commissioned Report on the Signs of Safety Model in Child Protection. NSPCC, London.

Cashmore, J., Kiely, P., 2017. Implementing and evaluating FGCs in the New South Wales experience. In: Burford, G., Hudson, J. (Eds.), Family Group Conferencing: New Directions in Community-Centered Child and Family Practice. Routledge, Oxon.

Caslor, M., 2011. The Metis DR/FE Project Evaluation. Building Capacity Consulting Services, Manitoba, Canada. https://www.metisauthority.com/. (Accessed 28 December 2019).

Cross, S., Hubbard, A., Munro, E., 2010. Reclaiming Social Work London Borough of Hackney Children and Young People's Services. Part one Independent Evaluation and Part Two Unpacking the Complexity of Frontline Practice – An Ethnographic Approach. Human Reliability Associates and the London School of Economics and Political Science, London.

de Shazer, S., 1985. Keys to Solution in Brief Therapy. Norton, New York.

Dijkstra, S., Asscher, J.J., Dekovic, M., Stams, G.J., Creemers, H.E., 2019. Randomized controlled trial on the effectiveness of family group conferencing in child welfare: Effectiveness, moderators and level of FGC completion. Child Maltreat. 24 (2), 137–151.

Edwards, D., 2018. Introduction. In: Edwards, D., Parkinson, K. (Eds.), Family Group Conferences in Social Work: Involving Families in Social Care Decision Making. Policy Press, Bristol.

Ferguson, H., 2014. What social workers do in performing child protection work: Evidence from research into face-to-face practice. Child Fam. Soc. Work 21 (3), 283–294.

Firmin, C., Eastman, A., Wise, I., Proschaka, E., with Holmes, D., Pearce, J., Wright, S., 2019. A Legal Framework for Implementing Contextual Safeguarding: Initial opportunities and consideration. Contextual Safeguarding Network. https://contextualsafeguarding.org.uk/assets/images/A-Legal-Framework-for-Implementing-Contextual-Safeguarding_190313_151714.pdf. (Accessed 9 November 2019).

Holmes, E., Miscampbell, G., Robin, B., 2013. Reforming Social Work: Improving Social Worker Recruitment, Training and Retention. Policy Exchange, London.

Holmgård Sørensen, T., 2013. Når Forældre Netværk Skaber Sikkerhed for Barnet: En Evaluering af 'Sikkerhedsplaner' I Arbejdet med Udsatte Børn Familier I Københavns Commune. Socialforvaltningen, Københavns Kommune.

Idzelis Rothe, M., Nelson-Dusek, S., Skrypek, M., 2013. Innovations in Child Protection Services in Minnesota – Research Chronicle of Carver and Olmsted Counties. Wilder Research, St. Paul, MN. www.wilder.org/. (Accessed 28 December 2019).

Jones, R., 2015. The end game: The marketisation and privatisation of children's social work and child protection. Crit. Soc. Policy 35 (4), 447–469.

Keddell, E., 2014. Theorising the Signs of Safety approach to child protection social work: positioning, codes and power. Child. Youth Serv. Rev. 47 (1), 70–77. https://doi.org/10.1016/j.childyouth.2014.03.011.

Love, C., 2017. Family group conferencing cultural origins, sharing and appropriation – a Maori reflection. In: Burford, G., Hudson, J. (Eds.), Family Group Conferencing: New Directions in Community-Centered Child and Family Practice. Routledge, Oxon.

Maclean, S., Finch, J., Tedam, P., 2018. SHARE: A New Model for Social Work. Kirwin Maclean Associates, Lichfield.

Maclean, S., Harrison, R., 2015. Theory and Practice: A Straightforward Guide for Social Work Students, fourth ed. Kirwin Maclean Associates, Lichfield.

Maclean, S., with Yusuf McCormack, P., and Surviving Safeguarding, 2019. Working Towards Accreditation: Putting the Pieces Together. Kirwin Maclean Associates, Lichfield.

Mason, P., Ferguson, H., Morris, K., Munton, T., Sen, R., 2017. Leeds Family Valued Evaluation Report. Children's Social Care Innovation Programme Evaluation Report 43. Department for Education, London.

Milner, J., O'Byrne, P., 2009. Assessment in Social Work, third ed. Palgrave MacMillan, Basingstoke.

Munro, E., 2011. The Munro Review of Child Protection: Final Report. A Child-Centred System. Department for Education, London.

Munro, E., Turnell, A., Murphy, T., 2016. You Can't Grow Roses in Concrete. Action Research Final Report. Signs of Safety Innovation Project. November 2014–March 2016. https://www.basw.co.uk/system/files/resources/basw_102921-2_0.pdf. (Accessed 11 November 2019).

Munro, E.R., Meetoo, V., Quy, K., Simon, A., 2017. Daybreak Family Group Conferencing: Children on the Edge of Care. Children's Social Care Innovation Programme Evaluation Report 54. Department for Education, London.

Pakura, S., 2004. The Family Group Conference 14-Year Journey: Celebrating the Successes, Learning the Lessons, Embracing the Challenges. www.iirp.org/article_detail.php?article_id=Mzg2. (Accessed 23 July 2010).

Pawson, R., 2006. Evidence-Based Policy: A Realist Perspective. Sage, London.

Rogowski, S., 2015. From child welfare to child protection/safeguarding: A critical practitioner's view of changing conceptions, policies and practice. Prac. Soc. Work Action 27 (2), 97–112.

Salveron, M., Bromfield, L., Kirika, C., Simmons, J., Turnell, A., 2015. Changing the way we do child protection: The implementation of Signs of Safety within the Western Australia Department for Child Protection and Family Support. Child. Youth Serv. Rev. 48, 126–139.

Sanders, M., 2019. Family Group Conferences – what does the evidence say? What Works for Children's Social Care. https://whatworks-csc.org.uk/blog/family-group-conferences-what-does-the-evidence-say/. (Accessed 11 November 2019).

Sheehan, L., O'Donnell, C., Brand, S.L., Forrester, D., Addis, S., El-Banna, A., et al., 2018. Signs of Safety: Findings from a Mixed-Methods Systematic Review Focussed on Reducing the Need for Children to be in Care. What Works Centre for Children's Social Care, London.

Shelley, P., Hitzel, S., Zgoda, K., 2016. Preventing Retraumatization: A Macro Social Work Approach to Trauma-Informed Practices and Policies. https://www.socialworker.com/feature-articles/practice/preventing-retraumatization-a-macro-social-work-approach-to-trauma-informed-practices-policies/. (Accessed 12 November 2019).

Skrypek, M., Idzelis, M., Pecora, P., 2012. Signs of Safety in Minnesota: Parent Perceptions of a Signs of Safety Child Protection Experience. Wilder Research, St. Paul, MN. https://www.wilder.org/wilder-research/research-library/signs-safety-minnesota-parent-perceptions-signs-safety-child. (Accessed 28 December 2019).

Tapsfield, 2003. Family group conferences: family-led decision making. Childright 195, 16–17.

The Who Cares Trust, 2015. Kinship Care. http://www.thewhocarestrust.org.uk/pages/kinship-care.html. (Accessed 14 February 2015).

Trowler, I., Goodman, S., 2012. A systems methodology for children and families social work. In: Trowler, I., Goodman, S. (Eds.), Social Work Reclaimed. Jessica Kingsley, London.

Turnell, A., Etherington, K., Turnell, P., 2017. Signs of Safety Workbook, second ed. Resolutions Consultancy Pty Ltd., East Perth.

Waterman, R.H., Peters, T.J., Phillips, J.R., 1980. Structure is not organization. Bus. Horiz. 23 (3), 14–26.

What Works Centre for Children's Social Care, 2018. Signs of Safety Information. https://whatworks-csc.org.uk/wp-content/uploads/Signs-of-Safety-information-sheet.pdf. (Accessed 8 November 2019).

15 SAFEGUARDING CHILDREN: THE ASSESSMENT CHALLENGES

MARTIN CHARLES CALDER

KEY POINTS

- Unravelling some of the challenges thrown up by the Framework for the Assessment of Children in Need and their Families (DoH et al., 2000).

- Examining some of the inherent contradictions within its structure.

- Examining some of the key recurring challenges that arise from serious case reviews, Ofsted inspections and contemporary research.

- Introducing how some of the emerging assessment frameworks and processes from elsewhere in the UK can be usefully harvested to enhance the chances of better outcomes.

- Considering a contemporary assessment process to structure assessments.

- Introduce a risk assessment dimension to the overly strengths-loaded current approach to practice.

INTRODUCTION

Good assessments in social work have always been needs led, although need can be understood differently by people and can become a 'contested' concept. Need is in most cases defined by others rather than as perceived by the person being assessed. This is the practitioner's dilemma: how to understand, consider and respond to the service user's view of their needs, whilst also acting within employers' requirements, using professional theories and with normative concepts of need in mind. Assessment should be a dynamic process which analyses and responds to the changing nature and level of need and/or risk faced by the child. A good assessment will monitor and record the impact of any services delivered on the child and family and review the help being delivered. Whilst services may be delivered to a parent or carer, the assessment should be focused on the needs of the child and on the impact any services are having on the child. Good assessments support professionals to understand whether a child has needs relating to their care or a disability and/or is suffering, or likely to suffer, significant harm. A good assessment will also ensure that the specific needs of disabled children and young carers are given enough recognition and priority. While the assessment is part of the overall child protection process, it is also an intervention and it is important that it is used as such (Calder, 2012). The purpose of assessment is to understand what it is like to be that child or young person (and what it will be like in the future if nothing changes).

RELATIONSHIPS AT THE HEART OF ASSESSMENT PRACTICE

Relationship practice is the heartbeat of assessment and engagement practice. It is emerging with different labels such as strengths-based, solution-focused and restorative approaches.

Restorative practice describes a way of behaving. It involves building and maintaining healthy relationships, resolving difficulties and repairing harm if there has been conflict between individuals or groups. It is about finding out what people can do and working with them to build on that. It does not mean that those supporting families should be stepping in to take control. Evidence shows that the futures of children and their families are brighter when those who support them work **with** and alongside them instead of making decisions **for** them or doing things **to** them.

It describes a way of being which threads through everything we do when we are communicating and resolving difficulties. Restorative approaches support those who work with children and families to focus on building relationships that create change. And it is worth bearing in mind that creating change sometimes needs people to be challenged as well as supported. That means moving from a culture focused on the problematic (i.e. assessing need). Instead, we are investing to create a stable confident workforce who can effectively manage uncertainty and risk and identify people's strengths and build on them to secure change and build resilience (Calder, 2020a).

Context Is Critical

There is a need to lay some solid foundations for all assessment practice, and this includes considering the ecological context within which the child and the family operate and the importance of relationships to enhance good outcomes, coupled with a clear outcomes driver from the child and family from the outset.

All assessments are context specific, and so it is imperative that we consider the systematic environment: the child needs consideration with the parents or carers, who have a wider family residing in an environment that embraces local demographics, as well as professional/system considerations. Assessment requires consideration of the mix of strengths and risks at each level and also, if they interact, with what effect. It is critical to gather information from multiple sources and to develop a full description of the life of the child from multiple perspectives. This assists with validating, clarifying or corroborating information, leading to more informed, comprehensive and accurate analysis and assessment. Identifying sources of information

should be a central part of your assessment plan. Key information sources should always be:

- **The child:** observing and interacting with the child in a way that is consistent with the child's age and stage of development and functioning is crucial to assess their presentation. Always try to engage with and speak to the child. If the child is preverbal, detailed information can be gained from observing the child, including their behaviour patterns and response or lack of response with each parent or caregiver, siblings and significant others.
- **Family and extended family:** information direct from the family should assist in gaining a view of the child's daily experience. A detailed family history identifies patterns of behaviour and abuse, relationships, significant events and a deeper understanding of how the family functions. Practitioners should also observe the interactions in the family and be aware of the strengths and types of relationships between family members, which can sometimes affect the validity and accuracy of the information provided. Contact should be made with non-resident parents, unless their whereabouts are unknown, with the aims of engaging them in the process and gathering and validating information. If a decision is made not to identify or engage a non-resident parent, the reason why this decision has been made must be clearly recorded. If, for example, there is a history of domestic abuse, any impact on the safety of family members must be accounted for in the assessment plan.

THE CHALLENGES OF USING THE FRAMEWORK FOR ASSESSMENT

The backbone of assessment expectations across the safeguarding spectrum revolves around the framework for the assessment of children in need and their families (DoH et al., 2000). This statutory guidance, issued to all agencies has not diminished the ongoing conflict about whether it is an exclusive social services framework or an inter-agency framework. Fuelled by premature governmental introduction, the emergence of the common assessment framework (CAF) to embrace other agencies had the side-effect of cultivating a 'them and us' scenario with many professionals believing that it was a means of building capacity for a growth in complex safeguarding cases within social care (Calder, 2020b). This was unfortunate as the emphasis should have been on how to pool resources to enhance collaboration by developing a common language, purpose and environment to ensure all the assessment focus was on enhancing the outcomes for children and young people we aim to safeguard.

Although the assessment framework was designed to standardise assessment practice, this has been impossible because:

- It was never a framework to guide assessment: it was at best a conceptual framework and a standardised means of recording.
- There was an expectation for assessments to be evidence-based and by implication, it required an appraisal of theory, research and practice wisdom to mould it to the individual context and family circumstances under consideration.
- There is disconnect between cases requiring assessment (with a higher threshold) and a framework that is therapeutically and strengths grounded. The assessment framework purposefully deleted reference to risk. This was both grounded in a misunderstanding that risk was a balance of risk and strengths and not purely deficit-focused, and was also at odds with an elevated threshold to mostly child protection, when risk removal and a therapeutic focus was of more use in a child in need/family support context. This was influenced, of course, by a paucity of frontline safeguarding authorships from social care (Calder, 2003a), which was alarmingly replicated in the ensuing review of child protection conducted by Eileen Munro (2011).
- It does not take into account the expanding definition of safeguarding, especially in the area of sexual abuse, and it does not capture the changing demographics and the need for further education and guidance for staff beyond Black families, as well as embracing religious considerations (Horwath and Lees, 2010). Safeguarding is a complex and contested term: it stands simultaneously as a high level concept capturing the state's aspirations for all children, whilst at the same time also functioning as an 'alert' button for speedy inter-agency coordination in response to a much smaller group of children at risk of significant harm.

- The common assessment framework, whilst designed to be holistic, has frequently been used primarily as a means of making a successful inter-agency referral into social care utilising the selected vocabulary from local threshold levels rather than the identification of need with a view to redressing it via supportive services.
- The assessment framework is punctuated with timescales, and this creates a salami effect with a narrow focus at the front door and an evolving span the longer the cases are open.
- Fostering and adoption, with its focus on family assessments, was never embraced and the significance of this has become more evident with more placements at home, with family and friends, and a greater use of special guardianship orders by the courts.

When there are efforts to use the assessment framework as the primary assessment structure, it has the potential to generate information that is not immediately relevant to the presenting concern, and this makes subsequent analysis and planning more difficult as workers struggle to separate the wood from the trees (Calder, 2020b). Some workers are directed that no assessment can be signed off if there is any blank box, and so this offers them a conflicting message between proportionate information collection and completion of all the form regardless of relevance to the presenting case (Calder, 2020c). Assessments should be proportionate and not performance dictated.

Inherent Contradictions

Several contradictions permeate the assessment framework. It says that assessments should run in parallel with actions and interventions, whereas the operational reality is that austerity has generated greater gatekeeping and needs are prioritised when they are acute, relegating accumulative concerns to secondary. Needs outstrip resources by 3 to 1 currently, and so workers must be clear about whether to meet three partially or one completely (Calder, 2003a).

There is an expectation that assessment is an ongoing process, not a single one-off event. The timescales accompanying the framework have introduced a very clear time-limit and caution exists about ongoing assessment as this has performance penalties. These relate to the business framework from government, which requires compliance with measurable outcomes in order to secure a good or outstanding grading or, conversely, punitive penalties if not secured (Calder, 2008). Conversely, the timescales, whilst useful in ensuring cases do not drift, do not necessarily capture or work with the reality that parents' problems are entrenched, and children require the chance to work at their own pace not dictated by standardised timeframes. Flexibility post Munro were aspirational, and local performance requirements has meant they have been maintained but with flexibility within but not at the end point.

There is an expectation that assessment should be grounded in evidence-based practice. The clarity that evidence should comprise the best of theory, research and practice wisdom is to be welcomed. The consequence of this is a challenge to access, absorb and apply the materials to individual cases when opportunities and costs as well as time are a barrier to this. There is also a need to acknowledge there is a different emphasis on evidence-based components across different professional groups, with some emphasising statistics (actuarial) rather than professional interpretation and use of judgment (clinical). The latter fuels a shift away from a standardised assessment approach given the need to tailor the evidence and collection of relevant information to individual cases. Such subjectivity can lead to a variance of assessment practice with a range from exceptional to dangerous A standardized approach results in families being pulled through regardless of presenting circumstances and, to counter this, requires moulding relevant evidence to make it case-specific. That stated, it is then a lottery on how individual workers tailor the assessment, drawing from a combination of the theory, research and their practice experience (Calder, 2020b).

The criteria for the appointment of a lead professional under the umbrella of the common assessment framework and the appointment of a key (social) worker at an initial child protection conference is the same: the need for an inter-agency plan. There is no clarity about the elements that comprise such plans and how you differentiate between the same plan at different levels. Clearly areas such as consent and compliance/cooperation play a key role (although perpetual lack of agreement about these terms persists within and across most agencies), as does the likelihood of the family moving to avoid surveillance where child protection systems remain substantially more responsive. The lack of any clarity about what constitutes significant harm (actual or likely) remains problematic as it is the mechanism that informs information exchange. Most thresholds are clearer when there is an incident, but children are harmed by exposure to accumulative events that make the trigger for action more subjective and contested. The timescales make the timing of the threshold judgement critical in terms of forcing a narrower focus, and challenges in practice toward proportionate and child outcomes focused decision-making are tempered organizationally as timeframe compliance remains the primary (Ofsted-fuelled) focus. Their persecution of practice is abusive and reflective of toxic parenting: high criticism and low warmth. This is part of a wider toxicity within which workers are operating (see Calder, 2016) and which impacts detrimentally on the centrality of cultivating relationships with the children and families with whom we work (Calder, 1995; 2003a).

Judicial decision making is now adding further challenges as the timescales for compliance with the 26-week deadline continues to slip, the uphill hurdle to overcome in being asked to make predictions without an adequate evidence-base or time, and a rejection of evidence premised on accumulative harm (human or parental rights predominate). There is also a driver towards a strengths-based approach which, whilst positive in engaging families and helping them plan for a brighter future, is jettisoning the most critical element of history (and understanding of) as it may throw up challenges to positivity. Strengths-based practice is not different to risk assessment practice: both have to examine positives and negatives and balance what this means as far as the child and young person is concerned; and both have to start with a history as a part of the journey, not just the here and now and the proposed future. Errors are not always in our control, but those that are have to be named and shared. Some practice is premised on an unwillingness to include agency history under an early help offer if the parents object. This is clearly an abdication of the need to capture the past to understand any hurdles they might bring to the future. Re-referral and re-registration become more evident as premature decisions are made based on cooperation not causal contribution, and over optimism that changes made will be sustained.

KEY RECURRING CHALLENGES ARISING FROM SERIOUS CASE REVIEWS, OFSTED INSPECTIONS AND CONTEMPORARY RESEARCH

The purpose of assessment is to understand what it is like to be that child or young person (and what it will be like in the future if nothing changes). Research inspections and inquiries indicate that children's voices are absent or minimised during assessments, the focus is on the parents rather than the child, and the use of language in reports is alienating. Several means of silencing children in assessments are identifiable and include:

- not reporting what was said,
- children being minor characters in the narrative,
- more weight being given to adult views when there are differences of opinion or conflicting accounts,
- presupposing what they might say,
- descriptions of children being limited only to how they respond or relate to their parents, or
- presenting their views as untrustworthy.

Involving children does work, however:

- Children feel listened to and taken seriously and this helps them to deal with difficult situations.
- When children are involved in decision-making and planning, the plans are more likely to be successful and services developed with the influence of children and young people are more likely to meet their needs.

Some of the lessons learned about involving children include:

- The more children participate in decisions that affect their lives, the more they develop confidence, competencies and aspirations which have a positive effect on their health and development, relationships within their family and community.

Good assessment has to counter the challenges to capture the relevant information via common outcome targets. Good practice involves the following (Table 15.1):

TABLE 15.1 Good Practice	
Building competence	By providing information so that children and young people can contribute meaningfully
	By giving time and explanations so that they can properly understand the issues and the process
	By being clear about what will be discussed and the likely consequences. Be straight about the boundaries of confidentiality
	By giving access to independent advocacy services if required
Practical considerations	Pay attention to venues and who will be present. Children should be involved in deciding who, when and where
	Provide interpreters if required
	Think about what tools and techniques you will use: preparation & planning
	Think about the use of new technologies
Create the right culture	Children are more likely to talk to people they know and trust – it takes time to build trust
	Feedback and discuss the outcomes, what happened
	Follow-up – do what you said you would do
	Be flexible in response to what children and young people say
Child-led assessments	Start with what is important to the child
	Go at the child's pace – gradually build a picture of their needs
	Attend to positives as well as negatives
	Forms/tick-boxes/checklists don't always work well with children

Recording is a continuing theme when cases go wrong. Time pressures, restrictions on use of phones to verbalize post-meeting key points for breach of data protection, and variance across staff on what is necessary to include is key. Logically, recording should provide any external reader the chance of understanding the information in context and then linking this to the analysis of what this means and a pathway to recommendations that bridges the different stages into a coherent whole. If done badly, the records become difficult to interpret. When we undertake a chronology, they are the foundations for identifying ongoing processes and patterns of harm. Workers are more inclined to record why they do things rather than why they do not. Recording requires clarification of what is deemed significant and, to this end, the emergence of clear factors for all agencies to use as a trigger to include have been helpful. The challenge is to get the originating agency to start the process rather than waiting for a crisis and then historical factors sought to contextualize it.

ENHANCING EXISTING ASSESSMENT STRUCTURES

Scotland modified the English triangle to capture the child as a core across all its domains and then to capture projected outcomes as supporting dimensions

(Fig. 15.1). Once this is achieved, then the ability to generate relevant questions to consider supporting the information required is made much easier.

This child- and outcome-focused framework was issued to and used by all professionals, thus creating a single assessment framework. It was then followed by a national risk assessment framework (Calder, Sneddon and McKinnon, 2012) that was designed to explicitly capture risk and indicate the relevant questions which evidence indicated require careful consideration in all assessments. It built on the earlier work carried out by the author around the risk diamond (Calder, 2004) (Fig. 15.2).

Eight well-being indicators have been identified as areas in which children and young people need to progress to do well now and in the future. The indicators allow practitioners to structure information which may identify needs and concerns and to structure planning for the child or young person. These eight well-being indicators are safe, healthy, active,

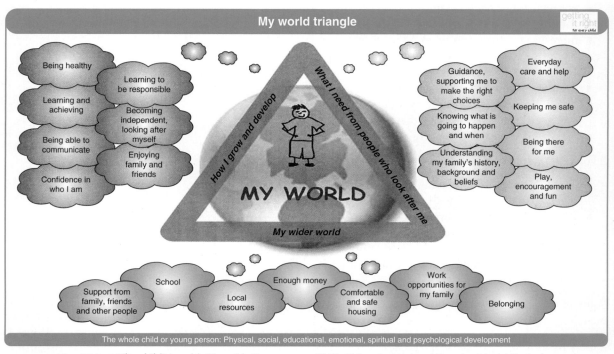

Fig. 15.1 ■ The child's world. (Scottish Government, 2010. Using the National Practice Model II: Gathering Information with the My World Triangle. 1st ed. [ebook] Edinburgh: Scottish Government)

achieving, nurtured, respected, responsible and included (SHANARI). Fig. 15.3 offers a useful visual reference point to bring this alive.

In Wales, the first childcare legislation, Social Services and Well-being (Wales) Act 2014, spans children and adult services. This takes one step further forward and enshrines outcomes as the starting point as well as the end point for all assessments. The approach puts people at the centre of their care and support planning. An outcomes-based approach is based on the following principles:

■ People are experts in their own lives.
■ They are best placed to tell you what is important to them and what gives them a sense of well-being, but they may need help to do this.
■ People want to do the things that matter most to them, in their own way.

■ People's strengths are important and need to be acknowledged.
■ We start by identifying what the person wants to achieve, and then thinking through how to achieve that outcome and agree a plan that helps them to do this.
■ The person's family, carers and local community can also contribute to this plan.
■ Meaningful conversations are central to understanding a person's outcomes.
■ A personal outcome is the picture the person paints of what it is they want to achieve.

A sense of well-being comes from things, such as:

■ relationships,
■ feeling loved,
■ being respected,

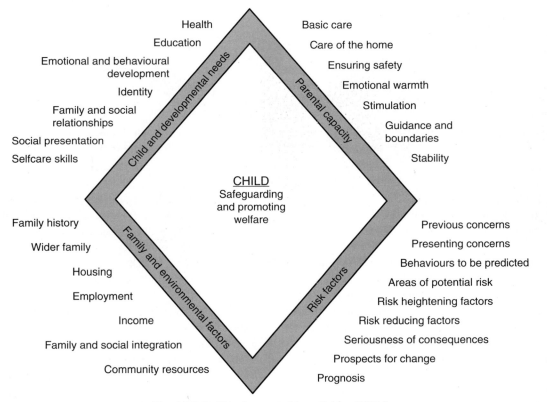

Fig. 15.2 ■ Risk diamond. (From Calder, 2004.)

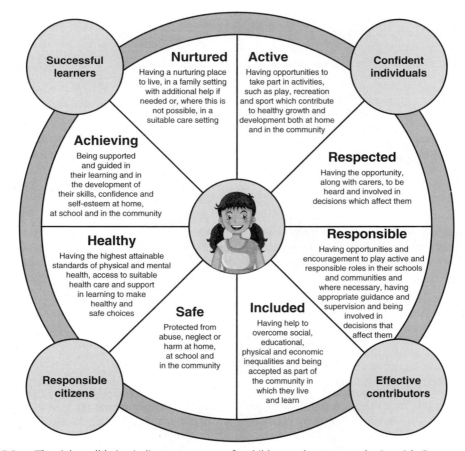

Fig. 15.3 ■ The eight well-being indicators necessary for children and young people. Scottish Government, 2010. Using the National Practice Model II: Gathering Information with the My World Triangle. 1st ed. [ebook] Edinburgh: Scottish Government

- having a sense of purpose,
- making a useful contribution, and
- the little things... that make life feel worthwhile.

The legislative sequence involves working through a number of steps as outlined in Fig. 15.4.

Personal outcomes describe what a person wants to achieve. These are realistic goals that the person receiving care and support, and their care worker or carer, can work towards. They are usually based around supporting the individual's well-being. Outcomes will vary from person to person and child to child because they are about what matters to that individual. A person is facing barriers to achieving their personal outcomes if something related to the individual's condition or circumstances, or something outside their control, is preventing them from meeting their outcomes. It is possible for individuals to have several low-risk elements which in themselves would not pose a threat to achieving personal outcomes, but the combination of risks and how they interact will result in a more serious threat. Positive risk taking is an essential part of everyday life which enhances independence and choice. Clearly with younger children a judgment on whether the individual is competent to assess the risks for themselves and can accept and bear those risks needs to be made. The greatest challenge is to balance between ensuring that the health and safety of vulnerable children is not put at risk and curtailing their choice, autonomy and independence.

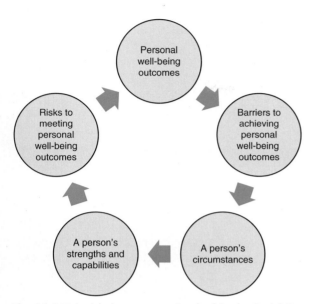

Fig. 15.4 ■ Legislative sequence involved in the Social Services and Well-being (Wales) Act 2014.

The skills, capacity, support and materials available to an individual from within themselves, their family and their community can be marshalled to meet their needs and promote their well-being. It is the function of the assessment to identify these personal resources, enable the individual to make best use of them, and maximise the contribution they make to achieving personal outcomes.

TOWARD A CONTEMPORARY ASSESSMENT PROCESS TO STRUCTURE ASSESSMENTS

Using the Stepwise model as a skeleton (Samra-Tibbett and Raynes, 2003), it can be extended to encapsulate the changing focus towards relationship, strengths-based and outcomes-focused practice into a contemporary assessment wheel (Fig. 15.5).

Outcomes

What outcomes do the child/young person/parents/workers/others feel should be achieved?
What are the barriers to achieving them?

Can resources within the family or externally be deployed to overcome the barriers?

Planning

This is often left out by the professionals as they feel pressured to get on with the task. This may be safe where they work together on a regular basis but is more concerning where they have never worked together beforehand. There needs to be a careful look at the information held already and what still needs to be gathered. There needs to be some agreement on channels of communication, as it is unrealistic for the social worker to expect to know everything at every stage of the process.

Issues to Keep in Mind When Starting Your Assessment – Supporting Reflective Practice

A thorough approach to assessment needs to take account of some key questions:

- What is getting in the way of this child or young person's well-being?
- Do I have all the information I need to help this child or young person?
- What can I do now to help this child or young person?
- What can my agency do to help this child or young person?
- What additional help, if any, may be needed from others?

Source of the risk:

- Who or what presents the danger/threat to the child's well-being?
- Where does the abuse occur – at home and/or in the wider community?
- What is the level of intent – is the abuse an act of commission or omission?
- Is the harm isolated to a single event or cumulative, reflecting more than one risk factor?
- What is the actual or likely impact of any harm?

Capacity of the parent/carer to effect the necessary changes:

- Does the parent have insight into self, child and the circumstances?
- Is there a shared understanding of professional concern/s by the family?

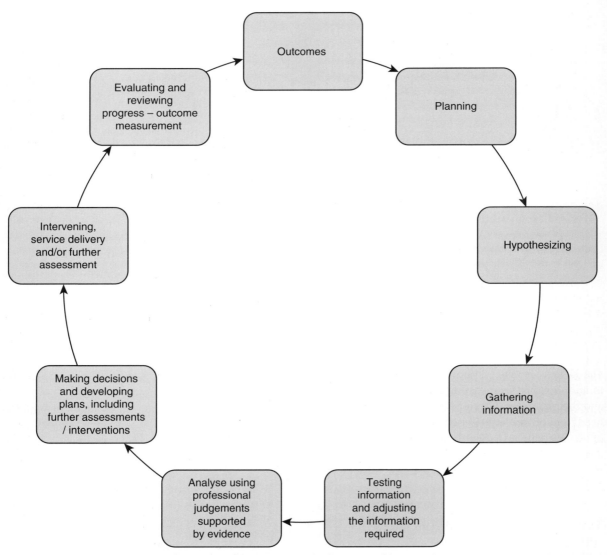

Fig. 15.5 ■ The assessment wheel. (From Calder, 2015.)

- What is the parents/carers understanding of the need for change – is change possible?
- Do they sincerely want to change?
- Are they able and willing to work with services to effect change?
- Do we have the resources to help address needs/ risk(s) and to build child and family resiliencies?
- How long is it likely to take to effect change?
- Can they maintain the change required?

These questions must assist us in planning the assessment – how we will gather enough information to be able to confidently answer them. We must then review the questions as we progress through to complete the assessment.

It is critical that the child is seen and that the objectives in seeing the child are clear:

- Record and evaluate her/his appearance, demeanour, mood state and behaviour
- Hear the child's account of allegations or concerns
- Observe and record the interactions of the child and her/his carers

- See and record the circumstances in which the child is currently living and sleeping and, if different, her/his ordinary residence
- Evaluate the physical safety of the environment including the storage of hazardous substances, (e.g. bleach, drugs)
- Ensure that any other children who need to be seen are identified
- Assess the degree of risk and possible need for protective action
- Meet the child's needs for information and reassurance

Seeing life from the child's point of view is critical. Messages from inquiries and Ofsted inspections include that the child was not seen frequently enough by the professionals involved or was not asked about their views and feelings (Calder, 2020b); agencies did not listen to adults who tried to speak on behalf of the child and who had important information to contribute; parents and carers prevented professionals from seeing and listening to the child; practitioners focused too much on the needs of the parents, especially on vulnerable parents, and overlooked the implications for the child; and agencies did not interpret their findings well enough to protect the child.

CLOSER LOOK: HYPOTHESIZING

This is defined in the dictionary as 'a starting point for an investigation'. There is evidence to show that workers sometimes begin the assessment with one hypothesis and gather evidence to support this. This can be dangerous as it forms a conclusion before the assessment has begun. The workers should consider all possible hypotheses, be open minded in gathering evidence and prioritise hypotheses only where there is clear evidence to do so. They need to take a step back from the early intervention in order to generate the maximum number of possibilities, so as not to shut down any avenue prematurely. The initial hypothesis is necessarily speculative and is used as the basis for gathering more information that will either confirm or refute it. It should embrace positive as well as negative possibilities. It should consider any available history and chronology to look at patterns and processes, as well as entertaining the possibility of change, and whether this is short- or long-term.

It is important to plan to include the children and this could include:

- How well do you know the child and to what extent do you know their views, wishes and feelings? This includes describing your relationship with them, how you think they perceive you, how often you have seen them and in what context – where and who else was present?
- Which adults (including professionals) know the child best? What is their relationship like, how well-placed are they to represent the child's views, what do they think are the child's key concerns and views?
- What opportunities does the child have to express their views to trusted or 'safe' adults? Does the child know how to access people? What would be the barriers, and what has been done to overcome any barriers and to ensure they know where to go if they want to talk to someone?
- How (if at all) has the child defined the problems in their family/life and the effects that the problems are having on them? This includes the child's perceptions and fears, and what they themselves perceive as the primary causes of pain, distress and fear. What opportunities has the child had to explore them?
- Has the child shared information, their views or feelings? In what circumstances has this occurred, and what, if anything, did they want to happen? This should only be stated if known and can be clearly demonstrated. Assumptions should not be made about a child's motivations for communicating something, nor should assumptions be made about their perceptions, views and wishes.
- What has been observed regarding the child's way of relating and responding to key adults such as parents and foster carers? Does this raise concerns about attachments? This would include describing any differences in the way the child presents with different people or in different contexts. Where conclusions are being drawn about a child's attachment, the reasons for such conclusions should be clearly demonstrated.
- What is your understanding of the research evidence in relation to the experiences this child is thought to have had and how they might affect them? For example, what are the likely or possible impacts on children who experience neglect, substance misuse, domestic violence, parental mental health, parental alcohol or substance misuse? This includes a consideration of potential harm, citing vulnerabilities along with resilience factors.

■ What communication methods have been employed in seeking the views, feelings and wishes of the child and to what extent have these optimized the child's opportunity to express their views? This includes consideration of whether equipment, facilitators, interpreters, the use of signs or symbols, play or story books could be helpful and whether the child's preferences are known.

■ How confident are you that you have been able to establish the child's views, feelings and wishes as far as is reasonable and possible for the child? This would include consideration of things that may have hindered such communication such as pressure from adults, time limitations, language barriers or lack of trust in the child-social worker relationship. How much sense are you able to make of the information you have?

Gathering Information

There is a tendency to gather too much information, which we need to guard against, as well as gathering irrelevant information. We may modify our original hypothesis many times as the new information is gathered from the family. It is not necessary to wait for a definitive hypothesis before intervening, as many times only the interventions themselves produce crucial information. Since the major purpose of a hypothesis is to make connections, how information is gathered is extremely important. The worker must take a neutral position and try not to imply any moral judgements or to align themselves with any one faction of the family. Change often comes about through the worker's ability to stand outside the family and gain a holistic view. The intervention is then geared at the most relevant of the presenting problems. In gathering information, it is helpful to keep the following questions in mind:

■ What function does the symptom serve in stabilising the family?
■ How does the family function in stabilising the symptom?
■ What is the central theme around which the problem is organised?
■ What will be the consequences of change?

Testing Information and Adjusting the Information Required

Different professionals will come together with information around levels of risk and potential and targets for change, and there needs to be some analysis about what evidence there is to either support or refute their views. Strategies for achieving change or the management of risk in the interim do need to be agreed, as do areas where gaps exist, and further information may need to be gathered. The following risk assessment checklist is helpful in identifying areas for testing out the information, and which leads us into the next block around deciding on the probability of future harm:

■ What is the nature of the concern?
■ What is the category of abuse?
■ Check out how your own attitudes and values will affect your responses.
■ Are there racial, cultural, linguistic or other issues that need consideration?
■ Are the injuries/incidents acute/cumulative/episodic?
■ When and how is the child at risk?
■ Did the injuries/incidents result from spontaneous actions, neglect or intent?
■ What are the parents/carers attitudes and response to your concerns? Explore why you think this is.
■ Is their explanation consistent with the injury/incident? If not, why not?
■ What does the child mean to the family? In what sense?
■ What are the child's views/needs/wishes?
■ What is the potential for change in the family?
■ Are incidents/injuries likely to reoccur?
■ How safe is the child? What are the possibilities? What is the probability? How imminent is the likely risk? How grave are the likely consequences? (Calder, 2003b)

Analysing Using Professional Judgements Supported by Evidence

Analysis involves the process of breaking down what is known about the complexity of a child and family's circumstances into smaller parts, to acquire a better overall understanding of what is or may be going on ('what is this information telling me?'). It requires consideration of the quality and character of the information collected, which is then sorted, weighted in terms of its significance and ultimately made sense of. Informed analysis will not only help determine the nature of current circumstances but also the potential likelihood of an event or series of events occurring/recurring.

Through the good use of analysis, practitioners may reach a more informed and insightful position whereby they can competently and confidently convey what it all means for the individual child, the adult carer(s), and the various relationships between each, as well as the services involved. Analysis should, thus, provide practitioners with a clearer picture of circumstances and inform future interventions that address need and manage/reduce risk for children and families.

Making sense of complex family and social situations is not an easy task. Analysis demands a thorough investigative approach on the part of practitioners, and it requires that they forensically and systematically examine circumstances and events to help understand:

- Why they may have arisen – the reasons, triggers, history?
- What they mean for the individuals and others involved – their significance and impact?
- How, if possible, they may be addressed – how best to manage, minimise and resolve?

Practitioners, therefore, need to reflect critically on all information gathered – its source, credibility, integrity, validity, whether it corroborates, challenges or contradicts the current assessment and analysis. They also need to be aware of any potential for bias and the difficulties of working solely based on information that is contested. Key consideration also needs to be given to the abilities of the parent/carer to protect, the known resilience and protective factors to and around the child that may help to better protect them, the impact of the identified risk factors on the child's future safety, and the capacity of the parents to effect any necessary changes in the timeframe commensurate with the child's age and development.

The Assessment Framework has a further checklist for the analytical stage:

- Is the assessment providing adequate evidence to analyse before making judgements leading to decisions about future actions?
- Is the worker distinguishing between fact and opinion?
- Is there reasonable cause to suspect that a child is suffering, or is likely to suffer, from significant harm?

- Has the assessment revealed significant unmet needs for support and services?
- If the decision is not to provide services, this is itself a decision. What is the next step?
- Is the worker able to evaluate evidence drawing on their understanding of theory, for example, child development?
- Is the worker drawing on knowledge of research?
- Is the worker informing the family (including the children) of the outcome and recommendations arising from the assessment?
- Is the supervisor ensuring that rigour and challenge form part of their supervision?
- Is the supervisor able to ask questions, to challenge and probe where necessary? This may mean asking obvious or unpopular questions.
- Is the supervisor encouraging both factual analysis and reflective practice?
- Is the supervisor able to address the areas of potential impact on the worker?
- Is there a supervisory agreement in place that allows for constructive challenge and feedback?
- Is the supervisor evaluating how the worker is currently making judgements?
- What is given priority and why?
- Which factors are marginalized and why?
- Which factors are causing most discussion and debate in terms of determining priority and why?
- What is this saying about their current practice?

(The Child's World: DoH, NSPCC and the University of Sheffield, 2000)

Calder (2017) developed an assessment questionnaire to mould use of the domains of the assessment framework (Fig. 15.6).

Important Areas to Look Out for When Carrying Out an Assessment

Serious incident case reviews repeatedly describe 'warning signs' that agencies have failed to recognise or take account of, or that should have acted as indicators that children and young people were at risk of serious harm. Examples include:

- Children and young people might be hidden from view; they are 'unavailable' when professionals visit the family.

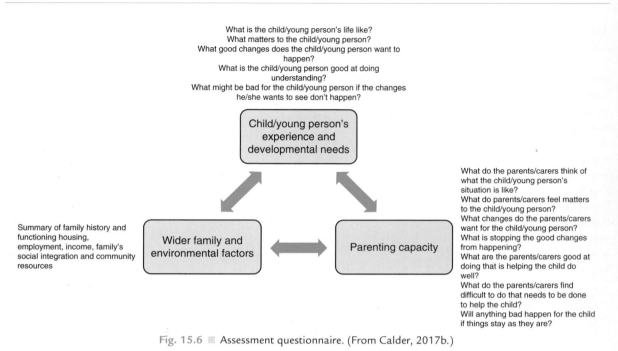

What is the child/young person's life like?
What matters to the child/young person?
What good changes does the child/young person want to happen?
What is the child/young person good at doing understanding?
What might be bad for the child/young person if the changes he/she wants to see don't happen?

Child/young person's experience and developmental needs

What do the parents/carers think of what the child/young person's situation is like?
What do parents/carers feel matters to the child/young person?
What changes do the parents/carers want for the child/young person?
What is stopping the good changes from happening?
What are the parents/carers good at doing that is helping the child do well?
What do the parents/carers find difficult to do that needs to be done to help the child?
Will anything bad happen for the child if things stay as they are?

Summary of family history and functioning housing, employment, income, family's social integration and community resources

Wider family and environmental factors

Parenting capacity

Fig. 15.6 ■ Assessment questionnaire. (From Calder, 2017b.)

- Children and young people who might be prevented from attending school or nursery or accessing healthcare or other services.
- Parents who do not cooperate with services, fail to take their children to routine health appointments and/or discourage professionals from visiting.
- Parents who appear to cooperate but do so only in a superficial manner.
- Parents who are consistently hostile and aggressive towards professionals and might threaten violence.
- Children and young people who are in emotional or physical distress but might be unable to verbalise this.
- Children and young people who are in physical pain (possibly from an injury) might be told to sit or stand in a certain way when professionals visit the family or might hide or otherwise disguise injuries.
- Children and young people who have gone missing/run away (with or without their families).

Concerns relating to actual or potential harm should never be ignored and are an indication that immediate intervention might be needed to ensure the protection of the child from future harm. The critical role of inter-agency chronologies to promote accumulative prospective harm is a very important option for workers. This is enhanced considerably when there are evidence-informed indicators that guide workers to the relevant information to include.

Making Decisions and Developing Plans, Including Further Assessments/ Interventions

This is where workers are asked to make decisions for the longer-term child protection plan. This requires them to review the way forward and may well include the potential for change within both the perpetrator and his family; the viability and focus of the necessary work; any mandate needed; any relaxation of contact restrictions and any family reconstitution. The assessment needs to move beyond the changes required to identifying whether change is possible and what motivation exists for change. Accompanying this must be some hope of reaching the goal, an ability to consider what has gone wrong and some opportunity for change in the situation. The plan should clearly set out the key outcomes that are required for the child, and all actions must be separately identified and linked to individual needs/risks. The plan should be set out in a systematic way that is achievable, accountable and accessible for all parties involved, including the child/family. Risk management planning must also be subject to regular review, which, where statutory involvement is present, will reflect statutory review requirements and timeframes where these exist.

Intervening, Service Delivery and/or Further Assessment

There should be a link between the decisions and plans and the availability of the identified resources. This may well be a source of tension and frustration where gaps and/or significant delays exist and pressures to dilute any resources strongly resisted. Sometimes plans struggle to be SMART where there is no clarity on the pull and pull combination of presenting issues, often seen in the dual disorder debate. Specialist or more specific and deep-dive assessments are frequently indicated in multi-problem scenarios.

Evaluating and Reviewing Progress – Outcome Measurement

It is important to establish what has worked and why. It is also important for workers to cross-check the outcomes formulated at the outset and examine which have been well met, why some may be met partially and why others may not have materialized. It is only with this information can workers and families understand what works and incorporate this into practice elsewhere.

Explicitly Reclaiming a Risk Assessment Dimension to Assessment Practice Across All Agencies

The following offer an explicit preliminary structure to wrap around the assessment triangle to ensure the focus is on child protection where necessary.

The Alleged Harm/Risk of Harm

- Circumstances and type of current harm – specific harm or multiple harms?
- Frequency/chronicity – the number of incidents, any pattern, is harm escalating?
- Severity – will the harm/risk of harm result in death, extensive injury, lasting significant damage, impact on child's development? Has severity increased over time?
- Recency and duration – when did incident/s occur? How long have any concerns been held?
- Likelihood of harm occurring in the future. Could impacts lead to significant harm?
- History – are there previous incidents of harm/previous allegations for similar issues/different issues? Repeated referrals to the department through both child concern report and notifications?
- If siblings, are there previous child protection concerns relating to them?
- Source of notifications – multiple sources alleging similar concerns/reports from professionals?
- If the harm is physical, describe the injury and location of the injury (for example, what part of the child's body). Describe any implements used to inflict the injury
- If the harm is emotional, detail statements made to the child, actions and circumstances, and behavioural indicators displayed by the child
- If the harm is sexual, determine access to the child by alleged person responsible
- If the harm is a result of neglect, include details of parental action/inaction and the resulting harms/conditions and risk of harms/conditions
- If harm is yet to occur, examine any risk factors
- Identity of alleged person/s responsible and relationship to child – more than one person responsible? Does the source of harm increase child's vulnerability to other persons responsible?
- Where relevant, what has been the previous pattern in relation to placement and reunification?

The Child

- Age of child – vulnerability and reliance on parent to meet all needs?
- Immediate safety of child – current whereabouts
- Culture and ethnicity – related child rearing factors, need for interpreter
- Disclosure (any statements made by the child about the alleged harm)
- Child's physical appearance – injuries and location, general – stature, hygiene
- Health and medical needs/issues – including infant prematurity, low birth weight, fetal alcohol syndrome, chemical dependency
- Special needs (includes intellectual/physical disabilities and developmental delays, e.g. Asperger's syndrome)
- Child's behaviour (for example, emotional or behavioural problems such as bed wetting, running away, self-harm, cruelty to children/pets, hypervigilance, school problems)
- Education – including attention/learning difficulties, disengagement, truancy
- Involvement with other services/community agencies/childcare/school
- Child's relationship with parents – level of attachment (secure/safe, insecure/avoidant/ambivalent/disorganized)
- Child's relationship with others – siblings, peers, carers – and quality of interactions/attachments
- Previous history of respite/out of home care placements
- Strengths and resiliency – coping mechanisms, identified support network, socially active, self-esteem and identity, life skills appropriate to age

The Parents

- Attitude, acknowledgment of and response to harm (for example, had medical treatment been sought?)
- Explanation of harm – is it consistent with the facts?
- Attachment to child and quality of relationship
- Perceptions and feelings about the child, expectations of the child
- Age and maturity of parents
- Any known child protection history during pregnancy – unborn child concerns
- Level of care provided to the child
- Previous requests for respite/placements
- Parenting patterns – discipline techniques
- Parent's own history of childhood abuse
- Relationship with alleged primary person responsible (if not the person responsible)
- Impediments to the parent's ability to act protectively (consider both in-home and out-of-home harm situations) – including court orders
- Domestic and family violence – is the child exposed to, or otherwise involved in, violent incidents in the home between household members?
- Substance misuse – current or historical use of alcohol/drugs, impacts of use on functioning/parenting; and details of any treatment received
- Mental health problems – including past or current treatment
- Physical/intellectual disability
- Criminal history as adult/youth justice history – e.g. assault/cruelty/substance misuse
- Stressors – financial, health, isolation, unemployment, accommodation, loss and grief issues, family law disputes, pregnancy
- Strengths and resiliency – supportive relationships (intra- and extrafamilial), emotional stability, self-awareness, ability to access resources, achievements
- Religious/spiritual beliefs and considerations for parenting practices
- Culture and ethnicity – related child rearing factors, need for interpreter

Social, Environmental, and Cultural Influences and Networks

- Presence of a person able **and** willing to protect the child
- Access to the child by the alleged person responsible/exposure to harm
- Physical environment (condition of the child's home – safe/hazards?)
- Household composition and quality of relationships including age and number of children in family
- Does the family receive supportive intervention from other agencies (counselling and community support agencies), have contact with other professionals (police, health, education)?
- Social environment/isolation – is the child/parent able to access out-of-home supports?
- Ability to access infrastructure – transport, schools, childcare, parks
- Mobility of family – housing related issues
- Financial/economic security, employment, income
- Cultural and ethnic influences – ability to maintain positive links in a respectful community environment; beliefs impacting on parenting

CASE STUDY 15.1: ASSESSMENT CHALLENGE

Social care received a referral indicating that a 7-year-old daughter was reported missing by her mother. Enquiries indicated that she was one of three children. The child was found within the hour, and it was concluded that it was the child playing hide and seek and the mother overreacted because she was new to the area and did not know her way around.

The mother did accept she was isolated and wanted to connect with people to support her settling into the new area. The move was driven by a wish to secure better private rented accommodation for her children with some garden space. The outcomes were seen as supportive and educational, and the children wanted to settle into schools and make friends.

Planning involved considering the additional needs of the 9-year-old whose behaviour was challenging his mother and also upsetting his siblings. It also involved educating the family about the known risk factors in the area – a busy motorway behind the house and also a probation hostel with known sex offenders' resident.

Workers did start to express some concerns about the mother's fluctuating engagement and the children not attending nursery or school on an increasingly regular basis. Whilst accepting the move was to secure a better base for the children to live, workers wanted to consider other reasons why they had moved. Could it be to avoid action in the previous authority? Were there problems in the adult relationships? Where was the children's father? And nothing was known about the extended family or friendship network.

Information was collected to test out these possible hypotheses, and it soon became clear that the mother had left a violent relationship as social care were concerned about the impact on the children that may trigger child protection concerns. A pattern of engaging with professionals to secure her own goals was established, and there were also concerns that the children had been tutored about what to say when spoken to by professionals. The presenting incident was also part of a longer pattern of concerns about neglect.

Information collection also indicated mother's health problems, and this included an alcohol dependency that seems to be connected to her exposure to domestic abuse. She was defined as vulnerable and needy in her own right, and her needs often outweighed those of the children.

The 9-year old was missing appointments with CAHMS, and his skin condition remained untreated. The 7-year old was popular at school but isolated at home. She was expected to care for her younger 3-year-old sister and take her to and from nursery.

Developmental checks indicated that all children remained broadly on target. The youngest children were very protective of their mother and adamant they would not be happy living elsewhere. They did not like their father or mum's last partner who they saw occasionally around the local shops. The eldest child presented with significant needs in their own right and struggled with being expected to help his mum when she was under the influence or exhausted.

Whilst they live in the same home, the impact on them individually was different. They required different responses, and this needed further exploration.

Any assessment only has a shelf-life for as long as the circumstances remain the same, and workers received information that the children were now refusing to go to school and that the mother was pregnant again and refusing to attend antenatal appointments or be seen by her GP despite her mental health becoming more unstable and her new partner being very controlling. Both the mother and the children had been seen with multiple bruises and were now evading all professional contact. The house was being used by known local drug dealers and users, and there was a deterioration in the house and its environs. The maternal grandparents have advised they will act as a monitor of the home situation as best they can and will not let their grandchildren be affected. Social care records indicate concerns about their parenting history including relevant convictions. The parents and grandparents refuse consent to use their history as part of the assessment and want no support at the present time. How does this change the focus of the assessment? For which child(ren)? Does the risk element need consideration using their history? Or should we simply walk away and await a call from the grandparents if concerns emerge?

REFLECTIVE QUESTIONS

- What are the pros and cons of starting and ending assessments with outcomes and planning?
- Which assessment challenges are in worker and manager's control and which are not?
- What are the differences between a strengths-based approach and a risk assessment approach other than the words used?
- Name five key elements that are required to translate a good assessment into a meaningful analysis and a connected plan.
- What do workers need to focus on to capture the child's lived experience?

CONCLUSION

The chapter has attempted to balance the challenges with the correctives as we strive to retain a child-focus throughout, and the enhancement of outcomes is key to helping repair any damage experienced as well as optimizing their individual potential. Workers do need to move from a standardized straitjacket to a more individually tailored approach that works around the presenting issues rather than against them. This is key to working genuinely alongside children and families, as well as fellow professionals, and pulling in the same direction. Assessment is the backbone of all our practice, and considerable reflection is required to ensure we embrace what works as well as jettisoning what does not work. The centrality of supervision in this process cannot be understated (Calder, 2020c).

REFERENCES

Calder MC (1995). Child Protection: Balancing paternalism and partnership. Br J Soc Work 25 (6): 749–766.

Calder, M.C., 2003a. The assessment framework: A critique and reformulation. In: Calder, M.C., Hackett, S. (Eds.), Assessment in Childcare: Using and Developing Frameworks for Practice. Russell House Publishing, Dorset, pp. 3–60.

Calder, M.C., 2003b. A Generic Framework for Conducting Risk Assessments. Keynote Presentation to a One-Day National Conference 'Risk Assessment: Developing and Enhancing Evidence-Based Practice'. TUC Congress Centre, London.

Calder, M.C., 2004. The integrated children's system: Out of the frying pan and into the fire? Child Care Pract 10 (3), 225–240.

Calder MC (ed.) (2008). Contemporary risk assessment in safeguarding children. Dorset: Russell House Publishing.

Calder MC, Sneddon R & McKinnon M (2012) Risk Assessment toolkit. Edinburgh: Scottish Executive.

Calder, M.C., 2012. Assessment: Contextual Challenges. OLM Briefing Paper.

Calder, M.C., 2015. Complex Assessments Masterclass. Thackley Hospital, Leeds.

Calder, M.C., 2016. Risk in Child Protection: Assessment Challenges and Frameworks for Practice. Jessica Kingsley, London.

Calder, M.C., 2017. Effective assessments in child care proceedings. In: Dixon, L., Perkins, D., Craig, L.A., Hamilton-Giachritsis, C. (Eds.), What Works in Child Protection: An Evidenced-Based Approach to Assessment and Intervention in Care Proceedings. Wiley-Blackwell, London.

Calder, M.C., 2017b. MARAF: Multi-agency Risk Assessment Framework. Calder Training and Consultancy Limited, Leigh.

Calder, M.C., 2020a. SRAF. Calder Training and Consultancy Limited, Lowton.

Calder, M.C., 2020b. Paralysis in Childcare Analysis: Causes, Consequences and Correctives. RHP, Dorset.

Calder, M.C., 2020c. Paralysis to Analysis in Childcare Work: A Workbook to Guide Frontline Workers. Calder Training & Consultancy Limited, Lowton.

Care Act 2014. https://www.legislation.gov.uk/ukpga/2014/23/contents/enacted.

Children and Families Act 2014. https://www.legislation.gov.uk/ukpga/2014/6/contents/enacted.

Department of Health, et al., 2000. Framework for the Assessment of Children in Need and Their Families. HMSO, London.

Equality Act (2010). https://www.legislation.gov.uk/ukpga/2010/15/contents.

Horwath, J., Lees, J., 2010. Assessing the influence of religious beliefs and practices on parenting capacity: The challenges for social work practitioners. Br J Soc Work 40 (1), 82–99.

Human Rights Act 1998. https://www.legislation.gov.uk/ukpga/1998/42/contents.

Munro, E., 2011. The Munro Review of Child Protection: Final Report, a Child-Centred System. The Stationery Office, London.

Samra-Tibbets, C., and Raynes, B., 1999. Assessment and planning. In Calder, M.C., and Horwath, J., (Eds.) Working for Children on the Child Protection Register: An Inter-agency Practice Guide. Aldershot: Arena, 81–117.

Scottish Government, 2010. Using the National Practice Model II: Gathering Information with the My World Triangle. 1st ed. [ebook] Edinburgh: Scottish Government.

The Rights of Children. https://www.ohchr.org/en/instruments-mechanisms/instruments/convention-rights-child.

The Rights of Persons with Disabilities. https://www.ohchr.org/en/instruments-mechanisms/instruments/convention-rights-persons-disabilities.

The Child's World, 1999. The Child's World: Assessing Children in Need Training and Development Pack. NSPCC, London.

16

CHILD PROTECTION LEGISLATION IN EMERGENCY SITUATIONS

KIM HOLT

KEY POINTS

- Emergency protection orders.
- Police protection orders.
- Alternative ways of handling emergencies: voluntary accommodation.

INTRODUCTION

Working with children and their families who are in crisis is arguably one of the most complex areas of work, even more so when in emergency situations. Although rare, there are circumstances where professionals need to intervene urgently in a child's life. Whenever such an intervention is considered, following the letter of the law and only acting in ways which the law permits are of utmost importance. Under article 8 of the Human Rights Act 1998 'Everyone has the right to respect for his private and family life [...] There shall be no interference by a public body with the exercise of this rights except such as is in accordance with the law.' Failing to act in accordance with the law when taking urgent action to protect a child would risk breaching the parents' and/or child's Human Rights.

This chapter therefore outlines the overarching legislative processes that govern emergency interventions in child protection. It also draws upon case law to provide further guidance on how to interpret and apply the law in practice.

CLOSER LOOK: THE ROLE AND FUNCTION OF CASE LAW

Case law (or judicial precedent) is law made by the courts and decided by judges. Judicial precedent operates under the principle of stare decisis which literally means 'to stand by decisions'.

Case law provides a record as to important disputes and disagreements in the application of the guidelines and provides guidance as to how to interpret and apply the guidelines going forward.

The chapter begins by introducing emergency applications. It then focusses more specifically on emergency protection orders (s. 44, Children Act (CA), 1989), powers of police protection (s. 46, CA, 1989) and then concludes by considering alternative ways of handling emergencies (via s. 20, CA, 1989). Importantly, in the absence of police protection (s. 46 CA, 1989) or a court order authorizing removal (s. 44 CA, 1989) or informed consent of a parent (s. 20 CA, 1989), the local authority is not entitled to remove a child from the care of a parent.

Safeguarding children is the responsibility of all relevant agencies and professionals, although the duty to investigate rests with the Local Authority. When risk to a child is high, this may necessitate action to remove a child from their family pending further assessment. The Courts provide a clear test that must be satisfied before a child is removed from the family. It is therefore imperative that professionals consider this test before any decision is made to remove a child (see Legal Test box).

LEGAL TEST FOR REMOVAL OF A CHILD FROM THEIR FAMILY

Case Law Example

The most recent decision regarding Interim Removal is set out in the following Court of Appeal Authorities in *Re C (A Child: Interim Separation) [2020] EWCA Civ 257* at [2]:

1. An interim order is inevitably made at a stage when the evidence is incomplete. It should therefore only be made in order to regulate matters that cannot await the final hearing, and it is not intended to place any party to the proceedings at an advantage or a disadvantage.
2. The removal of a child from a parent is an interference with their right to respect for family life under Art. 8. Removal at an interim stage is a particularly sharp interference, which is compounded in the case of a baby when removal will affect the formation and development of the parent–child bond.
3. Accordingly, in all cases an order for separation under an interim care order will only be justified where it is both necessary and proportionate. The lower ('reasonable grounds') threshold for an interim care order is not an invitation to make an order that does not satisfy these exacting criteria.
4. A plan for immediate separation is therefore only to be sanctioned by the court where the child's physical safety or psychological or emotional welfare demands it and where the length and likely consequences of the separation are a proportionate response to the risks that would arise if it did not occur.
5. The high standard of justification that must be shown by a local authority seeking an order for separation requires it to inform the court of all available resources that might remove the need for separation.

For the purposes of his decision in this case, the judge summarised it this way:

The test is whether the child's safety is at risk and, if so, any removal should be proportionate to the actual risks faced and in the knowledge of alternative arrangements which would not require separation.

In determining any application for interim removal, the court will apply the test in *Re C*. We will return to this point throughout the chapter.

EMERGENCY PROTECTION ORDERS

Emergency Protection Orders (EPOs) are covered in Section 44 (1) of the Children Act (1989):

(1) Where any person applies to the court for an order to be made, the order may be made if:
   (a) there is reasonable cause to believe that the child is likely to suffer significant harm if:
      (i) he is not removed to accommodation provided by or on behalf of the applicant; or
      (ii) he does not remain in the place in which he is then being accommodated.

An EPO lasts for 8 days (s. 45(1) CA89); although in exceptional circumstances, this may be renewed for a further 7 days (s. 45(5) CA89). It is important to note that in any application for interim removal of a child, the Court will apply the test in *Re C*, (see Legal Test box); a plan of removal will only be agreed by the Court if the child is at imminent risk of very serious harm and removal is both necessary and proportionate.

RESPONSIBILITY FOR TAKING EMERGENCY ACTION

The responsibility for taking emergency action rests with the local authority who encountered the child **(LA 1)** and has cause for belief this is an emergency scenario. If **LA 1 establishes** the child is looked after by, or is the subject of, a child protection plan in another authority **(LA 2)**, **LA 1** should consult **LA 2**. Only when **LA 1** explicitly accepts responsibility in writing is **LA 2** relieved of its responsibility to take emergency action.

The first course of action when considering emergency action is that the child is seen (this should be undertaken by a practitioner from the agency initiating the emergency action, usually the social worker). This is used to decide how best to protect the child and whether an application for an EPO is the most appropriate means of achieving this. One of the grounds for an EPO lies in the duty to investigate under s. 47 Children Act 1989. If during an investigation access to the child is unreasonably refused, the local authority may apply for an EPO (s. 44 (1)(b) CA89).

Following seeing the child (or being unreasonably refused access), the next step is to undertake a strategy discussion or meeting, involving as a minimum the social worker, manager and the police (Working Together, DfE, 2018). This discussion will consider the needs of the specific child, but also the needs of other children in the same household or in the household of an alleged perpetrator. The local authority should always consider whether an application for a child assessment order (s. 43 CA89) is more appropriate if the intention of the local authority is to undertake an assessment.

Accommodation, or rather where the child is going to remain living and with whom whilst an assessment is being undertaken, is perhaps one of the most pressing issues when the local authority is dealing with an emergency. The decision as to whether a child should remain living at home or be 'looked after' for a period will be based on an assessment of risk to the child. In applying the no order principle, the least restrictive option is for the child to remain living at home whilst an assessment is undertaken. The court also has the power to make an exclusion requirement to an EPO (s. 44A CA89): where there is reasonable cause to believe that, if the relevant person is excluded from the child's home:

- The child will not be likely to suffer significant harm or the local authority's s. 47 enquiries will not be threatened.
- There is someone else living there who is able and willing to give the child the care he or she needs.
- The person who will care for the child consents to the order being made.

The court can attach the exclusion requirement where the conditions are met, requiring the named individual to leave the home. The court can accept a formal undertaking from the named person to leave and stay away from the home; alternatively, the court can attach a power of arrest to the order.

When applying for the order, the social worker must have clear plans regarding the duration of the order, where the child should reside and any contact arrangements and with whom before an application is made. The emergency nature of this application is such that the social worker will need to have considered all these issues as within hours the child and his parents/carers will be seeking clarification on what will happen next. The situation will be highly charged and often acrimonious and not having a clear plan will only contribute to further distress for the child and his or her family.

It is good practice, where appropriate and safe to do so, to advise parents or those with parental responsibility to seek immediate legal advice when a decision has been made to apply for an EPO and always when an EPO is served. In exceptional circumstances an EPO may be made without giving notice to the parents (*ex parte*) – the court will allow the application to be made without all parties being in court. The decision to make an *ex parte* application must take account of the rights of the parent(s) as well as the child, although it is the welfare of the child that must remain paramount. The only justifiable reasons for not informing a parent/person with parental responsibility of an intention to make an application for an EPO is if to do so would put the child at further and imminent risk. There are important rules for applications without notice to be found in *Proceedings relating to children except parental order proceedings and proceedings for applications in adoptions placement and related proceedings (Family Procedure Rules (FPR) Part 12).* Where an EPO is made without notice, the applicant must serve a copy of the application on each parent/person with parental responsibility within 48 hours of the emergency order being made, unless the court directs otherwise. If the court refuses to make an order on an application without notice, it may direct that the application is made on notice (i.e. the application is granted, but the parents must be informed), in which case the application will proceed in accordance with r. 12.3 to r. 12.15.

Following the making of an EPO, the local authority remains under an obligation to consider less drastic alternatives to emergency removal. Section 44 imposes a duty on the local authority to keep the case under review daily to ensure the parent and child are separated for no longer than is necessary to secure the child's safety. A parent or person with parental responsibility may apply for a discharge of the EPO after 72 hours, providing that they were not present at the original hearing (r. 12.3). There is also the power to include an exclusion requirement in the EPO (s. 44A(1) CA89) where there is reasonable cause to believe that, if a person is excluded from a dwelling house in which the child lives, the child will not be likely to suffer significant harm (s. 44A(2) CA89). This means that in some circumstances the perpetrator will be removed from the home instead of the child.

Arrangements for 'reasonable contact' during the time the order is in force, required under s. 44(13) CA89, have to be needs-led and not resource-driven. In recent cases before the Court, members of the Judiciary have made it very clear to the local authority that contact arrangements have not been sufficient. Particularly for young children, arrangements for contact should be **no less than three times a week**. There have been numerous examples where local authorities have been advised that the care plan is **insufficient** in respect of arrangements proposed for contact between parents and siblings.

POLICE POWERS OF PROTECTION

There will be situations where the assistance of the police will be required in an emergency to remove a child to a place of safety. The police have to agree, and they need to be satisfied that the following grounds for taking this action are met, under Section 46(1) of the Children Act (1989):

Where a constable has reasonable cause to believe that a child would otherwise be likely to suffer significant harm, he or she may:

CASE STUDY 16.1: USING CASE LAW EXAMPLES - EPOS

Case law examples can help you to see how the law is applied in practice. Use the following case law examples to examine some legal precedents for the use of EPO's in practice.

GUIDING PRINCIPLES OF EPO'S

In the course of setting out a number of guiding principles in relation to EPOs, in *Re X Council v B (Emergency Protection Orders) [2006]*, Munby J held that: 'Separation is only to be contemplated if immediate separation is essential to secure the child's safety: "imminent danger" must be "actually established"'. Furthermore, he added that an application for an EPO should be approached with an anxious awareness of the extreme gravity of the impact of the making of such an order on the rights of both the child and family. Within this, the importance of independent representation to challenge this decision was highlighted in the late appointment of the family court advisor (FCA). It was regarded as unacceptable in an application for an EPO that the appointment of the FCA was **delayed by 10 days**. An EPO was a 'draconian' and 'extremely harsh' measure, requiring 'exceptional justification' and 'extraordinarily compelling reasons'. It should not be made unless the Family Proceedings Court is satisfied that it is both necessary and proportionate and that no other less radical form of order would promote the welfare of the child.

FUTURE HARM

The courts acknowledge that **in some cases removal on the basis on future harm is acceptable**, but **this must be based on the nature and gravity of harm.** The court should always consider the **least restrictive option** before ordering the removal of a child unless there are persuasive reasons to do so, as in the case of *Re O (A Child: Supervision Order: Future Harm) [2001]*. However, the premature removal of a baby based on future risk was severely criticized in *Re C and B (Care Order: Future Harm) [2001]*, and the court found there to be insufficient evidence in this case to warrant such action.

THE ABSENCE OF KNOWLEDGE

The absence of knowledge should never be the basis for the making of an EPO, nor should cases of either emotional abuse, sexual abuse or fabricated illness without specific evidence of immediate and direct risk of physical harm to the child. The case was followed in *Re X: Emergency Protection Orders* [2006] with further directions for emergency orders.

- Remove the child to suitable accommodation and keep him there; or
- Take such steps as are reasonable to ensure that the child's removal from any hospital, or other place, in which he is then being accommodated is prevented.

There is clear guidance provided to the police on how to exercise their powers (College of Policing, 2022). Police protection lasts for a maximum period of 72 hours (s. 46(6) CA89) and must be terminated as soon as the danger to the child has passed (s. 46(5) CA89). The police must take reasonable steps to inform the child, their parents, anyone else who has parental responsibility and the person the child was living with at the time of the removal of the action taken, the reason for it and the next stage (s. 46(4) CA89). The police officers' duties are to inform the local authority where the child is found and of where he ordinarily resides if the two are different (s. 46(3)(a)–(b) CA89). The police must also 'take such steps as are reasonably practicable to discover the wishes and feelings of the child' (s. 46(3)(d) CA89).

Police protection immediately triggers the duty to investigate (s. 47 CA89), which will involve the local authority considering whether to continue with the order and undertake an assessment of where the child should reside whilst any further assessments are being undertaken. If it is necessary and proportionate to either keep in or remove a child to a place of safety, a local authority should, wherever possible, and unless a child's safety is otherwise at immediate risk, apply for an EPO. Police powers to remove a child in an emergency should be used only in exceptional circumstances where there is insufficient time to seek an EPO, or for reasons relating to the immediate safety of the child (DoH, 2000, para. 5.51).

CLOSER LOOK: KEY CONSIDERATIONS WHEN CONSIDERING EMERGENCY INTERVENTIONS

1. Whether there is reasonable justification for an order interfering with the child's right to family life.
2. If there are any concerns, the court and local authority should take the least restrictive approach with alternatives explored before the option of removal taken. The local authority needs to consider whether there is clear established evidence of immediate risk of really serious harm or imminent danger, which cannot be reduced without removal of the child.
3. The court needs to be satisfied that the parents have been properly involved in the decision-making of the local authority or afforded the proper opportunity to make their case before a decision is made.
4. There may be extraordinarily compelling reasons which justify the removal of a child under an EPO.
5. An order for the assessment of a child is not in itself sufficient justification for removal.
6. Evidence in support of the removal of a child must be full, detailed, precise and compelling.
7. There need to be clear and detailed proposals for contact arrangements between the child and their parents.
8. The court will need all relevant documents, including child protection conference minutes, and will need to be satisfied that the parents have seen all relevant documents.
9. The court will seek evidence that the local authority has carried out a meaningful assessment of the family and the conclusions of the assessment. Where the local authority has not been able to obtain agreement to work with the family, the local authority will need to produce evidence of any attempts to obtain agreement from the parents. Refusal to cooperate with an assessment will not by itself justify the making of an EPO if other options can be employed and it is reasonable and safe to do so.

ALTERNATIVE WAYS OF HANDLING AN EMERGENCY (S. 20 CHILDREN ACT 1989)

If initial assessments indicate the child(ren) should be looked after for a short period outside of the family home, and there are no other relatives/friends who are able to fulfil this role, providing the person with parental responsibility for the child consents, the local authority can provide temporary and/or emergency accommodation under Section 20 of the Children Act (1989):

(1) Every local authority shall provide accommodation for any child in need within their area who

appears to them to require accommodation as a result of:

a. there being no person who has parental responsibility for him;

b. his being lost or having been abandoned;

c. or the person who has been caring for him being prevented (whether or not permanently, and for whatever reason) from providing him with suitable accommodation or care.

A looked after child may either be a child who is subject to a care order and the local authority has parental responsibility, or a child who is *accommodated* and parents retain parental responsibility. Although the route into being a looked after child may be significantly different, during the period they are looked after they will be entitled to regular reviews and, in both sets of circumstances, be visited by a social worker.

Diverting cases away from court with the use of s. 20 CA89 to accommodate a child may appear consistent with the principle of partnership working under the CA89 in achieving consensual solutions, but the parents may not have the opportunity to challenge the local authority and indeed may agree to accommodation rather than face the risk of a care order being made. Importantly, if used to either divert or resolve cases without judicial oversight, the evidence may never be properly challenged, and this may introduce additional delay for children. One study found that in nearly all cases children had at some stage been

---

CASE STUDY 16.2: USING CASE LAW EXAMPLES - THE MISUSE OF SECTION 20s

Common concerns about the misuses of Section 20s include excessively long use of Section 20 prior to care proceedings, pressuring parents to sign Section 20s, not explaining parental rights under Section 20 and obtaining Section 20s from parents lacking capacity. Use the following case law example to examine some of the case law regarding this practice.

CONSULTING PARENTS

In *Re G (Care: Challenge to Local Authority's Decision) [2003]*, Munby J held: '*The fact that a local authority has parental responsibility for children pursuant to s. 33(3)(a) of the Children Act 1989 does not entitle it to take decisions about children without reference to, or over the heads of the children's parents*'. In this case, Munby stated that the local authority **should not be entitled to remove a child without firstly properly consulting and involving the parent in the decision-making process**. Whilst it was acknowledged that the local authority had parental responsibility for the child, the parent **also shared parental responsibility**, and this should be **acknowledged and respected**.

PRECLUDE TO CARE PROCEEDINGS

In the case of *Re N (Children) (Adoption: Jurisdiction) [2015] EWCA Civ 1112*, paragraph 157, the President had been **critical of the use of section 20**. He stated: '*Section 20 may, in an appropriate case, have a proper role to play as a short-term measure pending the commencement of care proceedings, but the use of section 20 as a prelude to care proceedings for a period as long as here is wholly unacceptable. It is, in my judgment, and I use the phrase advisedly and deliberately, a misuse by the local authority of its statutory powers*'. The President re-stated the point he raised at paragraph 158 in *Re A (A Child), Darlington Borough Council v M [2015] EWFC 11*, para 100: '*There is, I fear, far too much misuse and abuse of section 20 and this can no longer be tolerated*'. **Section 20s should therefore not be used to replace care proceedings as a quick way for Local Authorities to remove children in favour of going through the appropriate procedures.**

UNACCEPTABLE USES OF SECTION 20S

The following are some examples of where Section 20s have clearly been misused by Local Authorities:

- *Re P (A Child: Use of S.20 CA 1989) [2014]*
- *Gloucestershire County Council v M and C [2015]*
- *Re AS (Unlawful Removal of a Child) [2015]*

accommodated under s. 20, *and* this had built in delay to the permanency planning for these children (Holt et al., 2013). Increasing attention is being paid by the judiciary to the misuse of Section 20s in practice.

Despite concerns about the misuse of Section 20s outlined previously, following increased judicial attention the message received by legal and social work professionals was to avoid the use of Section 20. In response, a number of commentators, including Masson (2017), have suggested that the use of Section 20 has been a source of support for families and is not a tactic to introduce delay for the child. Masson describes such judgments as disruptive with the intention to impact on practice. Whilst there are undoubtedly examples of where the use of Section 20 has been unacceptable, there are considerably more examples of where Section 20 has been used entirely appropriately and in the child's best interests.

Therefore, in summary, reflecting on the work of Packman et al. (1986) that pre-dates the CA89, but nevertheless raised questions about the voluntary accommodation of children in the context of child protection practice, whilst there may be good reasons for local authorities to accommodate children under s. 20 CA89, there is a need to regularly review these placements to ensure they continue to meet the needs of the child.

CONCLUSION

This chapter has outlined the appropriate steps to take in situations wherein children need emergency intervention to keep them safe. This is never the ideal approach; however, it is at times an unavoidable aspect of child protection work. This chapter has discussed the three core ways of taking emergency action: Emergency Protection Orders (s. 44, CA89), Powers of Police Protection (s.46 CA89) and Voluntary Accommodation (s. 20, CA89).

It is difficult to consider the future in the family court arena without first taking account of the immense pressure placed on the courts during the COVID-19 pandemic. In May 2022, The Children and Family Court Advisory and Support Service (Cafcass, 2022) report that there are currently 34,384 open active children's cases, which is 4248 (14.1%) more children's cases compared to March 2020 (at the start of the COVID-19 pandemic). These children's cases

involve 55,865 children. Compared to March 2020, there were 1627 *additional* open active children's cases in public law (13.5% increase) and 2621 *additional* open active children's cases in private law (14.5% increase). The implications for practitioners cannot be underestimated. The global pandemic that commenced in March 2020 has resulted in unprecedented challenges for both social workers and the Courts. The number of children and parents who are reporting mental health difficulties has increased significantly, with no corresponding availability of services to deal with these challenges. Whilst the numbers of children requiring protection is increasing, the Court's paramount consideration is the child or children in each individual case. Regardless of the volume of work for practitioners, the Court applies the same scrutiny in each and every case (Holt, 2021).

Although the legislative framework is largely effective, and the system generally works well, there is insufficient funding and resources to meet the needs of children and their families when they seek help, regardless of whether this is at an early stage or when they are in crisis and most in need of care and protection (Holt, 2016). Nonetheless poverty (predictions pre-pandemic suggested that there will be 5 million children living in poverty in 2020) and austerity measures; positioning early help and children in need services as a precursor to child protection rather than a statutory duty to provide a range of services (Dfe, 2018); differential regional use of legal orders; experience of families and practitioners working together and within systems as problematic; changing nature profiles of children and families seeking help (notably older children, children of different ethnicity, cases involving domestic violence, cases involving parental learning difficulties, cases of repeat care proceedings with women); and a mistrust between families, professionals, policy makers and the legislative system are clearly pivotal in understanding the care statistics and in developing systems to address the care crisis (Holt and Kelly, 2019).

The challenge for all professionals involved in child protection therefore is to improve decision-making in a timely manner with an obligation to provide improved access to justice for children (Judiciary of England and Wales, 2012, p. 4). The final report of the *Family Justice Review* (MoJ, 2011) and the Family

Justice Modernisation Programme (Judiciary of England and Wales, 2012) set in train a system that was designed to be quicker, simpler, more cost-effective and fairer, whilst continuing to protect children from risk of harm. Pivotal to achieving this aim is to ensure children remain the focus and are not lost amongst the competing needs and demands of adults. Parents and carers are clearly important and must be involved in the process, but decisions must be taken to protect children from harm at the earliest opportunity, and at times, this requires emergency action.

Fundamental to achieving change is to tackle inequalities with cross sector collaboration that addresses silo working, meeting increased demand for services, improving access to holistic care and support for children and their families (Holt, 2021).

REFLECTIVE QUESTIONS

- How can you combine emergency action to safeguard a child with working humanely with parents and carers?
- Reflecting on your own experiences of practice, how can you ensure that taking emergency action is a last resort?

REFERENCES

Cafcass statistics. https://www.cafcass.gov.uk/about-cafcass/our-data/. (Accessed June 2022).
Children Act 1989. Available at https://www.legislation.gov.uk/ukpga/1989/41/contents
College of Policing, 2022. https://www.college.police.uk/app/major-investigation-and-public-protection/investigating-child-abuse-and-safeguarding-children/police-response-concern-child
Department for Education, 2018. Working Together to Safeguard Children. HMSO, London.
Department of Health, 2000. Framework for the Assessment of Children in Need and their Families. HMSO, London.
Family Procedure Rules (FPR) Part 12.
Gloucestershire County Council v M and C [2015].
Holt, K., 2021. Technology, power and inequalities: Achieving a humane approach to the digital divide. J. Child Adolescent Ment. Health 26, 378–380.
Holt, K., Kelly, N., 2021. A personal and conceptual reflection on findings from serious case reviews during the period 1987-2018: Part I. J. Fam. Law 2021 (April), 543–548.
Holt, K., 2016. Child Protection. Palgrave, London.
Holt, K.E., Kelly, N., Doherty, P., Broadhurst, K., 2013. Access to justice for families? Legal advocacy for parents where children are on the "edge of care": An English case study. J. Soc. Welf. Fam. Law. https://doi.org/10.1093/bjsw/bcs168.
Holt, K., Kelly, N., 2019. Care in crisis – is there a solution: Reflections on the care crisis review 2018. J. Child Fam. Soc. Work.
Human Rights Act 1998. https://www.legislation.gov.uk/ukpga/1998/42/contents
Judiciary of England and Wales, 2012. The family justice modernisation programme: The third update from Mr Justice Ryder. March 2012. www.judiciary.gov.uk/Resources/JCO/Documents/Reports/family_newsletter3.pdf.
Masson, J., 2017. Disruptive Judgments. *Child and Family Law Quarterly*, 29(4), 401–422.
Ministry of Justice, 2011. Family Justice Review: Final Report. MoJ, London.
Packman, J., Randall, J., Jacques, N., 1986. Who Needs Care? Social-Work Decisions About Children. Basil Blackwell, Oxford.
Re A (A Child), Darlington Borough Council v M [2015].
Re AS (Unlawful Removal of a Child) [2015].
Re C (A Child: Interim Separation) [2020] EWCA Civ 257.
Re C and B (Care Order: Future Harm) [2001].
Re G (Care: Challenge to Local Authority's Decision) [2003].
Re N (Children) (Adoption: Jurisdiction) [2015].
Re O (A Child: Supervision Order: Future Harm) [2001].
Re P (A Child: Use of S.20 CA 1989) [2014].
Re X Council v B (Emergency Protection Orders) [2006].
Re X: Emergency Protection Orders [2006].

17

CHILD PROTECTION AND THE CRIMINAL JUSTICE SYSTEM

JOHN WILLIAMS

KEY POINTS

- Children and young people are entitled to the protection of criminal law.
- The criminal justice system supports children and young people to help them give their best evidence.
- Criminal courts have a duty to 'have regard' to their welfare – the Children Act 1989 paramountcy principle does not apply.
- A balance must be achieved between the accused's rights and those of children and young people as victims or witnesses.
- Testimony in court must meet the standards required by the law of evidence.
- Children and young people must be listened to and supported – agencies must work together.

INTRODUCTION

A challenge for the criminal justice system is to balance children and young people's welfare with the rights of the accused (Hoyano, 2001). For accused children and young people, how are their rights balanced against those of victims? This chapter explores how the criminal justice systems seeks to balance these interests. It discusses the role of criminal justice agencies (the police and the Crown Prosecution Service) and the role of social and health practitioners. Emphasis is placed on the courts, in particular the need to achieve the best evidence for trial. This involves helping children and young people giving evidence by mitigating the trauma. Special measures available for doing this are explained, as is the practitioner's role.

Special Measures

- Prerecorded interviews
- Live link cross-examination
- Pre-trial cross-examination
- Hearing evidence in private
- Screens
- Intermediaries
- Communication aids
- Removal of wigs and gowns

Children and young people applies to those under the age of 18 years.

Children and young people experience the criminal justice system in one of three ways:

1. As a victim
2. As a witness
3. As an accused

Children and young people are victims of many types of crime. Child sexual abuse is a major concern. For the year ending March 2019, police in England and Wales recorded 73,260 sexual offences where the data identified the child as the victim (National Statistics, 2020). Other offences include child abduction, trafficking, cruelty and neglect, and modern slavery. Children and young people may witness crimes at home and in public space. For children and young people in the third category, there has been a 10-year decline overall in the number of proven offences for this group. However, some crimes have seen an increase, for example knife crimes. In the year ending March 2022, 13,800 children received a caution or sentence. (National Statistics, 2023).

Alice's Story – NSPCC

Alice's story describes the experience of being a witness. Alice was abused by somebody known to the family, and it took her 10 years to disclose. She was interviewed by the police and social services but was scared to answer questions because she worried that she would not be believed. She says,

> *Going to court and being questioned about my evidence brought all my memories of the abuse straight back. I felt like my recovery was set straight back at the beginning again – it had a really big effect on me.*
> NSPCC (undated)

CHILDREN AND YOUNG PEOPLE AND THE CRIMINAL JUSTICE SYSTEM

Involvement in the criminal justice system means exposure to police investigations, including interviews. They may also encounter the Crown Prosecution Services (CPS), which decides whether prosecutions should proceed following police investigations. The child or young person will engage with lawyers and will be subject to examination and cross examination. They may have to give evidence against family members or known persons. Giving evidence is traumatic for children and young people as revictimisation by the experience may be as distressing as the abuse (Avery, 1983). Children and young people must be protected by the criminal law (HM Government, 2018, para 26; European Convention of Human Rights (n.d), article 2, 3, 6 and 8).

The police are one of the statutory safeguarding partners (Children Act 2004, s.16E; HM Government, 2018, pp. 62–63). Police powers and expertise complement local authority powers and duties. The CPS and the courts are equally important. Police investigations may lead to prosecutions; however, attrition rates between investigations and prosecutions are worrying. A study on case progression involving ex-police officers named resources as a factor, but not the only one. The tension between justice and what this means on individual and national levels also influence attrition. The best interest of the child or young person may conflict with the interests of justice (Krahenbuhl and Dent, 2017, p. 19). Practitioners should ensure that children and young people receive support and are listened to while making sure therapeutic work does not compromise criminal proceedings.

The criminal justice system is neither friendly nor accommodating. The welfare of children and young people is relevant, but not paramount. Children and young people as victims or witnesses are entitled to justice, albeit balanced with the accused's rights. Children and young people giving evidence often feel vulnerable – not only are they possibly victims of a crime or witnesses, but they are also exposed to a system designed for adults. Having a disability may add further complexity to the experience, for example, for those with intellectual disabilities, although their testimony may be accurate jurors tend to perceive their evidence as unreliable (Henry et al., 2011). Flin notes that pre-trial stress may lead to no prosecution because of children and young people's emotional unfitness to testify (Flin, 2008). Courts disempower victims and witnesses (Beckett and Warrington, 2015, p. 30). Pantell's American research found that:

> *(S)tudies have established that children experience anxiety surrounding court appearances and that the main fear is facing the defendant. Other fears include being hurt by the defendant, embarrassment about crying or not being able to answer questions and going to jail. The more frightened a child is, the less he or she is able to answer questions.*
> *Pantell (2017, p. 4)*

Minimising stress enhances the quality of the evidence, and the primary aim is to achieve best evidence (Ministry of Justice, 2020). Social care and health care practitioners must accept that the criminal justice system, while responding to children and young people's needs, is independent.

Where a child or young person is charged with an offence they must be treated in a way that takes account of age, levels of maturity, disability and intellectual and emotional capacity. Steps should be taken to promote their ability to take part in the proceedings. Where the offence attracts media attention, it is necessary to reduce feelings of intimidation and inhibitions as far as possible. In a case before the European Court of Human Rights brought by the child killers of James Bulger, the Court referred to psychiatric evidence that they could not take part in the proceedings. Representation by an experienced lawyer did not guarantee the right of an accused to participate in their trial. The UK had violated their human rights to a fair hearing (*T v UK* and *V v UK, 1999*).

Review of Literature and Research Findings

Plotnikoff and Woolfson's *Falling Short?* examines progress in responding to the needs of young witnesses since their earlier *Measuring Up* report (Plotnikoff and Woolfson, 2009; 2019). Using the experiences of policy makers and practitioners, it identifies what has worked and what has not. Porter explores from an American perspective the benefits of recorded interviews in minimising the trauma experienced by children and young people (Porter, 2018).

Andrews discusses the use of quantitative linguistic transcript analysis in assessing how children are questioned in forensic settings (Andrews, 2018). Elmi et al. examine the effects of legal involvement on the mental health and recovery of children and young people (Elmi, Daignault and Hébert, 2018). Hanna and Henderson, using Australian and New Zealand research, argue that many things diminish the quality of evidence, but in the right circumstances children can be effective and reliable witnesses (Hanna and Henderson, 2017).

Collins et al., 2017 found that intermediaries have positive implications for jury perceptions of testimony in court. Cooper's survey found the service has evolved. It has highs, in particular the satisfaction intermediaries find in being able to help witnesses. It has lows such as the failure of other professionals to understand the role and to engage with them (Cooper, 2014). A comparative review of the use of intermediaries in England and Wales, Northern Ireland and New South Wales concludes that further research is needed on their use and effectiveness (Cooper and Mattison, 2017).

Implications for Practice

Practitioners Should Remember

- Children and young people have the right to know what going to court involves.
- They have a right to support in preparing themselves.
- Those providing support must be aware of the restrictions in criminal cases.
- Two broad categories of therapeutic work can be undertaken prior to trial – counselling and psychotherapy. This work may be long term.
- Preparation for court may be undertaken to:
  - give the child or young person information about the legal process;
  - address any concerns the child or young person may have in relation to giving evidence; and
  - reducing anxiety.

Welfare is also a legal concept rather than purely a professional judgement (George, 2019). Under the Children Act 1989 the child's welfare is the paramount consideration when courts decide on their upbringing, property and income. The Social Services and Well-being (Wales) Act 2014 incorporates the paramountcy principle when defining well-being of children and young people (s.2(3)). The paramountcy principle applies in non-criminal proceedings and to social work and health care practitioners. Government guidance, *Working Together to Safeguard Children*, requires that:

> all practitioners should follow the principles of the Children Acts 1989 and 2004 that state that the welfare of children is paramount.
> **HM Government (2018, p. 9).**

A practitioner, if challenged in court (care proceedings, adoption, medical treatment, etc.) must justify their decisions in accordance with the paramountcy principle as it is the basis of judicial decisions.

However, in criminal proceedings, welfare is addressed in s.44(1) Children and Young Persons Act 1933, which says,

> (E)very court in dealing with a child or young person who is brought before it, either as . . . an

offender or otherwise, shall have regard to the welfare of the child or young person....

Although primarily applying to children and young people as offenders, for example for sentencing, the words 'or otherwise' include witnesses and victims. The duty is to 'have regard' which requires courts to do more than noting. In a case involving the 'have regard' duty in the School Standards and Framework Act 1998, Cobb J said that it was necessary:

to demonstrate that [the Governing Body] has considered and engaged with the Guidance, not ignored it, or merely paid lip service to it.

Reasons for departure should be given (*London Oratory School Governors case, 2015*, para 58). *Khatun v LB Newham (2004)* held the authority must take the Standards into account and give clear reasons for any departure. Although this is not a demanding duty, it is a legal one.

Criminal trials are adversarial and may involve discrediting witnesses. Orality is the foundation of adversarial trials which involves listening to testimony and observing demeanour (Ellison, 2003, p. 10). Some argue assisting a child or young people as witnesses undermines the accused's right under Article 6 of the European Convention on Human Rights to a fair hearing. Ho highlights the risk of unfairness to the accused if, for example, the assumption that evidence other than in open court is always convincing (Ho, 1999). However, the European Court accepts that the right to a fair hearing applies to the accused and witnesses. In Doorson, the Court said,

(P)rinciples of fair trial also require that in appropriate cases the interests of the defence are balanced against those of witnesses or victims called upon to testify.
Doorson (1996, para 70); Bates (1999)

This need to balance competing interests is recognised by courts in England and Wales (Hoyano, 2001).

Article 12(2) of the United Nations Convention on the Rights of the Child states that:

12(2) For this purpose [the right to express their views freely], the child shall in particular be provided the opportunity to be heard in any judicial and administrative proceedings affecting the child, either directly, or through a representative or an appropriate body, in a manner consistent with the procedural rules of national law.

The United Nations International Children's Emergency Fund (UNICEF) addresses human rights and helping children and young people giving evidence. The *Handbook on the Convention on the Rights of the Child* recognises the need to adapt courts to enable children to take part. Informality, design, dress codes, prerecorded interviews and separate waiting rooms should be introduced (Hodgkin and Newell, 2007, p. 156). This is a challenge to all criminal justice systems. In England and Wales progress has been made; whether it meets international human rights obligations is debatable. Research shows the criminal justice system does not always allow participation by children and young people (Plotnikoff and Woolfson, 2019).

THE CROWN PROSECUTION SERVICE AND THE DECISION TO PROSECUTE

Once the police complete their investigation, they decide if there is sufficient evidence to pass the files to the CPS. If they do, the CPS decides whether a prosecution goes ahead using what is known as the Full Code Test (Crown Prosecution Service, 2018).

The Crown Prosecution Service (CPS)

- The police provide the CPS with the evidence they have collected during their investigation.
- Decisions to prosecute are the responsibility of the CPS, which is independent of the police.
- The CPS may refer back to the police for clarification or further evidence.
- The CPS is responsible for applying to the court to use the special measures outlined below.
- The CPS does not decide guilt or innocence – they decide whether it is appropriate to prosecute.
- In deciding whether to prosecute, the CPS use the Full Code Test.

■ If the CPS do not prosecute, that does not mean that the child or young person has not been the victim of a crime – he or she may still need support.

There are two parts to the Full Code Test. Part 1 is whether the evidence is reliable and credible (para 4.8). Reliability and credibility may be compromised through fear and the intimidatory nature of courts, thus making prosecution less likely and denying victims their right to a fair hearing and effective remedy (Porter, 2018). Failure to prosecute may violate the European Convention on Human Rights right to private life (Article 8) which includes physical and psychological integrity *(X v Netherlands, 1985)*.

Part 2 requires that prosecution is in the public interest. The guidance names key elements of public interest:

1. The more vulnerable the victim, the more likely a prosecution is in the public interest.
2. Whether there is a position of trust between the suspect and the victim.
3. A prosecution is more likely if the offence was motivated by prejudice based on, for example, the victim's gender, age, ethic or national origin or disability.
4. Prosecutors must consider whether a prosecution is likely to have an adverse effect on the victim's physical or mental health bearing in mind:
   a. the seriousness of the offence,
   b. the availability of special measures (see below), and
   c. the possibility of a prosecution going ahead without the child or young person giving evidence (Crown Prosecution Service, 2018, para 4.14(c)).

Views expressed by victims or families about the impact of the offence should be considered. However, the CPS does not represent victims; it forms an independent view whether prosecution is appropriate (para 4.14(c)). Importantly, where a child or young person is known to social services, or has been in care, information about them is often available. This should not be used to disadvantage them;

prosecutors should address this if it becomes an issue. For example, the fact that the child or young person may have been 'in trouble' with the authorities should not influence the decision. Prosecutors must refer to the *Achieving Best Evidence Guidelines* (Ministry of Justice, 2022) Separate guidance on prosecuting sexual offences against children and young people requires early consultation between the police and CPS using the Rape and Serious Sexual Offences CPS Unit. Communication with victims must be age appropriate.

For both sexual and non-sexual offences, the *Code of Practice for Victims* sets out the minimum standards of service required for providing victims with case progression information (Ministry of Justice, 2020). Pre-trial therapy should be available, and neither the police nor the CPS should prevent this. The CPS guidance, *Provisions of Therapy for Child Witnesses Prior to a Criminal Trial,* stresses that therapy decisions depend on the paramountcy principle (Crown Prosecution Service, 2001). The CPS is not responsible for providing support but must ensure it is available. Support can be provided by organisations such as Victim Support, Rape Crisis England and Wales, and also Independent Sexual Violence Advisors (Crown Prosecution Service, 2017a).

The CPS and the Court and Tribunals Service published a joint protocol to fast track cases involving witnesses under 10 years; this helps to maximise recall and achieve best evidence (National Police Chief's Council, Crown Prosecution Service and HM Courts and Tribunal Service, 2018).

COMPETENCY, COMPELLABILITY, AND SWORN AND UNSWORN EVIDENCE

Legal Terms – Competence, Compellability and Sworn/Unsworn Evidence

■ Competency: the witness can lawfully be called to give evidence.
■ Compellability: The witness must attend court and give evidence, even if they object.
■ Sworn evidence: Normally evidence given in a court is sworn evidence which means that the

person swears an oath or makes and affirmation to tell the truth.

■ Unsworn evidence: In some instances, evidence may be given by a person who has not taken the oath nor affirmed.

Under s.53 Youth Justice and Criminal Evidence Act 1999 (the 1999 Act) children and young people are competent to give evidence whatever their age if they can understand questions asked of them as a witness and answer them in a way that can be understood. The party calling the child or young person must satisfy the court on a balance of probabilities (more likely than not) that they are competent *(R v Powell, 2006)*. Courts decide competency.

Competency

■ Although age is relevant, the decision depends on the individual child or young person.

■ The key issue is whether the child or young person can understand the questions and give intelligible answers.

■ In addressing this, the court should allow the witness to use intermediaries; they must treat the witness as receiving special measures which the court has approved (*R v. Watts* [2010] and *R v B* [2011]).

Under the 1999 Act, young people aged 14 years or older can give sworn evidence if they have 'sufficient appreciation of the solemnity of the occasion and of the particular responsibility to tell the truth which is involved in taking an oath' (s.55). Children under 14 years can give unsworn evidence; in criminal cases, this is treated as if given on oath (s.56). As a general rule, competent witnesses are compellable. Compelling an unwilling child or young person to attend court may lead to a change to a guilty plea by the accused. The defence may wait to see if all the prosecution witnesses turn up at the court; if they do, a guilty plea may follow.

CHILDREN AND YOUNG PEOPLE GIVING EVIDENCE AT TRIAL

In Crown Court cases child liaison officers liaise with the CPS about minimising distress and anxiety for children and young people attending court. For example,

they could use a separate entrance to minimise the risk of seeing the accused. Children or young people and support persons should have separate waiting areas. Ideally, children and young people should visit the court before trial to familiarise themselves with the environment. On the day of the trial, witnesses routinely must attend court at the same time and wait to be called (Fouzder, 2020). Liaison officers work with courts to minimise the time children and young people wait. Other matters include toilet and lunch arrangements. The need to support children and young people in the court environment is important (Morgan and Williams, 1993).

Following the recommendations of the Pigot advisory group which considered the use of pretrial video recordings, the 1999 Act changed the way children and young people give evidence in criminal trials (Pigot, 1989). The 1999 Act contains 'special measures' to assist children and young people to give best evidence (Bates, 1999). The CPS issued guidance for prosecutors (Crown Prosecution Service, 2020b).

The police and the CPS should discuss using special measures at an early stage. The police should provide the CPS with the following information:

■ the witness and their ability to give evidence;

■ whether the witness has other support needs;

■ the basis upon which the witness is eligible for special measures;

■ what special measures are needed?

■ the views of the witness on which special measures should be sought;

■ the appropriate individuals, such as an intermediary, to attend subsequent meetings between the prosecutor and the witness; and

■ whether the witness is receiving therapy (Crown Prosecution Service, 2020b).

Children and young people accused of crimes are treated harshly (Haydon and Scraton, 2000). The Children's Commissioner for England reports that a youth court was 'not a child friendly environment and is not meeting standards that we had hoped' (Pidd et al., 2019; BBC, 2018). It is questionable whether this complies with Article 6(3)(d) European Convention of Human Rights. Accused children and young people do not have the same access to special measures as victims or witnesses. The House of Lords and the European Court of Human Rights criticised this in the *R v. Camberwell Green Youth Court* (2005). In response, the 1999 Act was amended. An accused child or young person may use a live link (s.33A, 33B and 33C). Further amendments allow for the accused to access intermediaries, but a Criminal Practice Direction states:

There is however no presumption that a defendant will [have an intermediary] and, even where an intermediary would improve the trial process, appointment is not mandatory...The court should adapt the trial process to address a defendant's communication needs.
Lord Chief Justice (2015); see Hoyano and Rafferty (2017)

Achieving Best Evidence in Criminal Proceedings: Guidance on Interviewing Victims and Witnesses, and Guidance on Using Special Measures

The *Achieving Best Evidence in Criminal Proceedings* guidance identifies good practice when interviewing victims and witnesses and preparing them to give evidence. Although not legally binding, significant departure must be justified (Ministry of Justice, 2022, paras 1.1–1.2). Specialist training is available for police and social workers which includes how to interview children and young people. Given the evidential significance of a prerecorded video interview, practitioners should adhere to the guidance. It emphasises careful planning and clear objectives. Davies and Wescott, when discussing the earlier guidance, identified a tension arising from prerecorded interviews. Practitioners may regard them as the first step in a criminal investigation, an inquiry into whether a child or young person needs protection, or as and evidence-in-chief. They cannot be all three

as the aim is to gather evidence-in-chief for a trial (Davies and Westcott, 1999).

Prior to the interview, it is important to find out basic information on what has taken place to protect evidence, identify need for medical examinations, identify other witnesses and, if appropriate, arrest any suspect. However, this does not replace a formal prerecorded interview (paras. 2.4–2.6). Information gathering meetings enable practitioners to identify support needs. Therapeutic help can be given before giving evidence, and the CPS cannot prevent this. Those giving therapeutic support must follow the *Provision of Therapy for Child Witnesses Prior to a Criminal Trial: Practice Guidance* and inform the CPS of any proposed therapy, whether therapy is being provided or if it has already been provided. This allows the CPS to consider the impact on the criminal proceedings (Crown Prosecution Service, 2001, para 6.3).

Practitioners must avoid accusations of coaching the child or young person. In the case of *R v Momodou and Limani* (2005) the judge directed the jury that:

There is no place for witness training in our country, we do not do it. It is unlawful. A witness should give his or her own evidence, as far as practicable uninfluenced by what anyone else has said, whether in formal discussions or informal conversations.

It is acceptable for witnesses to familiarise themselves with court processes and procedures, but evidence should not be discussed. In *R v Richardson* (1971) the court said that statements or proofs of one witness should not be discussed with other witnesses.

Interviews should 'get an accurate and reliable account in a way which is fair, is in the witness's interests, and is acceptable to the court' (para 3.1). *Achieving Best Evidence* identifies four stages to the interview, as outlined Table 17.1.

TABLE 17.1

Four Stages of Interviewing Victims and Witnesses

Phase	Key points
Phase 1: Establishing rapport.	*Designed to settle the witness and relieve or reduce anxiety.* Rapport reduces stress and helps recall. Neutral questions unrelated to the offence are used which they can answer. This helps create a positive mood (para 3.8). Toward the end of this phase the witness should be advised to give a truthful and accurate account. As the video may be evidence, it is helpful if the court knows the witness is aware of the importance of telling the truth (para 3.18).
Phase 2: Free narrative account.	*To enable the child or young person to give an account in their own words.* The interviewer should initiate an uninterrupted free narrative account from the witness through an open-ended invitation (para 3.24). The witness should not be asked questions during their narration; these should be kept for later (para 3.26). Active listening is necessary, reassuring the witness that what they have said has been heard (para 3.28). The interviewer should avoid appearing too authoritative but should be confident and competent to reassure the witness that they can be relied on (para 3.29). The way the interview is conducted (e.g. overly authoritative) and the nature of the questions (e.g. suggestive or complex) influence the extent of unconditional positive responding (para 3.32). In many cases, (e.g. sexual abuse) witnesses may be reluctant to talk openly and freely. Interviewers can offer reassurance, (e.g. 'I know this must be difficult for you. Is there anything I can do to make it easier?'). It is acceptable to refer to a witness by their first or preferred name, but terms of endearment, verbal reinforcement and physical contact are inappropriate. This should not prevent physical reassurance by an interview supporter (para 3.33). If the witness says something requiring clarification, but is reluctant or unable to do so, it may be better to return to the point later in the interview rather than require an immediate response (para 3.34).
Phase 3: Questioning.	*To find out more about the alleged offence by asking questions that promote recall.* Outline what is expected of them at this stage (para 3.36). It may be necessary to leave a topic and return to it later if the witness becomes distressed – this may be necessary more than once (para 3.37). There are several types of question which vary in how directive they are. Questioning should start with open-ended questions and then, if necessary, specific-closed questions. Use forced-choice questions and leading questions only as a last resort (para 3.44). General guidance on each type of question is given in paras 3.45–3.64. Snow et al. found that open-ended questions may improve the coherence of the witnesses' statement (Snow, Powell and Murfett, 2009). The interviewer should not voice their suspicions to the witness or call them a liar: there may be an innocuous explanation for inconsistencies (para 3.68). The interviewer should ask only one question at a time and allow the witness to answer before asking a further question (para 3.69). Clearly indicate a topic change (para 3.71). Always check the witness has understood what is said to them (para 3.73).
Phase 4:	*To ensure that the child or young person has understood the interview and is not distressed.* If appropriate, interviewers should consider summarising what the witness has said, using their words as far as possible. This allows the witness to check the interviewer's recall for accuracy. The interviewer must tell the witness to correct them if they have missed anything out or got something wrong (para 3.80). Summarising the interview can lead to further recall. The witness should be told they can add new information (para 3.81). Regardless of the interview's outcome, every effort should be made to ensure that the witness is not distressed. Even if the witness has provided little or no information, they should not be made to feel they have failed or disappointed the interviewer. Praise or congratulations for providing information should not be given (para 3.85).

The guidance emphasises that:

Poor interviewers can cause children and vulnerable adult witnesses to provide unreliable accounts. However, interviewers who are able to put into practice the guidance on questioning in this document will provide witnesses with much better opportunities to present their own accounts of what really happened (para 3.84).

Children and young people must give their own account and, when they do, it must be the best quality evidence achievable and comply with the law of evidence.

SPECIAL MEASURES AVAILABLE FOR CHILDREN AND YOUNG PEOPLE

Giving Evidence in Court – Terminology

- Evidence-in-chief: in the case of a witness called by the prosecution, this is main testimony given before being cross examined by the defence.
- Cross examination: the witness is examined, in the case of a prosecution witness, by the defence who will seek to cast doubt on their evidence and elicit evidence favourable to their client.
- Re-examination: this follows cross-examination. The prosecution may question the witness only on matters arising out of the cross-examination.

The same process applies to witnesses called by the defence.

The following sections detail the special measures available under the Youth and Criminal Evidence Act 1999.

Prerecorded Video Interviews (s.27)

A prerecorded video interview is admissible in court as evidence-in-chief. If the recording was made when the child or young person was under 18 years, it is still admissible if they are 18 years by the time of the trial (s.21(9)). The Government's *Achieving Best Evidence* guidance on interviewing children and young people should be followed; failing to do so can lead to the evidence being inadmissible or edited (Ministry of Justice, 2022). There is a strong presumption that prerecorded interviews are admissible even if flawed. In deciding

on admissibility, the court considers matters such as the witness's age. Other evidence may show that the flaws in the recording do not undermine credibility. However, a substantial failure to follow the Guidance may result in children and young people going through the trauma of the interviews and having raised expectations only for the evidence to be inadmissible, which is often fatal to prosecutions.

Many English-speaking countries use prerecorded video interviews. Research shows advantages and disadvantages, particularly for prosecutors. Burrows and Powell's Australian research identifies challenges for prosecutors (Burrows and Powell, 2014). They found that jurors may feel less engaged with witnesses because it is different from seeing them in court. Despite a reminder by the judge that the jury is to treat the person as though they were in court, often they did not, and it is unclear what the effect was (Burrows and Powell, 2014, pp. 380–381). Prerecorded interviews risk a reduced sense of formality. Prosecutors felt that interviewers must be aware interviews can be used as evidence-in-chief at trial. Prosecutors stressed the importance of the solemnity of prerecorded interviews and that this could be achieved without compromising rapport or increasing feelings of threat, intimidation or stress. The quality of the equipment can compromise the clarity of the evidence, so it is necessary to work with the courts to ensure good quality equipment is available (Burrows and Powell, 2014, p. 382). A close shot of the interviewee helps the jury assess demeanour (Burrows and Powell, 2014, p. 385). If the sound quality is poor, subtitles may be added, although the leave of the court is most likely needed.

Burrows and Powell identify a risk that prerecorded evidence-in-chief leads to witnesses being unprepared for cross-examination. Children and young people may forget or re-interpret events which can be exploited by the defence in cross-examination. The child or young person will be unfamiliar with the question-and-answer process of the court, a feature of cross-examination (Burrows and Powell, 2014, p. 383).

The researchers do not argue against prerecorded interviews, nor did the participating prosecutors. Instead, they highlight issues needing attention to ensure they work in the interests of justice. They conclude:

(T)his study has provided valuable insight into the prosecution perspective on the usefulness of recorded interviews as evidence-in-chief. For recorded interviews to be useful and effective in providing reliable statements that are appropriate for use as evidence, continued collaboration is necessary between child developmental psychologists, investigators and prosecutors (Burrows and Powell, 2014, p.388).

Prerecorded interviews and special measures allow more cases to go to court. The CPS reports that between 2007–08 and 2016–17, convictions for child sexual abuse rose by 89% (Crown Prosecution Service, 2017b, p. 14).

Cross-Examination Via Live Link (s.24)

It may be possible for the child or young person to refresh their memory prior to the trial. Any written statement may be given to the witness ahead of the trial. Viewing a prerecorded interview will help the child or young person to re-familiarise themselves with their evidence and help them respond to cross-examination (*Safeguarding Children as Victims and Witnesses,* the Crown Prosecution Service, 2019).

Live links avoid children and young people appearing in open court by using remote testimony during cross-examination. If the prerecorded interview is inadmissible, the live link may still be used. The screen image of the child or young person must be visible to the judge or magistrate, the jury, at least one lawyer from each party, and any intermediary or interpreter for the witness. If live link facilities are unavailable at the trial court, the case can be transferred to one with the technology if possible. Failing that, screens should be considered.

Physical separation from the court using a neutral location has the advantage of removing the possibility of meeting the accused and family or removing the witnesses' fear of doing so. Court buildings are not child or young person friendly, and the physical environment may stress the witness and compromise their ability to give best evidence (Mcnamee, Molyneaux and Geraghty, 2012). Earlier indications suggested that many areas do not have video links separate from the courts. A 2018 protocol on national remote links sites states that they can be found in many different locations such as within the criminal justice system, victim or witness support groups, or local authority premises. (HM Courts and Tribunal Service et al., 2018). Practitioners will need to be aware of what is available in their area.

The CPS gives an interesting example of the use of live link testimony. Following a long period of abuse, a mother and her children fled the country. The abuse included repeated rape of the accused's sons. They agreed to give evidence, and arrangements were made to give it by live link from abroad. The court was cleared when the children gave evidence (Crown Prosecution Service, 2017b, p. 15).

Live link testimony was extended by s.51 Criminal Justice Act 2003 to allow witnesses, other than the accused, to give evidence remotely if the court is satisfied that it is in the 'interests of the efficient or effective administration of justice.' This differs from special measures; it may be available to practitioners with limited ability to attend court. The Coronavirus Act 2020 also extended the use of live link testimony during the crisis.

One other protection in the Youth and Criminal Evidence Act 1999 is protection from cross-examination by the accused in person for child complainants of, or witnesses to, sexual offences, offences of violence, cruelty, kidnapping, false imprisonment or abduction (ss.34–38).

Pre-Trial Cross-Examination or Re-Examination (s.28)

A recorded cross-examination or re-examination of children or young people made pre-trial and nearer the events surrounding the prosecution may be admissible as evidence in the Crown Court (Ewin, 2018). The government was initially reluctant to introduce these because of cost and necessary procedural changes. A precondition of their use is a s27 direction for a prerecorded interview. With court approval, prerecorded cross- and re-examinations are admissible if consistent with the interests of justice and if they achieve best evidence. Following pilot studies, a national roll out of this provision across England and Wales was completed in 2022. The evaluation of three pilot studies found that lawyers using s.28 cross-examinations felt witnesses were under less pressure; witnesses report being better able to recall events (Baverstock, 2016). The Ministry of Justice observed that this led to increased early guilty pleas and a reduced number of trials dropped because a witness does not turn up (The Inns of Court College of Advocacy, 2019).

Hearing Evidence in Private (s.25)

A feature of criminal trials is that they are held in open court in front of the public and media. However, under s.25 the courtroom may be cleared in sexual offences cases, or where somebody other than the accused may attend court to intimidate the witness. The special measures direction identifies who should be excluded (for example, the public). All but one nominated member of the press may be excluded; reporting restrictions can be imposed.

Section 37 of the Children and Young Persons Act 1933 also allows courts to direct that persons, other than court officers, the parties, the lawyers, and those directly concerned must be excluded during the witnesses' evidence. It applies to offences involving children and young people as witnesses in cases involving indecent or immoral conduct.

Screens (s.23)

The Court of Appeal has held that where there was fear of witness intimidation, evidence could be given out of sight of the accused *(R v Smellie, 1919)*. The argument against this is that accused people have the right to see their accusers. Section 23 follows Smellie by making screens a special measure available to children and young people. The witness must be able to see and be seen by the judge and jury, the lawyers and anybody acting as an interpreter or intermediary. In America, the routine use of screens is controversial; it is claimed that it breaches the Sixth Amendment to the Constitution, which gives accused people in criminal trials the right to confront witnesses, especially in cross-examination (Gershman, 2000).

Using an Intermediary (s.29)

A registered intermediary can be requested by the police or CPS to help witnesses with communication needs. Intermediaries are available throughout the criminal justice process, including the prerecorded evidence-in-chief stage, visits to the court and use of the live link for evidence-in-chief or cross-examination. To help the court, intermediaries may provide a written report outlining the witnesses' difficulties and identifying the questions they find problematic. In court, intermediaries communicate questions to witnesses and communicate answers to the court. The court must approve intermediaries, and they have a legal duty to perform their duties faithfully and not falsify what is said or make misleading statements.

Intermediaries

- The police or CPS may identify a child or young person who may need an intermediary as part of the investigation. The CPS will assess whether an intermediary is needed at the trial; if so, they will apply for an intermediary special measure.
- The earlier the involvement of an intermediary, the more likely their involvement will be successful.
- Intermediaries may well be needed if the child or young person seems unlikely to be able to recognise a difficult question or tell the questioner (who they see as a person in authority) they have not understood.
- Intermediaries ensure that the child or young person can give the best possible evidence, something that the criminal justice system demands.

The Victims Commissioner recommended that the role of registered intermediaries should be promoted and explained to judges as part of their training on special measures. She also recommended that the College of Policing should ensure that training of police officers should provide them with an understanding of the role (Victims' Commissioner, 2018, p. 383). It may also be helpful for social workers and other professionals working with children and young people to familiarise themselves with the role of the intermediary and be clear about the situations in which they may be required.

Communication Aids (s.30)

Communication aids can be used to overcome difficulties with understanding or answering questions. They can be used alongside an intermediary.

Removal of Wigs and Gowns (s.26)

Wigs and gowns, it is claimed, add something to the majesty of the law, but they can intimidate and add to the trauma. The practice arose of judges and lawyers removing wigs and gowns. This may now be part of a special measures direction.

The 'Primary Rule'

In determining whether special measures should be available for a child or young person the court, under what is known as the primary rule, must give a special measures direction which provides for:

- any prerecorded video evidence-in-chief (the witnesses' evidence used in court by the prosecution) must be admitted; and
- any other evidence given by witnesses must be via a live link rather than in open court (for example, cross examination) (s.24(1)–(3)).

The primary rule is disapplied if:

- the technology is unavailable in the court, or
- the court considers it is not in the interests of justice for the recording or part of it to be admitted – including where it is unreliable through non-compliance with the law of evidence, or
- the witness does not want to use special measures.

However, before disapplying the rule the court must be satisfied it would not diminish the quality of the evidence. In doing so it must consider the following:

- the child or young person's age and maturity.
- the child or young person's ability to understand the consequences of giving evidence without using prerecorded video and/or interactive link.
- any relationship between the child or young person and the accused.
- the child or young person's social and cultural background and ethnic origins; and
- the nature and alleged circumstances of the offence (s.21(4C)).

If the primary rule is disapplied because the witness does not want to use prerecorded or live video link evidence, the court must order that a screen is used for evidence in open court. However, screens will not be used if:

- the child or young person does not want to use them, and the court is satisfied that not using them does not diminish the quality of the evidence (having regard to the five factors listed previously); or
- the court is satisfied that screens would not maximise the quality of the evidence (s.21(4A)).

If video evidence is admissible under the primary rule, the child or young person must be available for cross-examination via video link. The court must consider whether other special measures should be available, namely communication aids, intermediaries, removal of wigs and gowns, or evidence in private. The court may then make a binding special measures direction.

In addition to the 1999 Act, courts can use their inherent powers to protect a witness. This can also support accused children and young people.

REFLECTIVE QUESTIONS

- How can I help children and young people giving evidence as witnesses or victims in criminal cases?
- How can I contribute to the discussions between the police and CPS on the use of special measures?
- How can I avoid allegations of coaching the witness if I am providing therapeutic support?
- What are the special training needs required for working with children and young people giving evidence?

CHILDREN AND YOUNG PEOPLE AS WITNESSES IN CRIMINAL TRIALS IN NORTHERN IRELAND

The Criminal Evidence (Northern Ireland) Order 1999 (1999 Order) is almost indistinguishable from the Youth Justice and Criminal Evidence Act 1999. As with the 1999 Act, it is based on the need to achieve the best evidence possible. The 1999 Order established a primary rule which follows the 1999 Act. Hayes and Bunting's small-scale study of the experience of young people pre- and post-trial identify that distress can continue post-trial, regardless of the outcome of the trial. In addition, delay adds to the stress and there is a need for prompt referrals to witness support schemes to achieve proper assessment and support. These findings equally apply to England and Wales (Hayes and Bunting, 2013).

CHILDREN AND YOUNG PEOPLE AS WITNESSES IN CRIMINAL TRIALS IN SCOTLAND

The Scottish Parliament passed the Vulnerable Witnesses (Criminal Evidence) (Scotland) Act 2019 (the 2019 Act). The 2019 Act builds on earlier legislation. Under the 2019 Act, children and young people under 18 years will, in the most serious cases, be allowed to have all their evidence prerecorded. Normally, this will be through a special measure referred to as 'evidence by commissioner'. This is subject to the proviso that its use would not significantly prejudice the interests of justice. Changes in Scotland were partly influenced by the pilot studies of prerecorded cross-examination in England and Wales.

Commissioner hearings were not originally intended as the main way of taking evidence from children and young people. Other special measures were used such as screens, live links and prerecorded evidence-in-chief (these are still available). A commissioner may be a judge, an advocate or other suitable person. Ahead of the trial they will hear the evidence of the child or young person; evidence will be given as normal in front of the commissioner. It will include evidence-in-chief and cross-examination; questioning must be in a language they can understand. A video recording of the hearing is played at the trial.

The Scottish Government has recently published the Bairns' Hoose standards based on the European model. (Health Care Improvement Scotland, & Care Inspectorate, 2023). This approach uses a multiagency centre where professionals from different settings work together to investigate suspect abuse and provide support in one physical centre. Integration is a key feature of this approach.

CONCLUSION

There is a need to address the concerns of the Children's Commissioner about the plight of children and young people who appear as the accused in criminal proceedings (Haydon and Scraton, 2000; Pidd et al., 2019). They deserve better protection.

Significant energy has been spent on supporting children and young people giving evidence in criminal proceedings as witnesses or victims. Special measures help achieve more prosecutions, although giving evidence remains traumatic. What more can be done? Initiatives, such as Children's Advocacy Centers in America and Barnahus in the Nordic countries, offer an innovative and integrated alternative. They coordinate the work of multidisciplinary investigation teams offering services for victims, including therapeutic support for children and families. The centres include social workers, school counsellors, paediatricians, medics, psychologists, psychiatrists, police, prosecutors and others working in the criminal justice system. This approach has much to commend it (Johansson, 2012; Rasmusson, 2011). It is encouraging that Scotland is actively looking at this approach.

Much has been achieved as shown by the case of a 2-year-old giving prerecorded evidence. This led to the accused pleading guilty before trial (Bowcott, 2017). However, more is needed.

CASES

R v. Camberwell Green Youth Court, ex parte D [2005] UKHL 4, [2005] 1 WLR 393; *SC v UK* (2005) 40 EHRR 10 (226)).

R Doorson v the Netherlands (App no 20524/92) ECHR 26 March 1996 (on the application of London Oratory School Governors) v Schools Adjudicator [2015] EWHC 1012 (Admin).

R v Powell [2006] 1 Cr App R 468.

R (on the application of Khatun) v Newham London Borough Council [2004] All ER (D) 386 *R v B* [2011] Crim L.R. 233.

X v Netherlands (1985) 8 EHRR 235.

R v Momodou and Limani [2005] EWCA Crim 177.

R v Richardson CACD ([1971] CAR 244.

R v Smellie (1919) 14 Cr App Rep 128.

R v. Watts [2010] EWCA Crim 1824.

T v UK and V v UK (1999) 30 EHRR 12.

FURTHER READING

Official Publications

Special Measures guidance. Although intended for a legal audience, it summarises special measures (Crown Prosecution Service, 2020b).

Therapy: Provision of therapy for child witnesses prior to a criminal trial is essential reading for practitioners providing therapeutic support (Crown Prosecution Service, 2001).

Working Together to Safeguard Children is again essential reading and places the role of the criminal justice system in a wider context (HM Government, 2018).

Practitioners must be familiar with the Ministry of Justice's Achieving Best Evidence in Criminal Proceedings: Guidance on interviewing victims and witnesses, and guidance on using special measures (Ministry of Justice, 2022).

Booklets Designed for Children and Young People

Going to Court: 5–11-year-olds, (2017)
Going to Court: 12–17 years olds, (2017)
(These booklets are designed to be read with an adult and provide a useful aid to discussion covering how evidence is given, what happens at trial, the use of special measures, and being asked and answering questions.)

Booklet Aimed at Parents, Carers, or People Going With Children and Young People to Court

Your Child is a Witness (HM Courts and Tribunal Service, 2017).

(It explains how they can help (if they are not implicated, and there is no conflict of interests), the role of intermediaries, going to court, the trial and post-trial, and any compensation available).

REFERENCES

Andrews, S.J., 2018. Assessing how child witnesses are questioned in forensic contexts using quantitative linguistic transcript analysis. SAGE Publications Ltd, London. https://doi.org/10.4135/9781526444189. (Accessed 22 August 2023).

Avery, M., 1983. The child abuse witness: Potential for secondary victimization. Crim. Justice J. https://www.ojp.gov/ncjrs/virtual-library/abstracts/child-abuse-witness-potential-secondary-victimization. (Accessed 22 August 2023).

Bates, P., 1999. Youth Justice and Criminal Evidence Act – the evidence of children and vulnerable adults, The. Child & Fam. LQ 11, 289.

Baverstock, J., 2016. Process Evaluation of Pre-Recorded Cross-Examination Pilot (Section 28). London. https://assets.publishing.service.gov.uk/government/uploads/system/uploads/attachment_data/file/553335/process-evaluation-doc.pdf. (Accessed 22 August 2023).

BBC, 2018. Vulnerable Witnesses 'Denied Help to Give Evidence' - BBC News. https://www.bbc.co.uk/news/uk-42689789. (Accessed 22 August 2023).

Beckett, H., Warrington, C., 2015. Making justice work. Bedford. http://uobrep.openrepository.com/uobrep/bitstream/10547/347011/1/MakingJusticeWorkFullReport.pdf. (Accessed 22 August 2023).

Bowcott, O., 2017. Two-year-old girl gives evidence in UK abuse case. https://www.theguardian.com/law/2017/oct/10/two-year-old-girl-gives-evidence-in-uk-abuse-case. (Accessed 22 August 2023).

Burrows, K.S., Powell, M.B., 2014. Prosecutors' perspectives on using recorded child witness interviews about abuse as evidence-in-chief. Aust N Z J Criminol. 47 (3), 374–390.

Collins, K., Harker, N., Antonopoulos, G.A., 2017. The impact of the registered intermediary on adults' perceptions of child witnesses: Evidence from a mock cross examination. Eur. J. Crim. Policy Res. 23 (2), 211–225 Springer.

Cooper, P., 2014. Highs and Lows: The 4th Intermediary Survey. King's University, London.

Cooper, P., Mattison, M., 2017. Intermediaries, vulnerable people and the quality of evidence: An international comparison of three versions of the English intermediary model. Int. J. Evid. Proof 21 (3), 351–370.

Criminal Evidence (Northern Ireland) Order 1999 (1999 Order). https://www.legislation.gov.uk/nisi/1999/2789/contents

Crown Prosecution Service, 2017a. Child Sexual Abuse: Guidelines on Prosecuting Cases of Child Sexual Abuse Crown Prosecution Service, London. https://www.cps.gov.uk/legal-guidance/child-sexual-abuse-guidelines-prosecuting-cases-child-sexual-abuse. (Accessed 22 August 2023).

Crown Prosecution Service, 2017b. Violence Against Women and Girls Report, 10th ed. Crown Prosecution Service, London. https://www.cps.gov.uk/sites/default/files/documents/publications/cps-vawg-report-2017_0.pdf. (Accessed 22 August 2023).

Crown Prosecution Service, 2018. The Code for Crown Prosecutors. https://www.cps.gov.uk/publication/code-crown-prosecutors. (Accessed 22 August 2023).

Crown Prosecution Service, 2019. Safeguarding Children as Victims and Witnesses. https://www.cps.gov.uk/legal-guidance/safeguarding-children-victims-and-witnesses (Accessed 22 August 2023).

Crown Prosecution Service, 2020a. Child Abuse (Non-Sexual) - Prosecution Guidance. The Crown Prosecution Service, London. https://www.cps.gov.uk/legal-guidance/child-abuse-non-sexual-prosecution-guidance. (Accessed 22 August 2023).

Crown Prosecution Service, 2020b. Special Measures. The Crown Prosecution Service, London. https://www.cps.gov.uk/legal-guidance/special-measures. (Accessed 22 August 2023).

Crown Prosecution Service, 2001. Therapy: Provision of Therapy for Child Witnesses Prior to a Criminal Trial. The Crown Prosecution Service, London. https://terapia.co.uk/wp-content/uploads/2020/05/Provision-of-Therapy-for-Child-Witnesses.pdf (Accessed 22 August 2023).

Davies, G., Westcott, H., 1999. Interviewing Child Witnesses Under the Memorandum of Good Practice: A Research Review. Policing and Reducing Crime Unit: Police Research Series. https://lx.iriss.org.uk/sites/default/files/resources/040. Research Review of the Memorandum of Good Practice.pdf. (Accessed 22 August 2023).

Ellison, L., 2003. The Adversarial Process and the Vulnerable Witness. OUP, Oxford.

Elmi, M.H., Daignault, I.V., Hébert, M., 2018. Child sexual abuse victims as witnesses: The influence of testifying on their recovery. Child Abuse Negl. 86, 22–32 Pergamon.

Ewin, R., 2018. Video recorded cross-examination or re-examination: A discussion on practice and research. J. Appl. Psychol. Soc. Sci. 4 (1), 22–38.

Flin, R., 2008. Child witnesses in criminal courts. Child. Soc. 4 (3), 264–283.

Fouzder, M., 2020. Be prepared to wait all day: HMCTS outlines court expectations. Law Society Gazette. https://www.lawgazette.co.uk/news/be-prepared-to-wait-all-day-hmcts-outlines-court-expectations/5103231.article. (Accessed 22 August 2023).

George, R., 2019. Matters of welfare and matters of law. J. Soc. Welf. Fam. Law 41 (3), 358–361.

Gershman, B.L., 2000. Child witnesses and procedural fairness. Am. J. Trial Advoc. 24. https://heinonline.org/HOL/Page?handle=hein.journals/amjtrad24&id=599&div=40&collection=journals. (Accessed 5 March 2020).

Going to Court: 5 -11 year olds, 2017. London. https://assets.publishing.service.gov.uk/government/uploads/system/uploads/attachment_data/file/708114/ywp-5-11-eng.pdf. (Accessed 22 August 2023).

Hanna, K., Henderson, E., 2017. Child witnesses in the criminal courts. In: The Palgrave Handbook of Australian and New Zealand Criminology, Crime and Justice. Springer International Publishing, Cham, pp. 421–435.

Haydon, D., Scraton, P., 2000. Condemn a little more, understand a little less: The Political context and rights implications of the domestic and European rulings in the Venables-Thompson case. J. Law Soc. 27 (3), 416–448.

Hayes, D., Bunting, L., 2013. 'Just be brave' – The experience of young witnesses in criminal proceedings in Northern Ireland. Child Abus. Rev. 22 (6), 419–431.

Henry, L., et al., 2011. Perceived credibility and eyewitness testimony of children with intellectual disabilities. J. Intellect. Disabil. Res. 55 (4), 385–391.

Health Care Improvement Scotland, & Care Inspectorate, 2023. Bairns' House: Final Standards. https://www.healthcareimprovementscotland.

org/his/idoc.ashx?docid=31b44a76-7c6c-48c2-95ce-e9f609eaca28&version=-1 (Accessed 22 August 2023).

HM Courts and Tribunal Service, NSPCC, CPS, 2018. National remote link sites protocol. https://www.cps.gov.uk/sites/default/files/documents/publications/Remote-Link-Sites-Protocol.pdf (Accessed 22 August 2023).

HM Courts and Tribunal Service, 2017. Your Child is a Witness. https://assets.publishing.service.gov.uk/government/uploads/system/uploads/attachment_data/file/708133/ywp-adult-eng.pdf. (Accessed 22 August 2023)

HM Government, 2018. Working Together to Safeguard Children. Stationery Office, London. https://assets.publishing.service.gov.uk/government/uploads/system/uploads/attachment_data/file/779401/Working_Together_to_Safeguard-Children.pdf (Accessed 22 August 2023).

Ho, H., 1999. A theory of hearsay. Oxford Journal of Legal Studies 19 (3), 403–420.

Hodgkin, R. and Newell, P., 2007. Implementation Handbook for the Convention On The Rights Of The Child: Fully revised 3rd edn. UNICEF, Geneva. https://www.unicef.org/reports/implementation-handbook-convention-rights-child (Accessed 22 August 2023).

Hoyano, L.C., 2001. Striking a balance between the rights of defendants and vulnerable witnesses: Will special measures directions contravene guarantees of a fair trial? Crim. Law Rev. 948–969. https://www.researchgate.net/publication/228183793. (Accessed 22 August 2023).

Hoyano, L., Rafferty, A., 2017. Rationing defence intermediaries under the April 2016 Criminal Practice Direction. Crim. Law Rev. 2, 93–105. https://ora.ox.ac.uk/objects/uuid:9211cffd-9d8d-47d2-8505-e3c49af0b5c3/download_file?file_format=application%2Fpdf&safe_filename=Rationing%2BDefence%2BIntermediaries.pdf&type_of_work=Journal+article (Accessed 22 August 2023).

Johansson, S., 2012. Diffusion and governance of "Barnahus" in the Nordic countries: Report from an on-going project. J. Scand. Stud. Criminol. Crime Prev. 13 (sup1), 69–84.

Krahenbuhl, S.J., Dent, H.R., 2017. The views of ex-police officers on child abuse case attrition in the United Kingdom. J. Interpers. Violence doi: 10.1177/0886260517744763.

Lord Chief Justice, 2015. Criminal Practice Directions 2015 [2015] EWCA CRIM 1567. https://www.judiciary.uk/wp-content/uploads/2019/03/crim-pd-amendment-no-8-consolidated-mar2019.pdf. (Accessed 22 August 2023).

Mcnamee, H., Molyneaux, F., Geraghty, T., 2012. Key Stakeholder Evaluation of NSPCC Young Witness Service Remote Live Link (Foyle).

Ministry of Justice and NPCC, 2022. Achieving Best Evidence in Criminal Proceedings: Guidance on Interviewing Victims and Witnesses, and Guidance on Using Special Measures. https://assets.publishing.service.gov.uk/government/uploads/system/uploads/attachment_data/file/1164429/achieving-best-evidence-criminal-proceedings-2023.pdf (Accessed 22 August 2023).

Ministry of Justice, 2020, Code of Practice for Victims of Crime in England and Wales. London. Available at https://www.gov.uk/

government/publications/the-code-of-practice-for-victims-of-crime (Accessed 22 August 2023).

Morgan, J., Williams, J., 1993. A role for a support person for child witnesses in criminal proceedings. Br. J. Soc. Work 23 (2), 113.

National Police Chief's Council, Crown Prosecution Service and HM Courts and Tribunal Service, 2018. A protocol between the National Police Chiefs' Council, The Crown Prosecution Service And Her Majesty's Courts & Tribunals service to Expedite Cases Involving Witnesses under 10 Years. London. https://www.judiciary.uk/wp-content/uploads/2015/03/police-cps-hmcts-ywi-u10-protocol-20180711.pdf. (Accessed 2 April 2020).

National Statistics, 2020. Child Sexual Abuse in England and Wales: Year Ending March 2019. https://www.ons.gov.uk/peoplepopulationandcommunity/crimeandjustice/articles/childsexualabuseinenglandandwales/yearendingmarch2019#child-sexual-abuse-recorded-by-the-police. (Accessed 27 October 2020).

National Statistics, 2023. Youth Justice Statistics 2021-2022. https://www.gov.uk/government/statistics/youth-justice-statistics-2018-to-2019. (Accessed 22 August 2023).

NSPCC (no date). Alice's story. https://www.nspcc.org.uk/what-is-child-abuse/childrens-stories/alices-story/ (Accessed 22 August 2023).

Pantell, R.H., 2017. The child witness in the courtroom. Pediatrics 139 (3). https://pubmed.ncbi.nlm.nih.gov/28219966/. (Accessed 22 August 2023).

Pidd, H., et al., 2019. Youth court system in "chaos", says children's commissioner. Guardian.

Pigot, T., 1989. The report of the advisory group on video evidence. Home Office, London.

Plotnikoff, J., Woolfson, R., 2009. Measuring up? Evaluating Implementation of Government Commitments to Young Witnesses in Criminal Proceedings. https://www.researchgate.net/publication/338503548_Measuring_up_Evaluating_implementation_of_Government_commitments_to_young_witnesses_in_criminal_proceedings. (Accessed 22 August 2023).

Plotnikoff, J., Woolfson, R., 2019. Falling short? A Snapshot of Young Witness Policy and Practice Full Report. NSPCC, London. https://www.nuffieldfoundation.org/wp-content/uploads/2019/12/Young-witnesses-in-criminal-proceedings_a-progress-report-on-Measuring-up_v_FINAL.pdf. (Accessed 22 August 2023).

Porter, M.L., 2018. From on the stand to on tape: Why recorded child victim testimony is safer, more effective, & fairer. UC Davis J. Juv. L. & Pol'y (27), https://sjlr.law.ucdavis.edu/archives/vol-22-no-1/JJLP-Vol22-Issue1-Porter.pdf.

Rasmusson, B., 2011. Children's advocacy centers (Barnahus) in Sweden. Child Indicators Research 4 (2), 301–321 Springer.

Safeguarding Children as Victims and Witnesses (no date). Crown Prosecution Service, London. https://www.cps.gov.uk/legal-guidance/safeguarding-children-victims-and-witnesses (Accessed 22 August 2023).

Snow, P.C., Powell, M.B., Murfett, R., 2009. Getting the story from child witnesses: Exploring the application of a story grammar framework. Psychol. Crime Law 15 (6), 555–568.

The Inns of Court College of Advocacy, 2019. Further Rollout of Pre-Recorded Cross-Examination - ICCA. https://www.icca.ac.uk/further-rowith-effect-from-3-june-2019-s-28-of-the-youth-justice-and-criminal-evidence-act-1999-yjcea-in-respect-of-s-16-assistance-for-witnesses-by-virtue-of-age-or-incapacity-is-in-force-in-the/. (Accessed 22 August 2023).

UK Government, 2017. Going to Court and Being a Witness: A Booklet. Stationery Office, London. https://assets.publishing.service.gov.uk/government/uploads/system/uploads/attachment_data/file/708093/ywp-12-17-eng.pdf. (Accessed 22 August 2023).

Victims' Commissioner, 2018. A Voice for the Voiceless: The Victims' Commissioner's review into the Provision of Registered Intermediaries for Children and Vulnerable Victims and Witnesses. London

Vulnerable Witnesses (Criminal Evidence) (Scotland) Act 2019 (the 2019 Act). https://www.legislation.gov.uk/asp/2019/8/enacted

Youth Justice and Criminal Evidence Act 1999. https://www.legislation.gov.uk/ukpga/1999/23/contents

18 DIRECT WORK WITH CHILDREN

MICHELLE LEFEVRE

KEY POINTS

- What is meant by direct work and what it looks like in child protection contexts.

- The importance of learning directly from children about their circumstances and concerns but why this may be challenging to achieve.

- The building of rapport and trust as a prerequisite for effective direct work.

- Skilled use of self and the organisational supports it requires.

- Play and activity-based assessment and intervention.

- A framework for child-centred direct work.

INTRODUCTION

Learning about children's experiences, thoughts and feelings is one of the most important tasks in child protection. Children are not passive objects of concern but important agents in their own lives who can provide vital insights into the harm they are facing. Their views and emotions should always be placed centre stage when decisions are being made and plans formulated. And yet we know that this remains an area of challenge for practitioners, who do not always feel skilled in engaging or communicating with children in unsafe situations. As a result, some children feel unheard and unsupported, and the risks they are encountering may not be fully appreciated.

Direct work offers a key pathway through which practitioners can gather information, elicit views, help children understand what is happening to them and provide support. The term refers not only to formal, planned work carried out over a number of sessions, but to everyday, impromptu or brief interactions with children on their own, in sibling groups or with their parents or carers present.

This chapter will clarify the role and place of direct work, explore what may lie beneath practitioner struggles and set out some principles and approaches which are proving helpful in child protection practice.

RIGHTS-BASED DIRECT WORK

The United Nations Convention on the Rights of the Child specifies that where a child's well-being and safety needs to be secured through legislative processes and services that provide care and protection, 'all interested parties shall be given an opportunity to participate in the proceedings and make their views known' (Article 9). 'Parties' in this context does not just mean adults; statutory services are also obliged to provide children with information in whatever format or media they require, to ensure children are able to express their views freely in all matters affecting them and to take their views into account (Articles 12 and 13). These principles of the Convention infuse all contemporary UK legislation, policy and guidance relating to child welfare and protection: professionals must see and speak to children, listen to what they say and take their views seriously (Scottish Government, 2014; Northern Ireland Department of Health, 2017; HM Government, 2018; Welsh Government, 2019). Such direct work ensures that children's wishes and feelings are taken into account, that matters are explained to them in a way that makes sense to them, and the child's own agreement to decisions and plans is achieved, as far as possible (HM Government, 2018, p. 48).

Rights-based direct work is not only a legal and ethical imperative, but of practical and therapeutic benefit. Decisions and plans that do not include the child's voice may lack vital information (HM Government, 2018). Children are also less likely to go along with plans that they feel ignore their concerns or fail to respect their wishes (Cossar et al., 2016). A child-centred assessment considers strengths, needs and risks from the child's perspective. Where there is the opportunity to engage with children's experiences and relationships through more open-ended direct work, professionals can learn from children themselves what their lives are like, what they are worried about and what they would like to happen. In this way, it may be possible to uncover the 'unknown unknowns' (Luft and Ingham, 1955) – important information that practitioners do not ask about because they are not aware it is even there.

Direct work is not psychotherapy; that is a more formal set of structures, processes and techniques conducted by a suitably qualified professional. However, direct work will be informed by therapeutic principles and may well have a therapeutic impact where it engages children in relationships of trust, helps them to express their emotions and enables them to process loss and trauma. Such opportunities are crucial for children who have been separated from their families and communities of origin following child protection concerns. Many are left with a sense of discontinuity between their past and present lives, resulting in uncertainty about who they are and what has happened (Harper, 1996). Where direct work is conducted by someone who moves between children's external social world of families, schools, peer groups, and placements, and their internal world of emotions, perceptions and aspirations, direct work is uniquely placed to help join the dots between children's inner and outer experiences (Schofield, 1998). Where a practitioner is involved consistently with a child over months or even years rather than days and weeks, this can provide the 'golden thread' that enables children to connect and make sense of their thoughts, feelings, experiences, relationships and events over space and time, and supports their heritage and identity (Care Inquiry, 2013, p. 14). Openings for such work may arise unexpectedly rather than being pre-planned – on a doorstep, in the car following contact or in the midst of a crisis meeting. Practitioners should seize the opportunity, tackling issues as they arise, as this may be the moment when a young person allows their defences to drop momentarily (Larkin and Lefevre, 2020).

THE VOICE OF THE CHILD

Common ethical and practical principles inform direct work (Lefevre, 2018), but specific knowledge and skills will be needed when child protection concerns have arisen. Public inquiries and serious case reviews have highlighted that professionals are not always successful in gaining children's trust, eliciting their views, listening to them or making sense of their experience (Care Inspectorate, 2016; Ofsted, 2011). Seeing children with their siblings and parents is an essential part of an assessment as it offers a window into family interactions and norms (Sidebotham et al., 2016). However, some children may be wary of speaking in the presence of a parent or carer, not only where they have been warned overtly not to, or even threatened, but where a parent's generally negative attitude towards professionals causes them to feel mistrust. Other children may not speak because they are protective of their parents, or their family's privacy.

There are numerous examples of serious problems arising when children have not been spoken with alone, to gain their perspective unmediated by other influences. Khyra Ishaq, a Black Muslim child in Birmingham, starved to death following a regime of cruelty and abuse at the hands of her mother and mother's partner. All the children in the household were severely malnourished, and concerns were raised by schools and health visitors. However, the children were seen only on the doorstep in the presence of their mother by police, education and social care workers, who did not pursue attempts to speak to Khyra or her siblings separately (Radford, 2010). Daniel Pelka, a White Polish boy, also beaten and starved to death, was 'invisible' to professionals, with 'no record of any conversation held with him by any professional about his home life, his experiences outside of school, his wishes and feelings and of his relationships with his siblings, mother and her male partners' (Locke, 2013, p. 71). Here, there was a sense that professionals had abrogated their responsibility, blaming their lack of dialogue with him on Daniel's youth and 'lack of confidence' in English. However, children's capabilities in communication are not a product of their individual competence but are interactionally driven. Mutual dialogue and meaning-making depend on the extent to which the professional creates a child-centred facilitating environment – that is, enables the child to feel safe and relaxed, and helps them to communicate in the language and modality which meets their needs and preferences (Lefevre, 2018).

These case reviews highlight the importance of communicating with children in their native or primary language, so they can represent and narrate their experiences, thoughts, feelings and wishes freely (Westlake and Jones, 2018). It is essential that interpreters become involved where necessary to facilitate such communication as there are numerous examples of serious risks to children being missed because the professionals relied on the parents to interpret and there was no separate verbal conversation with the child (Laird and Tedam, 2019). Disabled children, unaccompanied minors, and Black, Asian and minority ethnic children all have particular experience both of discrimination within wider UK structures and systems (Bhatti-Sinclair, 2011; Franklin, 2015) and of child protection systems failing to engage with them and understand their particular circumstances (Sidebotham et al., 2016). So, it is essential that services consider involving skilled intermediaries for interpretation with children where English is not their first language or using augmentative and alternative methods for children with learning disabilities, speech and language impairments (Brandon et al., 2020).

Communication can take almost double the length of time in such situations (Prynallt-Jones et al., 2018), so meetings, interviews and other encounters should always be planned with this in mind, including regular breaks. Although the extra time should be taken into account in workloads as a matter of course, this is not always practitioners' experience, and so they may find themselves needing to draw managers' attention to the additional time commitment that will be needed to fulfil their professional obligations to children – pointing

out the evidence from serious case reviews of harm to children where this has not happened can be helpful in arguing their case.

The serious case reviews cited earlier offer starkly obvious examples of inadequate communication, but other professional shortcomings may be more nuanced, given that adults do not always appreciate the indirect ways in which children convey their experience. 'Voice' encompasses more than just the information and views that children express directly and explicitly. Building a fuller picture requires us to attend to the whole of children's emotional, relational and bodily expression. The report of a significant case review conducted following the sexual abuse and neglect of a White Scottish sibling group whilst in the care of their parents (North Ayrshire Child Protection Committee, 2018) enables us to see the complexity of this (Case Study 18.1). The review was conducted because the child protection system as a whole had failed to identify and address risk to the children.

The report reveals that a whole range of factors had contributed to the poor practice in this situation, including role confusion across agency boundaries and inadequacies in communication between professionals and with the family. For example, police reports recorded the children as 'unaffected' by the domestic abuse in the family home. While the police had meant the children were not *physically* harmed during incidents, this had been misunderstood across the inter-agency system as meaning that the children were not adversely affected at all. When there are such shortcomings in interprofessional communication, as are reported in the majority of serious case reviews (Care Inspectorate, 2016; Sidebotham et al., 2016), it is even more essential that time is spent getting to know the children and building trust with them so that their experiences are better understood. An understanding of the situation from the perspective of the child can then be integrated with other sources of information.

DIRECT WORK AS AN INTERPERSONAL AND INTERPRETIVE ENDEAVOUR

The J Family Review shows that, just as vulnerable children often struggle to convey clearly what is important to them, practitioners may fail to appreciate

CASE STUDY 18.1 THE SIGNIFICANT CASE REVIEW OF THE J FAMILY

'There is a recurring theme throughout the progress of the case of a failure to both speak to and hear the children and to make best use of their non-verbal communication to address their wellbeing and safety. For some episodes children's words were reinterpreted or replaced by adults' phrasing and framing and the children's voices were lost or their presentations explained away too easily. For other episodes there were at best limited attempts to engage directly with the children and sometimes none, even in the context of concerns that should have triggered professional alarm ... As concern about the children's presentation grew, inappropriate assessment of their verbal contributions were made and their testimony was disregarded, for example, on the grounds of 'inconsistency'. Their non-verbal communication at these times was not considered ... There is also evidence of restricted and restricting interpretation across all agencies about what children's communication constitutes, especially with regard to the inclusion of behavioural indicators ... phrases such as [child's views] 'not known due to age and stage' continue to be used. Across the recording accessed for the case at the heart of this review there is very little evidence of the children's views being actively sought.'

(North Ayrshire Child Protection Committee, 2018, pp. 36–37)

what it is they are hearing or seeing. Not only were insufficient attempts made to speak directly with the J children, but even where conversations had occurred, practitioners did not treat these with care or respect. They ignored or reframed the children's words and dismissed their accounts as 'inconsistent', seemingly expecting that these very vulnerable children should be able to 'tell' directly and unproblematically about what had happened to them or what they would like to happen next. Such expectations may well be unrealistic, particularly for very young, unsafe, traumatised or disabled children (Franklin, 2015). Children in such circumstances may not have a conceptual understanding of their feelings and experiences, let alone the words to convey them. As the J review noted, 'They are unlikely to "know" and therefore disclose that they are being neglected, and may be waiting to be noticed and asked why they are unhappy' (North Ayrshire Child Protection Committee, 2018, p. 35).

So, although professionals should always try (and try hard!) to engage and communicate directly with children where there are child protection concerns, they must do so with the understanding that children will not always be able to give a coherent, linear or consistent narrative account of events, attributions nor their views on their situation – or at least not straight away (Marchant, 2013). A process of rigorous qualitative analysis is required to interrogate and synthesise all available information to start to make sense of children's inner and outer worlds.

A more nuanced and contextualised appreciation of the nature of communication is needed to inform direct work in such sensitive, contested and complex situations. Communication is never just a linear and purposeful transfer of verbal or written information from one person to another. Even among adults, words account for a minority of the conversational meaning formed (Remland, 2017). Eye contact, paralanguage (tone, volume and intonation), context, cultural competence and so on are all required to 'de-code' hidden or unconscious intentions and perspectives and to get beneath the surface of words (Hargie and Dickson, 2004). It is this complexity that can so often lead to miscommunications and misunderstandings. Careful and sensitised observation of a child in context is needed if the professional is to take in and consider the child's body language, affect, relationality, play and other behaviours. This is particularly so with preverbal or disabled children (Fleming, 2004).

This interpretive process is not one-way but, rather, interactional and intersubjective: both child and professional bring a range of feelings, thoughts, perceptions and intentions to their encounters, not all of which are intended or even within their full awareness. The nature of their relationship and the context of their interaction affects not only what the adult or child says and how they say it, but what the other hears and the meaning they take from it (Hargie and Dickson, 2004). Practitioners are not always able to find intelligible or appropriate ways of explaining difficult or sensitive issues, and this can compound children's confusion and uncertainty. Unconscious or disowned feelings and motivations may play a significant role (Ruch, 2013).

Children who have experienced abuse, problematic parenting and discontinuity of care bring their fear, uncertainty, anxiety, wariness and/or hostility to the direct work encounter (Knight, 2015). Neglectful or abusive parenting experiences may mean that some children are not used to adults really listening to, understanding and validating them, and they do not know how to begin to express themselves. Traumatised children may be hypervigilant to future risk, scrutinising the professional's body language and paralanguage, to evaluate the level of safety, and whether what they do or say will be understood, accepted and respected by the adult (Harris and Fallot, 2001). Some children may be frightened to speak, having been directly threatened with retribution to themselves or to loved ones if they disclose what is happening to them. Others may have taken on family scripts or unspoken rules about hostility to, or fear of, those who represent the authorities. Being compelled to talk before they are ready, or being asked intrusive questions, may recreate some of the dynamics of abuse and be re-traumatising for children, particularly following sexual abuse or exploitation. A grooming process which has sought to achieve children's compliance with sexual acts may leave children with feelings of guilt and shame and they may be motivated to hide what has happened from themselves or others, deliberately or unconsciously. Grooming, too, seeks to undermine the child's relationship with non-abusing parents and carers, with the result that the child can be drawn into the abuser's worldview and comes to trust neither family nor professionals (Cossar et al., 2013).

In such situations, professionals need to ensure the child feels they have been seen, heard, and understood, and that they are cared about. This requires practitioners to mentalize for the child (think about their state of mind) and to respond in an emotionally attuned manner (Fonagy and Allison, 2012). Practitioners need to constantly monitor and evaluate the mood and atmosphere to attune to what the child needs in that moment and respond in kind. This includes moderating their tone of voice, facial gestures and body language, responding in the same modality and degree of amplification as the child (e.g. through sound, gesture, play or words).

BUILDING RAPPORT, TRUST AND SAFETY

Moving straight into direct and focused conversations in assessment and intervention with children can be unhelpful both ethically and practically. As can be seen from the previous examples, pressing children about sensitive matters before they are ready may not only transgress the principle of nonmaleficence ('above all, do no harm') but may be counter-productive in causing children to become wary, even withdrawing completely. A slower-paced, child-centred approach, using the 'hundred languages of childhood' (Edwards et al., 1993) is preferable wherever possible. Informal and non-directive play, board or computer games (including virtual ones), and other activities such as talking about hobbies, going for a coffee or playing with pets can support the building of rapport and trust and act as a bridge to focused conversation (Lefevre, 2018). More focused exploration of difficult matters and expression of emotions and perceptions may be facilitated when a more metaphorical language, such as artwork, puppetry or stories, is used. These can all also act as what social pedagogy calls the 'common third', something for the worker and child or young person to focus on together that takes them away from the uncomfortable intensity of their interaction (Ruch et al., 2017).

How these processes play out in the real world can be explored through looking closely at real world direct work encounters. The excerpts in Boxes 18.1 and 18.2 are drawn from an unpublished study of social workers' practice with children in the context of child protection concerns that my colleague, Chris Hall, and I conducted with two local authorities in England. The research involves close scrutiny of video recordings of practitioners' conversations and interactions with children, usually conducted during home visits, and follow-up interviews with the children and social workers (separately) to learn about their perceptions of the recorded encounters. Box 18.1 describes interactions between social worker, Adeola, and 4-year-old Flora during the early stages of a home visit. At the time of recording, Adeola had been involved with the family for 3 months following concerns about neglect and the children having witnessed violence towards their mother from her (now ex-) partner. Adeola had visited regularly over this period, assessing risk and supporting the family. During each visit she would spend some time alone with Flora.

As soon as the recording begins, it is clear to the observer that Flora and Adeola were familiar with each other and their context, falling straight into playing and talking together. Their body language was suggestive of physical and emotional comfortableness

---

BOX 18.1

BEGINNING A DIRECT WORK ENCOUNTER

Flora and Adeola are sitting on the sofa. Adeola brings some activity sheets and colouring pens out of her bag, showing them to Flora. She gives Flora lots of eye contact as she carefully explains what is on each sheet and offers Flora choices:

ADEOLA: "Do you want to write or just do colouring? You can choose which one you want to do. Which one shall we start with? [points to one sheet]. Do you want to do one about a fabulous dream you have? So, do you remember your dreams sometimes? If you remember your dream, you can draw what happened. Or this one [shows another sheet]. You can write things that you are very, very good at, or sometimes things that make you feel silly. [laughs]

FLORA: Silly-h-h! [laughing]

ADEOLA: You want to do that one? Or do you want to do that, what makes you laugh and what makes you happy?

FLORA: Erm [.] I know! [bright tone] So make do happier one; erm, this one, this one!

As Adeola talks, Flora snatches at the papers and rifles through them, making sure she gets a good look at them. Adeola allows her to do this and smiles warmly at her. Flora kicks her legs around excitedly, grinning, and interrupts a lot to point at the sheets and ask questions. Once she has chosen, Flora grabs the papers and pens and runs across to the table to start drawing. Adeola moves to join her and they sit together, heads bent over Flora's drawing activity. At first, the talk while they draw is solely about Flora's picture. The pace is gentle. Adeola asks Flora whether or not she (Adeola) should join in with drawing, too. Flora shows how and where Adeola should add to the drawing. Their facial expressions, body language and tone of voice are characterised by mutual grinning, laughing and smiling – including with the eyes – a frequent turning towards each other, and warm tones of voice.

BOX 18.2

MOVING BETWEEN FREE PLAY AND FOCUSED CONVERSATION

Adeola makes suggestions about what they could talk about by pointing to different parts of the page.

ADEOLA: Maybe on one you could say what you like at school, what you like at the play centre, or what you like at home, so we can do that in a line like that [points]. And then here you can do what you like at the play centre, what you like at home, what you like at school. So you can talk about your friends, your teacher. So which one shall we start with first?

FLORA: This one.

Flora points to where 'school' had been indicated and so Adeola writes it down spelling out SCHOOL.

ADEOLA: Do you still like this school?

FLORA: Ye-e-ss. [uncertain tone]

ADEOLA: What's your teacher's name again?

FLORA: Miss X.

ADEOLA: And who are your friends, again?

Flora gives their names.

ADEOLA: You've got loads, good. And at home you go to daddy's today, innit?

FLORA: Mmm [mumbles].

ADEOLA: It's going to be what?

FLORA: [mumbles, unintelligible].

Flora turns away, focuses on drawing and ignores all further questions.

---

and they were attentive to each other's presence. Their growing relationship and the ethos for the work was fed through such interactions.

Such attention to the building of rapport and trust is an essential stage in direct work, a prerequisite of talk about more complex and private matters. Trust is most commonly built in three ways. First, a period of problem-free talk and play which progresses at the child's pace enables the child and worker to become familiar with each other in an unpressurised environment. The worker's approach will then be more attuned and responsive, as it will be informed by the child's needs and preferences. Second, the relationship is nurtured through the professional's skilled and congruent 'use of self' – being warm, friendly, open and caring towards the child. These are not distanced techniques, but rather real qualities in the practitioner that have been honed through self-awareness and self-reflection (Lefevre, 2018). Third, the worker needs to demonstrate their trustworthiness through being reliable, available, consistent, open and boundaried.

Many practitioners are 'time-poor' due to heavy workloads, or pressure to find information out from the child quickly in order to protect them, and it may be difficult in such circumstances for them to be child-led and to allow trust to build naturally – but the impact of this on a child's engagement in the work must be acknowledged. A realistic and honest report to a child protection conference or court in such circumstances should not say, *'Child was unable to give their view'* but, rather, *'The system/circumstances/practitioner's caseload did not allow the facilitating conditions to be built that might have enabled the child to give their view'.* Perhaps if such a transparent approach were taken, the system might begin to adapt to the child, rather than the other way around. Practitioners might be empowered to advocate for more time for their work through the 80/20 campaign which is being run by the British Association of Social Workers (https://www.basw.co.uk/what-we-do/campaigns/relationship-based-practice). The campaign is seeking to raise the profile of the benefits of relationship-based practice in social work and alert senior leaders and policy makers to their responsibilities in creating an effective and supportive context for practice, including through workload time, skilled training and reflective supervision.

Adeola had sought to make this encounter as child led as possible, offering Flora a range of options for the progression of the activity and creating a permissive atmosphere. This kind of empowering approach recognises the child's rights and nurtures her agency. The practical benefits were visible in the room: Flora appeared comfortable in the encounter and expressed her preferences confidently. It is likely that there were also therapeutic benefits. Children who have lived with chronic abuse and neglect, and/or in difficult and ongoing family circumstances, such as domestic abuse, may experience negative impacts on their psychological, physical, social, emotional or spiritual well-being that could persist into adulthood if trauma and adversity are not addressed (Knight, 2015). Direct work, even where the focus is assessment rather than therapy, offers nuanced and incremental opportunities for healing in every encounter, enabling the child to start to build a new, more positive theory of the world (Harris and Fallot, 2001).

This kind of relational direct work requires self-awareness and emotional availability in the practitioner, and an understanding of some of the deeper psychological and interactional processes that may occur between them. Professionals will inevitably bring their own emotional states and life experiences to their encounters with children, and any unresolved (possibly unconscious) issues may intrude on the encounter (Ruch, 2013). For example, when observing social workers visiting families due to child protection risks, Ferguson (2016) noticed that some practitioners seemed less able to emotionally attune to the children. They presented as 'detached', having become 'intuitively, cognitively and spiritually absent' in the direct work (Ferguson, 2016, p. 5).

Truly engaging with and comprehending children's pain, fear and distress can be intolerable for professionals at times. This will be compounded where the direct work takes place amid parental hostility, a tense, even threatening atmosphere in the family home, and a requirement to make difficult decisions in conditions of uncertainty. Practitioners can be pushed beyond the limits of their capacity to manage the child's emotional intensity, their own anxiety and the interactional complexity. Defence mechanisms, such as detachment, may kick in unconsciously to protect workers from being overwhelmed, but these also inure them from seeing, hearing, mentalizing and caring for a child who then becomes 'invisible', 'unthought' about, and not 'held in mind' by workers and systems (Ferguson, 2016, p. 5). Secondary or vicarious trauma may result, including burnout, compassion fatigue and the practitioner's own trauma histories being triggered (Taggart, 2018).

Importantly, Ferguson did not attribute such defence mechanisms or secondary trauma as solely due to shortcomings in the practitioner's training or skills, but rather as a normative response to highly distressing and complex work. A trauma-informed approach to practice does not only consider children's responses and behaviours as understandable and adaptive strategies to traumatic stress, but also the responses of professionals who are required to witness the pain and distress of children and young people over time (Knight, 2015). This indirect trauma can be reduced and contained by support built into a reflective practice system, including regular reflective supervision and space for practitioners to reflect upon their own relationship to interpersonal trauma (Ruch, 2013).

PLAY AS A FACILITATOR OF FOCUSED WORK

With the rapport built through the drawing activity at the beginning of the home visit, the scene was set for Adeola to build a bridge from the activity to more focused talk related to the aim of her visit: learning how Flora was experiencing life at home and school, and how her contact with her father was going.

This is a common example of how such conversations can go. Practitioners are keen to learn about particular areas of children's lives and interweave direct and focused questions in among the general chat and play-based activities. Sometimes they work, and children allow the conversation to unfold with the activity offering a soothing accompaniment. On other occasions, children use the activity as a way for them to avoid these focused questions. This is an important mechanism of escape for children as they may be very wary of the implications of the conversation and worried about breaching their family's confidentiality, particularly if they have been warned by a suspicious parent to be careful what they say. In my follow-up conversation with Adeola, she spoke of how she could sense Flora's rising tension at the probing questions. Like Flora, she had used the activity as a safe arena for retreat, gaining time to reflect on the impact on Flora of her questions and deciding when and how to move on. Knowing when to pursue a line of enquiry, and when to ease off, requires empathic attunement, with a sensitivity to the child's cues in the face of competing agendas.

As well as acting as a bridge, play may be the avenue itself for specific areas of exploration. A range of factors, including age, cultural heritage and gender identity, may influence children's interest in particular activities. It is important that workers do not pre-suppose what children might prefer but, wherever possible, provide a range of options that children can choose from. Ideally, practitioners will design focused activities around the child, drawing on their own creativity, but existing exercises and resources can provide helpful guidance and ideas upon which to build, particularly where workers have not yet built up their skills and confidence in this area of their practice. Sunderland (2018), for example, provides a photocopiable resource book containing a range of creative and interactive exercises and tools. Ecomaps – an approach to enabling children to sketch out their own subjective view of their family and community networks and supports – offer a basic framework upon which activities can be tailored to the situational requirements. At their most simple, ecomaps might just involve drawing lines and circles on a large piece of paper using size and colour to denote strength or quality of relationships. Including cut-out pictures, shapes such as buttons, or use of computer imagery can make the discussion of the image more dynamic, with the social worker or child moving them around to explore their social world (Lefevre et al, 2008). There are also some resources available that have been designed specifically for assessment in child protection, such as the 'words and pictures' storyboard (Hiles et al., 2008) and the 'three houses' model (Weld, 2008).

For children in the aftermath of very difficult circumstances, non-directive play can provide a space within which self-expression and exploration can take place at a symbolic level. In such circumstances, it is often unnecessary for workers to make direct connections between the play and the child's external world circumstances; the safe space in which children's play is supported and facilitated without interference or interpretation does the work. For other children, a focused and explicit activity might be more helpful. The child could be encouraged to engage in visual art, such as drawing or painting, to explore their concerns or wishes. Small figurines could be used to play out scenarios such as placement moves, or trips to the family court.

Stories are also an excellent way of exploring complex issues through metaphorical characters. These enable children to engage with the story's main theme gradually, either making their own connections or being helped to do so when the time is right (Sunderland and Armstrong, 2001). There are a number of books on the market exploring issues of relevance to child protection, such as those by CoramBAAF targeted at children in care or who have been adopted, with themes such as 'dealing with feelings' and 'moving to a new family'. However, more creative practitioners could have a go at writing a bespoke story which centres round similar contexts or experiences to those relevant for the child. Such stories can be very simple, and practitioners can illustrate them with photos or magazine images if they do not feel confident about illustrating them with their own drawings. An example of such a story is available in an e-learning course available from SCIE (Lefevre et al., 2008).

Remote contacts with children are becoming increasingly common, particularly in the aftermath of COVID-19, and it is equally important to ensure that these offer a safe and facilitative environment for direct work. Guidance has been issued by the Children and Family Court Advisory and Support Service (Cafcass) (2020) and the British Association of Social Workers (BASW) (2020) for direct work conducted virtually. Preparation tasks include ensuring that the parents or carers have given permission for remote working and have the available technology, that the worker is confident in the technical use of their equipment, and that the child has been able to make an informed choice about this form of contact. Some children may feel less comfortable with video calls, and for new contacts, it might be better to start with a phone introduction or a letter with a picture of the worker. The impact of parental presence during the call needs to be given careful thought. While some children may want or need support from the parent or carer to fully engage in the call, others may feel under pressure, particularly as the presence of a parent or carer might be hidden from the worker. So, it is always important to consider whether it is possible to safely conduct sensitive work in contexts of risk. Rapport building activities and conversational prompts will be more important than usual during video calls, and visual tools (which could be sent to the child in advance) may be particularly helpful. In all situations, careful attention needs to be given to observing the child's demeanour and affective state during the work and to ensuring that empathic support can be adequately conveyed through the screen, amplifying this verbally where necessary.

Whatever the approach, it is essential to go at the child's pace as far as possible and be sensitive to the strong emotional responses and relational connections that may be formed when undertaking direct work with children who have been harmed or are currently at risk. Practitioners should always try the activities out themselves in advance, carefully observe the child's affect and demeanour, ensure there is sufficient time to round off the session, and ensure that they or someone else is available for further support or reflection where painful issues have been triggered.

CONCLUSION

Fig. 18.1 offers a framework to inform direct work with children where there have been child protection

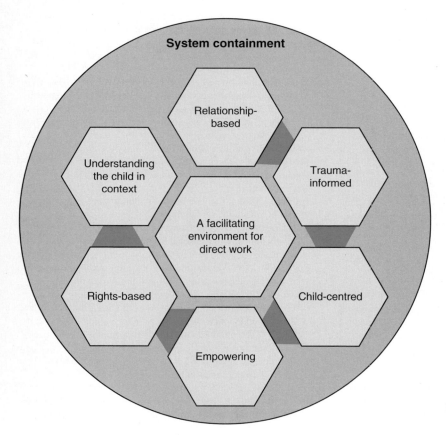

Fig. 18.1 ■ A facilitating environment for direct work.

concerns. It summarises the key points raised through this chapter setting out the key principles and approaches that should help practitioners provide a facilitating environment for direct work. A strong ethical stance is the bedrock of good practice, including a commitment to children's rights, to child-centredness and to strengths-focused practice. All children need to be understood as individuals with their own needs, views and subjectivities, but also as part of families and networks, and as social agents, who influence and are influenced by their social and cultural environment. For children who have experienced risk and harm, we must include a trauma-informed lens if we are to understand the impact of those experiences and respond empathically. All direct work, particularly with vulnerable children, will be most successful where it is carried out within an interpersonal relationship of trust and care. No worker is an island – the nature of this work can be demanding and distressing, and it is essential for child protection practitioners to be provided with psychological containment by their workplace, including through a supervisory relationship which offers a space for emotional reflection and validation.

REFLECTIVE QUESTIONS

- Think of an occasion as a child when an adult was supportive when you felt worried or unsafe. What did they say or do that was helpful? Did you feel you could trust them or talk to them? What learning is there from this situation that you would want to take into your work with children?

- If skilled direct work is as much about the person as what they do, how can you improve **you** so you become the kind of person children can communicate and engage with?

- Are you able to discuss the emotional and subjective aspects of your work in supervision? If not, how might you raise this with your line manager to start to change the way supervisory discussions happen and you can get what you need to stay safe and effective in your work?

REFERENCES

BASW, 2020. Practice guidance for Children and Families Social Work during Covid-19. https://www.basw.co.uk/practice-guidance-children-and-families-social-work-during-covid-19. (Accessed 5 August 2023).

Bhatti-Sinclair, K., 2011. Anti-Racist Practice in Social Work. Palgrave Macmillan, Basingstoke.

Brandon, M., Sidebotham, P., Belderson, P., Cleaver, H., Dickens, J., Garstang, J., et al., 2020. Complexity and Challenge: A Triennial Analysis of SCRs 2014-2017. Final report. Department for Education. https://assets.publishing.service.gov.uk/government/uploads/system/uploads/attachment_data/file/869586/TRIENNIAL_SCR_REPORT_2014_to_2017.pdf. (Accessed 29 May 2020).

Cafcass, 2020. Knowledge Bite: Using Skype and Other Forms of Video Conferencing for Interviews with Parents and Direct Work with Children. https://adcs.org.uk/assets/documentation/Cafcass_Knowledge_bite_video_conferencing_with_parents_and_children%28v2%29.pdf. (Accessed 29 May 2020).

Care Inquiry, 2013. Making not Breaking. Building Relationships for Our Most Vulnerable Children. Findings and recommendations of the Care Inquiry. https://thecareinquiry.files.wordpress.com/2013/04/care-inquiry-full-report-april-2013.pdf. (Accessed 29 May 2020).

Care Inspectorate, 2016. Learning from Significant Case Reviews in Scotland: A Retrospective Review of Relevant Reports Completed in the Period Between 1 April 2012 and 31 March 2015. Care Inspectorate, Dundee.

Cossar, J., Brandon, M., Bailey, S., Belderson, P., Biggart, L., 2013. "It Takes a Lot to Build Trust". Recognition and Telling: Developing Earlier Routes to Help for Children and Young People. Office of the Children's Commissioner, London.

Cossar, J., Brandon, M., Jordan, P., 2016. "You've got to trust her and she's got to trust you": children's views on participation in the child protection system. Child Fam. Soc. Work 21 (1), 103–112.

Edwards, C.P., Gandini, L. & Forman, G.E. (Eds.), 1993. The Hundred Languages of Children: The Reggio Emilia Approach to Early Childhood Education, Greenwich, CT: Ablex.

Ferguson, H., 2016. How children become invisible in child protection work: Findings from research into day to day social work practice. Br. J. Soc. Work 47 (4), 1007–1023.

Fleming, S., 2004. The contribution of psychoanalytical observation in child protection assessments. J. Soc. Work Pract 18 (2), 223–238.

Fonagy, P., Allison, E., 2012. What is mentalization? The concept and its foundations in developmental research. In: Midgley, N., Vrouva, I. (Eds.), Minding the Child: Mentalization-Based Interventions With Children, Young People and Their Families. Routledge, London, pp. 11–34.

Franklin, A., 2015. Voice as more than words: Involving children and young people with communication needs in decision-making. In: Ivory, M. (Ed.), Voice of the Child: Meaningful Engagement With Children and Young People. Evidence review. Research in Practice, Totnes, pp. 58–67.

Hargie, O., Dickson, D., 2004. Skilled Interpersonal Communication, fourth ed. Routledge, London.

Harper, J., 1996. Recapturing the past: Alternative methods of life story work in adoption and fostering. Adopt Foster 20 (3), 21–28.

Harris, M., Fallot, R., 2001. Envisioning a trauma-informed service system: A vital paradigm shift. New Directions For Mental Health Services 89, 1–22.

Hiles, M., Essex, S., Fox, A., Luger, C., 2008. The "words and pictures" storyboard: making sense for children and families. Context 97, 13–19.

HM Government, 2018. Working Together to Safeguard Children: A guide to Inter-Agency Working to Safeguard and Promote the Welfare of Children. https://www.gov.uk/government/publications/working-together-to-safeguard-children--2. (Accessed 29 May 2020).

Knight, C., 2015. Trauma-informed social work practice: Practice considerations and challenges. Clin. Soc. Work 43, 25–37.

Laird, S., Tedam, P., 2019. Cultural Diversity in Child Protection: Cultural Competence in Practice. Red Globe Press, London.

Larkin, R. and Lefevre, M., 2020. Unaccompanied Young Females and Social Workers: Meaning-Making in the Practice Space. Br. J. Soc. Work, 50(5), pp. 1570–1587.

Lefevre, M., 2018. Communicating and Engaging with Children and Young People: Making a Difference, second ed. The Policy Press, Bristol.

Lefevre, M., Richards, S., Trevithick, P., 2008. Using Play and the Creative Arts to Communicate with Children and Young People. Social Care Institute for Excellence, London. https://www.scie.org.uk/e-learning/communication-skills#module08. (Accessed 29 May 2020).

Locke, R., 2013. Serious Case Review into the Experience of Daniel Pelka: Independent Overview Report. Coventry Safeguarding Children Board, Coventry.

Luft, J., Ingham, H., 1955. 'The Johari Window, a Graphic Model of Interpersonal Awareness'. Proceedings of the Western Training Laboratory in Group Development. University of California, Los Angeles.

Marchant, R., 2013. How young is too young? The evidence of children under five in the English criminal justice system. Child Abus. Rev. 22 (6), 432–445.

North Ayrshire Child Protection Committee, 2018. Findings of a Significant Case Review - J Family. http://childprotectionnorthayrshire.info/cpc/media/2018/03/North-Ayrshire-SCR-Redacted-FINAL.pdf. (Accessed 29 May 2020).

Northern Ireland Department of Health, 2017. Co-operating to Safeguard Children and Young People in Northern Ireland. https://www.health-ni.gov.uk/publications/co-operating-safeguard-children-and-young-people-northern-ireland. (Accessed 29 May 2020).

Ofsted, 2011. The Voice of the Child: Learning Lessons from Serious Case Reviews. Ofsted, Manchester.

Prynallt-Jones, K.A., Carey, M., Doherty, P., 2018. Barriers facing social workers undertaking direct work with children and young people with a learning disability who communicate using non-verbal methods. Br. J. Soc. Work 48 (1), 88–105.

Radford, J., 2010. Serious Case Review Under Chapter VIII 'Working Together to Safeguard Children' In Respect of the Death of a Child: Case Number 14. Birmingham Safeguarding Children Board. https://northshropshe.files.wordpress.com/2015/07/khyra_ishaq_scr.pdf. (Accessed 29 May 2020).

Remland, M.S., 2017. Nonverbal Communication in Everyday Life, fourth ed. Sage Publications, Thousand Oaks, CA.

Ruch, G., 2013. "Helping children is a human process": Researching the challenges social workers face in communicating with children. Br. J. Soc. Work 44 (8), 2145–2162.

Ruch, G., Winter, K., Cree, V., Hallett, S., Hadfield, M., 2017. Making meaningful connections: Using insights from social pedagogy in statutory child and family social work practice. Child Fam. Soc. Work 22 (2), 1015–1023.

Schofield, G., 1998. Inner and outer worlds: A psychosocial framework for child and family social work. Child Fam. Soc. Work 3 (1), 57–67.

Scottish Government, 2014. National Guidance for Child Protection in Scotland. https://www.gov.scot/publications/national-guidance-child-protection-scotland/. (Accessed 29 May 2020).

Sidebotham, P., Brandon, M., Bailey, S., Belderson, P., Dodsworth, J., Garstang, J., et al., 2016. Pathways to Harm, Pathways to Protection: A Triennial Analysis of Serious Case Reviews 2011 to 2014. Department for Education, London.

Sunderland, M., 2018. Draw on Your Emotions, second ed. Routledge, London.

Sunderland, M., Armstrong, N., 2001. Using Story Telling as a Therapeutic Tool with Children. Speechmark Publishing Ltd, Brackley.

Taggart, D., 2018. Trauma-Informed Approaches with Young People: Frontline Briefing. Research in Practice, Devon.

United Nations Convention on the Rights of the Child. https://www.ohchr.org/en/instruments-mechanisms/instruments/convention-rights-child.

Weld, N., 2008. The three houses tool: Building safety and positive change. In: Calder, M. (Ed.), Contemporary Risk Assessment in Safeguarding Children. Russell House Publishing, Lyme Regis, pp. 224–231.

Welsh Government, 2019. Safeguarding Guidance. https://gov.wales/safeguarding-guidance. (Accessed 29 May 2020).

Westlake, D., Jones, R., 2018. Breaking down language barriers: A practice-near study of social work using interpreters. Br. J. Soc. Work 48 (5), 1388–1408.

19 WORKING WITH PARENTS (EDITOR'S INTRODUCTION)

LISA WARWICK ■ RACHAEL CLAWSON ■ RACHEL FYSON

Family structures are changing, and what constitutes 'family' is broader and more inclusive than ever before. Although most children live with their families throughout childhood, those families now come in many forms and embrace married parents, unmarried parents, cohabiting parents, same-sex parents, lone parents, stepparents and blended families. Whatever the family structure, working with parents or those in a parental role is a mainstay of child protection work. This chapter therefore explores what working with parents means for current practice.

The Children Act 1989 was a landmark piece of legislation and, despite various amendments, continues to provide the legislative bedrock of child protection in England and Wales. The Act is important not only for the introduction of the paramountcy principle in s.1(1), which recognises that in making any decision it must be the child's welfare that is of primary concern, but also for promoting the upbringing of children by their parents. The centrality of parents is there not only in associated guidance but also in s.1(5) – the 'no order' principle – which requires that working practices should minimise state interference and focus on maintaining family bonds. In 1998, the passing into law of Human Rights Act gave further support to parents through *Article 8: the Right to a Private and Family Life*. Article 8 is a qualified right, meaning that there are circumstances in which this right can be overruled in favour of other rights; this includes the absolute right enshrined in Article 3, which states that *No one shall be subjected to torture or to inhuman or degrading treatment or punishment*. The interplay of these two rights, alongside the legal framework of the Children Act 1989, means that child protection practice necessarily involves working with both the child and their parents or caregivers.

Although the Children Act 1989 continues to promote partnership working with parents, the political and practice climate shifted during the 2000s following the well-publicised deaths of Victoria Climbie in 2000 and Peter Connolly ('Baby P') in 2007, both in the London Borough of Haringey. Each of these deaths had a significant impact on child protection. Victoria's death, and the ensuing report by Lord Laming, led to new legislation and restructured services. Peter's death led to political pressure to change practice, resulting in sharp increases in referrals into children's social care, care order applications, and the number of children taken into care, with a concomitant increase in professional workloads. These cases also contributed to a growing climate of fear, cultivated by the media hounding of professionals involved in child protection work – particularly, but not exclusively, social workers. Practitioners, more than ever, feared 'getting things wrong'. Bureaucratical and managerial responses, and higher workloads, led to defensive practice. Coupled with the fear of failing to protect a child was an emerging view of parents as subjects of suspicion, rather than as individuals in need of support to care safely for their children.

Many parents experience the child protection process as harmful, not helpful. Those voluntarily seeking support may find few services available – and the services they can access are often already over-stretched.

There are relatively few services that focus on working with the trauma which often underpins problematic styles of parenting or which facilitate long-term therapeutic change. Support for children and families has fallen as preventative and early-help services have closed. High thresholds for accessing the services that remain mean that many vulnerable families do not receive support until they are in crisis. All too often a 'revolving door' of children's services has been created, in which support is only given when parents reach crisis point and is then withdrawn too soon, leading to further crisis and re-referral. At the same time, the blurred lines between neglect and poverty (discussed in Chapter 4) interact with the impacts of wider socioeconomic difficulties which influence the experiences and opportunities of both parents and children. All these factors need to be taken into account when working with parents.

Defensive and fearful practice has continued to influence approaches to child protection practice. This Handbook therefore advocates for a more humane approach to child protection, one that upholds the paramountcy principle but also works with, and not against, parents. It is recognised that humane and compassionate practice can be challenging when high caseloads combine with service cuts and difficulties with recruitment and retention of staff. However, the impact on parents of these same factors is also severe. This is outlined in Chapter 3 where Claire Western tells her own story – highlighting the need to understand child protection from the perspective of parents in order to achieve the best possible outcomes for children.

Although all parents are likely to find the involvement of child protection intimidating, some parents experience greater levels of scrutiny, stigma and discrimination. These parents are more likely to have their children removed, and they need independent advocacy support to ensure that their voices are heard within the child protection system. Child protection practice with some of these parents is reflected within this chapter. Working with these parents requires skilled and humane practitioners who can offer well-informed support that recognises the nuances of parental need as well as the needs of their children. With the right support, many of these parents *can* safely care for their own children.

Each section in this chapter outlines a stigma faced by a particular group of parents and sets out what professionals need to know in order to ensure that their practice is ethical, safe and humane. In Chapter 19a, Danielle Turney and Beth Tarleton explore the particular challenges facing *Parents with Learning Disabilities*, while in Chapter 19b, Kirsten Morley and Andrew Murphy outline an approach to *Working With Parents Experiencing Mental Distress* which ensures that the needs of child and parents are considered holistically. Both of these contributions consider the complexities of working across children's and adults' services and some of the difficulties this can cause.

The persistently gendered nature of child protection work, with mothers too often experiencing undue scrutiny of their parenting and fathers too often being excluded is discussed in Chapter 19c, where Caroline Lynch discussed the challenges faced by *Young Parents*, particularly those who have themselves spent time in care as a child. Lynch's contribution also pays careful attention to how the intersections of age and gender can impact on how parents are perceived and treated by services. Finally, in Chapter 19d, Karen Broadhurst, Claire Mason, Lisa Morriss and Bachar Alrouh draw upon their recent research to highlight the need for *Compassionate and Effective Practice with Parents at Risk of Repeat Removal of Their Children Through Care Proceedings*. In doing so they draw attention to the systemic injustices faced by these parents and the lack of support available to them.

REFERENCE

Children Act 1989. https://www.legislation.gov.uk/ukpga/1989/41/contents

19a

WORKING WITH PARENTS WITH LEARNING DISABILITIES

DANIELLE TURNEY ■ BETH TARLETON

KEY POINTS

- Parents with learning disabilities are reported as being overrepresented within the child protection system.

- Concerns about the welfare of their children are typically expressed in relation to neglect.

- Adults with learning disabilities are recognised as being 'vulnerable' themselves and may struggle with the complexities of everyday life.

- Mainstream services have been shown to lack experience and training in tailoring their responses to meet the needs of adults with learning disabilities when there are child protection concerns, and may struggle to provide a joined-up response that draws on both adult and children's services.

- This chapter draws on research findings to outline 'what works' when engaging effectively with parents with learning disabilities and proposes a relationship-based framework for practice based on the '6 Ts': time, trust, tenacity, truthfulness, transparency and a tailored response.

INTRODUCTION

Parents with learning disabilities are a group who may not have been particularly to the forefront of social work thinking in relation to child protection. For many years, policy directed that adults with learning disabilities, if not living with family members (typically their own parents), were likely to be living in institutional settings. However, with the moves towards de-institutionalisation and the closure of the old-style 'mental hospitals', the rights

of people with learning disabilities have moved into sharper focus. Now it is considerably more likely that an adult with a learning disability will be living in the community, perhaps in some form of supported housing, but with the assumption that they will be able to exercise many if not all of the choices about their lives that others enjoy – particularly in terms of establishing friendships, intimate relationships and parenting.

Adults with learning disabilities have typically been identified as 'vulnerable'; they may struggle with some of the complexities of everyday living and be experiencing a range of disadvantages. Studies suggest that as parents, they are overrepresented within child protection and court proceedings and at higher risk of having their children compulsorily removed from their care. Although we do not know precisely how many parents with learning disabilities are involved with child protection services as no records are kept identifying whether or not a parent has this diagnosis, it has been argued that 'there is a propensity for parents with learning disabilities to be over-represented in care proceedings' (Stewart et al., 2016, p. 21; see also Burch et al., 2019; Cox, Kroese and Evans, 2015; Hewitt, 2007). This chapter focuses on best practice with parents with learning disabilities when there are child protection concerns and looks at the role multidisciplinary family support can play in helping these families stay safely together. Unfortunately, most of the research focuses on mothers with learning disabilities, but an insight into the support needed by fathers can be found in Dugdale and Symonds (2018). (Videos for fathers can also be found at: http://www.bristol.ac.uk/

sps/wtpn/forparents/ and a link to video in the section on *Being a Dad*.)

We start the next section by briefly outlining what is known about the circumstances of parents with learning disabilities and the kinds of challenges they may face. We then go on to look at research findings in relation to the experiences of, and outcomes for, their children. Later, the focus is on understanding why and how parents with learning disabilities may come to the attention of child protection services before discussing how services can respond most effectively. We present a case study showing an example of good practice 'in action' using a 6-point framework for effective relationship-based practice, based on recent research findings.

WHAT DO WE KNOW ABOUT PARENTS WITH LEARNING DISABILITIES AND THEIR CHILDREN?

In this chapter we are focusing both on parents who have a diagnosed learning disability and those who have a milder level of impairment consistent with an assessment of learning *difficulty*. This is not always an easy distinction to make, but there are criteria for identifying and diagnosing a formal learning disability that may, in turn, have implications for access to social services, so it is an important distinction to be aware of. A learning disability is defined as:

> *A significantly reduced ability to understand new or complex information, to learn new skills (impaired intelligence); with a reduced ability to cope independently (impaired social functioning); which started before adulthood, with a lasting effect on development*
>
> *Department of Health (2001, p. 14)*

A learning disability is diagnosed when a person has an IQ of 69 or below; however, the IQ score typically gives an overall assessment, and an individual may well have varying levels of ability in relation to different activities, tasks and aspects of daily living.

Parents' needs are individual, but they often struggle with literacy, understanding abstract concepts such as time, organising routines and keeping their children

safe. They may also be experiencing a number of disadvantages, for example they may have mental health support needs, be unemployed and reliant on benefits, and/or be living with domestic violence and abuse (Cleaver and Nicholson, 2007; Darbyshire and Stenfert Kroese, 2012; Redley 2009). They face all of the stigma and possible harassment that any person with a learning disability commonly faces but may also encounter very negative social attitudes and assumptions about their capacity to parent well. Indeed, there is often a presumption that they can not or should not be able to parent at all. Parents often do not have a supportive social network or the help they need to develop their parenting knowledge and skills (Darbyshire and Stenfert Kroese, 2012; Emerson and Brigham, 2013; Tarleton, Ward and Howarth, 2006). For instance, if parents struggle with literacy, they will not be able to read most of the literature available on parenting – and they may have missed out on the experience of babysitting young children or being in situations where they have had the chance to learn about and/or take any responsibility for their care, before finding themselves in the position of being the primary carer for their own baby.

CLOSER LOOK: PARENTS' SUPPORT NEEDS

- Parents with a diagnosed learning disability would be classified as disabled under the Equality Act (2010) and entitled to 'reasonable adjustments' to the services they are receiving, for example from a local authority.
- Many parents have not been diagnosed as having a learning disability at the point where they come into contact with Children's Services.
- Diagnosis often occurs as part of the assessment process – perhaps as a result of a practitioner identifying that the parent is struggling, for example, with particular parenting tasks.
- Professionals should seek appropriate support from the Learning Disability team and/or request a cognitive assessment if appropriate, to understand whether a learning disability is a contributory factor in concerns regarding the welfare of the children (Burch et al., 2019; WTPN, 2014).
- It should be noted that there is **no** direct link between IQ and an individual's parenting ability when their IQ is above sixty (Tymchuk and Feldman, 1991).

- Parenting ability may be related to parents' difficulties with learning, but this has to be considered *along with* the challenges associated with their often poor socioeconomic status, lack of social networks and role models, and any additional physical and mental health support needs.
- A diagnosis may or may not be seen as beneficial by the parent – some parents may find it helpful and that it enables them to understand themselves and their experiences better, while others may feel shocked and not wish to engage with what is (still) perceived as a stigmatising label.

Parents With Learning Difficulties

As we have noted, in addition to the group of parents with diagnosed learning disabilities who may be eligible for support from Adult Services and Learning Disability Teams, there is also a large group of parents who have a milder impairment, often termed a 'learning difficulty'. These parents have an IQ of 70 or above but may struggle with many of the same issues as those with a diagnosed disability. However, they are less likely to receive support, for example from adult learning disability services where eligibility criteria screen out those with IQ of 70+. To try and reduce the risk of these parents 'falling through the cracks' between services, it is important to be aware that they could be provided with support under the Care Act (2014), so practitioners should ensure that this option is investigated.

Legal and Policy Framework

United Nations Conventions On:

The Rights of Children
- Article 18: States shall render appropriate assistance to parents in the performance of their child-rearing responsibilities

The Rights of Persons with Disabilities
- Article 23, respect for home and the family: States shall render appropriate assistance to persons with disabilities in the performance of their child-rearing responsibilities

Human Rights Act 1998
- Article 6: Right to a fair trial (includes family proceedings and the formal processes leading to court proceedings)

- Article 8: Right to family life
- Article 14: Right not to be discriminated against

Equality Act 2010
- Public sector/body duty to actively promote equality of opportunity (e.g. by making reasonable adjustments)

Care Act 2014
- Statutory responsibility for prevention and early intervention. Key details are contained in *Care and Support Statutory Guidance* issued under the Care Act 2014 by the Department of Health
- Care Act requires Local Authorities to provide information regarding services available
- Statutory Guidance p. 3, para 11.4(c): 'effective intervention at the right time can stop needs from escalating'
- Statutory Guidance p. 75, para 6.6: even if a person has needs that are not eligible at that time, the Local Authority must consider providing information and advice or *'other preventative services'*

Children and Families Act 2014
- In circumstances where parents may not have the capacity to engage fully with the process, all efforts must be made, such as working in partnership with adult services, to secure appropriate advocacy to ensure that Local Authorities actions are fully understood by parents (Court orders and pre-proceedings – for local authorities (DfE, 2014, p. 15, para 21)). (In fact, human rights case law requires steps to be taken to enable parents' 'full participation' in the process, not merely 'full understanding of LA actions'.)

Outcomes for Children of Parents With Learning Disabilities

The research evidence suggests that outcomes for children of parents with learning disabilities may be mixed. Collings and Llewellyn's (2012) literature review found that poorer outcomes for children of parents with intellectual disability (the term used in the study and found commonly in European and North American literature) were linked to poverty and poor social environments, associated with the parents' intellectual disability, rather than the parents' disability itself. However, Emerson and Brigham's (2014) UK study, adjusted for between-group differences related to low socioeconomic position, showed parental learning disability was associated with an increased risk of child developmental delay and speech and language problems, although not with child behaviour problems or frequent accidents or injuries. Hindmarsh et al.'s (2017) secondary analysis of data from waves 2 to 4 of the UK Millennium Cohort Study also found that children face a heightened risk of poor social-emotional well-being (at ages 3 and 5) and peer exclusion (by self-report) at age 7, while Wickstrom et al. (2017) found that at 7 years old, children of parents with intellectual disabilities in Sweden were at increased risk of injuries, violence and child abuse. Adult children of parents with learning disabilities discuss experiencing stigma, bullying and ostracism stigma associated with their parents' disability (Booth and Booth, 1998; O'Neill, 2011; Ronai, 1997; Traustadóttir and Sigurjónsdóttir 2005), while Lindblad et al. (2013) also note that children may experience later difficulties with relationships. More recently, Wołowicz-Ruszkowska and McConnell (2017, p. 482) discuss children experiencing a 'different, yet ordinary' life in which their parents were generally loving and supportive. Collings, Llewellyn and Grace (2017) add that children do not see their social worlds as restricted but as influenced, like all children, by a wide variety of things rather than just their parent/s' learning disability; they also note (again like all children) that they benefit from stable and supportive environments.

As this discussion indicates, not all the findings reported in the recent literature are positive. However, support from key adults who are interested in the child has been increasingly recognised in recent years as beneficial by and for children of parents with learning disabilities. This support can be from family, a family friend, a worker from a support service or a teacher but it should be continuous and responsive to the child's interests and social needs (Collings, Grace et al., 2017; Collings, Llewellyn et al., 2017; Faureholm, 2010; Gudkova, 2019; Lindblad, 2013). Collins, Grace and Llewellyn (2017) and Weiber et al. (2014) conclude that to promote best outcomes, children need individualised, tailored support.

CHILD PROTECTION, ASSESSMENT AND PRACTICE ISSUES

Typically, as noted earlier, when child protection concerns arise, they relate to neglect. Neglect is a complex area of practice (Tanner and Turney, 2003) and is discussed in more detail in Chapter 9; we will not repeat the discussion here but do want to draw out the more specific issues relating to neglect in the context of families where a parent has learning disabilities. While each situation is unique, the families who come into contact with Social Services typically present as complex 'cases' where it can be difficult to disentangle the different and sometimes competing concerns (Cleaver and Nicholson, 2007; Stewart et al., 2016). Issues include:

> parental or family characteristics (that can also present risks) including parental substance misuse, domestic abuse, and/or parental mental health problems; poor home conditions; or parental vulnerability to abusive adults in the community. In many cases, the child of concern to services already has older siblings or half siblings in care.
> **Burch et al. (2019, p. 5); see also Cleaver and Nicholson (2007)**

Challenges for Children's Services in Addressing Referrals Relating to Parents With Learning Disabilities

A number of issues may make it difficult for mainstream Children's Services professionals to respond effectively to referrals involving parents with learning disabilities (Cleaver and Nicholson, 2007; Feldman, 1998, 2004; Goodringe, 2000; Tarleton et al., 2006). These include:

■ Children and Families social workers may have little experience of working with parents with learning difficulties, and there is little evidence of them engaging support from Learning Disability professionals or of using specialist assessments (Cleaver and Nicholson, 2007).

■ Services may be unable to provide, and/or parents may not know about or feel comfortable accessing, family support services. This can lead to a situation where families are the focus of a number of low-level referrals before they meet the threshold for a response from the Child Protection team.

■ Lack of clarity and consistency amongst different professionals involved with the family about what constitutes good (or, indeed, 'good enough') parenting (Tarleton et al., 2006) – a common difficulty in situations of neglect more generally (Tanner and Turney, 2003).

- Lack of accessible information for parents.
- Lack of awareness of and/or access to specialist parenting assessments available for parents with learning disabilities (see later).
- Use of IQ levels as a proxy for parenting ability.

At the same time, Adult Learning Disability services may be facing their own challenges:

- strict eligibility criteria, usually IQ-related,
- lack of focus on parenting,
- perceived emphasis on adults' rights, or
- lack of knowledge/experience re child protection.

These separate sets of challenges can result in 'silo working' and a lack of joined-up thinking and planning in relation to parents with learning disabilities and their families, as represented in Fig. 19a.1.

But it is important, as with all referrals to child protection, that families receive an appropriate assessment to ensure that risks, needs and strengths are properly understood. Working with parents with learning disabilities, this first stage should involve careful consideration of the best way to approach the process. As noted previously, it may not be clear at the point of referral that a parent has a learning disability or difficulty, but if it is, then practitioners should consider using a specialist assessment approach such as McGaw's Parent Assessment Manual (PAMS), using the appropriate software. The PAMS should only be administered by someone who has been trained in its use, so practitioners involved in assessment should be aware of how to access this kind of specialised input. If it is thought that a parent may have a diagnosable learning disability, then a cognitive assessment should be sought (though please note the caveat on p. 2). This should assist the Children and Families practitioner to work in ways that address parents' strengths and to adapt their practice to mitigate the impact of parents' difficulties, where possible. For example, it may be that a parent has difficulties with time and with keeping appointments. Good practice might involve using visual aids to help them remember when a meeting

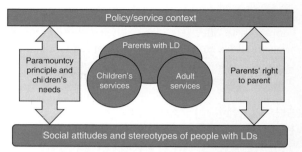

Fig. 19a.1 ■ How things are now. *LD,* Learning difficulties.

is due, sending text prompts and reminders to their phone, and so on.

If local authorities routinely use particular assessment packages (such as the Graded Care Profile for neglect), it is important to check that these are suitable when working with parents with learning disabilities as the language may not be accessible (Barlow et al., 2012; see also Johnson and Cotmore, 2015). Approaches such as Signs of Safety may be more useful as they allow issues to be framed in concrete and clear terms.

Good Assessment – a Summary of Key Points

Parents with learning disabilities have a right to fair and appropriate assessment. While the main principles of good assessment will apply (Turney et al., 2012), practitioners should additionally ensure they pay attention to:

- accessible communication (clear, simple language that avoids jargon),
- accessible information (e.g. 'easy read' format, or voice messages if parent struggles with literacy),
- a focus on strengths as well as difficulties and risk (start from what the parent/s can do),
- using specialised assessment formats (e.g. PAMS) if appropriate,
- home-based assessment where possible (familiar surroundings and household equipment),
- access to independent advocacy (to support the parents to engage with and understand concerns and processes, provide 'bridge' between parent and professionals, emotional support), and
- supporting skill development.

Observing these principles in practice will support practitioners to get the best understanding of a parent's strengths and support needs and to come to a fair assessment (WTPN, 2014). In this way, all avenues for support can be properly considered to ensure that children remain safely with their families wherever possible.

In the next section, we look at how parents can be supported to offer safe care to their children and the ways in which practitioners can intervene most effectively to promote best outcomes for both the children and their parents.

SUPPORTING PARENTS WITH LEARNING DISABILITIES WHERE THERE ARE CHILD PROTECTION CONCERNS – THE *GOOD PRACTICE GUIDANCE* AND THE '6TS' FRAMEWORK FOR PRACTICE

Research shows that with appropriately tailored support, the outcomes for children can be safeguarded and their welfare protected (Cleaver and Nicholson, 2007; McGaw and Newman, 2005; Tarleton and Porter, 2012; Tarleton et al., 2018; WTPN, 2009). English researchers McGaw and Newman , 2005, p.24 clearly stated that 'the main predictor of competent parenting is an adequate structure of professional and informal support' and that 'supporting families may require a combination of skilled support during crucial child developmental periods, more "low-level" but reliable support for lengthier periods and commitment to the family'.

However, before this kind of input can be provided, parents may need support to trust professionals and engage with services. Parents report that they are scared to engage with professionals as they fear their children will be removed from their care (Tarleton et al., 2006). Furthermore, they also perceive, as noted earlier, that there are unhelpful negative attitudes and stereotypes about parents with learning disabilities and may need to be convinced that their social worker will not start off with negative preconceptions of their capacity (Tarleton et al., 2006; Traustadottir and Sigurjonsdottir, 2010). So it is important that practitioners are honest about concerns but also able to identify strengths within the family or wider network that can be harnessed to address them. Parents also believe that they are expected to meet higher standards of parenting than other families. The involvement of an advocate from an early stage has been shown to be very beneficial in supporting parents'

engagement with and understanding of the child protection process (Tarleton, 2013).

Once trust has been developed, support may be needed to maintain an adequate standard of care. This support may need to start early (during pregnancy if possible) and be required for an extended period, changing over time to meet the developmental needs of the child. For some families, consistent, long-term engagement with services may be needed; for others, the availability of support on a more ad hoc basis may suffice but still be critical to maintain family functioning and meet the expectations of a Child Protection Plan, if one is in place. This support needs to be tailored to the individual and may be needed at certain times to teach new skills or over the longer term to compensate for skills/knowledge the parent does not have. This support should be provided by a multiagency team (Aunos and Pachos, 2013; Tarleton et al., 2006; Weiber et al., 2014) in line with local protocols and policies, as well as wider provisions advocating early intervention/support for families.

Part of the support provided to parents may include the use of parents' groups where parents can learn together and support each other (Coren, Ramsbotham and Gschwandtner, 2018; Gustavsson and Starke, 2017; Tarleton et al., 2006). However, parents with learning disabilities often struggle with standard parenting programmes which are not tailored to their learning needs. In recent years, two group parenting programmes, Triple P and the Mellow Futures programme from Mellow Parenting, have been adapted for parents with learning disabilities and have been shown to be beneficial (Glazemaker and Deboutte, 2013; Tarleton and Turner, 2016).

In England, the *Good Practice Guidance on Working with Parents with a Learning Disability* (DOH/DES 2007; WTPN 2016, WTPN 2021) provides a clear set of principles for effective practice. While the *Guidance* does not have statutory force, the previous (2016) version was endorsed by Sir James Munby, the (then) President of the Family Division in Guidance issued in April 2018 (https://www.judiciary.uk/publications/family-proceedings-parents-with-a-learning-disability/). As a result, judges involved in family proceedings involving parents with a learning disability should expect social workers and others to have a working knowledge of the GPG and be able to demonstrate that they have adhered to the principles it espouses and used them to support practice that is effective, fair and accountable. Similar guidance is also available in Scotland under the title *Supported Parenting: Refreshed Scottish Good Practice Guidelines for Supporting Parents with a Learning Disability* (SCLD, 2015). The *Good Practice Guidance* documents in both England and Scotland highlight the need for:

- Accessible information and communication. (This includes the provision of clearly written, easy read information as well as clear, straight-forward verbal communication. See https:// www.changepeople.org/blog/december-2016/ free-easy-read-resources for advice on easy in-formation or seek support from a Speech and Language therapist.)
- Clear and coordinated referral and assessment procedures and processes, eligibility criteria and care pathways.
- Support designed to meet the needs of parents and children based on assessments of their needs and strengths.
- Long-term support where necessary.
- Access to independent advocacy.

Additionally, the 'Supported Parenting' guidance (which has been endorsed by the Scottish Govern-ment) outlines the following principles:

- Support should be available from pre-birth on-wards.
- Support may need to be ongoing at every stage of the child's development.
- Support must be based on respect for the parents and for the emotional bond between the parent and child.
- Support should be for the family as a whole rath-er than individuals.
- Parents should be supported to be in control and to experience being competent.
- Support should focus on building strengths.
- Families are best supported in the context of their own extended families, neighbourhoods and communities.

These principles have been included in the Children and Young People (Scotland) Act 2014: National Guidance on Part 12: Services in Relation to Children at Risk of Becoming Looked After, etc.

The 6Ts Framework – Engagement and Support for Parents With Learning Disabilities

A recent study by Tarleton et al. (2018) investigated some specific examples of professionals working successfully with parents with learning disabilities where there were concerns about child neglect. The researchers investigated how professionals thought about the parents (i.e. their attitudes and assump-tions), what they understood about the neglect in context, and how they had adapted their practice to meet the parents' needs. Eight detailed case stud-ies of mothers and the support they received were developed, one of which has been adapted here to illustrate the 6Ts framework in practice. The case studies showed how the professionals understood and worked with the fact that the mothers had a learning disability and accepted that they were therefore likely to have on-going support needs – but that these could be addressed in ways that also allowed the children to remain safe. It was interesting to see that the profes-sionals appeared to share some basic assumptions in relation to the parents, taking a non-stigmatising and broadly strengths-based approach, while not falling into a naïve over-optimistic approach that minimised risk. The practice observed in the study was typi-cally seen to be in line with the principles of the GPG documents, although we discovered that a number of practitioners were actually unaware of this guidance. When asked about their approach, they related it back to what they understood to be core social work/ professional values.

The 6Ts framework (Fig 19a.2) drew together the key elements of this supportive and empowering approach that provided a foundation for a respectful but chal-lenging relationship-based practice that reached across the usual adult/children's services divide enabling the professionals to become a 'team around the family'. We explain each of the 'Ts' here.

Time: extra time is needed to get to know parents and communicate appropriately – in accessible

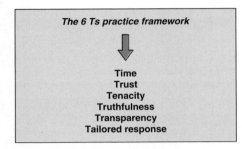

Fig. 19a.2 ■ The 6Ts practice framework.

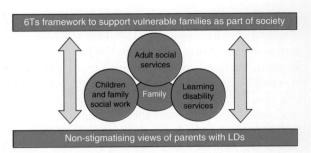

Fig. 19a.3 ■ Building an effective child protection response. *LDs,* Learning difficulties.

ways – with them. Parents may need more time than others to take on board information/new skills/knowledge. Parents may need support 'through time' – i.e. ongoing support in the long-term or recurrent periods of support, perhaps across the span of childhood.

Trust: parents and professionals need to be able to trust each other for the support to be effective; time is needed to develop this trust.

Tenacity: professionals 'sticking with' parents over the longer term, as necessary. This may include professionals working on issues with parents over a period of time or keeping in contact so that they can come back and teach new skills as required or help a parent to refresh their confidence/competence in particular situations.

Truthfulness: professionals need to be honest with parents in relation to both strengths and difficulties; they need to be truthful about the concerns they may have for an existing child or an unborn baby's welfare, and to convey these concerns in terms that the parent understands. And truthfulness needs to be a two-way street: practitioners need to be confident that parents will be honest with them, for example, if they do not think things are going well with their child/ren. Again, that capacity for truthfulness depends on developing the kind of trusting relationship that can be built through time.

Transparency: professionals and parents need to be really clear about what is happening and what needs to be done when and by whom, from first referral onwards. For example, midwives need to be clear with mothers why they are involving child protection or the learning disability team. Taking all these into account results in a:

Tailored response: understanding and working with parents in a way that works for them. Good communication is key to this. This response is often best provided by a multiagency team which needs coordination and leadership.

Fig. 19a.3 offers a way of showing how the elements we have discussed thus far can be brought together into a framework to enable an effective child protection response in situations involving parents with learning difficulties.

This section continues with a case study focusing on 'Janine' and the support provided to her that helped ensure the welfare of her daughter, Bella. The case study is a composite, based on the stories of three mothers who were involved in the research project mentioned earlier, which aimed at exploring examples of 'successful' practice with parents with learning disabilities (Tarleton et al., 2018); the stories have been combined to protect the anonymity of individual participants and to highlight how the 6Ts can underpin positive practice. The research was undertaken in areas where there were different forms of specialist parenting services for parents with learning disabilities; however, a specialist team is not necessary to put the 6T's into practice.

CASE STUDY 19A.1: JANINE AND BELLA

Janine is in her twenties and has mild learning difficulties. She is a single mother to her 4-year-old daughter, Bella. She has an older boy who was removed from her care when she was a teenager. He now lives with her mother due to concerns for his welfare as he was underweight and his father was violent towards Janine. Janine is supported by her sister, and there are currently no concerns regarding Bella's welfare. Janine came into contact with services again during her second pregnancy.

TIME AND TENACITY

Janine had had intermittent contact with the health visitor from her first pregnancy, who then arranged to be her health visitor again when she was pregnant the second time and then **remained involved with the family throughout. The health visitor** visited Janine very regularly (more than would usually be expected) throughout the 4 years. Even though there are now no concerns about Bella's welfare, Janine is still in frequent contact with the health visitor and knows she could ring the health visitor. Similarly, an early help worker who was involved throughout the assessment and Child in Need plan continued supporting Janine, for longer than she 'should', once the level of concern regarding the baby's welfare was reduced. The workers therefore ensured that they were in contact with Janine so that they were aware of difficulties at an early stage. Janine recognised that 'whenever I need help, they step in'.

TRUST AND TRUTHFULNESS

Initially Janine's family were concerned about her pregnancy and did not feel that they could offer much support as her mother was already caring for her elder son. However, the early help worker developed a good relationship with Janine's family and had what she described as some 'frank conversations'. Bella's social worker also made it very clear to the family that if family support was not available, when the baby was born Janine would need to be placed in a mother and baby unit to ensure that the baby had the care she needed. When the family understood the severity of the concerns, Janine's sister was able to become more actively involved and to offer support to Janine on a regular basis.

All of the workers involved with the family were honest with each other and with Janine regarding their serious concerns about Bella's welfare. Janine reported having **positive relationships** with all of the workers. She says they 'sat down and talked to me' and spelt out what they were concerned about, what she was expected to do and what support would be available to help her.

TRANSPARENCY

Janine was referred to an advocacy project, and the advocate supported her in meetings as she wished. He supported Janine to speak up for herself and ensured reasonable adjustments had been made to meet her communication needs. The **Signs of Safety approach** was used in Team Around the Child (TAC) and Child in Need (CiN) meetings to ensure Janine understood *what we are worried about, what's working well,* and *what needs to happen.* After Child in Need meetings, a slightly more formal easy read summary of the meeting was prepared and explained to Janine.

The workers were clear who was responsible for what. They kept in contact by phone and email in addition to attending the Team around the Child and then Child in Need meetings. All the professionals working with the family attended, as well as Janine and her family. Bella's social worker oversaw the work of the early help worker, whose views were also incorporated into the discussions and planning.

TAILORED RESPONSE

At the request of the social worker, while Janine was pregnant, a specialist assessment using the **Parent Assessment Manual** (PAMS) was undertaken by the specialist parenting services; this then informed the development of a detailed support plan which involved pre-birth teaching regarding practical parenting skills. A cognitive assessment was also undertaken, and the results of this assessment explained to the multiagency team by the clinical psychologist from the specialist parenting service so that support could be tailored appropriately for Janine. Midwives and the health visiting services provided a lot of input and **worked jointly** with the specialist parenting services and early help worker, often going on joint visits. The 'success' of this support was judged in relation to the professionals' concerns and goal-based targets included in the Child in Need plan. Janine was happy to have the support and to be taking care of Bella herself.

The support and teaching provided included pre-birth input on how to keep well in pregnancy, learning how to start parenting and keep her baby safe. This teaching of parenting skills by the health visitor and specialist parenting services was achieved through developing positive relationships, explaining using **'non-judgemental plain talk',** using 'easy resources', such as the 'My Baby 0-1' book from Change (2012), and practical teaching about looking after a baby. The health visitor explained how they prepared Janine to put the baby to bed:

> But with Janine we actually, you know, took a doll and took it into the sleep environment, and put it down in the cot, and showed her how to make the cot up, and what things to think about and so on, and were much more hands-on and practical with that.
> (HEALTH VISITOR)

When Bella was born, Janine was shown a video about breastfeeding and the breastfeeding coordinator spent **extra time** to support Janine to get Bella to latch on. Janine commented that workers helped her *'step by step and if I don't understand she'll say it again and again and again and again.'*

As Bella grew up, support was provided to ensure Janine understood Bella's emotional needs and to enable her to play appropriately with her. Janine was recognised as being *'grabby'* with the baby and missing Bella's cues, so she was shown 'The Social Baby video'. **Video interaction guidance** was also used to help Janine *'learn how to communicate with Bella'* and interact with Bella, building on examples of positive interaction. Psychological support was also provided for her mental health, to enable Janine to *'reflect on past experiences with her older child'* and to support her on-going contact with her son. Janine was also helped to develop necessary practical skills. For example, she was shown how to do her cleaning and supported with her finance and budgeting.

Janine has been attending **a college course** funded by Care to Learn, for parents with learning disabilities and young mothers, for 3 days a week for 3 years. Transport and a crèche are provided, and there is a high staff:parent ratio. Janine has learnt about childcare, literacy and numeracy and employability skills. A personal advisor provides individualised support to mothers. This course has provided Janine with a peer group, and she has made a close friend, thus expanding what was previously a very restricted social network.

REFLECTIVE QUESTIONS

- Have you worked with families in similar situations to Janine and Bella?
- Does your team/agency have any policy statements or protocols to support work with parents with learning disabilities? Is the *Good Practice Guidance* known and referred to?
- What are your thoughts about the support that was offered to Janine to help her to care successfully for Bella?
- What would you identify as features of 'successful' practice in this case?
- What are the challenges or barriers to 'successful practice', and how might they be overcome?

CONCLUSION

In this chapter, we have outlined the ways in which parents with learning disabilities are likely to come into the child protection system and some of the challenges that current practice can present in terms of fragmented responses, lack of understanding of the specific needs that parents with learning disabilities may have, alongside their experiences of more general disadvantage and social exclusion. But what we have seen from research, including the recent 'Getting Things Changed' study discussed earlier, is that good support provided in a timely way can be instrumental in keeping children safe – and that this support depends on effective multiagency working. Fig. 19a.3 shows how this might look. Debates about the balance between 'support' and 'protection' are not new and are currently reflected in discussion of the need for a 'social model' of child protection (Featherstone et al., 2018). We close by suggesting that such an approach is key to fair and effective work with parents with learning disabilities.

REFLECTIVE QUESTIONS

- What factors might lead you to think that a parent may have learning disabilities? Who/what additional services would you draw on, for advice and support?
- What are the main difficulties facing parents with learning disabilities?
- How can you incorporate the 6Ts approach into your own and/or your team's work with parents with learning disabilities?
- Can you identify procedures or practices within your own or your team's work that may be particularly challenging for parents with learning disabilities? How could ways of working be adapted to make them more accessible?

FURTHER READING

Good Practice Guidance documents

Scottish Consortium for Learning Disabilities (SCLD), 2015. Supported Parenting. SCLD, Glasgow. https://www.scld.org.uk/wp-content/uploads/2015/06/Supported_Parenting_web.pdf.

Working Together with Parents Network (WTPN), 2021. Update of the DoH/DfES Good Practice Guidance on Working with Parents with a Learning Disability (2007). University of Bristol, Bristol. FINAL 2021 WTPN UPDATE OF THE GPG.pdf (bristol.ac.uk).

Working Together with Parents Network, 2009. Supporting Parents with Learning Disabilities and Difficulties: Stories of Positive Practice. Norah Fry Research Centre, Bristol. http://www.bristol.ac.uk/media-library/sites/sps/migrated/documents/positivepractice.pdf.

Research Reports

Cleaver, H., Nicholson, D., 2007. Parental Learning Disability and Children's Needs. Jessica Kingsley Publishers, London.

Tarleton, B., Turney, D., Merchant, W., Tilbury, N., 2018. Successful Professional Practice When Working with Parents with Learning Difficulties. University of Bristol, Bristol. http://www.bristol.ac.uk/media-library/sites/sps/documents/wtpn/GTC%20SUMMARY%20REPORT%2016.5.2018%20designed.pdf.

Tarleton, B., Ward, L., Howarth, J., 2006. Finding the Right Support? A Review of Issues and Positive Practice to Support Parents with Learning Difficulties and Their Children. Baring Foundation, London. http://www.bristol.ac.uk/media-library/sites/sps/migrated/documents/rightsupport.pdf.

Website

The Working Together with Parents Network (wtpn.co.uk) provides support for professionals working with parents with learning difficulties and learning disabilities, and their children.

REFERENCES

Aunos, M., Pachos, L., 2013. Changing perspective: workers' perception of inter-agency collaboration with parents with an intellectual disability. J. Publ. Child Welfare 7 (5), 658–674.

Barlow, J., Fisher, J.D., Jones, D., 2012. Systematic Review of Models of Analysing Significant Harm. Department for Education: London.

Booth, T., Booth, W., 1998. Growing up with Parents Who Have Learning Difficulties. Routledge, London, UK.

Burch, K., Allen, V., Green, C., Taylor, V., Wise, S., 2019. Research on the Number of Children in Wales Placed into Care from Parents with Learning Disability and the Reasons behind Their Removal. Cardiff: Welsh Government, GSR report number 56/2019. https://gov.wales/parents-learning-disability-involvement-social-services.

Care Act 2014. https://www.legislation.gov.uk/ukpga/2014/23/contents/enacted.

Children and Families Act 2014. https://www.legislation.gov.uk/ukpga/2014/6/contents/enacted.

Children and Young People (Scotland) Act 2014. https://www.gov.scot/publications/children-young-people-scotland-act-2014-national-guidance-part-12/pages/3/.

Cleaver, H., Nicholson, D., 2007. Parental Learning Disability and Children's Needs. Jessica Kingsley Publishers, London.

Collings, S., Llewellyn, G., 2012. Children of parents with intellectual disability: Facing poor outcomes or faring okay? J. Intellect. Dev. Disabil. 37 (1), 65–82.

Collings, S., Grace, R., Llewellyn, G., 2017. The role of formal support in the lives of children of mothers with intellectual disability. J. Appl. Res. Intellect. Disabil. 30 (3), 492–500.

Collings, s., Llewellyn, G., Grace, R., 2017. Home and the social worlds beyond: Exploring influences in the lives of children of mothers with intellectual disability. Child Care Health Dev. 43 (5), 697–708.

Coren, E., Ramsbotham, K., Gschwandtner, M., 2018. Parent training interventions for parents with intellectual disability. Cochrane Database Syst Rev. 7 (7), CD007987. https://doi.org/10.1002/14651858.CD007987.pub3.

Cox, R., Kroese, B.S., Evans, R., 2015. Solicitor's experiences of representing parents with intellectual disabilities in care proceedings: Attitudes, influence and legal processes. Disabil. Soc. 30 (2), 284–298. https://doi.org/10.1080/09687599.2015.1005730.

Darbyshire, L., Stenfert Kroese, B., 2012. Psychological well–being and social support for parents with intellectual disabilities: Risk factors and interventions. J. Pol. Pract. Intellect. Disabil. 9 (1), 40–52.

Department of Health, 2001. Valuing People: A New Strategy for Learning Disability for the 21st Century. Department of Health, London.

Department of Health and Department for Education and Skills, 2007. Good Practice Guidance on Working with Parents with a Learning Disability. Department of Health and Department for Education and Skills, London.

Dugdale, D., Symonds, J., 2018. Fathers with Learning Disabilities: Experiences of Fatherhood and of Adult Social Care Services. http://www.bristol.ac.uk/media-library/sites/sps/documents/wtpn/FWLD%20SSCR%20Findings%204%20page%20summary%20FINAL.pdf.

Emerson, E., Brigham, P., 2013. Health behaviours and mental health status of parents with intellectual disabilities: Cross sectional study. Publ. Health 127, 1111–1116.

Emerson, E., Brigham, P., 2014. The developmental health of children of parents with intellectual disabilities: Cross sectional study. Res. Dev. Disabil. 35 (4), 917–921.

Equality Act (2010). https://www.legislation.gov.uk/ukpga/2010/15/contents.

Faureholm, J., 2010. Children and their life experiences. In: Llewellyn, G., Traustadottir, R., McConnell, D., Sigurjonsdottir, H. (Eds.), Parents with Intellectual Disabilities, Past, Present and Future. Wiley Blackwell, West Sussex.

Featherstone, B., Gupta, A., Morris, K., White, S., 2018. Protecting Children: A Social Model. Policy Press, Bristol.

Feldman, M.A., 1998. Preventing child neglect: Child care training for parents with intellectual disabilities. Infant and Young Child. 11 (2), 1–11.

Feldman, M.A., 2004. Self-directed learning of child-care skills by parents with intellectual disabilities. J. Infants and Young Child. 17 (1), 17–31.

Glazemaker, I., Deboutte, D., 2013. Modifying the 'positive parenting program' for parents with intellectual disabilities. J. Intellect. Disabil. Res. 57 (7), 616–626.

Goodringe, S., 2000. A Jigsaw of Services: Inspection of Services to Support Disabled Adults in Their Parenting Role. Department of Health, London.

Gudkova, T., Hedlund, M., Midjo, T., 2019. Supporting children of parents with intellectual disability: A scoping review. J. Appl. Res. Intellect. Disabil. 32, 737–749.

Gustavsson, M., Starke, M., 2017. Groups for parents with intellectual disabilities: A qualitative analysis of experiences. J. Appl. Res. Intellect. Disabil. 30, 638–647.

Hewitt, O. (2007), "What is the Effect on a Child of Having a Parent with Learning Disability?", Tizard Learning Disability Review, Vol. 12 No. 2, pp. 33–44. https://www.emerald.com/insight/publication/issn/1359-5474

Hindmarsh, G., Llewellyn, G., Emerson, E., 2017. The social–emotional well–being of children of mothers with intellectual impairment: A population–based analysis. J. Appl. Res. Intellect. Disabil. 469–481.

Human Rights Act 1998. https://www.legislation.gov.uk/ukpga/1998/42/contents.

Johnson, R., Cotmore, R., 2015. National Evaluation of the Graded Care Profile. NSPCC, London.

Lindblad, I., Billstedt, E., Gillberg, C., Fernell, E., 2013. An interview study of young adults born to mothers with mild intellectual disability. J. Intellect. Disabil. 17 (4), 329–338.

McGaw, S., Newman, T., 2005. What Works for Parents with Learning Disabilities? Barnardos, Ilford.

O'Neill, A.M., 2011. Average and bright children of parents with mild cognitive difficulties: The huck finn syndrome 20 years later. J. Appl. Res. Intellect. Disabil. 24, 566–572.

Redley, M., 2009. Understanding the social exclusion and stalled welfare of citizens with learning disabilities. Disabil. Soc. 24 (4), 489–501.

Ronai, C.R., 1997. On loving and hating my mentally retarded mother. Ment. Retard. 35, 417–432.

Scottish Consortium for Learning Disabilities (SCLD), 2015. Supported Parenting. SCLD, Glasgow.

Stewart, A., MacIntyre, G., McGregor, S., 2016. Supporting Parents with Learning Disabilities in Scotland: Challenges and Opportunities. Scottish Commission for Learning Disability, Glasgow.

Tanner, K., Turney, D., 2003. What do we know about child neglect? A critical review of the literature and its application to social work practice. Child Fam. Soc. Work 8, 25–34.

Tarleton, B., Porter, S., 2012. Crossing no man's land: A specialist support service for parents with learning disabilities. Child Fam. Soc. Work 17 (2), 233–243.

Tarleton, B., 2013. Expanding the engagement model: The role of the specialist advocate in supporting parents with learning disabilities in child protection proceedings. J. Publ. Child Welfare 7 (5), 675–690.

Tarleton, B., Turner, W., 2016. Mellow Futures Pilot Programmes in England and Scotland: Short Joint Report. School for Policy Studies, University of Bristol, Bristol. https://research-information.bris.ac.uk/files/94608706/joint_report_dayNovember_2016final.pdf.

Tarleton, B., Turney, D., Merchant, W., Tilbury, N., 2018. Successful Professional Practice when Working with Parents with Learning Difficulties. University of Bristol, Bristol.

Tarleton, B., Ward, L., Howarth, J., 2006. Finding the Right Support? A Review of Issues and Positive Practice to Support Parents with Learning Difficulties and Their Children. Baring Foundation, London.

Traustadóttir, R., Sigurjónsdóttir, H.B., 2005. Adult children of mothers with intellectual disabilities: Three life histories. In: Gustavsson, A., Sandrin, J., Traustadóttir, R., Tøssebro, J. (Eds.), Resistance, Reflections and Change: Nordic Disability Research. Studentlitteratur, Lund, Sweden, pp. 147–161.

Traustadottir, R., Bjorg Sigurjonsdottir, H.B., 2010. Parenting and resistance: Strategies in dealing with services and professionals. In: Llewellyn, G., Traustadottir, R., McConnell, D., Sigurjonsdottir, H. (Eds.), Parents with Intellectual Disabilities, Past, Present and Future. Wiley Blackwell, West Sussex, pp. 107–118.

Turney, D., Platt, D., Selwyn, J., Farmer, E., 2012. Improving Child and Family Assessments: Turning Research into Practice. Jessica Kingsley Publishers, London & Philadelphia.

Tymchuk, A.J., Feldman, M.A., 1991. Parents with mental retardation and their children: Review of research relevant to professional practice. Canadian Psychology/Psychologie Canadienne, 32(3), pp.486–496.

The Rights of Children. https://www.ohchr.org/en/instruments-mechanisms/instruments/convention-rights-child.

The Rights of Persons with Disabilities. https://www.ohchr.org/en/instruments-mechanisms/instruments/convention-rights-persons-disabilities.

Weiber, I., Tengland, P.A., Berglund, J., Eklund, M., 2014. Social and healthcare professionals' experiences of giving support to families where the mother has an intellectual disability: Focus on children. J. Pol. Pract. Intellect. Disabil. 11, 293–301.

Wickström, M., Höglund, B., Larsson, M., Lundgren, M., 2017. Increased risk for mental illness, injuries, and violence in children born to mothers with intellectual disability: A register study in Sweden during 1999–2012. Child Abuse and Neglect 65, 124–131.

Wołowicz-Ruszkowska., A., McConnell, D., 2017. The experience of adult children of mothers with intellectual disability: A qualitative retrospective study from Poland. J. Appl. Res. Intellect. Disabil. 30 (3), 482–491.

Working Together with Parents Network, 2009. Supporting Parents with Learning Disabilities and Difficulties – Stories of Positive Practice. Norah Fry Research Centre, Bristol. http://www.bristol.ac.uk/sps/wtpn/resources/.

Working Together with Parents Network, 2014. Parenting Assessments for Parents with Learning Difficulties. Norah Fry Research Centre, Bristol. http://www.bristol.ac.uk/sps/wtpn/resources/.

Working Together with Parents Network (WTPN), 2016. Update of the DoH/DfES Good Practice Guidance on Working with Parents with a Learning Disability (2007). University of Bristol, Bristol. http://www.bristol.ac.uk/media-library/sites/sps/documents/wtpn/2016%20WTPN%20UPDATE%20OF%20THE%20GPG%20-%20finalised%20with%20cover.pdf

Working Together with Parents Network (WTPN), 2021. Update of the DoH/DfES Good Practice Guidance on Working with Parents with a Learning Disability (2007). University of Bristol, Bristol. https://www.bristol.ac.uk/media-library/sites/sps/documents/wtpn/FINAL%202021%20WTPN%20UPDATE%20OF%20THE%20GPG.pdf

You and Your Baby 0-1. A guide to looking after babies in Easy Words and Pictures. Change: Leeds (www.changepeople.org)

19b

WORKING WITH PARENTS EXPERIENCING MENTAL DISTRESS

KIRSTEN MORLEY ■ ANDREW MURPHY

KEY POINTS

- Effective child protection work must involve consideration of parental mental distress; supporting the child involves also supporting parents.

- A child protection practitioner's role is not to diagnose mental distress, but to assess the impact that this distress may be having on the parents' daily functioning and ability to care for their child.

- The experience of parenting is likely to be more stressful for parents involved with social care services (Mellon, 2017).

- Many parents with whom practitioners work have experienced significant challenges in their own childhood and adolescence, and becoming a parent has the potential for such past experiences to be evoked and to cause distress (Siverns and Morgan, 2019).

- Relying on mental health diagnostic labels alone to make judgments about parenting capacity or risk is problematic.

- Asking clear, direct and sensitive questions to identify parental distress and the impact on children is important.

- Most parents who experience problems with their mental health are able to adequately care for their children, with the right support.

INTRODUCTION

Mental distress is a common human experience. Factors such as ethnicity, gender, trauma and poverty can affect people's likelihood of developing mental distress and the support they receive for it. Parenting is hard work and can lead to parental mental distress, especially when it evokes difficult memories and unresolved traumas from parents' past experiences. Child protection practitioners are likely to work with parents experiencing mental distress. Parental mental distress can affect parenting capability and have a significant impact on the well-being of children. However, child protection practitioners may not feel confident in identifying and discussing mental distress with parents. Some parents subject to child protection procedures have felt that their mental distress was not always recognised before interventions (Warwick and Morley, 2019). In addition, resource constraints mean that fewer parents with mental distress will receive specialist mental health services.

This chapter will explore what is meant by mental distress and its centrality as a concern for child protection practitioners. It will suggest practical advice on identifying and responding to parental mental distress, including suicidal thoughts. It concludes with guidance on eligibility and access routes to specialist adult mental health services.

WHAT IS MENTAL DISTRESS?

Terminology

In this chapter we will use the term 'mental distress' rather than 'mental illness' or 'mental disorders' to reflect a perspective that recognises wider social contexts and difficult life experiences including trauma and adversity (Tew, 2011). The social perspective we hold is not intended to be dismissive of a biomedical model; rather, to act as a counterbalance for practitioners wishing to use a holistic and trauma-informed approach.

Experiencing mental health difficulties is an ordinary part of life which does not usually require professional involvement. However, there are some occasions where practitioners may consider a parent to be presenting risks to themselves or to others (including their children) in connection with their mental distress, and it is this which we will consider in more detail. It is important to emphasise that a parent's experience of mental distress or a diagnostic label of mental 'disorder' alone does not indicate a need for professional safeguarding intervention.

Different experiences of parental mental distress may fall into one (or more) of the categories discussed. Child protection practitioners are most likely to encounter biomedical terms for mental distress based on the *Diagnostic and Statistical Manual of Mental Disorders* (DSM) (American Psychiatric Association, 2013), widely used by psychiatrists and clinicians, and these are included below, alongside more psychosocial groupings of distress. There is widespread debate about psychiatric diagnoses: some people find them helpful while others strongly reject them (see resource section later). Nevertheless, child protection practitioners will be working with people who have such diagnoses, and it is important to understand what they mean.

Psychiatric Label	What This Means
'Personality disorder' 'Depression' 'Bipolar Disorder'	Strong or overwhelming emotional states, of various kinds, that disrupt everyday life and prevent people from functioning.
'Obsessive-Compulsive Disorder'	Habitual and repetitive patterns of acting – for example, in relation to personal hygiene, or to do with safety and security – that create anxiety if they are not carried out.

Psychiatric Label	What This Means
'Schizophrenia' 'Schizo-Affective Disorder'	Experiences of seeing and hearing things that other people do not see or hear, or of holding beliefs that are considered by others to be unusual and extreme - (Cromby et al., 2013, p. 9)

Mental distress indicates a tipping point where difficulties with mental health start to become a problem in daily life. As Tew notes, '...the onset of mental distress marks a point on a continuum when particular experiences or patterns of response start to take over our overall functioning in a way that becomes problematic' (Tew, 2011, p. 88). Rather than focusing purely on symptoms, diagnosis and medical treatment, a social perspective on mental distress acknowledges factors that may have led to this crisis point, such as poverty, relationship breakdown or past experiences of trauma. Seeing a parent in the context of their life experiences and current social circumstances is crucial in forming a more balanced and thorough assessment of their own and their child's needs. Relying on diagnostic labels alone to make judgments about parenting capacity or risk is problematic.

CLOSER LOOK: THE POWER THREAT MEANING FRAMEWORK (PTMF)

- Developed as an alternative to more traditional models based on psychiatric diagnosis, the PTMF has a great deal of potential in social care work with families. The Framework integrates evidence from psychology, psychiatry, neuroscience, genetics, social work, other social sciences and trauma studies. It applies not just to people with a psychiatric diagnosis but to everyone. The Framework '...understands distress & troubling behaviour as the product of life experiences as they impact on people' (Cromby, 2018).
- The Framework '...summarises and integrates a great deal of evidence about the role of various kinds of power in people's lives; the kinds of threats that

misuses of power pose to us; and the ways we have learned as human beings to respond to threat. In traditional mental health practice, these threat responses are sometimes called "symptoms". The Framework also looks at how we make sense of these difficult experiences, and how messages from wider society can increase our feelings of shame, self-blame, isolation, fear and guilt' (BPS Overview document, 2018, p. 1).

■ The Framework uses a trauma-informed and narrative approach to ask four important questions: (i) 'What has happened to you?' (How is power operating in your life?), (ii) 'How did it affect you?' (What kinds of threats does this pose?), (iii) 'What sense did you make of it?' (What is the meaning of these experiences to you?), (iv) 'What did you have to do to survive? (What kinds of threat response are you using?) (Johnstone et al., 2018, p. 11).

■ 'A trauma-informed understanding of someone's distress is likely to focus on the impact of difficult events. What we call "symptoms" are better seen as "survival strategies" – creative ways of coping with emotionally overwhelming events and situations, which helped at the time, but may become a problem in their own right' (Johnstone and Watson, 2018).

THE PREVALENCE OF MENTAL DISTRESS IN THE GENERAL POPULATION AND PARENTS

Mental distress is common: it is estimated that at any given time, 17% of adults in England have experiences such as anxiety and low mood (McManus et al., 2016). 'Severe' mental 'illnesses' are less common, such as psychosis (<1% of population) and bipolar mood disorder (2% of population) (McManus et al., 2016). Mental distress can trigger stigma and discrimination, with 86% of mental health service users reporting discrimination in at least one aspect of their life; 40% had experienced discrimination related to being a parent (Mind, 2018).

Mental distress is not distributed evenly across society. Women are more likely than men to have a 'Common Mental Disorder': 19% compared to 12% of men (McManus et al., 2016). This discrepancy is greater for young women aged 16 to 24 years: 26% compared to 9% of men of this age. This may be partly due to a greater willingness in women to seek help, for example, by contacting their GP when they experience mental distress. In contrast, men may be more likely to respond to mental distress by using drugs and alcohol or risk-taking behaviour (Cromby et al., 2013). Men are more likely to drink hazardous levels of alcohol (McManus et al., 2016) and make up 95% of the prison population (Ministry of Justice, 2020). LGBTQIA+ people report higher levels of low mood and suicidal thoughts (Bachman and Gooch, 2018).

There are clear links between poverty, social inequality and mental distress. International comparisons show that countries like the UK with high rates of social inequality have higher incidence of mental distress (Pickett and Wilkinson, 2015). Unemployed people have higher rates of 'common mental disorder', and 66% of people in receipt of disability-related state benefits have a 'common mental disorder' (McManus et al., 2016).

Black women are more likely than White women to have a 'common mental disorder' (29% vs 21%), while Black men are significantly more likely than White men to be diagnosed with a 'psychotic disorder' (3.2% compared to 0.3%) (McManus et al., 2016). This finding has been replicated in research for 40 years. Hypotheses for this discrepancy include racist misdiagnosis (e.g. an expectation by mental health professionals that Black men will have psychosis) and the impact of lived experience of racism and disadvantage (Fernando, 2010). Less well known are other differential experiences relating to migration and cultural displacement, for example White Irish people in the UK have raised rates of mental distress, suicide and admission to psychiatric hospital (Fitzpatrick and Newton, 2005).

There are also discrepancies in access to mental health services. White British, female or middle-aged people are more likely to receive treatment in comparison to Black people (McManus et al., 2016). In addition, Black men are more likely to receive coercive treatment, with higher rates of detention in hospital under the Mental Health Act (NHS Digital, 2020).

Parental mental distress is common. Some 15% of dual-parent and 20% of lone-parent families include a parent with mental distress (Cleaver et al., 2011). It is estimated that up to 20% of women experience mental distress during pregnancy and the first year after childbirth (Bauer et al., 2014). Many child protection practitioners anecdotally report a high incidence of mental distress for the parents they work with. Research suggests that the prevalence of identified parental mental distress increases with the level of enquiry, with rates increasing through referral, assessment and Child Protection work (Cleaver et al., 2011). In Child in Need assessments under s17 Children Act 1989, parental mental health was identified as a factor at the end of 30% of assessments. The only factor more common was domestic violence (gov.uk, 2020). For Serious Case Reviews (SCRs), Brandon et al.'s (2020) analysis showed that 55% of SCRs reported parental mental health problems. They found that maternal mental health problems were much more common; this is likely to be due to under-identification of paternal factors. In general, there is far less research on fathers or male carers with mental distress (Cleaver et al., 2011).

WHY CHILD PROTECTION PRACTITIONERS NEED TO UNDERSTAND AND WORK WITH PARENTAL MENTAL DISTRESS

Consideration of parental mental health is an essential part of any child-centred assessment. The Framework for the Assessment of Children in Need and Their Families (DoH, 2000) presents (1) parenting capacity as one of the three key elements of thorough social care assessment, along with (2) family and environmental factors and (3) the child's developmental needs. Assessment of the impact of parental mental health issues is crucial when assessing a child under s17 of the Children Act 1989 and before making decisions about any action to protect children under s47 of this Act. Practitioners working with a child are also working with the family system around the child: the dynamics within the widening spheres of the child's 'micro, meso and macro system' (Bronfenbrenner, 1979) which also include parental experiences of poverty, discrimination, power/powerlessness and the impact of these on the family over time (Gupta et al., 2016).

Practitioners using a systemic approach are well aware of the symbiotic relationship of child and

parental mental health (Forrester et al., 2013), and good practice dictates that support for one is inevitably connected to the other. Having an understanding and awareness of the prevalence and impact of mental distress among parents, as well as strategies to support them and their child, is therefore essential. A commitment to early intervention in order to safeguard children's well-being also means identifying and supporting parents who may be struggling. A parent's mental health may affect their capacity to effectively parent a child and may also impact on the child's emotional environment. The role of child protection workers is not to assess the mental health of parents, but to evaluate the impact that their mental health may be having on their ability to adequately parent their child.

Parenting is hard work and often presents significant challenges, regardless of whether a parent experiences mental distress or not. Stressful life circumstances which were a strain before having children are likely to be heightened afterwards, and it is known that the experience of parenting is likely to be more stressful for parents involved with social care services (Mellon, 2017). The demands of parenting, including social, financial and emotional pressures, can magnify existing challenges, and it is often at this point where practitioners become involved. Many parents with whom practitioners work have experienced significant challenges in their own childhood and adolescence, and becoming a parent has the potential for such past experiences to be evoked and to cause distress (Siverns and Morgan, 2019). Some of the parents professionals work with have themselves had social care involvement in their life as children, with both positive and negative experiences of this. These experiences can understandably impact on parents' willingness and ability to successfully engage with practitioners (Featherstone et al., 2014).

Practitioners' involvement in parental mental health is unlikely to be required unless a parent's mental distress appears to be moving beyond their control to a point where this may impact considerably on their daily functioning or where there is clear evidence of risk to themselves or others. If this is the case, it is known that often only brief intervention from professionals may be required for the parent to regain their usual baseline. However, at other times a longer-term approach is needed to support the parent and child while stability is re-established (Duffy et al., 2016).

Multidisciplinary working is a key element of both short- and longer-term support, with clear communication between professionals and the family being crucial. Parents with lived experience of mental distress have also noted the importance of practitioners using a collaborative, strengths-based and transparent approach to their mental health and parenting support (Keddell, 2016) which we will explore further within this chapter.

Given the specialised nature of services, there has been a tendency for a 'silo' approach, where adult and children's needs are seen and treated as separate issues (Frost, 2017). In fact, there is a complex interplay between adults and children. Some of this has been indicated earlier, for example that the experience of parenting may in itself trigger mental distress through re-awakening of a parent's own traumatic childhood experiences. Falkov's Family Model (Falkov et al., 2020) suggests that there is an interaction between child and parental mental health; that not only can a parent's mental distress adversely affect a child's welfare, but that parenting can also trigger parental mental distress. Given this complexity, a 'Think Family' (Falkov et al., 2020) approach which sees children and parents' needs as interdependent and which requires a systematic approach to assessment and support is crucial. This will be supported by effective inter-agency working, especially where secondary mental health services are involved. It is worth noting that adult and children's social workers often have limited understanding of each other's roles and eligibility criteria, which in the past has proved to be an obstacle to effective interagency working (Duffy et al., 2016).

It is important to ask clear and direct questions about mental distress, using straightforward language. Some parents may readily volunteer information about their mental health, for example a diagnosis or contact with Adult Mental Health Services. Be mindful that willingness to disclose may be affected by the widespread stigma attached to mental distress and by previous contact with services. For instance, parents may fear that revealing their mental distress will lead to care proceedings or removal of children. People with previous coercive contact from mental health services, such as being detained under the Mental Health Act 1983, may also fear that disclosure may lead to further detention. Cultural factors may also affect willingness

CASE STUDY 19B.1: SERENA

Serena is 24 years old and the mother of three children aged 5, 3 and 18 months. When she was growing up, Serena's mother had serious problems with her mental health and misused alcohol. Serena's father was often verbally and emotionally abusive, and Serena describes this as a 'really difficult time'. Things were harder because the family had very little money, and social services had been involved in Serena's childhood due to concerns about the impact of her mother's mental health problems and domestic abuse perpetrated by her father. As an adult, Serena had experienced difficulties in personal relationships and, despite working long hours, was struggling to pay the bills and reliant on using food banks. She had been diagnosed with depression and anxiety in her late teens and began drinking heavily. Over time, concerns were flagged up by health professionals and school about her ability to adequately care for her children. Serena's oldest child, 5-year-old Holly, and her 3-year-old son Darius were taken into local authority care by social workers 2 years ago, and both now reside with adopted parents. Serena has no contact with them. Serena's youngest child Jordan is 18 months old and still lives with her. Child protection workers are currently involved in monitoring Jordan's welfare, and Serena is keen to keep Jordan in her care. She says she feels 'grief every day' for Darius and Holly, 'for losing them when I should have been helped to keep them with me' and feels that 'they just saw me as a bad mum, as an addict, when I needed help too'.

REFLECTIVE QUESTIONS

- What might have contributed to Serena's experience of mental distress?
- What else could have been done to support Serena whilst also keeping her children safe?
- How might you work with Serena and her children?
- How might practitioners identify parental mental distress?

and ability to discuss mental health. People from non-White Western cultures may have different conceptualisations of mental health, for example not recognising 'depression' as an experience (Fernando, 2010). Black British people may not talk about their mental distress because of a fear of stigma in their communities (Memon et al., 2016). It is important to acknowledge that it may take time for people to talk about their mental health. Being reassuring about your motivation for asking may help parents to talk about their mental health. Child protection practitioners will have to adapt their approach to each individual with mental distress dependent on the circumstances, rather than using a generic approach or 'tool'. It is important to look at the parents' situation from a systems perspective and use an open, relationship-based approach. The Mental Health Foundation has advice on language and ways of talking about mental health.

Parents may talk about their experiences of mental distress, but practitioners are also likely to observe potential signs of mental distress. Some possible signs are listed in the 'Possible Signs of Mental Distress' box. Asking sensitive questions based on your observations can be a way of raising the subject of potential mental distress with parents. Be mindful though that the practitioner's role is not to 'diagnose' through linking these signs to symptoms of a specific mental 'illness'. For child protection practitioners, a diagnostic label on its own is not necessarily useful. For example, words like 'depression' and 'anxiety' are used commonly by many people but may relate to very different experiences. What is important is identifying the impact the person's mental distress is having on their functioning and their ability to parent. Ask clearly what the term means for them and how it affects them day to day. For instance, 'You say you're depressed: can you tell me how this affects you?'

POSSIBLE SIGNS OF MENTAL DISTRESS

Note that some of these experiences are very common, (e.g. disturbed sleep), which in isolation may not always be a sign of mental distress without other evidence. Consider whether the experience is a change from the 'norm' for this person and is affecting their ability to carry out day-to-day activities and care for their child.

- Visible signs of emotional distress: e.g. crying, appearing withdrawn and worried, avoiding eye contact.
- Disturbed sleep: not enough or too much.
- Change in appetite: e.g. loss of interest in food. May be accompanied by weight loss or gain.
- Reduced ability to care for themselves and children: e.g. not washing, getting dressed etc., in someone who usually can do this.
- Lethargy and lack of motivation.
- Anxiety: this can be general, e.g. being anxious about many elements of life, or specific, e.g. being anxious about leaving the house, crowded places, etc. The manifestations of anxiety can feel more like physical health problems, for example sweating, chest pain, 'pins and needles' sensation on skin.
- Expressing unusual or what seems to be unlikely beliefs: e.g. that they are part of MI5 or are being pursued by government agents. Be mindful that some people express seemingly unlikely beliefs that may have a basis in truth.
- Hearing voices or seeing things which other people cannot hear or see.
- Be aware that the side effects of medication prescribed for mental distress can be similar to these signs. Many people who take psychiatric medication report side effects such as lethargy, nausea, disturbed sleep and weight gain. Note that these side effects may also affect people's parenting and ability to engage with support.

HOW TO RESPOND TO AND WORK WITH PARENTAL MENTAL DISTRESS

It has been suggested that along with a social model of mental health, a 'social model of child protection' is also required (Featherstone et al, 2016), moving beyond an individualised risk focus to consider adversities faced by parents themselves on a societal level. A key part of this approach relies on relationship building, and it is known that parents who experience mental distress appreciate support from workers who build trusting relationships with them and who acknowledge strengths as well as concerns (Buckley et al., 2011). However, any consideration of relationships also needs an honest approach which can acknowledge both the workers' potential to promote strengths and the power '...to diminish and destroy (including the power to 'shame')' (Featherstone et al., 2016, p. 14).

How to Respond to Someone You Think May Be Experiencing Mental Distress

- Child protection practitioners should be honest about what their role is with supporting mental distress, e.g. do not promise to be able to 'sort everything out'.

- If a parent has disclosed information about their mental distress, thank them and acknowledge that this might have been difficult to do.
- Focus on the impact of the mental distress on the parent and their children, rather than trying to link this to a diagnosis. For example, if someone hears voices, does this cause them distress? Does that distress affect their parenting, e.g. because they are distracted by what the voices are saying?
- Ensure that identifying the impact of the mental distress on their children is central. Does the parent's mental distress affect the child's emotional and physical well-being? For example, if someone feels depressed, does this affect their ability to show warmth and affection to their children and care for them?
- If someone has unusual beliefs or experiences, do not try to 'argue them away' by trying to prove they are imaginary. Try instead to focus on the emotional impact of the experience, e.g. 'it sounds like this really upsets you.'
- Allow people to talk about their mental distress before offering advice on managing it. Acknowledge the impact of mental distress on the person and the fact that they may not feel able to control this. For people experiencing significant depression, well-meaning advice to be more active and 'cheer up' may feel like a belittling of the impact of their distress.
- Despite this, practical, straightforward advice on managing mental health can be helpful. This could include encouraging a parent to develop some daily structure to help with motivation. The NHS self-help resources listed later may be helpful for some people.
- Encourage the parent to access support for their mental distress through their GP (see services section). If a parent refuses to see their GP and there are significant concerns, a practitioner could contact the GP with their concerns. The GP may then be able to contact the parent.

Young Carers

Children may take on the role of a carer for a parent with mental distress. This can have a significant impact on a child's well-being, especially if they have care responsibilities that are not suitable for their age. Young carers miss on average 48 school days a year and 68% have been bullied because of their caring role (Young Minds, 2021). It is crucial for practitioners to identify and offer support to young carers; the resources section at the end of the chapter has details of services.

HOW TO RESPOND IF A PARENT HAS SUICIDAL THOUGHTS

Thoughts of suicide are more common than many realise: 21% of adults report lifetime suicidal thoughts (McManus et al., 2016). It is therefore likely that child protection practitioners will encounter parents who are having thoughts of suicide. This is a complex area, and many practitioners worry if they ask about suicide they will 'make things worse.' Actually, this is unlikely – a conversation about suicide could help someone access the right support and assess the likelihood of harm. Some people may clearly disclose their suicidal thoughts; others may make ambiguous statements, or their behaviour may indicate potential suicidal thoughts. In situations where a practitioner is concerned that someone might be experiencing suicidal thoughts:

- Ask clearly and directly about suicide. If someone responds ambiguously, respond with a clear, closed question which avoids euphemisms. For example, ask 'are you having thoughts of ending your own life?' not 'will you do something silly?'
- If someone does talk about having suicidal thoughts, thank them for talking about this and reassure them that they have done the right thing in speaking about it. Many people with suicidal thoughts feel guilt. Explaining that these thoughts are more common than people think might help reassure them.
- Given the potential feelings of guilt, try not to increase this, for example by making reference to the possible impact suicide would have on family members.
- Ask more questions to find out more about the likelihood of them acting on the thoughts. Have they thought about potential methods, and if so, have they done any active planning towards this, such as collecting tablets? Active planning could indicate a higher risk of acting on the thoughts.

- Ask if the person has had these thoughts in the past and what helped then. Does the person have access to support currently, e.g. family members who can be with them?
- If a child protection practitioner is concerned there is a high risk of someone acting on their suicidal thoughts, consider supporting them to get referred to the Crisis Team through their GP or encourage them to go to the nearest hospital Emergency Department. In situations of immediate risk, consider accessing Emergency Services through 999.
- An excellent free online training course on suicide awareness and how to respond can be found at www.zerosuicidealliance.com/training.

WHAT SERVICES ARE AVAILABLE FOR PARENTS EXPERIENCING MENTAL DISTRESS?

In the UK, the main way of accessing NHS mental health support is through self-referral to Primary Care, usually through a GP. Support from Primary Care can include psychiatric medication, for instance antidepressant tablets, and brief 'talking therapies' such as cognitive behavioural therapy through the Improving Access to Psychological Therapies (IAPT) programme. The IAPT service can also be accessed through self-referral (the NHS website listed in the Further Reading section). People with more severe mental distress may be eligible for support from Adult Mental Health Services. Access is usually through a GP referral, not through self-referral. Adult Mental Health Services can involve support from psychiatrists, nursing, psychology and social care. In common with other public services, eligibility for services is focused on those most in need and may involve lengthy waiting times. This is particularly true of specialised therapeutic interventions, which can have long wait lists. However, people with urgent needs should be seen quickly, usually by Crisis Teams. For people who need immediate mental health support, including where there is immediate high risk of harm, consider using Emergency Services through 999. Emergency mental health assessments can be provided in NHS Emergency Departments. People whose mental distress is severe and are considered to be at significant risk of harm may be admitted to psychiatric hospital: 3.5% of those who use Adult Mental Health Services were admitted in 2020 to 2021 (NHS Digital, 2021). This requires a specialist assessment by Adult Mental Health Services.

When Might Support From Adult Mental Health Services Be Needed?

Signs that might indicate a need for Adult Mental Health services include:

- The support provided through Primary Care Services does not seem to be working, and there is a need for more specialist and intensive support.
- Someone's mental distress is causing significant risk of harm, either to themselves or others. This can include self-neglect, thoughts of suicide and significant self-harm.
- The mental distress has a major impact on a person's ability to function, for example a person's distress at the voices they hear is preventing them from eating or sleeping.

CASE STUDY 19B.2: SHANTELLE AND TOMMY

Shantelle is a 35-year-old woman of Jamaican heritage who lives with her 6-year-old son Tommy. Tommy has no contact with his father. Shantelle has a large extended family with five siblings. Shantelle has a difficult relationship with her siblings, accusing them of trying to control her and spying on her. Shantelle believes that she is under surveillance by the police and family members. She believes that the walls have had hidden CCTV cameras implanted in them when she leaves the house. Shantelle believes that she can be seen at all times in the house through the cameras. Shantelle is extremely distressed by these beliefs – some of the rooms have holes in the plaster where she has tried to search for and remove cameras. To avoid the cameras, Shantelle is sleeping with Tommy in a different room every night, sometimes waking him in the middle of the night to move to another room when she believes the cameras are filming them. Shantelle loves Tommy and says she wants to keep him safe from harm. She believes moving rooms makes him safer. Shantelle is still taking Tommy to school every day. His teachers have noted that he seems tired, but he is doing well at school.

REFLECTIVE QUESTIONS

- What is the potential impact on Tommy of Shantelle's mental distress?
- Shantelle believes what she is doing is keeping Tommy safe. How might you talk to her about the potential impact on Tommy?
- Do you think Shantelle is likely to seek a referral to adult mental health services? How might you help to do this?
- If adult mental health services start supporting Shantelle, what are the potential opportunities and challenges for multidisciplinary working between adult and child-focused services?

CONCLUSION

Mental distress is common, but is more prevalent amongst people experiencing poverty, social inequality and discrimination. Parenting is hard work and can lead to parental mental distress, especially when it evokes difficult memories and unresolved childhood trauma. Although many parents experience mental distress, this does not always affect a person's parenting capacity. Most parents with mental distress are able to care for their children well. However, for some parents their mental distress may significantly affect their functioning and ability to meet their children's needs. Parental mental distress is a factor in over half of Serious Case Reviews (Brandon et al., 2020).

For child protection practitioners, it is important to be able to identify and respond to parental mental distress. While being aware of psychiatric diagnoses and their meanings can be helpful, on its own a diagnosis does not identify the impact on ability to parent. A child protection practitioner's role is not to diagnose mental distress, but to assess the impact that this distress may be having on the parents' daily functioning and ability to care for their child. It is important to ask clear, direct and sensitive questions to identify parental mental distress. However, child protection practitioners should be mindful that some parents may be reluctant to disclose information about their mental health in fear that it will be used against them in care proceedings.

This chapter has suggested some practical ways that child protection practitioners can respond to parental mental distress, including suicidal thoughts. It is important to respond with care and compassion to parents when they discuss mental distress. It is crucial though that the impact of the mental distress on the child remains central. For some children, being a young carer has a significant impact on their development and well-being.

While specialist adult mental health services are available, not all parents experiencing mental distress will be eligible for these. Child protection practitioners can support the referral process, particularly at points of crisis. An attuned and informed child protection practitioner who sensitively supports parents with mental distress as part of their assessment, planning, implementation and evaluation of child well-being interventions can make all the difference.

FURTHER READING

Self-help resources: the NHS website has useful self-help guides on managing your mental health and includes information on mental health services and how to contact IAPT services in your area: https://www.nhs.uk/mental-health/talking-therapies-medicine-treatments/talking-therapies-and-counselling/self-help-therapies/.

Young Carers services and support: children may take on a caring role to support a parent with mental distress. The Young Minds website: https://youngminds.org.uk/find-help/looking-after-yourself/young-carers/) has advice and information on how to access support.

SCIE Guide 30: Think child, think parent, think family: a guide to parental mental health and child welfare: https://www.scie.org.uk/publications/guides/guide30/. This guidance from 2011 is still a useful overview of the Think Family model and how services can best support parents and children.

Trauma-informed approaches: Young Minds 'Adversity and Trauma-Informed Practice: A short guide for professionals working on the frontline'. Blue Knot – Trauma-Informed Practice Information.

NSPCC Resources: Parental mental health problems (https://learning.nspcc.org.uk/children-and-families-at-risk/parental-mental-health-problems) includes guidance and links to resources.

Royal College of Psychiatrists: Parental mental illness: the impact on children and adolescents: for parents and carers. https://www.rcpsych.ac.uk/mental-health/parents-and-young-people/information-for-parents-and-carers/parental-mental-illness-the-impact-on-children-and-adolescents-for-parents-and-carers.

Children's Commissioner (2018), "Are they shouting because of me?" Voices of children living in households with domestic abuse, parental substance misuse and mental health issues: https://www.childrenscommissioner.gov.uk/wp-content/uploads/2018/08/Are-they-shouting-because-of-me.pdf. Report on children's views of the impact on them of their parents' issues.

Suicide advice and resources: Papyrus aims to prevent suicide in people aged below 35: site has advice and resources for professionals. Samaritans offer support to people experiencing suicidal thoughts and have helpful guides on how to talk about suicide. Call Samaritans on 116 123.

Alternatives to Psychiatric Diagnosis and Social Perspectives on Mental Health:

The Power Threat Meaning Framework: https://www.bps.org.uk/power-threat-meaning-framework.

'A Disorder for Everyone': http://www.adisorder4everyone.com/links/.

Recovery in the bin: https://recoveryinthebin.org/.

Hearing Voices Network: http://www.hearing-voices.org/.

Social Perspectives Network: http://spn.org.uk/.

'Behind the label': https://www.behindthelabel.co.uk/.

Eleanor Longden 'The Voices in My Head'.

Icarus project resources: http://nycicarus.org/publications-media/.

REFERENCES

American Psychiatric Association, 2013. Diagnostic and Statistical Manual of Mental Disorders: DSM-5, fifth ed. American Psychiatric Association, Washington DC.

Bachman, C., Gooch, B., 2018. LGBT in Britain: Health Report. Stonewall, London.

Bauer, A., Parsonage, M., Knapp, M., Lemmi, V., Adelaja, B., 2014. The Costs of Perinatal Mental Health Problems. Centre for Mental Health, London.

Brandon, M., Sidebotham, P., Belderson, P., Cleaver, H., Dickens, J., Garstang, J., et al., 2020. Complexity and Challenge: A Triennial Analysis of SCRs 2014-2017. Department for Education, London.

Bronfenbrenner, U., 1979. The Ecology of Human Development: Experiments by Nature and Design. Harvard University Press, Cambridge, MA.

Buckley, H., Carr, N., Whelan, S., 2011. 'Like walking on eggshells': Service user views and expectations of child protection. Child Fam. Soc. Work 16 (1), 101–110.

Cleaver, H., Unell, I., Aldgate, J., 2011. Children's Needs – Parenting Capacity: The Impact of Parental Mental Illness, Problem Alcohol and Drug Use, and Domestic Violence on Children's Development, second ed. TSO, London.

Cromby, J., Harper, D., Reavey, P., 2013. Psychology, Mental Health and Distress. Palgrave Macmillan/Springer Nature, Basingstoke.

Cromby, J., 2018. An Alternative to Psychiatric Diagnosis? An innovative framework provides new ways of understanding mental health. Psychology Today https://www.psychologytoday.com/us/blog/the-bodies-we-re-in/201801/alternative-psychiatric-diagnosis (Accessed 22 August 2023).

Children Act 1989. https://www.legislation.gov.uk/ukpga/1989/41/contents

Department of Health, 2000. Framework for the Assessment of Children in Need and their Families. TSO, London

Duffy, J., Davidson, G., Kavanagh, D., 2016. Applying the Recovery Approach to the Interface between Mental Health and Child Protection Services. Child Care in Practice, Routledge.

Falkov, A., Grant, A., Hoadley, B., Donaghy, M., Bente, M., 2020. The Family Model: A brief intervention for clinicians in adult mental health services working with parents experiencing mental health problems. Aust N Z J Psychiatry 54 (5), 449–452 2020.

Featherstone, B., White, S., Morris, K., 2014. Re-Imagining Child Protection: Towards Humane Social Work with Families. Policy Press, Bristol.

Featherstone, B., Gupta, A., Morris, K., Warner, J., 2016. Let's stop feeding the risk monster: Towards a social model of 'child protection. Fam. Relatsh. Soc. 7 (1), 07–22. www.ingentaconnect.com/content/tpp/frs/pre-prints/content-pp_frs-d-15-00034r2.

Fernando, S., 2010. Mental Health, Race and Culture, third ed. Palgrave Macmillan, Basingstoke.

Fitzpatrick M and Newton J., 2005. Profiling mental health needs: What about your Irish patients? Br J Gen Pract, 55(519):739–40.

Forrester, D., Westlake, D., McCann, M., Thurnham, A., Shefer, G., Glynn, G., et al., 2013. Reclaiming Social Work? An Evaluation of Systemic Units as an Approach to Delivering Children's Services: Final Report of a Comparative Study of Practice and the Factors Shaping it in Three Local Authorities. University of Bedfordshire, Bedford.

Frost, N., 2017. From "silo" to "network" profession – a multi-professional future for social work. J. Child. Serv. 12, 174–183.

Gov.uk, 2020. Characteristics of Children in Need. https://explore-education-statistics.service.gov.uk/find-statistics/characteristics-of-children-in-need/2020#dataBlock-0247c828-2398-4d34-8b98-08d884b70554-charts (Accessed 19 March 2021).

Gupta, A., Featherstone, B., White, S., 2016. Reclaiming humanity: From capacities to capabilities in understanding parenting in adversity. Br. J. Soc. Work 46 (2), 339–354. https://doi.org/10.1093/bjsw/bcu137.

Johnstone, L., Boyle, M., with Cromby, J., Dillon, J., Harper, D., Kinderman, P., et al., 2018. The Power Threat Meaning Framework: Towards the Identification of Patterns in Emotional Distress, Unusual Experiences and Troubled or Troubling Behaviour, as an Alternative to Functional Psychiatric Diagnosis. British Psychological Society, Leicester. https://www.bps.org.uk/guideline/power-threat-meaning-framework-full-version.

Johnstone, L., and Watson, J., 2018. A Disorder for Everyone, https://www.mentalhealthtoday.co.uk/blog/disorders/a-disorder-for-everyone (Accessed 22 August 2023).

Keddell, E., 2016. Constructing parental problems: The function of mental illness discourses in a child welfare context. Br. J. Soc. Work 46, 2088–2103.

McManus, S., Bebbington, P., Jenkins, R., Brugha, T. (Eds.), 2016. Mental health and wellbeing in England: Adult Psychiatric Morbidity Survey 2014. NHS Digital, Leeds.

Mellon, M., 2017. Iriss., Child Protection: Listening to and Learning from Oarents Insight 39. https://www.iriss.org.uk/resources/insights/child-protection-listening-and-learning-parents.

Memon, A., Taylor, K., Mohebati, L.M., Sundin, J., Cooper, M., Scanlon, T., et al., 2016. Perceived barriers to accessing mental health services among black and minority ethnic (BME) communities: A qualitative study in southeast England. BMJ Open 6 (11). https://doi.org/10.1136/bmjopen-2016-012337.

Mind, 2018. Big Mental Health Survey 2017: Headline Findings. https://www.mind.org.uk/media-a/4368/mind-big-mental-health-survey-headlines-2017.pdf. (Accessed 26 May 2021).

Ministry of Justice, 2020. Statistics on Women and the Criminal Justice System 2019, available at https://www.gov.uk/government/statistics/women-and-the-criminal-justice-system-2019 (Accessed 22 August 2023).

Mental Health Act 1983. https://www.legislation.gov.uk/ukpga/1983/20/contents

NHS Digital, 2020. Mental Health Act Statistics, Annual Figures England, 2019-2020. https://files.digital.nhs.uk/99/3916C8/ment-heal-act-stat-eng-2019-20-summ-rep%20v1.1.pdf. (Accessed 11 June 2021).

NHS Digital, 2021. Mental Health Bulletin 2020-21 Annual report. Available at https://digital.nhs.uk/data-and-information/publications/statistical/mental-health-bulletin/2020-21-annual-report (Accessed 22 August 2023).

Pickett, K., Wilkinson, R., 2015. Income inequality and health: A causal review. Soc. Sci. Med. 128, 316–326.

Siverns, K., Morgan, G., 2019. Parenting in the context of historical childhood trauma: An interpretive meta-synthesis. Child Abuse Negl 98:104186.

Tew, J., 2011. Social Approaches to Mental Distress. Red Globe Press, British Association of Social Workers, UK.

Warwick, L., Morley, K., 2019. 'Trevi House: An Independent Evaluation'. https://nottingham-repository.worktribe.com/index.php/output/8135543/trevi-house-independent-evaluation-november-2019.

Young Minds, 2021. Young Carers. https://youngminds.org.uk/find-help/looking-after-yourself/young-carers/. (Accessed 3 June 2021).

YOUNG PARENTS

CAROLINE LYNCH

KEY POINTS

- Who young parents are and the challenges they face.
- The principles and importance of partnership working.
- Good practice in assessment and support for young parents.
- The needs and experiences of care experienced young parents.
- Exploring wider family and friends' network.
- Advice, information and advocacy for young parents.
- Post-removal support.

INTRODUCTION

This chapter explores child protection practice with young parents. Beginning by identifying who young parents are and the challenges they face, the chapter then explores partnership working, good practice in assessments and the particular vulnerabilities, stigma faced and needs of, care experienced young parents. This includes attention to exploring wider family and friends' networks, advocacy and post-removal support. Throughout the chapter key themes are repeated. First, young parents are often highly stigmatised in practice and as a result, receive higher rates of state intervention in relation to the care of their children. Second, core principles and legal duties apply no less to young parents than to other parents. Finally, resources made in collaboration with – and tailored towards – young parents are valuable for parents and practitioners alike

in understanding young parents' lived experiences and subsequently providing effective, humane and holistic support in practice.

WHO ARE YOUNG PARENTS?

The meaning of the term 'young parent' varies across local and national policies, strategies and guidance, as well as between services providing advice and support. Similarly, research has focussed on young people of differing ages and circumstance when examining young parenthood. This chapter therefore adopts a flexible interpretation of 'young parent'. Held in mind are young people experiencing pregnancy and parenthood in their teenage years and into early adulthood. Young parents are more likely to face increased scrutiny and are amongst those most harshly treated within the child welfare system (Ashley, 2021). Women who become mothers at a younger age are also more likely to experience recurrent sets of care proceedings in respect of their children (Broadhurst et al., 2015, 2017).

In 1999, a 10-year Teenage Pregnancy Strategy was launched in England. The foreword highlighted low expectations, poor contraception knowledge and 'mixed messages' as key factors underlying the under-18 conception rate at that time (Social Exclusion Unit, 1999). Reducing rates of conception for teenagers and the risk of teenage parents experiencing 'long term social exclusion' were the two main stated aims. The conception rate for women under 18 in England and Wales fell by 63% between 1993 and 2019 – from 42 per 1000 to 16 per 1000 women in that age bracket (Nuffield Trust, 2022).

Despite this downward trend, England continues to have one of the highest teenage pregnancy rates in western Europe (Nuffield Trust, 2022).

Young people with care experience are at higher risk of early pregnancy, often unplanned (Fallon & Broadhurst, 2015). In 2015, data provided by 93 local authorities in response to a Freedom of Information Act request revealed that 22% of female care leavers became teenage mothers – three times the then national average (Centre for Social Justice, 2015). Research analysing national level data about the care experienced population in both England and Wales highlights the vulnerability of care leavers in Wales to early parenthood and the removal of their children to adoptive placements (Roberts et al., 2017). Young fathers are often particularly marginalised during the involvement of child protection services and their strengths overlooked (Featherstone, 2013). This will be discussed in more depth later.

WHAT CHALLENGES DO YOUNG PARENTS FACE?

Young parents face the dual challenge of transitioning to adulthood *and* parenthood. They have complex and interconnected needs (Action for Children, 2017; Lynch, 2016) and can feel (and be) judged because of their young age and background, rather than by their parenting capacities. Younger parents often experience particular economic vulnerability, for example the national living wage is only available to those aged 23 years and over. A lack of accessible information or advice about benefit entitlements; barriers to remaining in education and training; and shortages of affordable or appropriate housing all disproportionately impact young parents. Childhood experiences including abuse, mental distress and homelessness may have implications for the resilience and resources of young parents, including whether they have supportive wider family and community networks to draw on. Past negative experiences of state services (e.g., education, health, police and social care) may further shape how young parents experience the child protection system and working with practitioners within it. Young parents may feel anxious and fearful of professional involvement with their children and such feelings may be heightened for those who are themselves care experienced (Chase et al., 2006; Maxwell, Proctor and Hammond, 2011).

Despite this nuanced picture, the needs and circumstances of young parents are often insufficiently and inconsistently recognised. Local protocols, service provision and professional practice often reflects limited consideration or understanding of young parents' experiences and needs, or how best to support them to keep their children safely in their care. Provision of tailored information and services for young parents is often limited, uneven or unknown (Lynch, 2016).

REFLECTIVE QUESTIONS

- Are you aware of the services available to young parents in your area? If not, spend some time researching the provision.
- Given what we know about the challenges young parents face, do you think the services available are sufficient?

PARTNERSHIP WORKING WITH YOUNG PARENTS

Partnership working is a core underlying principle of the Children Act (1989), with statutory guidance confirming that a *child-centred approach* means *working in partnership* with children and their families. Statutory guidance in England reminds us that:

children are best looked after within their families with their parents playing a full part in their lives unless compulsory intervention in family life is necessary.

Working Together (2018, p. 9)

These principles apply no less to young parents and their children. Local authority protocol documents should set out the specific processes that social workers should follow and how they will communicate with children and parents. How far, if at all, such local protocols are explicit in accounting for working with younger parents and their children varies.

Engaging young parents in reviews of key local policies, protocols and services is one crucial way in which local authorities can reflect on and improve practice. This is likely to be most effective when approached as a wider commitment to involving families in service and policy design and audit. Indeed, doing so responds to concerns set out in the *Care Crisis Review: Options for Change* report

(Ryan and Tunnard, 2018, pp. 45 - 46) that parents and families are 'rarely invited to contribute to service and policy development and provide feedback' and that there is a need to address this.

Practitioners seeking to be better equipped for working in partnership with young parents should engage with advice and information resources made in collaboration with – and tailored to – young parents. Some examples of helpful resources are included in the *further reading* section.

ASSESSMENTS: GOOD PRACTICE WITH YOUNG PARENTS

The parameters for high-quality social work assessment in England are laid out in Working Together (2018). The importance of building on strengths as well as identifying difficulties is made explicit. This is particularly important given research accounts of young parents feeling judged by their age, and of care experience being erroneously approached as an 'automatic risk factor' that should lead to child protection involvement (Lynch, 2016). Statutory guidance also emphasises the importance of social workers not waiting until assessments are complete to provide services and support it is already clear are needed (Working Together, 2018).

An updated draft of Working Together, launched for consultation by the Department for Education in July 2023 similarly does not include best practice guidance in respect of pre-birth child protection conferences (Department for Education, 2023). The need for

Good Practice Principles in Pre-birth Assessments

1. An assessment should start promptly once children's services are aware of the pregnancy. A decision about whether a pre-birth assessment is needed should be made within a day to decide whether an assessment is needed and what type of assessment it should be (Working Together, 2018, p. 33, para. 78).

2. The assessment report should be completed at least 4 weeks before birth to make sure there is enough time for parents to look at the assessment, ask questions and get legal advice:
   - This should be provided to parents (and their solicitors, if parents have them) as soon as it is complete.

3. An assessment should be updated regularly to make sure the plans for the baby continue to be relevant and best for them:
   - This should take into account relevant events that happen before and after the baby is born.

4. If children's services decide they need to apply to commence care proceedings once the baby is born, then:
   - The social work team should provide their legal department with all assessment reports and any other relevant documents. This should be at least 7 days before the mother's due date.
   - All court papers should be provided to the parents and their solicitors immediately. If they can be provided before the court has finished processing (issuing) the application, that can be done.
   - When the baby is born, children's services should send the papers to court promptly so the court can issue the case without delay.

Adapted from https://frg.org.uk/get-help-and-advice/who/parents-to-be/, 2022

effective pre-birth assessment work – and what this should look like – is, however, an issue picked up in case law, including in a decision involving young parents (Nottingham City Council v LW & Ors [2016] EWHC 11(Fam). In this decision, High Court Judge, Mr Justice Michael Keehan, set out good practice principles for conducting pre-birth assessments. The principles, combined with what Working Together does say regarding timeliness of decision-making about type of assessment, are highlighted in the Good Practice box. They may be noted and applied when working with young parents at a 'pre-birth' stage. Practitioners may also usefully draw on the Born into Care: Best practice guidelines for when the state intervenes at birth (Mason et al., 2023). The guidelines include a series of statements that local authorities and others can draw on, and adapt, to guide practice with parents and their unborn baby.

YOUNG FATHERS

Fathers can too often be overlooked, excluded or deprioritised in decision making about their children. Young fathers specifically are often viewed as a risk rather than resource, together with being viewed as 'hard to reach', which serves to stigmatise and place the onus for engaging with services firmly on them (Neale and Davies, 2015). Young age and previous care experience increase fathers' likelihood of experiencing recurrent care proceedings in relation to their own children (Philips et al., 2021), and Local Government and Social Care Ombudsman decisions continue to highlight the exclusion of fathers from assessment processes (see reference list). Case law provides an example of poor communication and exclusion from child protection conferences amounting to a breach of one father's human rights (see SW & TW (Human Rights Claim: Procedure) (No1) [2017] EWHC 450 (Fam)). Against this backdrop, practitioners must be mindful of such wider systemic issues as well as reflect on their own assumptions and prejudices to work humanely with young fathers. Practitioners should be clear about their duties to engage young fathers, including where there is opposition to their involvement, and note that relevant statutory guidance does not define parent in terms of whether they hold parental responsibility for their child. Overlooking young fathers in turn has implications for drawing on the potential resources

and supports that may be available for the child from within the wider family and friends network.

It is important that young fathers have the opportunity and support to understand social workers' concerns, including the chance to challenge these if they think concerns are not based on clear, reliable or up-to-date information. Assessments should provide opportunities for young fathers to demonstrate changes made, their strengths and how they can develop these further. Encouraging fathers to think through who may be able to provide up-to-date insights into their current situation is important. Examples may include close relatives and friends, mentors or advocates. Clear understanding of practice options where there are risks to manage in relation to the involvement of a parent in a meeting is essential, for example considering the use of 'split' child protection conferences. Recent research sheds light on the some of the impacts of the COVID-19 pandemic on young fathers and provides insights regarding use of digital and face-to-face means of supporting and working with them (Tarrant et al., 2021, 2020). Reviewing key messages from research regarding working with young fathers, listening to the accounts of young fathers involved in the child welfare system and taking opportunities to develop links with organisations specialising in supporting fathers are three practical strategies for strengthening individual and team practice (see suggestions for further reading and resources).

EXPLORING THE WIDER FAMILY AND FRIENDS' NETWORK

Exploration of the maternal *and* paternal family and friends' network should occur early on (from Early Help, or Child In Need if applicable) to identify *timely* support for the family and potential alternative carers (whether short, medium or long term) if children cannot safely remain with their parent(s). The Public Law Outline makes it clear that assessments relating to the child 'and/or family and friends of the child' should be available to the court at the start of the proceedings (except for in emergencies) and should therefore be some of the earliest work undertaken.

Services such as family group conferences (FGCs), which identify sources of familial support and help to coordinate it, are important for young parents. Indeed, FGCs are foregrounded as an effective way to explore the strengths and resources of the wider family network both in statutory guidance concerning kinship care (Department for Education, 2011 at para 2.8 and 4.34-5) and work prior to court proceedings (Department for Education, 2014 at para 24). Statutory guidance states that local authorities should consider referring families to FGC services if they believe there is a possibility the child may not be able to remain with their parents, or in any event before a child becomes looked after, unless this would be a risk to the child (Department for Education, 2014 at para 24). Best practice guidance about working with families prior to court proceedings was issued by the Public Law Working Group and states that one purpose of a legal planning meeting should be to identify family members who can be consulted to offer support or be assessed as alternative carers. The guidance refers to early use of an FGC (or similar locally developed model) stating that it 'is essential unless there is good reason why this is impracticable' (Public Law Working Group, 2021 at para 19(f)).

CLOSER LOOK: FAMILY GROUP CONFERENCES (FGCs)

A family group conference (FGC) is a **family-led** decision-making meeting. It brings together the whole family and others who are important to the child. Together, at the family group conference, they make a plan for the child. The process is supported by an independent coordinator who helps the family prepare for the FGC. Children are usually involved in their own FGC, often with support from an advocate. It is a voluntary process.

An FGC may take place where practitioners who know the child have raised concerns or where a family is asking for more support. The family group conference should address the problems identified. The aim is to agree a plan to address those challenges, led by what the family think will help.

Family group conferences are based on the idea that if families are properly supported, they will make safe, relevant plans for their children. They are different because:

- It is the family who make the decisions.
- In other meetings the plan is made by practitioners who sometimes consult with some of the family.
- A family group conference takes place at a time and a place to suit the family, which may be outside of office hours.
- Wider family members and friends are invited.
- Children are invited and should be supported to play an active role. A family group conference will always involve private family time.

Focussing on support for young parents with care experience is particularly important when considering evidence regarding how the care system too often breaks relationships for young people (Care Inquiry, 2013). One successful model specifically designed to support young people with care experience is **Lifelong Links** (see Lifelong Links box).

CLOSER LOOK: LIFELONG LINKS

Lifelong links is an approach that aims to ensure that children in the care system have positive support networks around them during their time in care and into adulthood. The model includes tools and techniques for Lifelong Links coordinators to search for and find family members (known or unknown to the young person) and other adults (such as former foster carers or teachers) who care about the young person.

This network is then brought together in a Lifelong Links family group conference to make a life-long support plan with, and for, the young person. The local authority should integrate the Lifelong Links plan into the young person's care plan and social workers should work with the young person and their support network during their childhood and transition to adulthood. Independent evaluation has found that Lifelong Links led to an improved sense of identity for young people, greater stability in their care placement and more social connections. Longer term study found improvements in placement stability and in children's mental health and well-being associated with Lifelong Links.

Modified from https://frg.org.uk/get-help-and-advice/top-tips-and-templates/, 2022

SPECIALIST INFORMATION, ADVICE AND ADVOCACY

The power inequalities between state and parent are acute in the context of compulsory intervention under the child protection framework. The availability of publicly funded legal advice is often very limited when child protection conferences are convened. Low remuneration rates under the legal aid scheme means fewer high street legal aid firms are in a position to take on cases at this early stage. The extent of the advice and assistance that it is possible to provide under the legal aid rate is also limited. Similarly, demand for specialist advice and advocacy provided by voluntary sector organisations is high (and may outstrip supply). As public bodies, local authority children's services departments must take account of a person's rights under the European Convention of Human Rights. This includes making sure that procedures for decision-making about children's lives are fair (Human Rights Act, 1989) and involve children and parents. This includes whether individuals have been able to challenge decisions. Thinking through what needs to be in place so a young parent can meaningfully take part in child protection processes from an informed position is key. Whether a young parent's involvement is, or has been, fair is something that should always be actively examined and reflected upon.

Independent specialist advice and advocacy can help parents to participate in local authority planning processes from an informed position. With an understanding of their rights and options, how to navigate complex child welfare system processes, raise concerns and pursue challenges, young parents are more likely to be well placed to work in partnership. Government guidance recognises that advocacy support for parents may be an important part of helping families to work with children's services at an early stage. It identifies advocacy as an important part of making sure the actions that children's services take are understood by parents (Department for Education, 2014).

In relation to child protection conferences, social workers have a specific responsibility to ensure parents understand the *purpose* of a child protection conference and *who will be there* (Working Together, 2018, p. 48). They also should 'give information about advocacy agencies and explain that the family may bring an advocate, friend or supporter' to child protection conferences (Working Together, 2018, p. 44). This requirement falls somewhat short of requiring this to be arranged and funded. It does, however, reflect that practitioners should ensure they have an understanding of national and local services and resources available for parents, including young parents. Taken together with the principles of partnership working referred to earlier, understanding what advocacy support a young parent may wish to draw on, what may assist them and being familiar with what is on offer is a critical part of early-stage work. While parental advocacy services for young parents tend to be localised and sparse, pockets of specialised service provision do exist. There are many benefits to independent advocacy.

If a decision is made to refuse a young person the opportunity to bring a particular supporter or advocate, the reasons for this should be very clearly explained

> ## CLOSER LOOK: ADVOCACY SUPPORT
>
> What can an advocate support a young parent to do?
> - Prepare for meetings with social workers
> - Understand their rights, options and how child protection planning and decision-making works
> - Reflect on why social workers are concerned about their child
> - Support the young parent to think through safe plans for the child, which may include alternative care within the family
> - Feel emotionally supported and more confident to participate
> - Ask the social worker questions
> - Speak up, get their voice heard by practitioners and their point of view across
> - Reach agreements/negotiate with social workers
> - Challenge social workers or others in a constructive way
> - Record and remember what has been said and agreed so that they can plan what to do next
>
> Family Rights Group, 2021 'Working with an advocate'

and confirmed in writing. It is important this is done so the young parent can understand the objection and consider whether they need to challenge the decision. The more vulnerable the young person feels and the more serious the child protection concerns and decisions to be made, the less reasonable it is likely to be to refuse input from an advocate or supporter. The advocacy needs and entitlements of a young parent will also vary depending on whether they have any additional needs under the Equality Act 2010 – for example, a physical disability, or a learning disability.

In such cases, drawing on relevant best practice guidance, having an awareness of equality duties and the need to make reasonable adjustments will be important too. There is, for example, guidance on good practice during the child protection process when working with parents with learning difficulties or disabilities (Working Together Parenting Network, 2021, p. 27).

PLANS FOR CARE EXPERIENCED YOUNG PEOPLE, PLANS FOR THEIR CHILDREN

Young people who are care experienced are more likely to experience early parenthood compared to peers who have not been looked after in the care

LEAVING CARE SUPPORT

A young person who has been looked after for 13 weeks or more since they were 14, including for at least one day after their 16th birthday will be entitled to leaving care support. Depending on their age, whether they are presently looked after or have already left care, such young people will variously be 'eligible', 'relevant' or 'former relevant' children (see Sections 23A, 23C and 24 of the Children Act 1989). The law requires that young people falling into those categories should have a pathway plan (up to the age of 25 years).

Some care experienced young people will not have been looked after in the care system for the necessary 13 weeks (and one day beyond their 16th birthday) to be eligible for legal care support. However, those in that situation who are aged between 16 and 20 should still be **befriended** by the local authority. The local authority *may* provide additional assistance. This group of 'qualifying' young people includes, for example, young people who left the care system because a special guardianship order was in place, and they remain under that order (or did until they turned 18).

system (Fallon & Broadhurst, 2015). Care experienced young parents are also more vulnerable to experiencing recurrent care proceedings (Broadhurst et al., 2015, 2017; Philips et al., 2021) and having their children removed to adoption (Roberts et al., 2017). Local authorities have legal duties to provide some groups of care experienced young people with help to support them in moving into adulthood and independence. From the outset, practitioners should hold in mind the **seven corporate parenting principles** set out in the Children and Social Work Act (2017). These must always be considered when supporting young people who are looked after or leaving the care system. These principles do not cease to apply because a young person becomes a parent.

Pathway plans should set out what will be done to support young people with their health and development, education, training and employment, contact with family and managing money. In practice, pathway plans may fail to consider the support that a care leaver needs as a young parent. Too often there is a lack of connectively between plans formulated to support the care experienced young parent as a young person

leaving the care system and the plans in place for their child.

Statutory guidance applicable to child protection work emphasises the importance of all assessments for a child being coordinated so that 'the child does not become lost between the different organisational procedures' (Working Together, 2018). Yet there is no specific guidance from the government about coordinating and linking the assessment of need and resulting pathway plan for a young person with any child protection planning being undertaken in respect of their child. Nevertheless, practitioners will want to consider from an early stage how to work across teams and services most effectively. This includes considering with the young parent what role their personal adviser might have in supporting them within the child protection processes and meetings regarding their child. Where the young parent is still looked after, they may have an advocate whose role in assisting the young person can be explored. Young parents will have views and expectations about how they wish to be supported and about how information might be shared and discussed.

In parallel, it will be crucial to ensure that a young parent has information and support to understand their rights and options in respect of the child protection processes and as a young person leaving care. For example, government regulations require that pathway plans are reviewed every 6 months; however, young people have the right to request a review of their plan at any time. A young parent may want and need their pathway plan to be reviewed as pregnancy progresses and following the birth to ensure the plan works for them. How this is linked with or is coordinated with development and review of a child protection plan for their child will be relevant.

POST-REMOVAL SUPPORT

Local authorities in England and Wales are required to take reasonable steps to reduce the need to bring care proceedings and other types of court proceedings that might lead to children being in their care (Children Act 1989, schedule II, paragraph 7). The need to provide support to young parents who have

CASE STUDY 19C.1: HELENA

Helena is 20 years old and expecting her first child in 4 months. She has been told that a pre-birth child protection conference will be arranged for her baby because of concerns about her being a 'care leaver' and not having any support from her family. Helena doesn't want to go to this meeting alone. She hasn't had any advice about how to prepare for it.

Helena is living in semi-independent accommodation, a studio flat. She lived with foster carers until she was 17 and was looked after from age 7. She doesn't have any contact with her own parents but talks fondly about her aunt who lives an hour away that she sees regularly. She refers to her cousins too and their young children.

Helena is enrolled at college but has been nervous about speaking with her tutors and peers about her pregnancy and is uncertain about how to do this. Helena missed some classes recently due to maternity appointments and meetings with her social worker. She wants to complete her course before the baby arrives and thinks she could do this if she could just make it to college. She would like to enrol onto the next stage of her college course but thinks no one wants her to focus on college once the baby is born. She's heard the college has a creche but assumes she wouldn't have enough money to pay for that. The social worker for her unborn baby has said she must prioritise attending child protection meetings and assessments appointments, otherwise there will be concerns about her commitment and 'engagement'.

Helena has a pathway plan, but the last time she spoke to her personal adviser he explained this was 'separate' from the plan for her baby. He said he would try to talk to the social worker but needed to focus on the pathway plan rather than the plans for the baby. In meetings about her baby, no one has mentioned Helena's pathway plan or her personal adviser.

---

already experienced the removal of a child is arguably one important aspect of working to attend to this duty. Beyond the legal framework itself, there is a wider recognition that a humane child welfare and family justice system does not simply engage in repeated removal of children from parents with no provision made to support them either to address underlying difficulties or the effects of experiencing the removal of a child. In practice, availability of services and funding for post-removal support is often challenging.

Even where a child is to be removed from their parent there is a clear benefit to the child of the parent having the support they need to address their difficulties as well as the trauma of losing a child. This is not least in relation to the plans for future contact and the future relationships between child and birth parent. Where the young parent is owed care leaving duties, pathway planning may provide a route to post-removal support, given that pathway plans should include focus on education and health needs and wellbeing more generally. It is also important to ensure that following the conclusion of proceedings, parents have copies of key paperwork including the final court orders, care plans, copy of the court judgment and key assessments including those that set out recommendations for any therapeutic and other work.

Keeping abreast of recent exercises to map availability of post-removal support services and drawing on these is sensible. Accounts of the experiences and insights of parents who have had their children removed may be of use to practitioners to understand the impact of removal on young parents and its legacy for their future parenting as well as for their feelings about working with practitioners in the future. There are rich examples of lived experience accounts in a range of formats – articles, blogs, vlogs and similar (see Further Reading for examples).

REFLECTIVE QUESTIONS

- What role might a young person's personal adviser have in supporting and advocating for them in the context of child protection involvement with their child?
- How do the plans for the young person's education, training, health and accommodation account for their current, or pending, young parenthood?
- How might development and review of a young person's pathway plan and development and review of plans for their child need to work together?

CONCLUSION

Working with a young parent requires tailored practice, but it is also important to retain focus on the core principle of working in partnership, the statutory requirements for good assessment and exploring wider family and friends networks. These apply no less to young parents. In all work with young parents, practitioners must be mindful of the pitfalls of stereotyping and assuming that young age equates to heightened risk. Practice that starts from the position of understanding the specific challenges that young parents may face (and why), and with a familiarity of local and nationally available resources for young parents, is likely to be more effective. Advice materials developed by – and for – young parents have a central role in enhancing practitioner knowledge and understanding, including ensuring familiarity with the parents' rights and options.

It is crucial for practitioners to be aware of the heightened risk of early parenthood for care experienced young people and the higher risk of experiencing intervention with their children and removal. Understanding the interface of the duties owed to the young person as a looked after child or young person leaving care and their rights as a parent within child protection processes should be part of the baseline knowledge for working effectively and in partnership with young parents. This includes the interface of pathway planning and the development of plans in respect of the young person's child.

REFLECTIVE QUESTIONS

- What should practitioners consider when working with young parents in a child protection context? Consider this both in terms of the parent and their children.
- What kind of practice helps or hinders young parents in working with practitioners?
- What advice and support may young parents need to navigate the child protection system?

FURTHER READING

Care to Learn: https://www.gov.uk/care-to-learn.

Family Rights Group young parents website: https://frg.org.uk/get-help-and-advice/who/young-parents/.

Family Rights Group blogs and vlogs from young parents involved with the child welfare system: https://www.frg.org.uk/ypa/blogs.

Just for Kids Law young parent animation: https://www.justforkidslaw.org/news/animated-film-if-i-could-talk-me.

REFERENCES

Action for Children, 2017. The Next Chapter: Young People and Parenthood. https://media.actionforchildren.org.uk/documents/the-next-chapter.pdf.

Ashley, C., 2021. Speech at Family Rights Group Seminar 'How Can Partnership with Families Run through Family Support and Child protection Systems and Practice?' https://frg.org.uk/news-blogs-and-vlogs/news/seminars-looking-at-what-reforms-are-needed-to-our-child-welfare-system/. Direct youtube linkhttps://youtu.be/DA_RvD9zWa8.

Broadhurst, K., Alrouh, B., Yeend, E., Harwin, J., Shaw, M., Pilling, et al., 2015. Connecting events in time to identify a hidden population: birth mothers and their children in recurrent care proceedings in England. Br. J. Soc. Work 45 (8), 2241–2260.

Broadhurst, K., Mason, C., Bedston, S., Alrouh, B., Morriss, L., McQuerrie, T., et al., 2017. Vulnerable Birth Mothers in Recurrent Care Proceedings: Final Main Report. University of Lancaster. Centre for Child and Family Justice Research, Lancaster. http://wp.lancs.ac.uk/recurrent-care/files/2017/10/mrc_final_main_report_v1.0.pdf.

Care Inquiry, 2013. Making Not Breaking: Building Relationships for Our Most Vulnerable Children. https://www.adoptionuk.org/Handlers/Download.ashx?IDMF=85fe35ed-2c73-4ba8-83e5-5396d34969a7.

Centre for Social Justice, January 2015. Finding Their Feet: Equipping Care Leavers to Reach Their Potential. http://www.centreforsocialjustice.org.uk/publications/finding-their-feet.

Chase, E., Maxwell, C., Knight, A., Aggleton, P., 2006. Pregnancy and parenthood among young people in and leaving care: what are the influencing factors, and what makes a difference in providing support? J. Adolesc. 29 (3), 437–451.

Children Act 1989. https://www.legislation.gov.uk/ukpga/1989/41/contents

Children and Social Work Act, 2017. https://www.legislation.gov.uk/ukpga/2017/16/contents/enacted

Department for Education, 2011. Family and Friends: Statutory Guidance for Local Authorities. https://www.gov.uk/government/publications/children-act-1989-family-and-friends-care.

Department for Education, 2014. Volume 1 Child Act 1989: Court Orders and Pre-proceedings. https://www.gov.uk/government/publications/children-act-1989-court-orders--2.

Department for Education, 2023. Draft: Working Together to Safeguard Children 2023. Available at: https://consult.education.gov.uk/child-protection-safeguarding-division/working-together-to-safeguard-children-changes-to/

Equality Act, 2010. https://www.legislation.gov.uk/ukpga/2010/15/contents

Fallon, D., Broadhurst, K., 2015. Preventing Unplanned Pregnancy and Improving Preparation for Parenthood for Care-Experienced Young People. Coram, London.

Family Rights Group, 2021. Working with an advocate. https://frg.org.uk/get-help-and-advice/top-tips-and-templates/

Featherstone, B., 2013. Working with fathers: risk or resource? In: Ribbens McCarthy, J., Hooper, C., Gillies, V. (Eds.), Family Troubles: Exploring Change and Challenges in the Family Lives of Children and Young People. The Policy Press, Bristol, pp. 315–326.

Human Rights Act, 1989. https://www.legislation.gov.uk/ukpga/1998/42/contents.

Local Government and Social Care Ombudsman decision: Gloucester County Council (21 003 170) and London Borough of Sutton (21 0009 765). https://www.lgo.org.uk/decisions.

Lynch, C., 2016. Young Parents Involved in the Child Welfare System. Family Rights Group, London.

Mason, C., Broadhurst, K., Ward, H., and Barnett, A., 2023. Born into Care: Best practice guidelines for when the state intervenes at birth: https://www.nuffieldfjo.org.uk/resource/born-into-care-best-practice-guidelines-and-other-resources

Maxwell, A., Proctor, J., Hammond, L., 2011. 'Me and my child': parenting experiences of young mothers leaving care. Adoption and Fostering. 35 (4), 29–40.

Neale, B., Davies, L., 2015. Hard to Reach? Rethinking Support for Young Fathers. Following Young Fathers Briefing. Paper No. 6.

Nottingham City Council v LW & Ors [2016] EWHC 11 (Fam).

Nuffield Trust, 2022. Teenage Pregnancy. https://www.nuffieldtrust.org.uk/resource/teenage-pregnancy.

Philip, G., Bedston, S., Youansamouth, L., Clifton, J., Broadhurst, K., Brandon, M., et al., 2021. 'Up against it'. Understanding Fathers' Repeat Appearance in Local Authority Care Proceedings. Research Project Report. www.cfj-lancaster.org.uk/app/nuffield/files-module/local/documents/Up_Against_It_Full_Report.pdf.

Public Law Working Group, 2021. Best practice guidance: Support for and work with families prior to court proceedings. https://www.judiciary.uk/wp-content/uploads/2021/03/Prior-to-court-proceedings-BPG-report_clickable.pdf

Roberts, L., Meakings, S., Smith, A., Forrester, D., Shelton, K., 2017. Care-leavers and their children placed for adoption. Child. Youth Serv. Rev. 79, 355–361.

Ryan, M., Tunnard, J., On behalf of Family Rights Group Review Team, June 2018. Care Crisis Review: Options for Change. https://frg.org.uk/product/the-care-crisis-review-options-for-change/.

Social Exclusion Unit, 1999. Teenage pregnancy: Report by the Social Exclusion Unit presented to Parliament by the Prime Minister by command of Her Majesty, June 1999.

SW & TW (Human Rights Claim: Procedure) (No1) [2017] EWHC 450 (Fam).

Tarrant, A., Way, L., Ladlow, L., 2021. Tarrant (2021): Supporting at a Distance: The Challenges and Opportunities of Supporting Young Fathers through the COVID-19 Pandemic, FYFF Briefing Paper Three. https://followingyoungfathersfurther.org/asset/working-papers.

Tarrant, A., Way, L., Ladlow, L., 2020. From Social Isolation to Local Support: Relational Change and Continuities for Young Fathers in the Context of the COVID 19 Crisis, FYFF Briefing Paper Two. https://followingyoungfathersfurther.org/asset/working-papers.

Working Together Parenting Network, 2021. Update to the Good Practice Guidance on Working with Parents with a Learning Disability. University of Bristol. https://www.bristol.ac.uk/media-library/sites/sps/documents/wtpn/FINAL%202021%20WTPN%20UPDATE%20OF%20THE%20GPG.pdf.

Working Together to Safeguard Children, 2018. Statutory Guidance on Inter-agency Working to Safeguard and Promote the Welfare of Children. Department for Education. https://www.gov.uk/government/publications/working-together-to-safeguard-children--2.

19d

COMPASSIONATE AND EFFECTIVE PRACTICE WITH PARENTS AT RISK OF REPEAT REMOVAL OF THEIR CHILDREN THROUGH CARE PROCEEDINGS

KAREN BROADHURST ■ CLAIRE MASON ■ LISA MORRISS ■ BACHAR ALROUH

KEY POINTS

- Why it is imperative to reduce recurrent care proceedings.
- Statistics on the scale of parents' repeat appearances in care proceedings.
- Shortfalls in mainstream social work practice and what needs to change.
- Essential elements of compassionate and effective practice when involved in repeat proceedings.

INTRODUCTION

Care proceedings are issued for children in England and Wales under s31 of the Children Act 1989 where there are concerns about actual or likely significant harm. A number of outcomes of care proceedings are possible, but the family courts can make life-changing decisions regarding parental rights and the care of children, including placing children in out-of-home care or with adopters. In this context, an issue that has attracted considerable interest is how to work compassionately and effectively to prevent parents' repeat appearances in care proceedings. For any parent, the removal (or curtailment) of parental rights constitutes a major form of loss; however, where parents experience repeat removal of their children, through care proceedings, losses are multiple. This loss is felt by parents, but also siblings, grandparents and wider kin networks.

This chapter starts by introducing the statistical landscape regarding repeat removals, outlining what needs to change – and what is effective – in contemporary practice. Following this, the chapter focusses on the impact of multiple disadvantage and trauma, which many parents who experience repeat removals in respect of their children have experienced in their early lives. This includes a particular focus on material disadvantage, stigma and isolation. The chapter concludes by outlining suggestions for good practice in terms of supporting parental identity beyond child removal, subsequent pregnancies, and the legal rights and entitlements of parents who have experienced multiple removals.

PARENTS IN REPEAT CARE PROCEEDINGS: THE STATISTICS

A focus on parents in repeat care proceedings has gathered pace since 2015, when the first research was published which uncovered the scale of mothers' repeat involvement in care proceedings based on full-service population data (Broadhurst et al., 2015). A sizeable proportion of mothers (1 in every 4 mothers) who have had a child removed from their care in England and Wales were found to be at risk of returning to court

(Alrouh et al., 2022; Broadhurst et al., 2015, 2017). Two 'types' of recurrent pathways were noted. Some mothers returned to court because the reunification of a child had broken down and fresh care proceedings were issued. However, by far the largest proportion of recurrent mothers returned to court following the birth of a new baby. It is the latter group of mothers who are commonly described as caught in a cycle of 'repeat removals'.

Broadhurst and colleagues also uncovered the high number of new-born and very young babies subject to care proceedings, in cases where a child had previously been removed from mothers (Broadhurst et al., 2015). Given this finding, the *Born into Care* series (Broadhurst et al., 2018a) was developed, which reported considerable regional disparities in intervention at birth, with the highest rates of new-born care proceedings concentrated in areas of high deprivation (Alrouh et al., 2019; Doebler et al., 2022). Published by the Nuffield Family Justice Observatory, the series has also uncovered high rates of mental health need in mothers and fathers and emergency health service use (Griffiths et al., 2021; Griffiths et al. (2020)).

The literature on 'repeat removals' has focused largely on mothers; however, an important body of literature has confirmed fathers' appearances in repeat care proceedings (Bedston et al., 2019; Philip et al., 2020). This research has also drawn attention to recurrent couples. However, it is harder to quantify how many fathers are linked to children in repeat care proceedings because fathers who do not have parental responsibility will not automatically be joined to cases.

Overall, these statistics indicate the need for a concerted preventative agenda given that repeat appearances in care proceedings are far from unusual for mothers and fathers. Qualitative enquiry has uncovered the dire human costs of repeat removal of children including exacerbation of mental health difficulties (Broadhurst et al., 2017; Morriss and Broadhurst, 2022). In addition, recurrent care proceedings are costly for local authorities and the family courts.

REFLECTIVE QUESTIONS

- Why do you think parents who have already experienced their children being removed are at risk of having subsequent children removed?
- What do you need to be mindful of in your practice when working with parents who have had previous children removed?

PRACTICE SHORTFALLS: WHAT NEEDS TO CHANGE?

In England and Wales, parents have historically had few avenues of support following the removal of their children through care proceedings. Aside from short-term counselling for birth parents whose children have been adopted (Cossar and Neil et al., 2010), there is no formal legislative mandate on services in England or Wales to provide help for parents' own rehabilitation – even if this has been recommended by the courts during care proceedings (Broadhurst et al., 2017; Cox et al., 2012). The same shortfalls in services beyond permanent child removal are reported in a range of jurisdictions with similar child protection systems (Grant et al., 2011, 2014; Taplin and Mattick, 2014; Wise, 2021). However, the statistical discovery of recurrence, together with support for mothers to speak out about their experience (Broadhurst et al., 2017; Boddy and Wheeler 2020; Mason et al., 2020; Morriss and Broadhurst, 2022), has challenged the perceptions of the public regarding the factors that lie behind repeat family court involvement. In particular, empowering women with lived experience to contest stigmatised identities and share the multiple barriers they face to recovery has prompted practice pioneers to recognise the legitimacy of women's claims for better service provision. Since 2015, services have begun to recognise that terminating involvement with mothers and fathers, beyond the removal and placement of children, is short-sighted and requires practice change. The fact that a high proportion of repeat court proceedings concern new-born babies is also glaringly at odds with the emphasis within the Children Act 1989 on supporting children's upbringing within their birth families, as well as obligations within Part III of the Act to provide family support.

PRACTICE DEVELOPMENTS: COMMON ELEMENTS OF EFFECTIVE PRACTICE

Multiple new practice initiatives have developed to help parents avoid repeat care proceedings. New services work with parents following the removal of their children or during a subsequent pregnancy (Boddy and

Wheeler 2020; Cox et al., 2017, 2020; Roberts et al., 2018). Many services have been focused on women, but more recently, services have extended their reach to include fathers and wider family networks. New services mark a departure away from an overly child-centred discourse, which historically has served to erode the entitlements of parents within children's services. As practice developments begin to mature, a wealth of new knowledge has been generated which can, and should, inform greater roll-out of service provision. Overall, evaluative evidence is that services are far more successful in preventing parents' appearances in care proceedings than standard local authority social work practice (Boddy and Wheeler 2020; Cox et al., 2020).

Although service developments differ, the six core themes listed in the Closer Look box are common and essential ingredients of effective practice to prevent parents' becoming involved in a very negative cycle of repeat care proceedings.

CLOSER LOOK: SIX ESSENTIAL FEATURES OF EFFECTIVE PRACTICE

1. Recognition of long-standing disadvantage and complex trauma in the lives of parents
2. Recognition of material disadvantage and support to overcome difficulties of housing and poverty
3. An understanding of the impact of stigma and isolation, resulting from child removal
4. Support for parental identity beyond child removal
5. Provision of timely, sensitive and sufficiently intensive support in the context of a further pregnancy
6. Support to access legal rights and entitlements

Parents in Recurrent Care Proceedings: Multiple Disadvantage and Complex Trauma

A consistent finding from research and evaluative evidence is that parents who experience repeat removal of children have themselves experienced multiple adversities in their own childhoods (Broadhurst et al., 2017), which include spending time in public care. The most reliable evidence regarding care experience is for birth mothers in England, with research and evaluation data indicating that between 40% and

50% of birth mothers have been in care themselves as children (Broadhurst et al., 2017; Boddy and Wheeler 2020). However, for both mothers and fathers, childhoods characterised by instability in caregiver arrangements and loss, coupled with socioeconomic hardship are common. This knowledge has led new services to adopt the concept of 'complex trauma' as a unifying way of understanding parents' difficulties, which include challenges in their engagement with professionals. This knowledge also supports the emphasis within multiple projects on longer-term trauma informed relational practice, as the vehicle for change (Boddy and Wheeler 2020; Mason et al., 2020).

The concept of complex trauma (variously referred to as developmental trauma or complex trauma disorder) refers to difficulties that arise as a result of prolonged exposure in childhood to neglect or harms within the care-giver relationship. Proponents of complex trauma draw a distinction between time-limited or event-specific trauma captured by the diagnostic category PTSD (posttraumatic stress disorder) and the complex symptomatology of trauma that results from enduring exposure to multiple stressful events and experiences (Briere and Lanktree, 2012; Cloitre et al., 2009; Herman, 1992; Kisiel et al., 2016; Van der Kolk, 2005). Of particular relevance to parents in care proceedings is an understanding that chronic exposure to stress in the context of *interpersonal dependence* (Van der Kolk, 2005) can result in multiple adult difficulties. Here the literature on adverse childhood experiences (ACE) is also important, as ACE are associated with vulnerabilities across the life course (Felitti et al., 1998). This is not to suggest that difficult childhoods *determine* poor outcomes for adults; however, multiple adversities in childhood certainly do little to foster adult well-being. Recent research, which has sought to advance thinking about ACE, makes the case for far greater attention to parental mental health in particular (Lacey et al., 2022; Morriss and Broadhurst, 2022).

Individuals whose childhoods lack the necessary security of consistent care giving coupled with material hardship are considered to struggle in their adolescence and adult lives with trust, emotional regulation and low self-esteem. Individuals exposed to chronic stress in their own childhoods are also considered to be more at risk of secondary harms, including conflict and domestic abuse. Although there is considerable critique of the medicalised language associated with complex trauma, there is no doubt that *recognition* of parents' difficult childhoods and feeling let down by the State is an important element of effective and respectful practice with parents. In addition, consistent and flexible relational practice can, over time, help parents to develop a sense of trust where this has previously been eroded in both their personal relationships and relationships with professionals (Mason et al., 2020; Turney, 2012). Although professionals have rarely experienced the kind of multiple and enduring disadvantages parents described, professionals can still serve as 'allied others' (Denzin and Lincoln, 2008) by listening to and recognising parents' own articulation of need and providing compassionate help. Such relationships can be pivotal in reframing parents' expectations of both themselves and others.

Applying the Concept of Complex Trauma in Practice: Engagement

Bringing a complex trauma lens to professional intervention with parents who have experienced disadvantage directs practitioners to pay far more attention to parents' social histories and requires a highly skilled therapeutic response which recognises that parents may not feel able to readily engage with professional services and require a sensitive, persistent and proactive approach to relationship building (Broadhurst et al., 2018b; Mason et al., 2020). Parents' difficulties are better understood as complex adaptations to trauma, developed over the life course, and which can present particular challenges in terms of both giving and receiving help. When we apply learning from the literature on complex trauma, resistance can be viewed as an adaptive response where childhoods have instilled little confidence in the capacity of others to meet their dependency needs. Problematic parent–professional dynamics should not be simply seen as intentional acts of resistance, rather parents understandably struggle with trust, particularly if children have previously been removed from their care (Broadhurst et al., 2017; Mason et al., 2020). Working with parents who have histories of complex trauma requires a highly informed approach, with practice attuned to

the developmental roots of parents' difficulties and service histories.

From this standpoint, there is a fundamental mismatch between social work services that typically monitor difficulties and offer short-term practical assistance and the needs of these parents. New service developments (see Practice Examples later) invest heavily in the process of active engagement, understanding that it takes time and sensitivity to overcome barriers to help and build trust with families. Services ensure small caseloads for practitioners, affording the time and space for intensive therapeutic engagement with parents. This allows the relationship with the practitioner to be at the centre of the intervention.

Sequencing Intervention and Building Personal Agency

There is a general consensus that intervention needs to be sequenced and progressive for parents with histories of exposure to complex trauma. Parents can feel easily judged and overwhelmed by professional demands, particularly where they are signposted to multiple services without sufficient care in understanding parents' practical and emotional difficulties in engaging with services. The work of Ford et al. (2005) provides a useful framework for considering a staged approach to intervention. Ford and colleagues conceptualised effective help as comprising three phases: (1) symptom reduction and stabilization, (2) processing of traumatic memories and emotions, and (3) life integration and rehabilitation after trauma processing. This understanding has now helped shape a number of service developments (Boddy and Wheeler 2020; Mason and Wilkinson, 2021). At the heart of new practice initiatives is a careful and compassionate approach to engagement, which recognises the need to incrementally build personal agency and trust in helping relationships.

Therefore parents are unlikely to respond well to a case management approach in which the social worker simply acts as a broker of other services. Signposting these parents to services that offer short-term parent education or domestic violence programmes alone will do little to meet parents' complex needs. Psycho-educative programmes that compartmentalise and deal separately with presenting symptoms, for example, substance misuse or mental health problems or conflictual intimate relationships, fail to grapple with the complex underlying causes of parents' difficulties or to understand links between problems. Proponents in favour of a trauma-informed approach argue that unless the core problem of complex trauma is addressed, it is highly likely that problems will simply persist or re-emerge.

Material Disadvantage

A trauma-informed approach is, however, best blended with a deep appreciation of the material and economic disadvantage parents face (Boddy and Wheeler 2020; Broadhurst and Mason, 2020; Doebler et al., 2022; Lacey et al., 2022). Successive evaluations of service evidence the widespread economic insecurity in women's lives (Boddy and Wheeler 2020). Not only are women at the sharp edge of a more restrictive social safety net, in addition mental health difficulties and a general lack of confidence make it difficult for parents to navigate benefits systems. Material disadvantage can lead to the accumulation of debt which can overwhelm parents with few resources to find a way out of chronic debt. Actual or risk of homelessness is everpresent in the lives of parents with limited material resources who frequently have significant rent arrears. As Boddy and Wheeler 2020 write, the practitioner therefore plays a critical role in helping women navigate housing systems, secure their full entitlement to welfare benefits and manage debt.

Parents who find themselves appearing as respondents in care proceedings have often made an earlier transition to parenthood than their peers in the general population (Alrouh et al., 2022; Broadhurst et al., 2017). Parents bring the legacy of difficult childhoods to parenthood, but with fewer resources to manage the challenges of first-time parenting. Broadhurst and Mason (2020) refer to this population of birth parents as having fragile and restricted social statuses. Parents have fewer options in terms of employment opportunities, are often reliant on welfare benefits or are in low paid and insecure employment (Phillip et al., 2020). Once a child is removed from parents' care, parents can face further losses of income and housing. Parents living in social housing are at risk of losing their home due to the under-occupancy penalty (also known as the 'bedroom tax') which was introduced as part of the Welfare Reform Act 2012 (Morriss, 2018). Of course, further losses are likely to increase parents' resort to drugs and alcohol, or other self-harming behaviours.

The lack of attention to economic insecurity in everyday social work practice has been widely observed by critics (Featherstone et al., 2014, 2021; Gupta, 2017). Social workers do not intend to ignore poverty – rather the wider socioeconomic context of their practice limits options in terms of tackling the material hardship of lives. A rigorous review of the international literature on the relationship between poverty, child abuse and neglect by Bywaters et al. (2018) underscores the critical importance of addressing poverty in the lives of children and families. Poverty should not be treated as an incidental issue – rather poverty and financial insecurity compound and are part and parcel of the challenges parents face within statutory services.

Stigma and Isolation

It is important to recognise the *social* as well as psychological consequences of child removal. The loss of a child on account of safeguarding concerns is a highly stigmatising form of loss that isolates parents from others. The work of Morriss (2018) has been influential in drawing attention to the pervasive nature and impact of stigma, which is experienced in multiple settings and over time, when children are removed by the courts from parents' care. For mothers, daily routines are profoundly interrupted, and the loss of children is all too visible within informal networks and neighbourhoods. Women struggle to explain the absence of their children and are estranged from communal environments such as playgroups or schools, or other informal settings (Broadhurst and Mason (2020); Morriss, 2018). Broadhurst and Mason (2020) document the ways in which the trauma of child removal in the absence of support exacerbates risk in other aspects of women's lives, both in terms of the immediate psychosocial crisis that follows the loss of a child, and in the longer-term. Therefore, creating opportunities for connection between women who have experienced child removal is a powerful form of helping, which reduces isolation and provides women with some comfort that they are not alone in their experience. Morriss (2018) refers to the importance of a 'maternal commons' in describing the positive impact of collective group experience for women living apart from their children. A number of services which aim to prevent child removal now offer therapeutic group work to parents and train parents to serve as peer mentors, empowering other parents on their journeys to change (see Practice Example later).

Support for Parental Identity Beyond Child Removal

A consistent complaint from mothers who have had children removed from their care is that professionals do not recognise that women self-identify as mothers although children are not in their care. When children are removed from parents' care, they may live with other family members or friends, or with foster carers, or may be adopted. However, parents do not want to lose their own sense of strong connection to their children despite this separation. Birthdays, Mother's Day, Father's Day and Christmas are profoundly difficult for parents living apart from their children. For parents living apart from their children removed to public care or adoption, grief is complicated. As Morriss (2018, p. 7) writes on children who are adopted: 'mothers are unable to follow the customary grief rituals of bereavement as their child has not died but is alive, but somewhere unknown'. Living apart from children is particularly difficult to resolve for all parents, but when separation is involuntary and there are restrictions placed on contact (or parents have no direct contact), parents describe lives in limbo, as they wait to be reunited with their children in the future.

It is vital that services support parents to maintain contact with their children, where this is possible, and work to improve the quality of this contact. For parents who have experienced repeat sets of care proceedings, their children may live with different caregivers which makes contact arrangements more complicated and challenging. As previously discussed, financial hardship can also mean that parents struggle to cover transport costs to visit their children and feel unable to offer their children the kind of financial security that is typically provided by foster carers or adoptive parents.

Subsequent Pregnancies

For parents who have experienced the removal of a child, a new pregnancy brings considerable anxiety. This anxiety is compounded if services are not offered at a timely point in pregnancy or with sufficient sensitivity to parents' understandable fears that their new baby will also be subject to involuntary removal. Based on national data, evidence is that local authorities act more swiftly and are more likely to issue care proceedings at birth if there is a history of a previous removal (Alrouh et al., 2019; Broadhurst et al., 2015). Therefore parents face an up-hill struggle to convince services of change. Broadhurst et al. (2017) found that although many birth mothers sought help early in pregnancy, pressures on services meant that help was offered very late in pregnancy, leaving mothers with insufficient time to demonstrate change. Moreover, an assumption among some is that mothers will conceal their pregnancies if they are known to children's services. Recent research from Griffiths et al. (2020) based on 1000 mothers in care proceedings in Wales challenged such assumptions, noting that mothers were only marginally later than a matched comparison group in terms of notifying antenatal services of a new pregnancy. So how can services help mothers who are pregnant and have a history of previous child removal?

> ### CLOSER LOOK: SUPPORTING PREGNANT MOTHERS WHO HAVE A HISTORY OF PREVIOUS CHILD REMOVAL
>
> 1. Respond early to a new pregnancy (first trimester)
> 2. Provide practical help and advocacy to enable parents to stabilise lives, for example, by obtaining adequate housing and access to welfare benefits
> 3. Proactively support access to mental health services
> 4. Proactively explore with parents resources within the wider family network that can support parenting at an early point in pregnancy
> 5. Provide space for parents to share feelings, which may include considerable anger and mistrust, about the removal of a previous child
> 6. Be clear and transparent about local authority expectations and check out understandings
> 7. Ensure timely birth planning between local authority and children's social care services, ensuing wherever possible that mothers have a partner or other birth companion

New draft guidelines co-produced with families and professionals by Mason et al. (2022) provide detailed advice on how to work inclusively in pregnancy and how to work sensitively with parents and the wider kin network if safeguarding action is to be taken at birth.

Legal Rights and Entitlements

Access to robust legal advice and representation is vital for all parents whose children are at risk of care proceedings. However, for parents with a history of child removal, effective legal advocacy is essential given what is known empirically about high rates of infant removal at birth within repeat proceedings. In previous work, we described parents' anxieties about whether a history of removal would prejudice both the local authority and court's decision making in the context of a new set of proceedings (Broadhurst and Mason, 2017). A family court history is never spent, and while family courts must always consider a change of circumstances, a history of child removal will also be part of any social work chronology. Moreover, for parents who have previously experienced care proceedings and child removal, their anxieties about the family courts are typically heightened on account of prior negative experience. Consistent evidence is that the family court process is very difficult for parents to follow and legal representation is highly variable (Broadhurst et al., 2017; Harwin et al., 2022; Hunt, 2010). Particularly in pre-proceedings, there is deep concern about the funding of legal aid and sufficiency of legal advocacy (Public Law Working Group, 2021). Parents' difficulties in understanding complex legal terminology and procedures are very well documented in the published research literature (Lindley, 1994; Broadhurst et al., 2022). Moreover, parents have reported that the presence of a robust advocate or trusted support worker in child protection meetings can change how parents are treated by other professionals (Boddy and Wheeler 2020).

When care proceedings are issued at birth, particular considerations apply. Legal advocacy is vital defence against unwarranted state intervention – and in the immediate postpartum period, the vulnerability of mothers seriously undermines their ability to participate fairly in care proceedings (Broadhurst et al., 2022). When babies are deemed at risk at birth, social workers and the family courts must carefully balance the protection of the baby, with the imperative to act in ways that are proportionate and fair. However, there is widespread international disquiet about care proceedings at birth, given the potential breaches of parents'

Article 6 and 8 rights (Human Rights Act, 1998). Under Article 6 of the Human Rights Act, parents have the right to a fair trial in care proceedings. Under Article 8, local authorities must have respect for the right to family life, regarding both parent and child. Recent research evidence has drawn attention to the increasing volume of care proceedings issued at birth and raised questions about the reliability of hasty decisions for babies, but also the ability of parents to contest removal at short notice (Broadhurst et al., 2022; Chill et al., 2003; Pattinson et al., 2021).

The Closer Look box lists considerations which help to support parents' legal and procedural rights.

CLOSER LOOK: SUPPORTING PARENTS LEGAL AND PROCEDURAL RIGHTS

- Proactively support parents' access to information about where they can obtain legal representation and ensure parents understand their legal rights.
- When parents are invited to a preproceedings meeting, provide time for parents and parents' lawyers or other representatives to ask questions about local authority concerns; carefully check out parents' understanding and offer more time for clarification.
- If the local authority plans to issue care proceedings, as far as possible, parents need to be given sufficient time to see their own solicitor, who is key in ensuring parents' meaningful participation in care proceedings.
- In cases of care proceedings at birth for infants, effective liaison with maternity hospitals and ensuring sufficiency in mother and baby placements can avert the need for urgent care proceedings in the immediate postpartum period. Wherever possible, mothers should not be expected to attend court within hours or a few days of giving birth.

Practice Example: Intensive Relationship-Based Approach to Prevent Repeat Removal

There are a range of new services which work with women, and in some cases with fathers and wider networks. Practitioners have small caseloads and can therefore take a trauma-informed relationship-based approach to practice. Services offer intensive support to help mothers cope with the pain of child removal and work with mothers to prevent further removals. Projects work to build emotional resilience, confidence and self-esteem, and help women develop supportive informal networks. Some services place considerable emphasis on peer mentoring and group work as powerful ways of engaging women and role-modelling recovery from adverse experiences. Services also support women's access to a range of health and well-being services, including sexual and reproductive health services. Some services also support women's access to legal advocacy and help women to engage with contact arrangements when their children are in care or are adopted. Successive evaluation reports evidence marked improvement in women's lives and a reduction in subsequent care proceedings (Boddy and Wheeler 2020; Cox et al., 2020; Roberts et al., 2018, Leigh and Wilson, 2020).

CONCLUSION

To conclude, although England and Wales record high rates of parents' repeat appearances in care proceedings, compassionate and effective practice can prevent the repeat removal of children. The essential ingredients of effective helping must focus on engagement, but also the social costs (stigma) of child removal and economic hardship in the lives of this population of parents. Moreover, legal representation must be of sufficient quality and intensity such that parents can realise their legal rights. Scaling up practice approaches which have proven to be effective in reducing parents' involvement in repeat care proceedings remains critical (Alrouh et al., 2022) given continued demand on the family courts and the huge personal costs for families.

REFLECTIVE QUESTIONS

- What does the concept of complex trauma refer to and why is this useful for social workers seeking to prevent parents' involvement in care proceedings?
- How do we breakdown isolation and stigma for parents whose children have been removed from their care?
- Why is effective legal representation for parents with a history of repeat removal of children vitally important?

FURTHER READING

Broadhurst, K., Alrouh, B., Yeend, E., Harwin, J., Shaw, M., Pilling, M., et al., 2015. Connecting events in time to identify a hidden population: Birth mothers and their children in recurrent care proceedings in England. Br. J. Soc. Work 45 (8), 2241–2260 (open access).

The British Association of Social Workers (BASW) has published an antipoverty guide for practice. Available at: https://www.basw.co.uk/what-we-do/policy-and-research/anti-poverty-practice-guide-social-work.

Mason, C., Wilkinson, J., 2021. Services for parents who have experienced recurrent care proceedings: Where are we now? Findings from mapping of locally developed services in England – Research Report. .

Mason, C., Broadhurst, K., Ward, H., Barnett, A., Holmes, L., 2022. Born into care: Draft best practice guidelines for when the state intervenes at birth. .

REFERENCES

Alrouh, B., Abouelenin, M., Broadhurst, et al., 2022. Mothers in Recurrent Care Proceedings in England and Wales: Where Are We Now? Nuffield Family Justice Observatory, London.

Alrouh, B., Broadhurst, K., Cusworth, L., Griffiths, L.J., Johnson, R.D., Akbari, A., Ford, D., 2019. Born Into Care: Newborns and Infants in Care Proceedings in Wales. Nuffield Family Justice Observatory, London.

Bedston, S., Philip, G., Youansamouth, L., Clifton, J., Broadhurst, K., Brandon, M., et al., 2019. Linked lives: Gender, family relations and recurrent care proceedings in England. Child. Youth Serv. Rev. 105, 104392.

Boddy, J., Wheeler, B., 2020. Recognition and justice? Conceptualizing support for women whose children are in care or adopted. Societies 10 (4), 96 1–21.

Briere, J.N., Lanktree, C.B., 2012. Treating Complex Trauma in Adolescents and Young Adults. SAGE, London.

Broadhurst, K., Alrouh, B., Yeend, E., Harwin, J., Shaw, M., Pilling, M., et al., 2015. Connecting events in time to identify a hidden population: Birth mothers and their children in recurrent care proceedings in England. Br. J. Soc. Work 45 (8), 2241–2260.

Broadhurst, K., Mason, C., 2017. Birth parents and the collateral consequences of court-ordered child removal: Towards a comprehensive framework. Int. J. Law Policy Fam. 31 (1), 41–59.

Broadhurst, K., Mason, C., Bedston, S., Alrouh, B., Morriss, L., McQuarrie, T., et al., 2017. Vulnerable Birth Mothers and Recurrent Care Proceedings. Final Main Report. Centre for Child and Family Justice Research, Lancaster.

Broadhurst, K., Alrouh, B., Mason, C., Ward, H., Holmes, L., Ryan, M., et al., 2018. Born Into Care: Newborns in Care Proceedings in England. Nuffield Family Justice Observatory, London. https://www.nuffieldfjo.org.uk/resource/born-into-care-newborns-in-care-proceedings-in-england-final-report-october-2018.

Broadhurst, K., Mason, C., Webb, S., 2018. Birth mothers returning to court: Can a developmental trauma lens inform practice with women at risk of repeat removal of infants and children. In: Shaw,

M. (Ed.), Justice for Children and Families: A Developmental Approach. Cambridge University Press, Cambridge.

Broadhurst, K., Mason, C., 2020. Child removal as the gateway to further adversity: Birth mother accounts of the immediate and enduring collateral consequences of child removal. Qual. Soc. Work 19 (1), 15–37. https://doi.org/10.1177/1473325019893412.

Broadhurst, K., Mason, C., Ward, H., 2022. Urgent Care proceedings for new-born babies in England and Wales – Time for a fundamental review. Int. J. Law Policy Fam. 36 (1):ebac008. https://doi.org/10.1093/lawfam/ebac008.

Bywaters, P., Brady, G., Bunting, L., Daniel, B., Featherstone, B., Jones, C., et al., 2018. Inequalities in English child protection practice under austerity: A universal challenge? Child Fam. Soc. Work 23 (1), 53–61.

Children Act 1989. https://www.legislation.gov.uk/ukpga/1989/41/contents

Chill, P., 2003. Burden of proof begone: The Pernicious effect of emergency removal in child protective proceedings. Fam. Court Rev. 41, 457.

Cloitre, M., Stolbach, B.C., Herman, J.L., van der Kolk, B., Pynoos, R., Wang, J., Petkova, E., 2009. A developmental approach to complex PTSD: childhood and adult cumulative trauma as predictors of symptom complexity. J. Trauma. Stress 22 (5), 399–408.

Cossar, J., Neil, E., 2010. Supporting the birth relatives of adopted children: How accessible are services? Br. J. Soc. Work 40 (5), 1368–1386.

Cox, P., 2012. Marginalized mothers, reproductive autonomy, and repeat losses to care. J. Law Soc. 39 (4), 541–561.

Cox, P., Barratt, C., Blumenfeld, F., Rahemtulla, Z., Taggart, D., Turton, J., 2017. Reducing recurrent care proceedings: Initial evidence from new interventions. J. Soc. Welf. Fam. Law 39 (3), 332–349.

Cox, P., McPherson, S., Mason, C., Ryan, M., Baxter, V., 2020. Reducing recurrent care proceedings: Building a local evidence base in England. Societies 10 (4), 88. https://doi.org/10.3390/soc10040088.

Denzin, N., Lincoln, Y., 2008. "Introduction". In: Denzin, N., Lincoln, Y., Smith, L.T. (Eds.), Handbook of Critical and Indigenous Methodologies. Sage, London. 2008.

Doebler, S., Broadhurst, K., Alrouh, B., Cusworth, L., Griffiths, L., 2022. Born into care: Associations between area-level deprivation and the rates of children entering care proceedings in Wales. Child. Youth Serv. Rev. 141, 9.

Featherstone, B., White, S., Morris, K., 2014. Re-imagining Child Protection. Policy Press, Bristol, UK.

Featherstone, B., Gupta, A., Morris, K., Warner, J., 2018. Let's stop feeding the risk monster: Towards a social model of child protection. Fam. Relatsh. Soc. 7 (1), 107–122.

Felitti, V.J., Anda, R.F., Nordenberg, D., Williamson, D.F., Spitz, A.M., Edwards, V., et al., 1998. Relationship of childhood abuse and household dysfunction to many of the leading causes of death in adults. The Adverse Childhood Experiences (ACE) Study. Am. J. Prev. Med. 14 (4), 245–258. https://doi.org/10.1016/s0749-3797(98)00017-8.

Ford, J.D., Courtois, C.A., Steele, K., Hart, O.V.D., Nijenhuis, E.R., 2005. Treatment of complex posttraumatic self–dysregulation. J. Trauma. Stress 18 (5), 437–447.

Grant, T., Huggins, J., Graham, J.C., Ernst, C., Whitney, N., Wilson, D., 2011. Maternal substance abuse and disrupted parenting: Distinguishing mothers who keep their children from those who do not. Child. Youth Serv. Rev. 33 (11), 2176–2185.

Grant, T., Graham, J.C., Ernst, C.C., Peavy, M.K., Brown, N.N., 2014. Improving pregnancy outcomes among high-risk mothers who abuse alcohol and drugs: Factors associated with subsequent exposed births. Child. Youth Serv. Rev. 46, 11–18. https://doi.org/10.1016/j.childyouth.2014.07.014.

Griffiths, L.J., et al., 2021. Born Into Care: One Thousand Mothers in Care Proceedings in Wales: A Focus on Maternal Mental Health. Nuffield Family Justice Observatory, London.

Griffiths, L.J., et al., 2020. Born Into Care: One Thousand Mothers in Care Proceedings in Wales – Maternal Health, Wellbeing and Pregnancy Outcomes. Nuffield Family Justice Observatory, London.

Gupta, A., 2017. Poverty and child neglect – the elephant in the room? Fam Relatsh Soc. 6, 21–36.

Harwin, J., Golding, L., 2022. Supporting Families After Care Proceedings: Supervision Orders and Beyond: Parental Perspectives on Care Proceedings, Supervision Orders and Care Orders at Home. Department for Education. https://assets.publishing.service.gov.uk/media/62441b7bd3bf7f32b5aa0662/Harwin_Report_on_Parental_Perspectives.pdf

Herman, J., 1992. Trauma and Recovery. Basic Books, New York, USA.

Human Rights Act, 1998. https://www.legislation.gov.uk/ukpga/1998/42/contents

Hunt, J., 2010. Parental Perspectives on Family Justice System in England and Wales: A Review of Research. Nuffield Foundation, Oxford.

Kisiel, C.L., Fehrenbach, T., Torgersen, E., Stolbach, B., McClelland, G., Griffin, G., Burkman, K., 2014. Constellations of interpersonal trauma and symptoms in child welfare: Implications for a developmental trauma framework. J. Fam. Violence 29 (1), 1–14.

Lacey, R.E., Howe, L.D., Kelly-Irving, M., Bartley, M., Kelly, Y., 2022. The clustering of adverse childhood experiences in the avon longitudinal study of parents and children: Are gender and poverty important? J. Interpers. Violence 37 (5–6), 2218–2241. https://doi.org/10.1177/0886260520935096.

Leigh, J., Wilson, S., 2020. Sylvia's story: Time, liminal space and the maternal commons. Qual. Soc. Work 19 (3), 440–459.

Lindley, B., 1994. On the Receiving End: Families' Experiences of the Court Process in Care and Supervision Proceedings Under the Children Act 1989. Family Rights Group, London.

Mason, C., Taggart, D., Broadhurst, K., 2020. Parental non-engagement within child protection services. How can understandings of complex trauma and epistemic trust help? Societies 10 (4), 93. https://doi.org/10.3390/soc1004009.

Mason, C., Wilkinson, J., 2021. Services for Parents Who Have Experienced Recurrent Care Proceedings: Where Are We Now? Research in Practice, Dartington.

Mason, C., Broadhurst, K., Ward, H., Barnett, A., Holmes, L., 2022. Born Into Care: Developing Best Practice Guidelines for When the State Intervenes at Birth. Nuffield Family Justice Observatory, London. https://www.nuffieldfjo.org.uk/resource/

born-into-care-developing-best-practice-guidelines-for-when-the-state-intervenes-at-birth.

Morriss, L., 2018. Haunted futures: The stigma of being a mother living apart from her children following state-ordered court removal. Soc. Rev. Monographs 66 (4), 816–831.

Morriss, L., Broadhurst, K., 2022. Parental Mental Health and Care Proceedings: Towards an Agenda for Change. Centre for Child and Family Justice Research, Lancaster.

Pattinson, R., Broadhurst, K., Alrouh, B., Cusworth, L., Doebler, S., Griffiths, L.J., et al., 2021. Born Into Care: New-Born Babies in Urgent Care Proceedings in England and Wales. Nuffield Family Justice Observatory, London.

Philip, G., Bedston, S., Hu, Y., Youansamouth, L., Clifton, J., Broadhurst, K., et al., 2020. 'Up Against It': Fathers and Recurrent Care Proceedings Final Report. Nuffield Foundation, London, UK.

Public Law Working Group, 2021. Recommendations to Achieve Best Practice in the Child Protection and Family Justice Systems. https://www.judiciary.uk/publications/message-from-the-president-of-the-family-division- publication-of-the-presidents-public-law-working-group-report/. (Accessed 12 November 2021).

Roberts, L., Maxwell, N., Messenger, R., Palmer, C., 2018. Evaluation of Reflect in Gwent, Final Report. https://orca.cardiff.ac.uk/id/eprint/123258/1/Reflect%20report%20published.pdf.

Taplin, S., Mattick, R.P., 2014. The nature and extent of child protection involvement among heroin-using mothers in treatment: High rates of reports, removals at birth and children in care. Drugs Alcohol Rev. 34 (1), 31–37. https://doi.org/10.1111/dar.12165.

Turney, D., 2012. A relationship-based approach to engaging involuntary clients: The contribution of recognition theory. Child Fam. Soc. Work 17, 149–159.

Van der Kolk, B.A., Roth, S., Pelcovitz, D., Sunday, S., Spinazzola, J., 2005. Disorders of extreme stress: The empirical foundation of a complex adaptation to trauma. J. Trauma. Stress 18 (5), 389–399.

Wall-Wieler, E., Roos, L.L., Bolton, J., Brownell, M., Nickel, N.C., Chateau, D., 2017. Maternal health and social outcomes after having a child taken into care: Population-based longitudinal cohort study using linkable administrative data. J. Epidemiol Com. Health 71 (12), 1145–1151. https://doi.org/10.1136/jech-2017-209542.

Wall-Wieler, L., Roos, L.M., Brownell, M., Nickel, N., Chateau, D., Singal, D., 2017. Suicide attempts and completions among mothers whose children were taken into care by child protection services: A cohort study using linkable administrative data. Can. J. Psychiatry 63 (3), 170–177.

Wise, S., 2021. A Systems Model of Repeat Court-Ordered Removals: Responding to Child Protection Challenges Using a Systems Approach. Br. J. Soc. Work 51 (6), 2038–2060. https://doi.org/10.1093/bjsw/bcaa031.

20

SAFEGUARDING IN EDUCATIONAL SETTINGS

MIKE CULLERN ■ MARY TESSA BAGINSKY

KEY POINTS

- The policy context of schools' role in child protection.
- The role of the designated safeguarding officer.
- Development and implementation of the *Keeping Children Safe in Education* guidance.
- Safeguarding in residential schools.
- Engaging schools in a multiagency response to child protection.
- Thresholds.
- Managing disclosures and referring to social services.
- Role of schools in early help.
- Child-on-child abuse.
- The facilitators and barriers for schools working with other agencies.
- Safe recruitment practice.
- Allegations against staff.
- The changing nature of problems encountered in schools.

THE POLICY CONTEXT OF SCHOOLS' ROLE IN CHILD PROTECTION

Schools' role in child protection and safeguarding has been closely intertwined with increasing awareness of child abuse and an increased role for government in developing relevant policies, leading to an emphasis on agencies working together to protect children. The first iteration of *Working Together to Safeguard Children* (Department of Health et al., 1999) appeared over 20 years ago. It set out how all agencies and professionals should work together to promote children's welfare and protect them from abuse and neglect. Since then the document has been updated and reshaped but continues a tradition that had started many years earlier, of agencies collaborating to keep children safe. This chapter deals with the role of maintained schools in England in doing just that, but independent schools have similar responsibilities, as do schools in the other three countries of the United Kingdom.[1] It sets out the policy context alongside the role of schools in a multiagency approach to child protection and what needs to be in place to support that work.

Recent research has looked at the role of schools in a multiagency response to safeguarding and child protection (Baginsky et al., 2022). The two-and-a-half-year study was confined to England and provided a wide ranging review from the perspective of experts in the field, as well as those working in local authority education and social care services, the then Local Safeguarding Children's Boards and schools. The areas explored below draw on this work, particularly on the data collected from the 58 case-study schools, and draw some comparisons with a similar study conducted nearly 15 years previously (Baginsky, 2007).

THE ROLE OF THE DESIGNATED SAFEGUARDING LEAD

In keeping with the Children Act (1989), the Department of Education and Science (1988) and then the

---

[1]Each nation has its own laws and guidance that sets out the responsibilities of schools.

405

Department for Education and Employment (1995) produced statutory guidance for schools that included the appointment of designated teachers for child protection. The then local education authorities began to keep lists of these teachers and to provide training, initially using dedicated government funding. However, it was the Children Act 2004 that made it a statutory requirement for a range of organisations, including schools, to have a designated or 'named' person for safeguarding children and young people.

Keeping Children Safe in Education (Department for Education (DfE), 2020) sets out the minimum statutory standard for the role of designated safeguarding lead within schools, with some revision since the document's introduction in 2015. This person should be a senior staff member from the leadership team, be sufficiently trained and hold the status and authority within the school to fulfil the functions of the role. The document advises that is best practice that schools appoint a deputy safeguarding lead(s) able to support the designated lead and ensure the continued coordinated response to safeguarding matters in the absence of the designated lead.[2] The serious case review following the death of Daniel Pelka (Coventry Local Safeguarding Children's Board, 2013) highlighted the need for schools to have coordinated leadership in the response to all safeguarding and child protection matters.

The role holder takes lead responsibility for the response to safeguarding and child protection matters, both strategically and operationally. This includes the implementation and review of policy and procedures related to the safeguarding of children, identifying children in need of early help, holding oversight of multiagency referrals, contributing to the multiagency child protection response, raising awareness and supporting school staff to fulfil their safeguarding responsibilities and ensuring that concerns for the welfare of children are accurately and securely recorded.

In reality, the role can at times feel as if it is one of firefighting, dealing with multiple emergencies simultaneously. In the past, the primary role of teachers was to educate children, but it now requires a multifaceted skill set, from mediator to social worker. Some schools

have now moved away from appointing a member of teaching staff simply because of the demands on the role, and instead they have appointed those with previous safeguarding experience who are able to devote their full attention to managing the challenges.

A key finding in both the Daniel Pelka (Coventry Local Safeguarding Children's Board, 2013) and Child J (Whiffen, 2017) serious case reviews was a lack of understanding of the significance of concerns reported by staff which was, in part, a failure in robust recording mechanisms. In many schools electronic recording systems designed specifically to monitor safeguarding and welfare issues have been introduced to allow staff to report concerns in a timely manner and facilitate the drawing together of information that would be needed when making a referral. A primary role of the designated safeguarding lead is to not only record incidents of concern but to analyse critically the significance of repeat concerns and explanations provided by parents and carers.

DEVELOPMENT AND IMPLEMENTATION OF THE *KEEPING CHILDREN SAFE IN EDUCATION* GUIDANCE

In September 2004, government guidance, *Safeguarding Children in Education* (Department for Education and Skills, 2004) set out the specific duty on all those in education to safeguard and promote the welfare of children. While the guidance emphasised the need for all staff to share the view that the safeguarding of children may best be undertaken by proactively making detailed arrangements to provide a safe environment within educational settings, it made clear that, within the wider remit of safeguarding and promoting the welfare of *all* children, there remained a need for education staff to identify those *individual* children who are suffering or may be likely to suffer significant harm and for appropriate action to be taken. These two aspects of the duty placed upon education staff – to safeguard all children and to protect individual children from harm – remain coterminous. Over the years this guidance has been updated regularly. The child should always be at the centre of the safeguarding response, ensuring that children are listened to and have a voice which is captured throughout child protections records. The

---

[2]See Annex B of *Keeping Children Safe in Education* (DfE, 2020) which clearly sets out the minimum requirements for the role.

response should be led by the needs of the child and be empathetic to the child's lived experience when there are concerns that they are at risk of harm.

The many versions of *Keeping Children Safe in Education* (KCSIE) (latest DfE, 2020), which are the successors of *Safeguarding Children in Education,* provide guidance for schools on how they should safeguard and promote the welfare of their pupils. The guidance applies to all schools and colleges and does not distinguish between type of school:

> *(whether) maintained, non-maintained or independent schools (including academies, free schools and alternative provision academies), maintained nursery schools and pupil referral units.*
>
> *DfE (2020, p. 3)*

It emphasises the importance of schools embracing and embedding safeguarding practices into every aspect of school life. These areas include, for example, how a school deals with bullying and racist behaviour, how school staff support those pupils with specific medical needs, how the school monitors the effectiveness of its security system and how it monitors the safety and welfare of those pupils who are on work experience placements. Over the years it has been updated to include subjects which were not in earlier iterations such as female genital mutilation, radicalisation and county lines. [3]

Part 1 of KCSIE focuses on how all school (and college) staff fulfil their safeguarding duties and so should be read by everyone. It makes clear that all staff must be aware of the school's child protection policy, behaviour policy, staff behaviour policy, safeguarding response to children who go missing from education, and the role of the designated safeguarding lead (including the identity of the designated safeguarding lead and any deputies). They must receive appropriate and regular safeguarding and child protection training which must cover the skills that all school staff need to respond to the imperatives covered within 'safeguarding', as well as those needed to recognise the potential for harm. Staff should understand the spectrum of risks to children that include not solely risks within the familial home, but contextual safeguarding matters such as criminal and sexual exploitation, which may appear in many forms that are different from those previously associated with child abuse and neglect. In addition all staff must be aware of their local early help process and understand their role in it; be aware of the process for making referrals to children's social care and for statutory assessments under the Children Act 1989; and know what to do if a child tells them they are being abused or neglected.

Part 2 of KCSIE deals with the responsibilities of governing bodies, proprietors and management committees to manage safeguarding arrangements. As with Part 1, the various iterations of the guidance reflect changes and policy priorities that have implications for schools and colleges. In 2018 this included updated guidance on children missing from education, peer on peer abuse and greater emphasis on the need for information sharing. In the 2019 version the development of multiagency safeguarding arrangements, replacing local safeguarding children boards (LSCBs) from September 2019, and the new Ofsted inspection framework were amongst the important additions. When the multiagency safeguarding arrangements were announced following the Wood Review (2017) of LSCBs, education was not named as one of the statutory partners[4], and concern was expressed that this would marginalise schools and minimise their contribution. The 2019 version of KCSIE (DfE, 2019) recognised this concern and makes it clear that the partners will work with relevant agencies to safeguard and promote the welfare of local children:

> *...locally, the three safeguarding partners will name schools and colleges as relevant agencies and will reach their own conclusions on how best to achieve the active engagement of individual institutions in a meaningful way.*
>
> *DfE (2019, p. 20)*

Alongside KCSIE, the DfE also publishes a Data Protection Toolkit for Schools (DfE, 2018) which is also regularly updated and provides advice on all aspects of data protection within an educational setting. The

---

[3]Where drug gangs from cities expand their operations to smaller towns, exploiting children and vulnerable people to sell drugs.

[4]The three statutory partners are the local authority, health and the police.

Data Protection Act 2018 and General Data Protection Regulation do not prevent the sharing of information for the purposes of keeping children safe. Fears about sharing information must not be allowed to stand in the way of the need to promote the welfare and protect the safety of children, and governing bodies and proprietors should ensure that relevant staff have due regard to the data protection principles (see DfE, 2020, paragraphs 82–88).

SAFEGUARDING IN RESIDENTIAL SCHOOLS

In April 2020, the Independent Inquiry into Child Sexual Abuse published *Safeguarding children from sexual abuse in residential schools* (Roberts et al., 2020). For the purposes of the inquiry the definition of a residential school was mainstream residential settings which includes independent or private schools, state boarding schools and residential schools for children with special education needs and disabilities (SEND). The inquiry was set up in 2015 to consider the extent which state and non-state settings had failed in their duty to protect children from sexual harm, with the aim to make recommendations for change.

One of the key findings of the inquiry was residential schools face distinct and complex challenges to prevent and respond to incidents of child sexual abuse effectively (Roberts et al., 2020, p. 101). A complexity being that staff spend a significant amount of time with children in their care and professional boundaries can become blurred often due to the 'in loco parentis' role that staff have within residential schools. It can be a challenge for schools to manage the balance between encouraging independence at the same time as safeguarding children in an environment that is both their home and school.

The guidance set out in *Keeping Children Safe in Education* and *Working Together to Safeguard Children* is equally applicable to residential schools as it is to non-residential settings. Schools should consider the additional vulnerability of children living away from home, and it is vital that they focus on their pastoral offer to children. The elevated caring role of residential staff can increase the complexity in the dynamic between staff and children. Schools need to ensure that they create environments where children feel safe, listened to and have a voice to raise concerns.

Staff training should cover all aspects of safeguarding but reflect the additional complexities of safeguarding children in residential settings. Children may be at increased risk of peer on peer abuse or exploitation, and training should equip staff to recognise and respond as is necessary. There should be clear expectations on staff and pupil behaviour, and all staff should be clear about their safeguarding responsibilities as well as the school's procedures to escalate concerns. Allegations against staff should be dealt with swiftly and in line with statutory and local guidance, and focus should be placed on the need to safeguard resident children and staff whilst investigations are undertaken.

ENGAGING SCHOOLS IN A MULTIAGENCY RESPONSE TO CHILD PROTECTION

In the 1960s the importance of inter-agency collaboration was officially recognised in several reports, including one from the Central Advisory Council for Education Report in 1967 and the Committee on Local Authority and Allied Personal Social Services Report in 1968. Nevertheless inquiries into child deaths over the subsequent 20 years frequently contained references to the failure of professionals to collaborate (see, for example, London Borough of Brent, 1985 and London Borough of Greenwich, 1987). A piece of legislation that is over 30 years old remains the key to providing guidance to agencies on cooperation. The Children Act 1989 is the principal legislative framework for recognising and responding to abuse and neglect. It introduced the concept of 'significant harm' where 'harm' is defined as ill treatment or the impairment of health and development and is the threshold that justifies intervening in family life to act in the best interests of children. One of the challenges and complexities of the legislation is that there is no absolute standard to judge what constitutes significant harm. It may be one single, serious incident, or it could be the result of ongoing harm that damages a child's physical and/or emotional development. The Act placed inter-agency working at the heart of the remit for social services (see Anning et al., 2006, p. 5) with

Section 27 placing a duty on education, housing and health services to cooperate with each other.

The guidance that accompanied the implementation of the Children Act (1989), *Working Together Under the Children Act 1989* (Home Office et al., 1991), not only identified specific tasks for teachers and school nurses, but it also set the context for joint working between schools and the then social services departments. Circular 10/95 (Department for Education and Employment, 1995) not only clarified the responsibility for child protection within education departments, schools and colleges but also gave guidance on links with other agencies involved in the protection of children. Subsequently the Education Act (2002) gave schools a statutory duty to promote and safeguard the welfare of children. The 2002 legislation was directly related to the death of Lauren Wright in May 2000. Although the inquiry into her death (Norfolk Health Authority, 2002) found other agencies to be at fault, the child protection arrangements in Lauren's school were deemed to be wholly inadequate. Staff had failed to follow guidance which until this point was not a statutory requirement. However, the biggest reorganisation of children's services in England followed the death of 8-year-old Victoria Climbié at the hands of her aunt and the aunt's partner where, in a report by Lord Laming (2003), it was stated that inter-agency communication systems had again failed. Structural reforms of children's services that followed were intended to support a more joined up approach to the protection of children, with local authorities required to amalgamate their education and children's social services department under one director responsible for children's service.

In September 2004, government guidance, *Safeguarding Children in Education* (DfES, 2004), set out the specific duty on all those in education to safeguard and promote the welfare of children. While the guidance emphasised the need for all staff to share the view that the safeguarding of children may best be undertaken by proactively making detailed arrangements to provide a safe environment within educational settings, it made clear that, within the wider remit of safeguarding and promoting the welfare of *all* children, there remained a need for education staff to identify those *individual* children who are suffering or may be likely to suffer significant harm and for appropriate action to be taken. These two aspects of the duty placed upon education staff – to safeguard all children and to protect individual children from harm – remain coterminous. Over the years this guidance has been updated regularly.

THRESHOLDS

Staff working in education have an important part to play in preventing, recognising and responding to the abuse and neglect of children. The identification of children at risk and the sharing of information is a key part of the child protection process. In the year April 2018–March 2019, there were over 650,000 referrals to children's social care, and 20% came from school or other education services (DfE, 2019b).

The term 'threshold' refers to the point at which the local authority's Children's Social Care are likely to accept a referral for an intervention with a child, young person or their family. Local authorities produce their own local threshold document. These documents are intended for all professionals working with children and families to provide guidance both where they may have a concern about a child and how thresholds inform which referrals are accepted by children's social care. The referral route into children's services is usually by telephone in a multiagency safeguarding hub (MASH) or directly to a team in children's social care. Research conducted by one of the authors in the early years of this century (Baginsky, 2007) found some authorities used a generic call centre where referrals were sifted before being passed to social workers. Schools disliked them because they thought the process introduced delays and often left them unclear as to who was handling the referral. Call centres that dealt with child protection concerns alongside reports of failing drains and potholes seem to have disappeared. In the recent study schools were less critical of the processes they used to make referrals, but as in the earlier study, they did not always think they received a timely response. Although it could be irritating if the referral was not deemed to be urgent by the receiving agency, schools were more concerned when they were left with the impression that the referral was a cause for concern, but the response was not immediate. If a school was asked not to allow a child to go home until they had heard from a social worker, and that call did not come before then end of the school day, it left the school staff unsure of their right to detain the child while not wanting to put him or her into any danger. In reality, schools have no legal basis to hold a child in school if the parent wishes to remove them. However, schools can find it useful to make it explicit in their child protection policy circumstances when the school may be asked to safeguard a child on school site until social care arrive. This helps set the foundation of dialogue with parents when the school has been asked to detain the child. In circumstances which become hostile or a parent does attempt to remove their child, the school are within their right to call the police for assistance should the safeguarding concern warrant it.

There is a further complication around referrals and thresholds which has implications for a multiagency working, and this is the disconnect between training which teachers may receive and the criteria in place in children's social care for accepting referrals. From observing the child protection training that some designated teachers received, it was clear that the emphasis was on the signs that might indicate a child was suffering abuse and on the reporting of concerns to the social worker. The terms 'significant harm' and 'child in need' are fundamental to the Children Act 1989 but were rarely explored or explained in training. Within the Children Act 1989, there is no definition of risk; child protection is constructed in terms of 'significant harm'. There are no absolute criteria on which to rely in judging what constitutes significant harm, and it is dependent on an assessment of risk and thresholds.

> ...the point at which behaviour is defined as abusive. Furthermore, they represent the point beyond which one set of actions relevant to one stage of the child protection process is superseded by those of a successive stage.
>
> **Little (1997, p. 28)**

The threshold document is crucial. One of the topics which causes many problems for schools is the disconnect they often perceive between what they thought thresholds should be and their experiences. While most authorities in the recent study said that the threshold document was a key component of the safeguarding training for designated safeguarding leads,

awareness of its importance and even its existence varied considerably across the schools.

MANAGING DISCLOSURES AND REFERRING TO CHILDREN'S SOCIAL CARE

For most children, school is a place of safety. School should be an environment where children have a voice and feel safe to express their wishes and feelings and disclose what is worrying them. It is equally important that all staff receive adequate safeguarding training to ensure that they are aware of their role and responsibilities in the safeguarding of children and are aware of the indicators of abuse. Regardless of the school's geographical location or pupil demographic, staff should hold the attitude of 'it could happen here', (DfE, 2020). In recent years, the expectations on all staff on their role and responsibility in the safeguarding of children has increased. An example is the mandatory duty placed on teachers to report known cases of female genital mutilation to police which came into effect in 2015. Further to this, staff now need to be alert to not only risk of harm in familial settings, but risk to children in contextual situations.

It is not the role of school staff to investigate suspected abuse of children but rather to ensure that children are listened to, that what they are disclosing is taken seriously, that disclosures are recorded accurately and that they understand the procedures in the school for immediate escalation of concerns. It is important that staff do not promise children confidentiality and that staff are transparent about their role and responsibility to keep children safe.

In most circumstances, the responsibility of referring to children's social care would form part of the role for the designated safeguarding lead. Part 1 of *Keeping Children Safe in Education* (2020) highlights the need for all staff to be aware of the processes for making referrals. As part of all staff safeguarding training, schools should ensure that staff are aware of the local procedures for referring concerns.

Staff should be aware that, where a decision has been taken not to escalate concerns to social care by the school, staff can still make a referral to social care if they believe the child to be at risk of harm. The designated safeguarding lead should continue to support and oversee this process.

Disclosures and suspicions of harm should be referred to children's social care immediately and where a child is deemed to be at imminent risk, the police. Schools should be aware of local child protection thresholds and the mechanisms for referring into children social care, as well as the procedures to challenge and escalate when they feel that decisions made by partner agencies are not being made in 'the child's best interests' and a child remains at risk of harm (HM Government, 2018).

ROLE OF SCHOOLS IN EARLY HELP

In the previous study (Baginsky, 2007), schools were anxious to play their part in a collaborative approach to safeguarding children but were often confused by the threshold for action by social services and by the definition of what constituted 'at risk of significant harm' and 'a child in need'. Social workers wondered why schools did not make direct referrals to services in the community which might be able to help families, while schools were unaware of when they could make such a referral and did not believe they had the knowledge of available providers. In recent years attention has again focused on intervening early in a family's problem to stop it escalating to the point where it requires a statutory intervention.

Where a family agrees to an early help assessment it will involve all professionals involved with the family to decide on the right combination of support. If there is a school-aged child, school staff will be expected to contribute and even lead on the assessment process. Some schools have a range of services based on site or available to them and usually found involvement less demanding than small schools without similar access. Most authorities have an Early Help service, although the size and remit does vary enormously. In some areas there is a full range of services on offer, while in others it may consist of an advice service to point families and professionals towards sources of support. In the recent study (Baginsky et al., 2022) concerns were expressed by schools that early help was being used not for families' benefit, but to keep cases away from children's social care; and that where families failed to engage it only served to delay the time when a statutory intervention would be required. These concerns were aggravated when any voluntary agencies and local authority services they had previously used disappeared as a result of budget cuts.

CHILD-ON-CHILD ABUSE

The role of school in early intervention is not limited to the ability to identify familial need but extends to contextual safeguarding, working on the basis that prevention is equally as important as responding to concerns of harm. In June 2021, Ofsted undertook a review of sexual abuse in schools between children in the wake of the Everyone's Invited website (https://www.everyonesinvited.uk/) where current and previous pupils shared their experiences of harmful sexual behaviour in school, their perception of cause and effect and a school's response to these concerns. The review's findings demonstrated that the prevalence of child-on-child abuse was both significant and complex across all schools visited. Children spoke of experiencing both non-contact and contact forms of harm from their peers, whether directly or indirectly, and it was evident that online and social media played a large role in facilitation of harm. There was a striking disparity between the experiences of girls compared with that of boys. Children were more likely to tell a friend or parent than an adult within the school.

Ofsted emphasised the importance of having a 'zero-tolerance' approach to child-on-child abuse, for schools to re-enforce what is acceptable and unacceptable behaviour, and to create an environment where pupils feel safe to talk about abuse. It was evident that in some schools, pupils' perceptions of the prevalence of harmful behaviour did not align with that of school staff and highlighted the need for a whole school approach to recognising and responding to behaviours and language which children deemed 'commonplace'.

A robust Relationships, Sex and Education (RSE) curriculum designed to teach children about their rights and those of others, as well as about the nature of healthy relationships, prepares them for life both inside and outside of school and plays a key role in the prevention of harmful behaviour between children. The ability to prepare, identify and respond to problematic behaviour early before it escalates is an essential aspect of a school's safeguarding response to child-on-child abuse.

The safeguarding landscape in each school can differ depending on the demographic of the pupils who attend. Deprivation is not necessarily an indicator that children are more or less likely to experience harmful behaviour from their peers, and what Ofsted referred to an 'affluent neglect' was significant for children in those schools who may previously not have considered their pupils to be at risk. In areas with high levels of domestic violence, schools may find it even more challenging to counter children's perception of healthy relationships and acceptable behaviour between peers. It is evident from the experiences of children and adults posted on the Everyone's Invited website that many had experienced some form of harmful sexual behaviour in their school regardless of the school's perceived status.

It is acknowledged that this area of safeguarding and early intervention is complex and is not solely the responsibility of schools to tackle. It requires a multiagency response that is both preventative and reactionary when there are concerns of harmful behaviour between children. Sexual Violence and Sexual Harassment in Schools and Colleges (DfE, 2021) was updated in response to the Ofsted review and highlighted the importance of the multiagency safeguarding partners, including children's social care, having a range of comprehensive and effective services in place to address needs early.

THE FACILITATORS AND BARRIERS FOR SCHOOLS WORKING WITH OTHER AGENCIES

In the same recent study (Baginsky et al., 2022) staff in education and children's social care responding to a survey agreed that 'clear thresholds' and 'good quality safeguarding training' were the key to them working effectively together. They were also in agreement that 'workforce stability in children's social care', 'clear and transparent assessment processes', a 'designated Lead Profession and/or clarity about professional responsibilities', 'data and information sharing' and 'regular meetings between schools and children's social care' were essential components. There was similar agreement that the absence of these items set barriers in the way of close working relationships.

The landscape of state-maintained education has changed considerably with a rapid increase in the number of academies since 2010, weakening local authorities' ability to manage those areas which remain its responsibility such as child protection. In August 2020, 57% of schools were maintained by local authorities with the remaining state funded schools holding academy status.[5] However, only one in ten of those in education thought these arrangements stood in the way of strengthening collaborative relationships across agencies in relation to child protection, although nearly one in three of those in children's social care thought they did.

SAFE RECRUITMENT PRACTICES

The murder of two 10-year-old girls, Jessica Chapman and Holly Wells, in 2002 by Ian Huntley, a school caretaker, highlighted the deficits in the vetting procedure that had allowed him to get this job. After he was convicted, it emerged that he had been investigated in the past for sexual offences and burglary, but he had still been allowed to work in a school as the investigations had not resulted in a conviction. An independent inquiry was conducted by Sir Michael Birchard (2004), and one of his recommendations was anyone working with children should be vetted before working with them.

The primary purpose of safer recruitment practices is to prevent those who may be unsuitable or pose a risk to children from working in a school environment. Whether employing to a permanent role, agency staff or volunteer, schools should adhere to safe recruitment practices as set out in Part 3 of *Keeping Children Safe in Education 2020*, and within the best practice nonstatutory guidance issued by the Safer Recruitment Consortium, updated in May 2019.

Governing bodies, proprietors and senior leaders should ensure that schools have robust recruitment and staff behaviour policies in place and that those undertaking the recruitment of staff have been sufficiently trained in safe recruitment practices. The schools commitment to the safeguarding of children should be evident throughout the employment process, from advertisement through to interview, as a deterrent to those who may pose a risk of harm to children.

The suitability of prospective employees or volunteers should be scrutinised through checks and evidence obtained via criminal records checks (DBS), barred list checks, prohibition checks, references

---

[5]https://www.gov.uk/government/publications/open-academies-and-academy-projects-in-development

and during the interview process. Particular attention should be made to any gaps in employment, inaccuracies or conflicting information which may be an indicator that a person may not be suitable for appointment due to previous safeguarding concerns. Any arising matters should be resolved satisfactorily prior to appointment.

All schools and colleges must maintain a single central record (SCR) which evidences the pre-appointment checks undertaken for all staff and the dates which the checks were carried out. *Keeping Children Safe in Education 2020* sets out the minimum information which must be recorded for all staff members.

ALLEGATIONS AGAINST STAFF

In recent years there have been several high-profile cases related to the harm of children in a school setting. In 2012 North Somerset Safeguarding Children's Board published a serious case review into the sexual harm perpetrated by Nigel Leat, a primary school teacher who was convicted of multiple offences related to children (Craddock, 2012). In 2013 East Sussex released a serious case review following the conviction of Jeremy Forrest for abduction and sexual offences related to a secondary age female pupil (Harrington, 2013). These cases are a stark reminder of the importance for staff conduct policies and robust and swift responses when concerns about a person's behaviour towards a child becomes apparent.

Working Together to Safeguard Children 2018 and Part 4 of *Keeping Children Safe in Education 2020* set out criteria of an allegation and the procedures which should be followed whilst managing the allegation process. It is important to note that the application of the guidance extends beyond teaching staff to any staff member working within a school who may come into contact with children.

The allegations criteria are:

- behaved in a way that has harmed a child, or may have harmed a child;
- possibly committed a criminal offence against or related to a child;
- behaved towards a child or children in a way that indicates he or she may pose a risk of harm to children; or

- behaved or may have behaved in a way that indicates they may not be suitable to work with children.

The fourth criteria, 'behaved or may have behaved in a way that indicates they may not be suitable to work with children', is an addition to the most recent *Keeping Children Safe in Education* and reflects the need to consider transferable risk, for example being arrested for assault or drugs offences. While it may not relate directly to the harm of children, it may raise concerns about their suitability to work with children.

Schools should ensure that they create an environment where children feel safe to talk about what worries them, including what happens during the school day. Children in general are vulnerable because of the power imbalance between them and adults, but this dynamic can become more complicated and embedded when considering the power imbalance between a child and their teacher who is a trusted adult.

Staff need to be alert to behaviour of colleagues which may be inappropriate and outside of school policy and understand the duty to report concerns. The North Somerset and East Sussex serious case reviews highlighted a key theme that staff observed behaviour which made them feel uncomfortable or knew was not appropriate but failed to act sooner. It can be a challenge for staff who have worked together for a number of years not to normalise behaviour of colleagues which step outside the boundaries of appropriate. Schools should ensure that they are constantly reminding staff of the expectations on conduct and what to do if they are concerned.

Staff should report concerns immediately to the headteacher or the designated safeguarding lead and if the allegation is against the headteacher, the chair of governors. Schools should create an environment for staff where they feel confident to challenge poor and potentially harmful practice and escalate in line with school policy. Ultimately, staff should hold a 'it could happen here' attitude to all forms of abuse, including risks to children during the school day.

Any concern related to a staff member which may fall into the allegations criteria should be referred to the Local Authority Designated Officer (LADO) immediately. The role of the LADO is not to investigate, but rather to coordinate and hold oversight of the investigation and to steer it to an outcome as set out in *Keeping Children Safe in Education* (DfE, 2020). Dependant on the severity of the allegation, the investigation may be led by police, social care, the employer or may be a combined multiagency team.

Staff who are the subject of an allegation can find the process extremely stressful. Schools should have effective support mechanisms in place, and any immediate actions to safeguard should be proportionate and as neutral as possible while the investigation takes place. Responses to allegations should be fair, timely and proportionate. In reality, investigations led by Police can become protracted due to the complexity of a criminal investigation when compared to investigations considered on a balance of probability, led by social care or the employer. This is where it normally becomes vital that schools have robust support in place for staff throughout the process.

THE CHANGING NATURE OF PROBLEMS ENCOUNTERED IN SCHOOLS

It was evident in the recent research study (Baginsky et al., 2022) that schools across the age spectrum were dealing with subjects that were proving particularly challenging and which were placing children and young people at risk. There was a range of issues linked with poverty and austerity including housing and food poverty and the difficulties schools faced in dealing with them but also the problems they encountered in recognising and distinguishing neglect. There was also what seemed to school staff to be an escalating level of alcohol and substance abuse, domestic violence and poor mental health amongst many parents, much of which impacted on, or were also problems experienced by, young people. In two of the five areas where the research was conducted, there were significant levels of gang affiliation, as well as criminal and sexual exploitation. Although the incidence of these had increased, more experienced teachers admitted that these had long been problems but had not always attracted a response from children's services or the police. The reporting that followed the uncovering of the Rotherham child sexual exploitation scandal (Jay, 2014), as well as the number of young people killed and injured as a result of knife injuries and the media

attention on county lines, had made it more likely although not inevitable that they would get a response to these concerns.

There were, however, two areas which had not been mentioned in previous research. These were the impact of the use of social media and radicalisation, both of which had attracted additional training. The use of mobile telephones in schools divided opinion. In some schools they were used and valued to supplement curriculum activities, but they were also associated with grooming, bullying and gang activity.

Concerns arising from radicalisation, from the right wing and from Islamists, were not common, but when they occurred, the experience had a significant impact, with teachers reporting uncertainty about their interpretation of indicators as well as fears over alienating members of the school and local community. However, in all the instances reported to the researchers, schools were very positive about the support they had received from their local authorities and from the police.

With increasing frequency, schools are often at the forefront of the multiagency response to critical incidents. A critical incident can be defined as a significant event which results in trauma, serious injury or the fatality of a pupil(s) or staff member on school premises, or it could relate to an incident which takes place in the wider community and causes significant disruption to the functions of the school. Incidents which result in serious injury or fatality, such as a stabbing, can be extremely overwhelming and distressing for pupils, staff and the wider community. Schools need to plan how they will respond to the immediate presenting incident and the wider and long-term impact on the school community. Partnership working with Police, social care and health colleagues will be vital to support the school to manage situations effectively and support children and staff.

Each local authority will have their own guidance on the response to emergency and critical incidents. Schools should familiarise themselves with local procedures and incorporate into their safeguarding policies. Critical incidents can often be sudden and school staff should know the internal school procedures, reporting mechanism and their role as part of a multiagency response.

CONCLUSION

Over recent years there has been an increasing focus on the role of schools in the safeguarding of children. The move by the Department for Education to shift the bulk of guidance from *Working Together to Safeguard Children* and move to a stand-alone document, *Keeping Children Safe in Education,* is testament to the vital role schools play in the child protection arena. Whereas *Working Together* provides the guidance to schools on the role they play within the multiagency, *Keeping Children Safe in Education* has become the 'go-to' document for education settings.

Multiagency working can at times feel fragmented and following rejected social care referrals, schools can feel that they are often left to safeguard children in isolation. Although the focus in serious case reviews, such as Daniel Pelka and Child J, can often cast light on when school arrangements have failed to adequately safeguard children, what we hear less of are the success stories and how schools often go above and beyond to ensure that children within their care are safe.

This has never been more evident than now. At the time of writing this chapter, the world finds itself in the middle of a pandemic. Schools have stepped up to the forefront of the multiagency to ensure that children are safeguarded when the task has faced unprecedented challenges (Baginsky, 2020). During the lockdown periods, the majority of schools were able to remain open for children of keyworkers and those deemed vulnerable. Schools held sight of the children not attending school by making regular contact, children entitled to free school meals continued to be fed, and schools extended their offer to children who had become vulnerable due to the impact of the pandemic. All this has been achieved when government guidance has been regularly changing and reactionary.

The importance of multiagency collaboration has never been more evident than now. During this pandemic period, there has been a positive shift in how agencies pull together to share information, focus on the needs of the child and greater support between partners to meet the needs of children (Baginsky, 2020). This was all achieved in a short period of time. The question for partner agencies is, how do we hold on to these achievements as we move out of the pandemic?

What has become evident is that schools play a pivotal role on the frontline to keep children safe.

KEY POINTS

- Induction and regular child protection training should equip staff with the skills and knowledge to fulfil their safeguarding responsibilities to children.
- All staff should understand their role in the evolving landscape of contextual safeguarding.
- School staff play a key role in the multiagency approach to safeguarding children and should hold a 'it could happen here' attitude to all forms of harm to children.
- The child's voice and 'lived experience' should be at the centre of the schools safeguarding response.
- Schools should have robust policies and procedures for safe recruitment and the management of allegations against staff.

USEFUL WEBSITES

https://learning.nspcc.org.uk/research-resources – The NSPCC website contains access to professional resources on child protection, classroom resources, national serious case reviews and access to safeguarding training.

www.isi.net – The independent school inspectorate provides guidance to schools, pupils and parents on the independent school's inspection framework and guidance on the role and responsibilities to safeguard children.

www.gov.uk/topic/schools-colleges-childrens-services/safeguarding-children—The central government website page where schools and staff can access statutory guidance on safeguarding children in schools or other settings, multiagency working arrangements and safeguarding in specific circumstances.

www.safeguardinginschools.co.uk – Andrew Hall is a specialist education safeguarding consultant, and his website contains useful resources and regular updates on safeguarding matters as well as access to training and materials.

www.londoncp.co.uk – The London Child Protection Procedures set out both the multiagency core procedures and practice guidance for the response to child protection concerns. These procedures are adopted across all London boroughs. Nationally, schools should look to procedures set out locally by their partnership boards.

REFERENCES

Anning, A., Cottrell, D., Frost, N., Green, J., Robinson, M., 2006. Multi-Professional Teamwork for Integrated Children's Services. Open University, Buckingham.

Baginsky, M., 2007. Schools, Social Services and Safeguarding Children: Past Practice and Future Challenges. NSPCC, London.

Baginsky, M., 2020. Keeping Children and Young People Safe During a Pandemic: Testing the Robustness of Multiagency

Child Protection and Safeguarding Arrangements for Schools. King's College London, London.

Baginsky, M., Driscoll, J., Purcell, C., Hickman, B., Manthorpe, J., 2022. Protecting and Safeguarding Children in Schools. Policy Press, Bristol.

Birchard, M., 2004. The Birchard Inquiry Report. TSO, London.

Central Advisory Council for Education, 1967. Children and their Primary Schools (Plowden Report). HMSO, London.

Children Act, 1989. https://www.legislation.gov.uk/ukpga/1989/41/contents

Children Act, 2004. https://www.legislation.gov.uk/ukpga/2004/31/contents

Committee on Local Authority and Allied Personal Social Services, 1968. Report on the Committee on Local Authority and Allied Personal Social Services (Seebohm Report). Cmnd 3703. HMSO, London.

Coventry Local Safeguarding Children's Board, 2013. Daniel Pelka Serious Case Review. Coventry Local Safeguarding Children's Board, Coventry.

Craddock, M., 2012. Serious Case Review Re Abuse of Pupils in a First School. North Somerset Safeguarding Children Board, Weston-Super-Mare. North Somerset.

Data Protection Act, 2018. https://www.legislation.gov.uk/ukpga/2018/12/contents/enacted

Department for Education, 2015. Keeping Children Safe in Education. Department of Education, London.

Department for Education, 2018. Data Protection Toolkit for Schools. Department of Education, London.

Department for Education, 2019. Statistics: Children in Need and Child Protection. Department for Education, London.

Department for Education, 2020. Keeping Children Safe in Education. Department of Education, London.

Department for Education, 2021. Sexual Violence and Sexual Harassment Between Children in Schools and Colleges: Advice for Governing Bodies, Proprietors, Headteachers, Principals, Senior Leadership Teams and Designated Safeguarding Leads. Department for Education, London.

Department for Education and Employment, 1995. Circular 10/95. HMSO, London.

Department of Education and Science, 1988. Working Together for the Protection of Children from Abuse: Procedures within the Education Service (Circular 4/88). Department of Education and Science, London.

Department for Education and Skills (DfES), 2004. Safeguarding Children in Education. DfES-0027-2004. London.

Department of Health, Department for Education and Employment and Home office, 1999. Working Together to Safeguard Children: A Guide to Interagency Working to Safeguard and Promote the Welfare of Children. TSO, London.

Education Act, 2002. https://www.legislation.gov.uk/ukpga/2002/32/contents

Harrington, K., 2013. Serious Case Review. Child G. East Sussex. Lewes: East Sussex Local Safeguarding Children Board.

HM Government, 2018. Working Together to Safeguard Children. A Guide to Inter-Agency Working to Safeguard and Promote the Welfare of Children. HM Government, London.

Home Office, Department of Health, Department of Education and Science and Welsh Office, 1991. Working Together Under the Children Act 1989: A Guide to Arrangements for Interagency Co-operation for the Protection of Children from Abuse. London: HMSO.

Jay, A., 2014. Independent Inquiry into Sexual Exploitation in Rotherham 1997-2003. Rotherham, Rotherham.

Laming, H., 2003. (Cmnd5730). The Victoria Climbie Inquiry; Report of an Inquiry by Lord Laming. TSO, Norwich.

Little, M., 1997. The Re-focusing of Children's Services. In Parton, N. (ed) Child Protection and Family Support. London: Routledge.

London Borough of Brent, 1985. A Child in Trust: The Report of the Panel of Inquiry into the Circumstances Surrounding the Death of Jasmine Beckford. London Borough of Brent, London.

London Borough of Greenwich, 1987. A Child in Mind: Protection of Children in a Responsible Society — The Report of the Commission of Inquiry into the Circumstances Surrounding the Death of Kimberley Carlile. London Borough of Greenwich, London.

Norfolk Health Authority, 2002. Summary Report of the Independent Health Review into the Death of Lauren Wright. Norfolk Health Authority, Norwich.

Relationships, Sex and Education (RSE). https://www.gov.uk/government/news/relationships-education-relationships-and-sex-education-rse-and-health-education-faqs

Roberts, E., Sharrock, S., Yeo, A., Graham, J., Turley, C., Kelley, N., 2020. Safeguarding Children from Sexual Abuse in Residential Schools. Independent Inquiry into Child Sexual Abuse, London.

Safer Recruitment Consortium, 2019. Guidance for Safer Working Practice for those Working with Children Young People in Education Settings. V2. Safer Recruitment Consortium. https://www.saferrecruitmentconsortium.org/.

Wiffen, J., 2017. Serious Case Review Re Child J. Nottingham City Safeguarding Children Board, Nottingham.

Wood, A., 2017. Wood Report: Review of the Role and Functions of Local Safeguarding Children Boards. Department for Education, London.

21

SAFEGUARDING CHILDREN IN HEALTHCARE CONTEXTS

MARIA CLARK ■ LOUISE ISHAM

KEY POINTS

- Medical indicators of abuse.
- Under-nutrition and failure to thrive.
- Safeguarding children in hospital.
- Key health professionals who play a role in child safeguarding.
- Managing disclosures and referring to social services.
- Employment practices (DBS) and allegations against staff.
- Future directions and conclusion.

INTRODUCTION

Children are vulnerable to abuse within and outside of healthcare contexts, and at additional risk of harm if they have physical or mental disabilities, impairments, learning disabilities or lack capacity to make informed decisions about their care (NHS England, 2017, 2019). Health professionals routinely undertake physical, social, emotional and mental health examination in hospital settings, and also in primary care, community clinics, schools, prisons and in domestic home environments. In the United Kingdom (UK) the National Health Service (NHS) is the largest public sector employer of healthcare staff who have a duty of care to safeguard their patients from harm (HM Government, 2018, 2004). The Child Protection-Information Sharing (CP-IS) project in England is an example of rapid digital efforts to share information securely between health and social care in order to protect vulnerable children at risk of maltreatment and abuse (NHS Digital, 2020a,b).

Recent serious case reviews identified that health professionals routinely undertook multiple types of assessment of children at serious risk of harm, often without responding appropriately to signs of abuse (Brandon et al., 2020; Department for Education, 2020; Sidebotham et al., 2016). Indeed, decades of learning from high profile cases, including Victoria Climbie, Kyra Ishaq, Daniel Pelka and Child G, show that poor communication systems weaken individual efforts for collaborative working, particularly between health and social work/care (Hudson, 2005). Everyday practice is still characterised by 'silo' working in close vicinity, but not effective sharing of information (Sidebotham et al., 2016; Taylor and Corlett, 2007). Over the past 10 to 20 years, however, evident legal trends emphasize greater collaborative working with and by health professionals (HM Government, 2018, 2004). Alongside the new CP-IS, the National Network of Designated Healthcare Professionals (NNDHP) shows increased recognition of child safeguarding and well-being functions beyond those working in designated specialist roles. Implementation of the 'common assessment framework' (LCC, 2020) is showing promise in some regions, alongside proactive procurement of health visiting leadership for the Healthy Child Program (HCP) (Local Government Association, 2019).

Furthermore, safeguarding supervision and training is accessible to health professionals, working in a variety of trauma-informed roles, working within and outside of the NHS (Hudson, 2005; Oral et al., 2016).

In this chapter we cover some of the key aspects of safeguarding in healthcare contexts in England and explain the role and structures of child protection processes for those working within and alongside the NHS.

MEDICAL INDICATORS OF ABUSE

Medical work is primarily concerned with clinical recognition of signs and symptoms of disease and recovery from illness. Disease prevention includes early detection and action to address social determinants of health inequity (WHO, 2010). The impact of adverse childhood experiences (ACEs) on poor health outcomes is increasingly recognised (Chandon et al., 2020; Hughes et al., 2017), particularly the impact of trauma and child abuse (Sperlich et al., 2017). Medical indicators of child abuse are complex and should involve paediatric examination when abuse is suspected or disclosed, including assessment for physical, emotional and sexual abuse, and neglect. Examination is an opportunity to assess the child's health and well-being while gathering evidence about injury through observation and forensic sampling.

Physical Injury and Trauma

Top to toe child medical examination is necessary to assess for signs of physical injury. Physical indicators of abuse include infant and child head or brain injury. The National Institute for Health and Care Excellence (NICE) outlines the key priorities for medical examination (NICE, 2019), including neuroimagery to differentiate multi-mechanism injuries that could signal abusive head trauma (AHT). Hsieh et al. (2015) showed that subdural haematoma, cerebral ischaemia retinal haemorrhage, skull fracture and intracranial injury were found to be indicative of AHT. Retinal haemorrhages and rib fractures suggested abusive head trauma in children under 3 years of age, with compounding clinical features including intracranial injuries, apnoea, seizure, head or neck bruising (Maguire et al., 2011) and inhalation of foreign bodies (Passali et al., 2010).

Poor oral health, such as frequent dental carries, poor gum health and premature loss of teeth, is recognised as an 'early' indicator of neglect, given the sensitivity of the teeth and mouth area in infants and children. Left untreated, dental disease and poor oral hygiene can have a number of negative, often 'hidden' physical impacts on children, including persistent pain and discomfort, acute and chronic infection, loss of appetite and subsequent reduction in body weight, and loss of sleep, resulting in disrupted attention for play and learning (Harris, 2018). In addition, the face, neck and mouth region are the most common sites of physical (including sexual) injury to children (Kellogg, 2005). It is important that all professionals recognise that poor oral health is often caused by socioeconomic factors, such as poor diet and nutrition or difficulties accessing dental care, particularly when there are costs to treatment (Heads, 2013). Similarly, interprofessional working is critical in this area, and this is increasingly recognised within the dentistry community (Harris, 2018); however, there remains limited knowledge and confidence amongst health and social work professionals to explore children's oral health and assess potential signs of domestic violence and abuse and neglect (Bradbury-Jones et al., 2019; Bradbury-Jones, 2016c).

New and emerging threats to children and adolescents include child criminal exploitation, sexual exploitation, knife crime, financial or commercial exploitation also related to drug crimes (county lines) and radicalisation. The multiple threats may intersect and child perpetrators of crimes may be victims too. Midwives, health visitors and designated safeguarding specialists are especially well placed to identify and respond to children in need and to mobilise intercollegiate partnership working in the crucial early years of child development (Royal College of Nursing (RCN), 2019). There is an equally urgent need to address intersecting problems associated with serious crime; gang and knife-related injuries are rising across the UK, increasingly involving healthcare professionals in treating physical injuries in acute hospital settings. Malik et al. (2020) reported that knife-injuries constitute 12.9% of trauma workload in urban emergency care and that violence recidivism and intoxication are common. The authors called for targeted violence reduction interventions across health, social care and law enforcement, noting that 13.9% of injuries treated involved serious harm from machetes.

Case reviews of 'child abuse linked to faith and belief' (CALFB) or ritual abuse show physical injury and trauma, compounded by emotional and psychological abuse sometimes associated with accusations of 'witchcraft'. Bruising, knife wounds or scarring on limbs may be present on medical inspection or examination. There may be emergency hospital admissions involving expunging herbal substances found in body orifices (eyes, ears, and genitalia). Bite marks and emaciation may be present, or not, and like the other signs, require holistic medical, psychological and social assessment for CALFB (FGM Centre, 2018; Noorazma et al., 2006).

Sexual Abuse

Cutland (2019) outlined the scope of medical examinations where there are concerns about child sexual abuse (CSA). She noted that the majority of children who are known to police and social services regarding CSA are not referred for medical examination. Reasons for this are poorly understood. It is surmised that there may be beliefs that forensic material is unlikely to be obtained or that the examination will cause further distress and harm to the child. Children who were examined, on the other hand, reported that the examination was positive, helping them to evidence their case for support. In these cases, medical examination can help obtain evidence of CSA (such as semen or DNA or anogenital physical findings of CSA) or of other categories of injury outside the anogenital area; signs of abuse more broadly, identifying sexually transmitted infections, blood-borne diseases such as HIV and other infections, or the need for emergency contraception, early identification of pregnancy, and other unmet physical and mental health needs. In parallel, mental health risk assessments are vital for assessing self-harm and suicidal ideation.

Presentations of suspected CSA include the following (The Royal College of Paediatrics and Child Health (RCPCH), 2015 cited by Cutland, 2019, p. 7):

- Health – Pregnancy in a child under 16 years of age.
  - Sexually transmitted infection.
  - Anogenital trauma with an absent or implausible explanation.
- Behavioural – Harmful sexual behaviour.
  - Self-harm, anxiety and other mental health presentations.
  - Psychosomatic symptoms.
- Other – Siblings of victims of CSA.
  - A child living with an adult who poses a risk to children or is in contact with a sexual offender.

Guidelines on paediatric forensic investigations (RCPCH, 2017) outline elements of good practice including high quality photo documentation and familiarity with evidence-based guidance about the signs, for example when a child has perceived or actual medical problems such as recurrent vulvovaginitis. It is crucial that any doctor (paediatrician or forensic physician) who undertakes a forensic assessment of a child who may have been subjected to sexual abuse must have particular skills and the ability to communicate comfortably with children and carers about sensitive issues.

Neglect and the Emotional Impact of Chronic Trauma

Cumulative harms usually refer to more than one traumatic incident, resulting in chronic trauma (Bryce, 2019; HM Government, 2022). Weightman et al. (2012) quantified the cumulative harms associated with poor health of children within impoverished families and concluded that the intergenerational effects of social disadvantage on child health outcomes is indisputable. Domestic violence, substance misuse and mental ill health feature, alongside unemployment, poor educational attainment and chronic illness across the life-course. A recent briefing from an analysis of reviews from 2014 to 2017 highlighted the importance of identifying and responding to neglect, in the context of poverty, with attention to a child's physical, mental and emotional well-being in the family nexus (Brandon et al., 2020). UK health polices aim to better equip healthcare staff to identify and respond to the social determinants of health (NHS England, 2017, 2019; Public Health England, 2016). Potential signs of neglect include noticing an unusually silent or distressed child with development delay and behavioural problems, an unkempt infant or child living with food poverty, or dental caries. These issues may arise from benign neglect circumstances and/or compound other concerns about child health and social development.

Introduction to the Case Scenario

We derived the following composite case from serious case reviews and practice. While this situation is unique, the case represents some of the common risk factors encountered in assessment of children vulnerable to abuse or suffering maltreatment. From birth, infants may have had contact with midwives, neonatal nurses, children's nurses, health visitors, social workers and Child and Adolescent Mental Health Services (CAMHS).

In this chapter, the case is used to illustrate the role of health professionals in identifying and assessing medical indicators of potential abuse suffered by a young infant child on a child protection plan. The case involves physical injury and professional concerns regarding a looked after infant in a complex family situation.

CASE STUDY 21.1: HILDA, NANCY AND YVETTE

Nancy is 16 and has given birth recently to Hilda, aged 6 months. Hilda presented to the Accident & Emergency department of a local hospital following a reported child choking accident. The event involved Nancy's scarf, which had reportedly lodged in Hilda's mouth while she slept in her cot. Hilda's mother, Nancy, accompanied her to the hospital, with her foster carer, Yvette, whom she lives with. Yvette reported that she had popped in to say goodnight to Nancy and noticed Hilda was blue and struggling to breathe. Yvette reported that she had picked the baby up, pulled the scarf out of her mouth and performed resuscitative first aid. She directed Nancy to call an ambulance. The paramedics arrived promptly and reported that the baby was breathing but pale and floppy, with a rapid heart rate and reduced oxygenation. Hilda was responsive to stimulation. Paramedics were concerned about the impact of hypoxia (oxygen deficit) on Hilda during the choking episode, and they were unclear about the nature of the accident. Hilda was transferred to hospital by ambulance.

The initial physical health assessment focuses on immediate lifesaving needs, and it is the quality of the proximal relationships that suggest whether child safety and health is at risk within the family nexus (Bronfenbrenner & Morris, 1998; Ermond, 2019). Determining whether the choking episode was accidental or not relies upon thorough, accurate reporting of the physical injuries (Henderson, 2016; Hseih et al., 2015). In Hilda's case, emergency aid was appropriately sought and good history-taking enabled robust assessment of the physical state of the infant during and after the event. Holistic top to toe physical assessment of a child, under a protective care order, may involve many health and social care professionals, including the paediatric

and emergency care medical and nursing staff, neuroimaging and child social work (Mitchell, 2018).

ASSESSING MEDICAL INDICATORS OF ABUSE

The four categories of abuse are embedded within 'working together' guidance on multiagency assessment of risk of harm (Department for Education, 2018). We privilege physical health assessment here as a means towards establishing risk factors that may incorporate assessment for mental and/or emotional harms, sexual harms and neglect. Pain and injury are features of physical child abuse, and it is important to remember the presenting medical issue may be the tip of the iceberg (Brandon et al., 2020). Following the paramedic emergency response to child choking, Hilda's general health needs were assessed, according to her infant age (appropriate to her stage of development) and to identify any signs of child maltreatment (NICE, 2020). The NICE 2020 quality standard for identifying and responding to child abuse and neglect provides a framework for health professional and allied staff to involve parents and carers in assessment. This standard summarised the need for consistent support provision to those involved in parenting children and young people, including foster carers and other agencies involved. NICE (2013) produced several quality standards for maintaining health and well-being of looked after children and young people. Across these standards health professionals have a duty to ensure that all aspects of children's and young people's health needs are met by working in collaboration with partner agencies. Assessing the quality of the parenting relationship in the context of suspected harm or abuse is complex and requires attention to numerous medical indicators of abuse.

UNDERNUTRITION AND FAILURE TO THRIVE

Failure to thrive (FTT) is a medical term (Kessler, 1999) with psychosocial implications (Dubowitz and Black, 2018, p. 1). It is described as:

> less than expected growth over time during the first 3 years of life when tracked on appropriate growth charts for children of the same age and sex.... However, the definition varies between different healthcare providers, and the criteria used to diagnose the condition must be specified. FTT can be a pejorative term. Under-nutrition is a descriptive term for poor growth and is preferred because it is more specific than FTT; it does not compound the possible failure parents may feel due to their infant's poor growth.

Dubowitz and Black (2018) explain that the diagnosis requires assessment of growth within normative parameters relative to birth weight, familial trends and feeding patterns (weight; length/height, and head circumference over time). The authors advise that while medical and psychosocial indicators are relevant, extensive medical tests are usually not advised. Hospitalisation is reserved for severe cases. The authors concur that undernutrition can occur at all socioeconomic levels. Medical assessment and diagnosis of gastrointestinal disorders might be relevant and needs to incorporate assessment of dyadic feeding behaviour and responsiveness (Jameson et al., 2018). Early intervention is crucial to holistic child health needs assessment (Early Intervention Foundation, 2020; RCPCH, 2020).

SAFEGUARDING CHILDREN IN HOSPITALS

In England, the NHS Long Term Plan (LTP) (NHS, 2019c) set out the role and responsibilities for health professionals to ensure 'everyone gets the best start in life'. New Sustainability and Transformation Partnerships (STPs) and Integrated Care Systems (ICSs) comprise local NHS organisations working together with local councils and others, to develop and implement 5-year strategies for improving population health through collaborative cross-boundary working. Safeguarding children is a professional duty of care in all

CASE STUDY 21.2: A FOCUS ON FAILURE TO THRIVE

In this scenario, Hilda's growth was imperative to establish whether she was maintaining her birth weight and feeding well, or beginning to show the medical signs of what is currently commonly referred to as FTT (indicated by undernutrition over a period of time) (Kuczmarski et al., 2000). Lord Laming's review (Laming, 2013) and others (Brandon et al., 2020, Sidebotham et al., 2016) persistently showed child emaciation and starvation in serious case reviews. In this case, full body examination should ascertain whether malnourishment is present and establish any bruising or injuries to body parts. Examination of Hilda's skeletal system, limbs, torso and orifices will help assess for abrasions, marks, tears, discolouration and any unexplained injuries that may require further investigation.

Hilda's skin colour and body temperature were also measured to help gather medical evidence of her overall health and the physical impact of the harms endured during the asphyxia (choking) event she suffered. Regular nursing monitoring of her vital signs, including her blood pressure, respirations and peripheral oxygenation, contributed to the holistic physical assessment and clinical investigations. This helped form a collaborative medical and nursing narrative of child health, allowing related psychosocial explanations to inform her care plan and emerge over time, in conversation with her mother, foster carer and the wider child protection team and network.

NHS provider contexts, and it is a strategic driver in local and national Clinical Commissioning Groups (CCGs) (HM Government, 2018; Department for Education, 2018; Hood et al., 2017).

Safeguarding children in hospital requires multiple roles and resources, including acute 'A-E' assessment of fast deteriorating child health in ambulatory domiciliary and in-patient neonatal units (Rogers and Nurse, 2019). When a child choking situation at home involves emergency admission to hospital, other indicators of child vulnerability and risk should involve notification to local emergency safeguarding procedures (Jameson et al., 2018).

In a health service, the paramedic team are often first responders in the domiciliary home. Their observations about the immediate environment are crucial, and they may have to consider whether the local A&E or field hospital is the appropriate route for child medical assessment.

Immediate referral to the Multi-Agency Safeguarding Hub (MASH) team will instigate telephone triage (and perhaps virtual consultations) to determine the best pathway to appropriate medical care. Following the ambulance transfer to hospital, healthcare professionals will need to assess the child while noting parental and carer responsibilities and behaviours in caring for the child, including foster care and/or kinship care. Assessing extrafamilial relationships and arrangements that impact upon the child's lived experience is vital to safeguarding in hospitals to ensure the child is protected.

Key Healthcare Professionals Who Play a Role in Child Safeguarding

Health professionals and healthcare contexts are fast diversifying, representing multiple disciplines. Doctors, nurses, midwives and allied health professionals dominate – the latter including pharmacists, speech and language therapists, physiotherapists, diagnostic radiographers, radiotherapists, occupational therapists, operating department practitioners, psychologists, counsellors, dentists and others (Public Health England, 2016; RCN, 2019). Good hospital care relies upon information sharing with other agencies, including the GP in primary care, who should be able to signpost to any specialist healthcare professionals involved such as the Family Nurse Practitioner (FNP) in some localities. FNPs in the UK are a less utilised resource but are often involved in caring for adolescent mothers and families with high health and social needs (FNP, 2020). Medical doctors and nurses represent multiple specialisms, including primary care, paediatrics and child health, acute medicine, surgery, rehabilitation, maternity services and community and public health. Healthcare support workers and assistants, who often have regular and close contact with children, also work within and outside of the NHS, social care and voluntary sector. Within the statutory sector, midwives, health visitors, nursery nurses, school nurses, family support workers and child and adolescent mental health workers often work in child protection. Specialist safeguarding roles include named nurses and doctors for child protection and child deaths and paediatricians for sexual violence (RCN, 2019).

Vulnerable children require health professionals to be aware of their safeguarding responsibilities, embedded in professional, regulatory codes of practice. Over the past 20 years, NHS workplace policies and operational procedures routinely recommend general safeguarding training for all staff, and specialist provision for staff working in services with close and regular contact with children and families. Child safeguarding skills and competencies for healthcare staff are also informed by NICE (2015, 2020) as well as specialist guidance published by Public Health England (2016, 2019). There is a plethora of guidance, much of which is specific to healthcare disciplines and the contexts in which they practice. Recent updates include safeguarding guidance for general practice reporting (NHS England, 2019), identifying and preventing child female genital mutilation (NHS England, 2018), child sexual exploitation (NHS England, 2017a,b) and guidance for mental health services in preventing radicalisation (NHS England, 2017c).

Although safeguarding children is everybody's responsibility, some healthcare staff are especially involved due to their early point of contact with pregnant women and children. Midwives, neonatal nurses, health visitors and paediatrician roles are vital to early detection and recognition of children at risk of harm and in need. Designated safeguarding roles for doctors and nurses complement such roles and provide better intercollegiate linking between hospital, primary care and community settings. Working across adult and child protection services is vital to coordinated information sharing and responses to hospital admissions and discharge planning. In Table 21.1, we summarise the role of six of the principal healthcare professionals involved with child welfare and safeguarding work.

Managing Disclosures and Referring to Social Services

Legal and procedural frameworks underpin healthcare responses to disclosures about children at risk of or experiencing abuse. NICE provides a range of standards for health and social care, including guidance on how to identify and manage child abuse and

TABLE 21.1			
Key Healthcare Professionals Who Play a Role in Child Safeguarding			
Role	**Overview of Role**	**Where Do They Work?**	**Role Within Hospital and Community Safeguarding**
Midwives	Midwives are responsible for the care of pregnant mothers and babies up until 28 days following childbirth, when their statutory duties cease. At this point, they usually hand over care to the health visitors. Although their contact is relatively short-term, they often offer intensive health promotion and welfare support to ensure their safeguarding responsibilities are realised.	In hospital (usually on dedicated maternity and neonatal wards) and in community settings (e.g. within a GP surgery or primary care clinic). Some community midwives carry out outreach work, visiting women and families at home	Midwives tend to play an important, albeit often time limited, role in the multidisciplinary safeguarding team. However, some midwives are employed in specialist roles, involving regular monitoring and supervision of vulnerable women and children, including those experiencing domestic violence and abuse (PHE, 2019) and women with problematic substance misuse. These specialist midwives often play a key role in multidisciplinary teams and tend to support women and babies for longer than hospital based and community midwife colleagues.
Neonatal nurses	Neonatal nurses specialise in caring for premature infants. Prematurity and low birth weight are indicators of health risk, suggesting small babies are likely to have poorer health outcomes across their life-course.	In hospitals, usually on specialist wards	Neonatal nurses can and do identify families who present with potential indicators of abuse and neglect as well as identifying parents whose behaviours might make those babies more vulnerable to abuse and neglect. Their role in assessing the health needs of vulnerable infants is also vital to multiagency information sharing.
Health visitors (HVs)	In the UK, health visiting is a universal service for children and families from 0 to 19 years with a particular focus on the under fives. One important aspect of health visitors' work is to carry out, by statutory requirement, five developmental assessments of children, from 28 weeks in pregnancy to 30 months (PHE, 2017). They run regular 'drop-in' child health clinics in communities and primary care, to enable families to seek parenting advice, non-medical prescribing for minor ailments and the recommended 'Healthy Start' vitamin supplementation.	In the community, both within clinic settings and visiting children and families at home. HVs will also liaise with school nurses (SNs): [SNs in England cover large geographical areas/ caseloads for population health]	Health visitors are nurses and/ or midwives with additional qualifications. They draw on psychological and behaviour theories to guide work on supporting parents with issues such as feeding, sleeping, toileting issues and bonding. Health visitors play a vital role in supporting the transition to parenthood and in promoting perinatal and postnatal mental health. They provide enhanced and specialist services to populations with additional health or social needs (e.g. women and children with disabilities or complex illnesses, looked after children, asylum seeking and homeless populations, teenage parents, etc.). HVs deliver, supervise and delegate child development assessment and universal child health services though the Healthy Child Programme in the UK.

Continued

TABLE 21.1
Key Healthcare Professionals Who Play a Role in Child Safeguarding—cont'd

Role	Overview of Role	Where Do They Work?	Role Within Hospital and Community Safeguarding
Paediatricians	Paediatrics is a specialist area of medicine, dealing with the medical needs of infants, children, and young people in primary, secondary and tertiary care.	In community (often specialist clinic) and hospital settings	Paediatricians play a key role at several important processes associated with child protection and safeguarding: for example, leading a medical assessment of a child when there are concerns about physical or sexual abuse, and assessing the health needs of children in care. When a child has complex or ongoing health needs, a paediatrician may be a core member of the inter-agency team around the child.
Designated nurses for safeguarding	Named and designated nurses for child protection (England, Wales and Northern Ireland) work in many specialties and have additional interests in and responsibilities for safeguarding children.	In hospital or community settings	The Royal College of Nursing (RCN) characterises the role as: provides safeguarding, child protection expertise and leadership throughout health and multiagency partnerships. The designated safeguarding role is distinct, and there are efforts to protect the position due to a lack of sustained investment in the designated nurse programme nationally.
Designated doctors for safeguarding	Like nurses, named and designated doctors for child protection (England, Wales and Northern Ireland) work in many specialties and have additional interests in and responsibilities for safeguarding children. Their roles are summarised in the intercollegiate competency framework (RCN, 2019).	Designated doctors' roles often bridge hospital and community services	Designated doctors take a lead responsibility for child welfare and safeguarding issues and play a key role within healthcare teams on such matters. They receive additional training and are likely to have considerable experience working with children with additional needs and/ or in safeguarding contexts.

neglect (NICE, 2020). NHS England Safeguarding provides resources to help professionals work together to protect children and young people (and adults) from harm. Reports and rapid reviews include those associated with child criminal exploitation, sexual exploitation, female genital mutilation, modern slavery, county lines, human trafficking and domestic violence and abuse. The NHS England Safeguarding app raises professional awareness of safeguarding requirements, including how to make a social services referral. Managing disclosures of child abuse or exploring the risk of it taking place requires health professionals to undertake sensitive conversations. Developing confidence to undertake such conversations and refer to

social services requires training, education and skill, drawing on research-informed practice frameworks that encourage cross-sectoral and specialist support for intersecting problems, such as domestic violence and abuse (Bradbury-Jones et al., 2016a,b,c; Bradbury-Jones et al., 2017). An added dimension of complexity in such situations are professionals' different conceptualisations of, and ways of addressing risk and safety in, children and young people's lives.

In the NHS, the new CP-IS system links IT systems across health and social care, sharing basic information about children subject to child protection plans or who are children in care. Identified by their NHS number, the CP-IS is endorsed by the Care Quality Commission

(CQC) and included in the 2019 NHS Standard Contract for providers of unscheduled and scheduled care. This is a relatively new national programme in the UK, aiming to share relevant data between children's social care and unscheduled health care settings in order to protect children at risk of harm. Its success is dependent on good operational use of the technologies across sectors (NHS Digital, 2020b).

Allegations Against Staff and Employment Practices (DBS)

It is not unusual for allegations against staff to be made during child protection, sometimes involving parental or carer counterclaims and/or medical litigation (NHS England and NHS Health Improvement, 2013a). The management of risk is based on assessment of claims about harm and abuse. Definitions of harm can be found in NHS England and NHS Healthcare Improvement (2013) guidance on *Safeguarding Children and Young People, Adult Safeguarding: Roles and Competencies for Health Care Staff* (2018) and the Care Act (2014). The Francis Inquiry recommended a statutory duty to be open with people when things go wrong. This 'Duty of Candour' is regulated by the CQC and triggered by a 'notifiable safety incident' for any 'unintended or unexpected incident that has occurred in respect of all service users during the provision of a regulated activity' (NHS England and NHS Improvement, 2013b).

Safeguarding against organisational or institutional abuse perpetrated by healthcare staff is a less explored area of child protection. Should a member of healthcare staff be considered to pose a risk to children (or might have committed a criminal offence against one or more children), the Working Together (HM Government, 2018) guidance stipulates that information must be shared with the Local Authority Designated Officer (LADO). To protect the public, health professionals are subject to routine checks on entering NHS and social care employment. The statutory scheme for undertaking the checks is administered by the UK government Disclosure and Barring Service (DBS) (UK Government DBS, 2013). The DBS checks are important to identifying people barred from undertaking regulated activity with children and adults. Intelligence checks provide evidence at the time. Gibson (2020) reminded that even if a person's DBS check is satisfactory, it does not mean they do not pose a future risk. Employers should refer to Schedule 3 of the Health and Social Care Act (2008) (Regulated Activities) and Regulations (2014) which stipulates what information is required for people appointed for the purpose of regulated healthcare activity.

FUTURE DIRECTIONS

The way UK health professionals respond to childhood trauma, abuse and inequality has shifted over the past 10 years. Influenced by strategic guidance, digitisation, partner disciplines (such as social work), emerging research and innovation in health systems internationally, the NHS is embracing new ways of thinking about and responding to disadvantaged and 'vulnerable' children. We set out two examples of this changing approach: (1) Public health approaches to tackling violence and abuse; and (2) Trauma-informed care. Although these are not in themselves 'safeguarding' systems, the concepts and techniques that they encompass are likely to shape how health professionals working in a variety of roles identify, respond to and support children who are at risk of harm in all practice settings.

Public Health Approaches to Tackling Abuse and Violence

Safeguarding children in healthcare contexts is gaining ground as a public health and NHS priority in England (NHS England, 2017a,b,c, 2019a,b,c). The public health approach to violence – encompassing domestic violence, serious violent crime and child abuse – is foregrounded on the assumption that violence is not inevitable, it can be prevented and interventions, especially in childhood, can make a real difference to people's lives. The public health approach also stresses that violence is a major cause of ill health, poor well-being and is closely linked to social inequalities (Bellis et al., 2012). Adopting a public health approach is characterised as thinking about violence in a similar way to an infectious disease, recognising that there are complex, intersecting factors that affect the infection's spread. Effective prevention and minimisation of harm requires good-quality evidence and the coordinated involvement of multiple public services, including health, police and social care (HM Government, 2022). Public health approaches also tend to emphasise the importance of working with and alongside communities, adopting a collaborative approach and challenging narratives that normalise or accept violence.

Over the past 10 years, the approach has been an increasingly common feature of health policy and practice. Led by successful initiatives in Scotland, particularly in relation to knife and gang-related crime, it is gaining momentum across England and Wales (HM Government, 2022). In 2019, the UK government announced that a legal duty will be placed on public bodies to work together to prevent and reduce serious violence. However, it remains unclear how the policy will be practically implemented and how the focus of police work can be shifted to tackling the root causes of inequalities and cultures of violence, rather than criminalisation alone.

Trauma-Informed Care

There has been a movement across different parts of the devolved NHS to embed a 'trauma-informed' approach, for example in health services for children with mental health problems, children in care, and forensic and therapeutic services for children and adults who have experienced sexual abuse. A trauma-informed approach asks the question, 'what has happened to you?' rather than 'what is wrong with you?' (Sweeney et al., 2018). As a result, trauma-informed practitioners work with people in a holistic way, communicate with thoughtfulness and compassion, and are willing and able to engage with complexity. Key dimensions of a trauma-informed approach include enabling people to talk about their lives, problems and strengths in their own words; responding to people with insight and empathy; offering support that is timely, holistic and person-centred; and consistently checking and seeking to understand a person's needs throughout their care or treatment (Wilton and Williams, 2019). The adoption of trauma-informed approaches indicates that healthcare systems are increasingly trying to identify and respond to children and adults' life-course experience of harm – which may include abuse, inequality or trauma – and this step-change may support interprofessional working

with families where there are child protection concerns (Reeves, 2015; Sperlich et al., 2017). However, there are evident challenges to rolling out this way of working amongst professionals who tend to use more clinical and diagnosis-orientated approaches and may not work within a 'system' that is itself trauma-informed.

CONCLUSION

Health professionals are increasingly aware of the intergenerational, contextual safeguarding factors that impact on their roles, reflecting real world complexity and challenges for healthcare (Brandon et al., 2020; Department for Education, 2020; Firmin, 2020). In this chapter, we have highlighted the roles of some of the key healthcare professionals regularly involved in child welfare and safeguarding. Their roles are complex and varied; however, we focused on three of the principal contexts in which health professionals may become involved in safeguarding: (1) identifying and responding to medical indicators of abuse, (2) concerns about a child's potential failure to thrive and (3) safeguarding children in hospital. Hilda and Nancy's journey serves as a way of exploring the legal and procedural impacts on one family's experiences of the intersection between health and safeguarding in NHS contexts. Here, we emphasise the importance of partnership working at every point of contact with children and families with healthcare services and suggest greater attention to the embodied relational nature of child abuse as it may emerge across the life-course. The following reflective questions aim to help the reader consider their role, recognising social factors that increase the likelihood of harm to children.

REFLECTIVE QUESTIONS

The following reflective questions aim to help the reader consider the embodied nature of child experience, recognising the social factors that increase the likelihood of harm to children in complex care relationships. We encourage discursive practice within and outside of healthcare, considering multiagency research and responsibilities for safeguarding children from harm.

- What type of cumulative harms are likely to adversely impact upon health across the life-course?
- Why is it important to identify and assess child weight and height during routine physical examination?

■ What medical and clinical investigations might be incorporated into health assessment for an infant admitted to hospital with a suspected abusive injury or trauma?

■ What is the protective role of midwives and health visitors in safeguarding children from abuse?

■ What protective support can health professionals provide to help support a looked after child following an adverse health incident or event?

FURTHER READING

- Institute of Health Visiting: https://ihv.org.uk/.
- NHS England Safeguarding: https://www.england.nhs.uk/safeguarding/.
- NHS Digital: https://digital.nhs.uk/services/child-protection-information-sharing-project.
- National Institute for Health and Care Excellence (NICE): https://www.nice.org.uk/.
- Public Health England: https://www.gov.uk/government/publications/healthy-child-programme-rapid-review-on-safeguarding.
- Royal College of Nursing: https://www.rcn.org.uk/get-involved/forums/children-and-young-people-staying-healthy-forum/communities/safeguarding-children-and-young-people.
- Royal College of Paediatrics and Child Health: https://www.rcpch.ac.uk/sites/default/files/2019-08/safeguarding_cyp_-_roles_and_competencies_for_paediatricians_-_august_2019_0.pdf.

REFERENCES

Bellis, M., Hughes, K., Perkins, C. and Bennett, A., 2012. Protecting People, Promoting Health - A public health approach to violence prevention in England. [online] Department of Health. https://assets.publishing.service.gov.uk/government/uploads/system/uploads/attachment_data/file/216977/Violence-prevention.pdf

Bradbury-Jones, C., Clark, M., 2016a. How to address domestic violence and abuse. Nurs. Times 12, 1–4 online issue.

Bradbury-Jones, C., Clark, M., 2016b. Intimate partner violence and the role of community nurses. Prim. Health Care, Online issue 26 (9), 42–47. https://doi.org/10.7748/phc.2016.e1184.

Bradbury-Jones, C., Clark, M., Parry, J., Taylor, J., 2016c. Development of a practice framework for improving nurses' responses to intimate partner violence. J. Clin. Nurs. https://doi.org/10.1111/jocn.13276.

Bradbury-Jones, C., Taylor, J., Clark, M., 2017. Abused women's experiences of a primary care identification and referral intervention: A case study analysis. J. Adv. Nurs. 73 (12), 3189–3199. https://doi.org/10.1111/jan.13250.

Bradbury-Jones, C., Isham, L., Morris, A.J., Taylor, J., 2019. The "neglected" relationship between child maltreatment and oral health? An international scoping review of research. Trauma, Violence, & Abuse 22 (2), 265–276.

Brandon, M., Sidebotham, P., Belderson, P., Cleaver, H., Dickens, J., Garstang, J., et al., 2020. Complexity and Challenge: A Triennial Analysis of Serious Case Reviews 2014-2017. Department for Education, London.

Bronfenbrenner, U., Morris, P.A., 1998. The ecology of developmental process. In: Damon, W., Lerner, R.M. (Eds.), Handbook of Child Psychology, Vol. 1: Theoretical Models of Human Development. vol. 1, fifth ed. Wiley, New York, pp. 992–1028.

Bryce, I., 2019. Cumulative harm: Chronicity, revictimisation, and developmental victimology. In: Bryce, I., Robinson, Y., Petherick, W. (Eds.), Child Abuse and Neglect. Academic Press, Cambridge, MA, pp. 151–173. https://doi.org/10.1016/B978-0-12-815344-4.00009-X.

Care Act, 2014. https://www.legislation.gov.uk/ukpga/2014/23/contents/enacted

Cutland, M, 2019. The Role and Scope of Medical Examinations When There are Concerns About Child Sexual Abuse. Centre of Expertise on Child Sexual Abuse. www.csacentre.org.uk (Accessed 23 April 2023).

Chandon, J.S., Keerthy, D., Okoth, K.O., Gokhale, K.M., Raza, K., Bandyopadhyay, S., et al., 2020. The association between exposure to childhood maltreatment and the subsequent development of functional somatic and visceral pain syndromes. eClinicalMedicine 23:100392.

Department for Education and the Department for Health and Social Care, 2015. Promoting the Health and Wellbeing of Looked-After Children: Statutory Guidance on the Planning, Commissioning and Delivery of Health Services for Looked-After Children. https://www.gov.uk/government/publications/promoting-the-health-and-wellbeing-of-looked-after-children--2. (Accessed 29 February 2020).

Department for Education, 2018. Working Together to Safeguard Children – A Guide to Inter-Agency Working to Safeguard and Promote the Welfare of Children. Department for Education, London. www.gov.uk/government/uploads/ system/uploads/attachment_data/ file/729914/Working_Together_to_Safeguard_Children-2018.pdf. (Accessed 29 February 2020).

Department for Education, 2020. Complexity and Challenge: Triennial Analysis of Serious Case Reviews 2014-17. Department for Education, London. https://www.gov.uk/government/publications/analysis-of-serious-case-reviews-2014-to-2017.

Dubowitz, H., Black, M., 2018. Failure to thrive. Summary. BMJ Best Practice. https://bestpractice.bmj.com/topics/en-gb/747#referencePop2. (Accessed 19 October 2020).

Early Intervention Foundation, 2020. Adverse Childhood Experiences: What We Know, What We Don't Know and What Should Happen Next. https://www.eif.org.uk/files/pdf/adverse-childhood-experiences-report.pdf. (Accessed 24 February 2020).

Ermond, A., 2019. Health for all Children, fifth ed. Oxford University Press, Oxford.

Family Nurse Partnership (FNP), 2020. FNP adapt. Family Nurse Partnership. https://fnp.nhs.uk/. (Accessed 19 October 2020).

Firmin, C., 2020. Contextual Safeguarding and Child Protection: Rewriting the Rules. Routledge, London. https://doi.org/10.4324/9780429283314.

Gibson, K., 2020. NHS safeguarding – back to basics (1 of 3). FutureNHS Collaboration Platform. https://future.nhs.uk/. (Accessed 15 October 2020).

Heads, D., 2013. Dental caries in children: A sign of maltreatment or abuse? Nurs. Child. Young People 25 (6), 22–24.

Henderson, R., 2016. Choking and Foreign Body Airway Obstruction. Professional Reference Article Patient. https://patient.info/doctor/choking-and-foreign-body-airway-obstruction-fbao. (Accessed 29 February 2020).

Harris, J.C., 2018. The mouth and maltreatment: Safeguarding issues in child dental health. Arch. Dis. Child. 103 (8), 722–729.

Health and Social Care Act, 2008. https://www.legislation.gov.uk/ukpga/2008/14/contents

HM Government (Gov.uk), 2022. Serious Case Reviews; Analysis Lessons and Challenges. https://www.gov.uk/government/publications/serious-case-reviews-analysis-lessons-and-challenges

HM Government, 2018. Serious Violence Strategy. HMSO, London. https://assets.publishing.service.gov.uk/government/uploads/system/uploads/attachment_data/file/698009/serious-violence-strategy.pdf. (Accessed 29 February 2020).

HM Government, 2004. Children Act 2004. HMSO, London. http://www.legislation.gov.uk/ukpga/2004/31.

Hood, R., Price, J., Sartori, D., Maisey, D., Johnson, J., Clark, Z., 2017. Collaborating across the threshold: The development of interprofessional expertise in child safeguarding. J. Interprof. Care 31 (6), 705–713.

Hseih, K.L.-C., Zimmerman, R.A., Kao, H.W., Chen, C.-Y., 2015. Revisiting neuroimaging of abusive head trauma in infant and young children. Am. J. Roentol. 204, 944–952 2015.

Hudson, B., 2005. Information sharing and children's services reform in England: Can legislation change practice? J. Interprof. Care 19 (6), 537–546.

Hughes, K., Bellis, M., Hardcastle, K., Sethi, D., Buthchart, A., Mikton, C., 2017. The effect of multiple adverse childhood experiences on health; a systematic review and meta-analysis. The Lancet (Public Health) 2 (8), 356–366.

Jameson, M., Fehringer, K., Neu, M., 2018. Comparison of two tools to assess dyad feeding interaction in infants with gastroesophageal reflux disease. J. Spec. Pediatr. Nurs. 23 (1). https://doi.org/10.1111/jspn.12203.

Kellogg, N., 2005. Oral and dental aspects of child abuse and neglect. Clinical Report. Pediatrics 116 (6), 1565–1568.

Kessler, D.B., 1999. Failure to thrive and pediatric undernutrition: Historical and theoretical context. In: Kessler, D.B., Dawson, P. (Eds.), Failure to Thrive and Pediatric Undernutrition. Paul H. Brookes Publishing, Baltimore, MD, pp. 3–18.

Kuczmarski, R.J., Ogden, C.L., Guo, S.S., et al., 2002 May. 2000 CDC growth charts for the United States: Methods and development. Vital Health Stat 11 (246), 1–190.

Laming, L., 2013. The Victoria Climbie Inquiry. http://dera.ioe.ac.uk/6086/2/climbiereport.pdf. (Accessed 21 February 2020).

Leeds City Council (LCC), 2020. The Common Assessment Framework. https://www.leeds.gov.uk/children-and-families/common-assessment-framework.

Local Government Association, 2019. Health Visiting; Giving Children the Best Start in Life. https://www.local.gov.uk/health-visiting-giving-children-best-start-life.

Maguire, S.A., Kemp, A.M., Lumb, R.C., Farewell, D.M., 2011. Estimating the probability of abusive head trauma: A pooled analysis. Pediatrics 128, e550–e564 2011.

Malik, N.S., Munoz, B., deCourcy, C., Imran, R., Kwang, C.L., Cehembumroona, S., et al., 2020. Violence related injuries in a UK city; Epidemiology and impact on secondary care resources. EClinicalMedicine 20. https://doi.org/10.1016/j.eclinm.2020.100296.

Mitchell, W., 2018. NHS Great Glasgow and Clyde Paediatric Guidelines: Recognition and Management of Maltreatment in Infants (Children Under the Age of 1). https://www.clinicalguidelines.scot.nhs.uk/ggc-paediatric-guidelines/ggc-guidelines/child-protection/recognition-and-management-of-maltreatment-in-infants-children-under-the-age-of-1/. (Accessed 29 February 2020).

National FGM Centre, 2018. Mardoche Yembi: Advice for professionals. National FGM Centre, London. http://nationalfgmcentre.org.uk/calfb/. (Accessed 9 November 2020).

National Institute for Health and Care Excellence (NICE), 2013. Looked-after Children and Young People (QS31). https://www.nice.org.uk/guidance/qs31/resources.

National Institute for Health and Care Excellence (NICE), 2019. Head injury: Assessment and Early Management. Clinical guideline [CG176] NICE. https://www.nice.org.uk/guidance/cg176.

National Institute for Health and Care Excellence (NICE), 2020. Child Abuse and Neglect Overview NICE. https://pathways.nice.org.uk/pathways/child-abuse-and-neglect.

NHS Digital, 2020. (a) Child Protection – Information Sharing Project NHS Digital. https://digital.nhs.uk/services/child-protection-information-sharing-project.

NHS Digital, 2020. (b) DCB1609: Child Protection – Information Sharing NHS Digital. https://digital.nhs.uk/data-and-information/information-standards/information-standards-and-data-collections-including-extractions/publications-and-notifications/standards-and-collections/dcb1609-child-protection-information-sharing.

NHS England, 2017a. Child Sexual Exploitation: Advice for Healthcare Staff. https://www.england.nhs.uk/publication/child-sexual-exploitation-advice-for-healthcare-staff/.

NHS England, 2017b. Guidance for Designated Professionals Safeguarding Children and Child Protection Information Sharing (CP-IS). https://www.england.nhs.uk/publication/guidance-for-designated-professionals-safeguarding-children-and-child-protection-information-sharing-cp-is/.

NHS England, 2017c. Guidance for Mental Health Services in Exercising Duties to Safeguard People from the Risk of Radicalisation. https://www.england.nhs.uk/publication/guidance-for-mental-health-services-in-exercising-duties-to-safeguard-people-from-the-risk-of-radicalisation/.

NHS England, 2018. Female Genital Mutilation: Standards for Training Healthcare Professionals. https://www.england.nhs.uk/publication/female-genital-mutilation-standards-for-training-healthcare-professionals/.

NHS England, 2019a. NHS England Safeguarding: Annual update 2018/2019. https://www.england.nhs.uk/publication/safeguarding-annual-update/.

NHS England, 2019b. Safeguarding Children and Vulnerable Adults: General Practice Reporting: Supporting Documents. https://www.england.nhs.uk/wp-content/uploads/2015/07/B0818_Safeguarding-children-young-people-and-adults-at-risk-in-the-NHS-Safeguarding-accountability-and-assuran.pdf.

NHS England, 2019c. The NHS Long Term Plan. (Accessed 29 May 2023). www.longtermplan.nhs.uk

NHS England and NHS Improvement, 2013a. (Updated 2019) Managing Safeguarding Allegations against Staff: Policies and Procedures. https://www.england.nhs.uk/wp-content/uploads/2019/09/managing-safeguarding-allegations.pdf.

NHS England and NHS Improvement, 2013b. (Updated 2019) Safeguarding Children, Young people and Adults at Risk in the NHS: Safeguarding Accountability and Assurance Framework. https://www.england.nhs.uk/wp-content/uploads/2015/07/safeguarding-children-young-people-adults-at-risk-saaf.pdf.

NICE, 2015. Children's Attachment: Attachment in Children and Young People who are Adopted from Care, in Care or at High Risk of Going into Care NICE Guideline [NG26]. https://www.nice.org.uk/guidance/ng26. (Accessed 28 November 2020).

NICE, 2020. Child Abuse and Neglect Overview. NICE Interactive Pathway [NG76]. https://pathways.nice.org.uk/pathways/child-abuse-and-neglect. (Accessed 28 November 2020).

Noorazma, S., Shahrom, A.W., Suhani, M.,N., 2006. Identification of perpetrator by metric analysis of bite marks: A case report. J. Forensic Med. Toxicol. 23 (2), 29–32.

Oral, R., Ramirez, M., Coohey, C., et al., 2016. Adverse childhood experiences and trauma informed care: The future of health care. Pediatr Res 79, 227–233. https://doi.org/10.1038/pr.2015.197.

Passàli, D., Lauriello, M., Bellussi, L., Passali, G.C., Passali, F.M., Gregori, D., 2010. Foreign body inhalation in children: An update. Acta Otorhinolaryngol Ital. Feb 30 (1), 27–32.

Public Health England, 2016. Health Matters; Giving Every Child the Best Start in Life. https://www.gov.uk/government/publications/health-matters-giving-every-child-the-best-start-in-life/health-matters-giving-every-child-the-best-start-in-life.

Public Health England, 2017. Review of Mandation of the Universal Health Visiting Service. https://assets.publishing.service.gov.uk/government/uploads/system/uploads/attachment_data/file/592893/Review_of_mandation_universal_health_visiting_service.pdf.

Public Health England, 2019. A Whole-System Multi-Agency Approach to Serious Violence Prevention: A Resource for Local System Leaders in England. PHE Publications, London. https://assets.publishing.service.gov.uk/media/5e38133d40f0b609169cb532/multi-agency_approach_to_serious_violence_prevention.pdf

Reeves, E., 2015. A synthesis of the literature on trauma-informed care. Issues Ment. Health Nurs. 36 (9), 698–709.

Rogers, A., Nurse, S., 2019. Child protection in the neonatal unit. J. Neonatal Nurs. 25, 99–101.

Royal College of Nursing, 2019. Safeguarding children and young people: Roles and competencies for healthcare staff. In: Intercollegiate Document, fourth ed. Royal College of Nursing. https://www.rcn.org.uk/professional-development/publications/pub-007366. (Accessed 27 November 2020).

Royal College of Paediatrics and Child Health, 2017. State of Child Health Report. https://www.rcpch.ac.uk/state-of-child-health. (Accessed 1 March 2020).

Royal College of Paediatrics and Child Health, 2020. The State of Child Health in the UK. https://stateofchildhealth.rcpch.ac.uk/.

Sidebotham, P., Brandon, M., Bailey, S., Belderson, P., Dodsworth, J., Garstang, J., E., et al., 2016. Pathways to Harm, Pathways to Protection: A Triennial Analysis of Serious Case Reviews 2011 to 2014. Department for Education, London.

Sperlich, M., Seng, J.S., Li, Y., Taylor, J., Bradbury–Jones, C., 2017. Integrating trauma–informed care into maternity care practice: Conceptual and practical issues. Journal of Midwifery & Women's Health 62 (6), 661–672.

Sweeney, A., Filson, B., Kennedy, A., Collison, L., Gillard, S., 2018. A paradigm shift: Relationships in trauma-informed mental health services. BJPsych Adv. Sep 24 (5), 319–333. https://doi.org/10.1192/bja.2018.29.

Taylor J, Corlett J, 2007. Health practitioners and safeguarding children. In Wilson K, James A (Eds). The Child Protection Handbook. Third edition. Baillière Tindall, London, 301–317.

UK Government Disclosure, Service, Barring, 2013. DBS Checks; Detailed Guidance. https://www.gov.uk/government/collections/dbs-checking-service-guidance--2.

Weightman, A.L., Morgan, H.E., Shepherd, M.A., et al., 2012. Social inequality and infant health in the UK: Systematic review and meta-analyses. BMJ Open 2:e000964. https://doi.org/10.1136/bmjopen-2012-00096.

Wilton, J., & Williams, A. Engaging with Complexity: Providing Effective Trauma-Informed Care for women. Centre for Mental Health, Mental Health Foundation and Health and Well-being Alliance. https://www.centreformentalhealth.org.uk/sites/default/files/2019-05/CentreforMH_EngagingWithComplexity.pdf.

World Health Organisation, 2010. EPHO: Health Promotion including Action to Address Social Determinants and Health Inequity World Health Organisation (Europe). World Health Organisation, Geneva. https://www.euro.who.int/en/health-topics/Health-systems/public-health-services/policy/the-10-essential-public-health-operations/epho4-health-promotion-including-action-to-address-social-determinants-and-health-inequity.

SAFEGUARDING IN SPORT AND LEISURE

NICK SLINN ■ MICHELLE NORTH

KEY POINTS

- The key roles that sport plays in the lives of children in the UK.
- The diverse structure and organisation of sport and the implications for safeguarding arrangements.
- The core safeguarding standards which exist for sections of the sport sector.
- Ways in which sport presents specific safeguarding challenges, as well as opportunities to promote children's welfare.
- The key factors child protection professionals need to clarify when responding to safeguarding concerns arising within, or linked to, sports settings.

INTRODUCTION

With millions of young people taking part in sport and physical activity every week across the UK, it is essential that those working with children within Social Care recognise and understand the significant part that the sector can play in a young person's life. Involvement in sport can improve children's physical and mental health, and help develop social skills and network. For many children it provides an outlet from difficulties elsewhere in their lives and offers opportunities to develop meaningful relationships with positive adult role models. However, there have been a number of cases where adults have used sport as a vehicle to access and harm children which

have recently come to the attention of the press and court systems. See for example the non-recent abuse cases in football, the identification of a bullying culture in British Cycling and the widespread sexual abuse by Larry Nasser in US Gymnastics (see British Cycling, 2017; BBC, 2018; NPCC, 2018). Perpetrators are drawn to the sports environment much as they are to residential institutions, religious settings or education establishments which facilitate access to children and young people. These high-profile cases have driven a greater appreciation of the significance and relevance of the sports sector on the part of statutory agencies tasked with safeguarding children.

Sport is increasingly playing a positive part in providing a safe environment for young participants. And, over the past 20 years, the sector in the UK has worked hard to develop safeguarding structures and practices to ensure children and young people are protected from harm and abuse. This is not solely about identifying and responding to people who pose a risk to children; it also involves adopting preventative measures that can help identify and respond to any wider welfare concerns that children may face in any context, for example peer bullying and mental health concerns.

Increasingly government and other sectors recognise sport's potential to engage harder to reach communities and address wider societal issues (e.g. obesity, knife crime and antisocial behaviour). Over recent years high level strategies for sport and physical activity have reflected this. For example, Sport

England's 2021–31 strategy looks to tackle a range of social issues including inequality, and promotes increased access to sport and physical activity through GPs to address a range of physical and mental health issues (Sport England). There has also been increased focus on alternative, non-traditional sports and activities (e.g. parkour, parkrun or dancing for fitness), as a means to engage more inactive people.

SPORT AND PHYSICAL ACTIVITY STRUCTURES IN THE UK

The way youth sport and activity is structured and delivered is very diverse. It extends from informal community-based activities (sometimes delivered by a single individual), through to organised club, league and competition structures, to elite level international sport. Activities take place in a variety of environments from public spaces, schools and leisure centres to purpose-built facilities and private spaces.

Generally, better regulated and supported clubs (for example operating within a National Governing Body structure) are more likely to have robust safeguarding arrangements in place than may be the case in smaller, independent groups. However, regardless of the organisational context of activities, no sport activity, in its own right, is inherently safe or good for children. This is entirely dependent on the way the activity is planned and delivered. Individuals and organisations providing opportunities for children and young people must ensure they have implemented appropriate safeguarding arrangements in order to reduce risk, create a positive environment and promote a lifelong interest in sport and activity (DfE, 2018).

There is no regulatory body for sport that governs safeguarding. However, in the UK, as part of the Sports Councils' funding requirements, sports organisations that receive funding are required to comply with sport specific safeguarding standards for their respective nation. For Wales, Northern Ireland and England, the Child Protection in Sport Unit (CPSU) is funded to oversee overall compliance at a governing body level with the standards. Children 1st provide a similar service in Scotland.

Arrangements need to include safe recruitment; processes to respond to suspected abuse within and outside the sports context; clear standards of behaviour (codes of conduct) and linked disciplinary systems; safeguarding training appropriate to individuals' roles; and clear communication with all stakeholders (including children and parents).

The following table provides information about some of the range of sports and physical activity providers, and organisations that support them, across the UK. It describes their key roles and summarises their main contributions to safeguarding children.

Type of Organisation	Key Roles	Safeguarding Responsibility
Home Nation (HN) Sports Councils (Sport England, Sport NI, Sport Scotland, Sport Wales)	Establish and implement HN sport and activity strategies. Oversee the distribution of funding to sports bodies. Principally concerned with supporting sport and increasing participation at community level.	Establishing minimum safeguarding requirements for funded organisations. Directly fund other organisations to support the sector in fulfilling safeguarding responsibilities.
UK Sport	Strategically invests funds into Olympic and Paralympic sport. Focused on elite sport at national and international level.	Establishing minimum safeguarding requirements for funded organisations. Directly fund other organisations to support the sector in fulfilling safeguarding responsibilities.

Type of Organisation	Key Roles	Safeguarding Responsibility
Sports' National Governing Bodies (NGBs) (e.g. The Football Association, GB Taekwondo, The Welsh Rugby Union)	Effectively govern their respective sports. Establish rules, structures, leagues and competitions, and performance pathways. Provide support to clubs, coaches, officials and participants.	The way NGBs operate is varied, and in safeguarding terms this is often linked to whether or not they receive funding: a) NGBs in receipt of funding from HN sports councils or UK Sport (funded NGBs) are required to comply with their respective HN safeguarding standards or framework, and to work towards embedding safeguarding policies and practices at all levels in the organisation. They will have trained safeguarding leads and centralised systems for managing criminal records checks and responding to safeguarding cases. b) Recognised but non-funded NGBs will have met a number of basic requirements set by the HN sports councils, including some around safeguarding. However, they are not required to comply with the respective sports safeguarding standards or frameworks. c) These and other non-funded NGBs do not receive sports council or UK Sport funding and are therefore less likely to have robust (or sometimes any) safeguarding arrangements in place.
Support Partners (e.g. Institutes of Sport, Sport Resolutions, British Athletes Commission, Activity Alliance)	Funded by central funding bodies to provide a wide range of specialist services to support (usually) funded NGBs and/or individual athletes.	Organisations in receipt of funding from HN sports councils or UK Sport are required to comply with their respective HN safeguarding standards or framework, with a particular focus on the safeguarding implications of partnership working.
Active Partnerships (APs)	These exist in England only. They are organisations that work strategically in a locality (often a county area) to support sport and delivery partners to help get the nation active.	These are funded by Sport England and are subject to the same safeguarding requirements as funded sports. APs facilitate access to safeguarding training locally, provide or signpost to safeguarding resources, guidance and advice, often link to local statutory agencies, and provide information about local safeguarding services and contacts. APs commission and fund activity deliverers and are required to set and monitor clear safeguarding standards as part of their contracts with these clubs and organisations.

Continued

Type of Organisation	Key Roles	Safeguarding Responsibility
Unregulated and unaffiliated sports organisations, clubs and deliverers	These may be stand-alone activities, individual providers, businesses or small charities. They will not have a regulating or affiliating body, and may therefore have no source of advice, oversight or support.	Although in principle there should be appropriate safeguarding arrangements in place, often this is not the case. Children and young people engaging in activities in this context can be particularly vulnerable in the absence of appropriate safeguards or processes to respond to concerns that arise.
Venues	These are where sport and other activities takes place and can include school sites, public areas, leisure facilities and specialist clubs or facilities. Venues may be stand-alone businesses, owned and run by Local Authorities or linked trusts, or operated by large, national leisure businesses.	Safeguarding standards and implementation vary greatly. Currently there are no formal safeguarding standards applicable to venues. A particular issue relates to whether and how venues apply safeguarding requirements for third parties using or hiring facilities to provide activities for children. However, some venue operators opt to apply their own (varied) minimum safeguarding requirements to third party facility hirers who provide activities for children.
Clubs, coaches and activity deliverers	This is where and how children and young people typically engage with sport and other activities. These may be regulated or licenced by NGBs with robust safeguarding arrangements and requirements, or stand-alone arrangements outside the jurisdiction of any overseeing body.	Clubs and individuals affiliated to funded NGBs should comply with a wide range of safeguarding requirements and are supported by the NGB in implementing these and responding to concerns. Clubs should have safeguarding officers, clear reporting processes, codes of conduct for a range of stakeholders, and links to disciplinary and safeguarding systems operated by their NGB. Unregulated, unaffiliated activities may have few or none of these arrangements in place and pose the greatest challenge to statutory agencies seeking to address reported safeguarding concerns.
NSPCC Child Protection in Sport Unit (CPSU)	CPSU's mission is to build the capacity of sports to safeguard children and young people in and through sport and to enable sports organisations to lead the way in keeping children safe from harm.	Lead agency in promoting and driving safeguarding in sport across the UK. Established sports safeguarding standards in England, Northern Ireland and Wales, and oversee their implementation. Provide access to sport and physical activity orientated safeguarding guidance, resources and training.

SPORTS SAFEGUARDING ARRANGEMENTS

As in other sectors, any individuals or organisations involved in the provision of sport and physical activity for children and young people are required by legislation and guidance to have safeguarding arrangements in place. These should include systems both to prevent harm to children and to respond to any concerns or incidents that arise. This responsibility exists regardless of the size and structure of the organisation or the nature of the activity. In England, the Working Together to Safeguard Children (2018) statutory guidance specifically references sports clubs and organisations and requires funded sports' National Governing Bodies (NGBs) to comply with the NSPCC (2015) *Standards for Safeguarding and Protecting Children in Sport*. This demonstrates how government and statutory agencies are beginning to understand the size and influence of the sector.

Fig. 22.1 demonstrates the relationship between safeguarding legislation, guidance and sports' policies and procedures.

The UK's Code for Sports Governance was launched in 2017 and includes a requirement for all bodies seeking government and National Lottery funding (typically NGBs) to address safeguarding along with other integrity issues, (e.g., antidoping, match fixing, discrimination and organisational corruption).

In all four Home Nations (HNs) the Sports Councils have supported the development and implementation of sector wide safeguarding standards for sport. These are (Fig. 22.2):

1. UK Sport & Sport England (2017): A Code for Sports Governance
2. NSPCC (2015): Standards for safeguarding and protecting children in sport (England)
3. Irish Sports Council & Sports Council of Northern Ireland (2013): All Ireland safeguarding framework (N Ireland)
4. Sport Scotland (2017): Standards for child wellbeing and protection in sport (Scotland)

The format, design and application of these standards differ slightly across the Home Nations; however, they essentially include the same core safeguarding principles, policies and practices as required by legislation. While they are promoted to, and available for, any sports organisation, they are most rigorously applied to those bodies receiving funding from the respective sports councils.

All four UK sports councils and UK Sport have facilitated and funded the development and provision of sport specific safeguarding support. In England, Wales and Northern Ireland this has principally been through funding to the NSPCC's CPSU and in Scotland through the Children 1st Safeguarding in Sport team. This support includes access to consultation and advice,

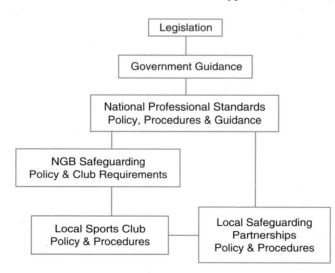

Fig. 22.1 ■ National Framework for Safeguarding & Protecting Children

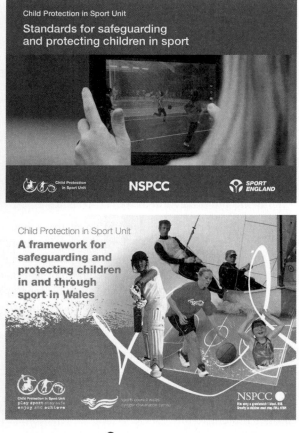

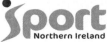

Club framework for safeguarding standards in sport

Fig. 22.2 ■ Sports Councils of Home Nations.

access to sport specific safeguarding training, and the development of safeguarding resources and policy templates for organisations, clubs and individuals. Increasingly, there is funding being provided to a wider range of support organisations to assist the sector with safeguarding, child protection and case management.

One of the most high-profile reviews into abuse in sport has been undertaken by Clive Sheldon QC who looked into the number of non-recent sexual abuse cases in football and produced the independent Sheldon Report into these allegations The Football Association (thefa.com). The publicity around the non-recent abuse in football resulted in a review of sports organisations' arrangements, and a range of government departments and sports met to consider the safeguarding landscape in sport. A range of challenges and concerns were identified. These included sports coaches (unlike teachers) not being included in the Police, Crime and Sentencing Bill (2021), which was to address the abuse of young people ages 16 and 17 years by those in positions of trust (NSPCC, 2021); inconsistency in safeguarding practices when schools deploy sports coaches or link to sports clubs; the additional vulnerability of participants who are young elite, disabled and of Black and minoritized ethnicity; and independent, community sport and activity providers and clubs (a particular issue within parts of the martial arts community). Independent providers often have little motivation or support to effectively address safeguarding in the same way that funded sports bodies do. This can mean that practice standards (supervision ratios, safer recruitment and technical qualifications) can all vary widely. In response to this, the government indicated a willingness to consider extending the duty of care legislation (Police, Crime and Sentencing Bill 2021) to include sports coaches. Sport England supported the introduction of a voluntary Safeguarding Code for Martial Arts (NSPCC, 2015), primarily to encourage unregulated instructors and clubs to meet minimum safeguarding requirements. The following case study demonstrates some of the challenges and concerns highlighted by the review.

SPORT SPECIFIC SAFEGUARDING CONSIDERATIONS

There are a number of characteristics of the sports and activity sector that statutory safeguarding agencies should be aware of when responding to safeguarding or child protection concerns. These will have an

CASE STUDY 22.1: ALLEGATIONS OF ABUSE

Consider identical allegations of abuse being made against two coaches. The first volunteers in a club affiliated to and supported by a funded sports NGB, the other in a small, independent, unaffiliated sports club. Here are some practice implications for statutory agency staff dealing with this case:

	Affiliated to funded NGB	Small independent organisation
Clear safeguarding policy and process for responding to concerns	Yes	Possible but unlikely
Identified, trained club safeguarding/ welfare officer	Yes	Possible but unlikely
NGB safeguarding lead to support and/or manage the case (includes investigation and risk assessment once statutory agency actions are completed)	Yes	No
NGB disciplinary process to facilitate temporary suspension and prevent individual seeking work in another affiliated club	Yes	No
Information sharing protocol to facilitate communication to key individuals	Yes	Possible but unlikely
Recording and information storage processes	Yes	Possible but unlikely
Competent (club or NGB) contact for police, Local Authority Designated Officer (LADO) or social worker to link and liaise with	Yes	Possible but unlikely

Unless a club/organisation has clear safeguarding reporting and an identified, trained safeguarding lead, it is difficult for professionals to be confident about sharing information or discussing concerns with anyone within the club. Without these structures in place, statutory agency staff may be constrained (in light of data protection considerations) about whether or how they can share concerns with anyone involved. The absence of robust disciplinary policies and processes may make it difficult to rely on a club taking appropriate protective action (e.g. suspension). A loose organisational structure presents challenges for a Local Authority Designated Officer (LADO) wishing to establish and ensure an appropriate response to allegations about the coach and raises serious concerns about the club's ability to prioritise children's safety.

---

impact on the sports organisation or club's response to concerns and capacity/ability to work effectively with statutory agencies.

Volunteers. Sport and physical activity, particularly at community level and sports events and competitions where the majority of children and young people engage in it, is predominantly organised and delivered by (mainly adult) volunteers. An estimated 6.2 million (13% of UK's population) volunteer in sport and physical activity in some capacity – many of these in relation to activities for children and young people (Geoff-Nicols et al., 2004). It is agreed across the sector that without the support of volunteers, organised sport in the UK would not be able to happen.

While this should not affect organisations' safeguarding responsibilities, often a fear overstretching volunteers can inhibit requirements placed on them – in terms of their time, roles and responsibilities, and costs. Examples include difficulties implementing requirements to attend regular safeguarding training, or a failure to apply as rigorous an approach to safe recruitment of some volunteers as would be required for paid staff. In addition, the way in which many volunteers become involved with clubs can be a gradual and evolving process, meaning that a parent, for instance, may start simply helping out with some minor practical tasks, but end up with a much wider and substantial role that may include responsibility for children – all without a formal recruitment or suitability checking process ever having been considered or applied. This has proved to be a route used by a number of individuals who were clearly motivated to abuse children (Harthill and Lang, 2018).

Sports ethos and culture. There are many examples of approaches to the delivery of sport at all levels that do not prioritise the welfare or voice of young participants. These may reflect and sustain power relationships (particularly between coaches and athletes) that can be open to abuse; encourage dependence on an individual (coach) for progression in the sport or team membership; promote a 'win at all cost' attitude; discourage self-expression and challenge; and silence or disarm parents. Significant strides have been made to counter these approaches in some sports, for example, Rugby Football League (rugbyleague.com). However, issues are still evident across the sector – leaving many young people vulnerable to poor coaching practice, manipulation, grooming or abuse. For example concerns about the widespread and damaging culture within many parts of gymnastics across the globe resulted in the independent review into the sport in the UK (About the Whyte Review).

Spectators. Spectators, often more specifically parents, have been identified in many sports as presenting a safeguarding challenge. A number of sports have launched campaigns to address the issues (e.g. Parents In Tennis: How To Support Your Child | LTA).

While the involvement of parents and their support (emotional, practical and financial) and encouragement plays a significant part in most children's participation in these activities, many sports also struggle to manage the less positive aspects of some parents' behaviour which can and does have a deleterious effect on their own child and other children, the activity providers and sometimes the club itself. Poor (often aggressive) side-line behaviour, a refusal to leave coaching to the coaches, an over-emphasis on winning at the expense of enjoyment, placing unrealistic (sometime damaging) expectations on their children, and vicariously seeking to achieve in sport through their children are all problems reported by the majority of sports organisations. Many sports have introduced codes of conduct for spectators/parents, and a number have devised more sophisticated rules and arrangements to limit the negative impact of badly behaved spectators, while promoting the positive influence of the majority. One example of this is the Football Association's Respect programme (2018) which provides very clear guidelines on what is expected from spectators.

Hazing Rituals and 'Banter'

Sport in particular often features other harmful forms of behaviour that are still too often accepted by coaches, athletes and parents. Particularly in college and university contexts, these include some team or squad initiation rituals (also called 'hazing') that can include high levels of alcohol, humiliation, sexual assault or physical harm. Hazing often takes place in secret and is sometimes denied by the sports organisers who do not want to acknowledge the impact of these types of behaviours. On the lower end of the spectrum there is an acceptance of 'banter' (from peers and adults) which in other context would often constitute harassment, verbal abuse or bullying.

The primary challenge is to ensure that participants and delivers of activities understand the negative impact of certain behaviours. Organisations codes of conduct and links to safeguarding and disciplinary procedures need to include safeguarding concerns arising from hazing and other harmful behaviours.

The FA Respect Programme aims to ensure clubs create a fun, safe and inclusive environment. It includes practical resources (policy templates, handbook and posters) to create an open safeguarding culture at club level. It offers free training courses and clear codes of conducts to help people understand the expectation around behaviours and clear reporting processes to address any issues that arise (Respect - Get Involved | The Football Association (thefa.com)).

Variety of deliverers and context. Sports and activities are provided and delivered in a wide variety of different ways and contexts, and this can make it difficult for external agencies to clarify and navigate the environment when responding to safeguarding concerns. Clubs, coaches or instructors (terminology also varies across sports) may be affiliated to or licenced by a governing body with sound safeguarding arrangements (e.g. in football or rugby) or be more loosely linked to a less well organised body with few policies or procedures in place, for example a group of parents who offer opportunities for their own and other local young people to go cycling on a regular basis. What starts as an informal arrangement for their own children may develop over time into what might be perceived to be a more formal club – though without any consideration or provision of safeguarding arrangements. Activity deliverers may be sole traders (e.g. a single coach) or larger businesses (e.g. a private gym or climbing wall), and activities may take place in public spaces (municipal pitches or skateparks) or leisure centres, private clubs, schools or purpose-built facilities. Each aspect has implications for the way in which children are safeguarded, how concerns may be reported (internally and to statutory agencies) and the degree to which robust arrangements are available to address poor practice and implement recommendations from safeguarding professionals.

Transitions. As in other aspects of children's lives, transitions in sport represent potential points of vulnerability and require additional consideration. In addition to moving up through different age groups, many young athletes also need support to successfully manage their journey along the talent pathway (i.e. moving from involvement for fun, through more structured competition or league levels, to competing at county, national or international levels). Shifts from engaging in a children/young person's environment to a competitive adult one poses a number of safeguarding challenges. The move from competing or participating alone to undertaking formal roles within the sport (e.g. volunteering, officiating or coaching) also

need care and consideration – particularly in that these young people are effectively moving into positions of trust for others that requires support.

Talented and elite young athletes. Much of the early research into child protection within sport focused on the performance end of the sports pathway. There is considerable evidence to state that talented athletes (particularly those at pre-peak, pre-national squad level) are at significantly higher risk of abuse and poor practice than others. Reasons for this include greater dependence on a coach who may well have helped them achieve success (and may hold the key to further progression); coaches often having significant influence over a wide range of the athlete's life (e.g. diet, lifestyle, training regime, free time); significant travel away with the coach – often without family; operating in a highly competitive, adult-orientated environment; limited contact with wider support networks and friendship groups; and the sacrifices (time or money) the young person and parents have made to reach this position. These factors may increase opportunities for abuse, reduce the support network around a young person and encourage the acceptance, tolerance or recognition of potentially harmful practices and behaviours (e.g. over training, or training whilst injured) (CPSU, 2021).

Disabled young athletes. As in wider society, disabled young sports people are additionally vulnerable to abuse and bullying, and for many of the same reasons. While this is a factor that all sports and activity providers should be aware of and address, it is of particular relevance to those operating at the high-performance level of sport. The safety and well-being of elite disabled athletes should be prioritised because this group may be vulnerable in terms of both their disability and their elite status (Jones et al., 2012; Sullivan and Knutson, 2000; Vertommen, 2016).

Mental health. Growing public awareness of issues relating to poor mental health have helped highlight this within the context of sport. Increasing numbers of athletes are describing the negative impact that aspects of their involvement in sport have had on them. There are clearly some aspects of some sports delivery that may actually trigger mental health problems (e.g. an overemphasis on weight or body shape may lead to disordered eating or body dysmorphia). Sometimes experiences or messages received through sport have exacerbated pre-existing conditions (e.g. depression, anxiety, OCD), and for some young people with existing conditions the issue for sports organisers and deliverers is how to accommodate any additional support required (CPSU, 2020).

Engaging hard to reach groups. Sport and physical activity is increasingly being used as a mechanism and resource to identify, reach and engage with particular groups of children and young people for a range of purposes well beyond simply engaging in the activity. These include addressing knife crime, social isolation and obesity. In almost every instance, these groups have also been correctly identified as being particularly vulnerable in safeguarding terms. This increases the responsibility of activity organisers and deliverers to recognise these additional factors and implement safeguarding arrangements appropriate to the needs of particular groups.

An example of this is the Dame Kelly Holmes Trust Transforming Young Lives programme. The organisation uses sport and physical activity and believes all young people must have an equal opportunity to be the best versions of themselves. They work to equip young people with the positive behaviours and mindset they need to tackle the disadvantages they face due to inequality in their everyday lives. They deliver transformational programmes designed to improve their well-being, help them build healthy relationships and unlock the confidence, self-esteem and resilience needed to achieve in education, work and life.

Another example at a strategic level is Sport England's strategy – Tackling Inactivity and Economic Disadvantage.

Adults involved in multiple sports. Unlike many other employment sectors (including education), sport affords opportunities for individuals to be involved in a number of different activities, in a number of different roles, perhaps in different counties or countries, and on a variety of different sites or venues. This means that when dealing with an adult about whom concerns have been expressed, care must be taken to establish the full extent of the individual's involvement in any sport or activity, and in any capacity. We would recommend that professionals ask very direct questions to determine where they work or volunteer – both as a job and their leisure time. If there are clear indications that the individual is involved in sport, identify

organisations, for example Active Partnerships, that may be able to help identify where the individual may be working. Failure to do so may leave significant numbers of children or young people at risk and mean that those responsible for these children in other sports/contexts are not provided information to help safeguard them.

Take the case of Gemma, for example. Gemma is a level 2 netball coach, having achieved the necessary qualifications through the netball NGB. She coaches two junior teams at Cloystone Netball Club, a local NGB-affiliated club and member of the local league. During school holidays Gemma operates her own junior netball coaching academy with two colleagues (both level 1 qualified). These activities take place on several school sites and at a local leisure centre. She is also a martial artist (a Korean form of karate) – achieving black belt status at the karate club operating out of a privately owned gym where she is also an instructor. Recently the club has been commissioned to provide activities for pupils at a nearby private school.

Were a safeguarding referral to be made about Gemma's behaviour towards a child at Cloystone Netball Club, for example, investigating professionals would need to establish the full range of wider contexts in which she operates or has operated. This includes what children's activities she is/has been involved with, when she undertakes these and where/for whom to ensure any investigation covers all potential victims, and that this wide range of organisations are appropriately informed. A focus solely on children within the netball club would therefore be too limited and could potentially miss a much wider group of vulnerable children.

Sports organisations operating across the UK. Agencies tasked with investigating child protection need to be aware that although many organisations (e.g. Squash Wales, or Swim England) operate within only one of the HN, and therefore need to address only one set of safeguarding legislation, guidance and arrangements, some (e.g. GB Wheelchair Basketball, or the England and Wales Cricket Board) span more than one country or the whole UK. Consequently, these organisations have to navigate a wider range of safeguarding and child protection arrangements. Legislation, statutory structures and even safeguarding terminology vary across the UK, making reporting routes more complicated, creating practical problems for sports officials tasked with referring and managing concerns across these borders. Differences across the UK in eligibility criteria for, and language around, criminal records checks are just one challenge to negotiate when operating across HN borders. The first port of call would be the NGB if the sport is known; alternatively contact the CPSU for support and advice.

Away trips and events. Sport involves young people's involvement in trips and events on a regular basis – often to distant venues (UK and overseas) and often overnight. Events can include inter-club or inter-school competitions, county events, national or international training camps or competitions. The reason in highlighting this as a unique characteristic is to recognise the inbuilt safeguarding risks associated with these activities in terms of travel, overnight stays and levels of supervision. Although sport has come a long way, the sports organisations often look to Ofsted guidance for ratios on supervision that would be adequate in the context of the education sector. Due to the nature of sport activities and events, organisers need to plan for illness (staff and children), injuries and down-time (i.e. non-competition or training time) – along with the specific needs of the young people they may be taking to an event. They also need to factor in the nature of the activity involved, where it is taking place and the suitability of the responsible adults. This involves planning to ensure adequate numbers of suitable supervising adults, and proactively considering and addressing any additional needs or vulnerabilities on the part of the participants.

Poor Practice. Sports organisations frequently separate out the concept of poor practice from abusive practice. Poor practice refers to any behaviours that fail to comply with a club or organisation's stated code of conduct to which the individual should have been required to commit, for example, smoking in front of children or using physical exercise as a punishment. Clearly behaviours that constitute abuse are also poor practice, but these would be referred and responded to by appropriate statutory agencies who should advise the organisation of appropriate steps to take. Many sports bodies state that the majority of safeguarding concerns reported to them relate to incidents of poor practice (below the threshold for statutory involvement), and most have in place safeguarding and disciplinary processes to manage cases of poor practice. While many cases never reach the threshold for referral to statutory agencies, poor practice spans behaviours that are clearly harmful or potentially harmful to children and may be the seedbeds or grooming processes that facilitate the commission of much more seriously abusive behaviours.

POSITIVE CONTRIBUTIONS TO SAFEGUARDING

Notwithstanding these additional characteristics, the sport and physical activity sector can also make a significant positive contribution to safeguarding young participants. The implementation of safeguarding policies and practices at all levels in many organisations means that many thousands of adults have received sports-orientated safeguarding training to help recognise and respond to concerns about young people. Arrangements to prevent abuse (e.g. safer recruitment, codes of conduct, disciplinary processes, etc.) have no doubt contributed to the creation of much safer environments across swathes of the sports landscape. Indeed many NGBs report a marked increase not only in the numbers of concerns being identified within their activities, but also in the numbers of concerns arising in children's homes or the wider community that are being identified within sport and passed on to statutory agencies for action.

CPSU's experience of working with and supporting a range of sports bodies, together with advising LADO's, police officers and other professionals, has identified a number of key points that are useful when statutory agencies are responding to concerns involving sport and physical activity. These are summarised in the Sports Safeguarding Checklist box.

Sports Safeguarding Case Checklist for Professionals

In addition to information that will be sought as a matter of standard good practice when dealing with safeguarding concerns, professionals involved in sport-linked cases should consider:

■ It is worthwhile establishing whether any person of concern has (or has had) any involvement or role in any junior sports or similar activities. Many individuals would consider their involvement in sport as merely a pastime or hobby rather than their main employment, and so would not necessarily volunteer this information without being asked the question directly.

If so:

- What is/are the role/s of the person of concern within that club/organisation (particularly related to contact with or responsibility for a particular child or other children and young people)?
- What is their sports role and relationship to any child/children allegedly harmed or at risk?
- Are the individuals (and/or the club/organisation) affiliated, registered with, licenced by or otherwise linked to a wider umbrella body (e.g. an NGB)?
- If so, does this body have in place robust safeguarding arrangements (e.g. code of conduct for coaches, participants and clubs) and a trained safeguarding Lead Officer with responsibility for responding to or managing safeguarding concerns? Has the individual been subject to a safer recruitment process including criminal records checks (where eligible), references etc? This body may hold relevant current and non-recent information about the individual and may operate the mechanism for suspending the individual (temporarily or permanently) from involvement with children during or after any investigation.
- If this is a stand-alone club or deliverer, are there any safeguarding arrangements in place (including a safeguarding or welfare lead, a clear safeguarding process, and systems for managing concerns appropriately and confidentially)?
- Is the person of concern linked to or operating within any other sports activities (e.g. in another sport or activity altogether) or in any other contexts (e.g. coaching within a school, providing holiday activities on behalf of a local council, offering individual coaching on a private basis)?
- Is it clear where any activities undertaken by this person take place (e.g. sports clubs, leisure centres, schools), and does this have potential safeguarding implications?
- Has consideration been given to sharing information about the concerns under investigation with the full range of other relevant sports-based organisations?
- Which bodies require information about the investigation process or outcome in order to inform their disciplinary or safeguarding process and take steps to safeguard children or young people in their care?

The positive links between physical activity and physical and mental well-being are increasingly being recognised and used by other sectors (e.g. Health), and access to activities for these purposes (rather than purely for sports sake) are being actively promoted. Additionally the profile of sport is also being used to engage with harder to reach groups (e.g. youths involved in gangs, knife crime or county lines activities) in order to achieve wider social change and benefits. There is increased collaboration between statutory agencies (in England, particularly LADOs) and sports organisations when safeguarding concerns arise about children or those in positions of trust.

CONCLUSION

The sports sector comprises significant numbers of individuals, and clubs and organisations of very different sizes and types. This means that there is no single model for the way in which safeguarding is prioritised or implemented. There are significant differences in the robustness of arrangements, for example within clubs supported by funded NGBs and those operating independently, so it is essential that safeguarding professionals are aware of the particular challenges and issues to consider (described in this chapter) when involved with concerns linked to sport. Large sections of the sector have made positive strides in safeguarding practice, but there are still significant gaps and shortfalls, even within well-regulated sports, as several recent high-profile cases demonstrate.

Despite these challenges, sound policies and safeguarding training rolled out across the sector have resulted in significant numbers of referrals of concerns identified by sports people that arise both within and importantly outside the sports context. The sector offers opportunities for safeguarding agencies to communicate and engage with huge numbers of children, young people and their parents. There are a range of organisations operating at different levels within the sector that support the development and implementation of safeguarding at activity delivery level and can often provide advice, support or information to professionals dealing with cases.

SOURCES OF INFORMATION AND SUPPORT FOR STATUTORY AGENCIES

Club/Group/Organisation Website

- Club safeguarding policies and procedures, codes of conduct etc
- Any club affiliation to wider body (e.g. NGB)
- Coaches operating within the club
- Welfare or safeguarding leads or officers
- Contact information, including to welfare or safeguarding officers
- Process for reporting safeguarding concerns

NGB or Other Affiliating Body Website

- Overarching safeguarding policies, procedures and guidance (including what is mandatory for affiliating clubs/coaches)
- Details of reporting procedures, including contact details for the wider organisation's safeguarding lead
- Safer recruitment, qualification, safeguarding and disciplinary records for individual coaches

  (See https://thecpsu.org.uk/help-advice/deal-with-a-concern#contact-your-national-governing-body)

Active Partnerships (Aps) (England)

- Information about local sports network and structure, including many local sport and activity providers
- Sources of support (e.g. training and guidance) available to local clubs, organisations and coaches
- Access or signposting to sports safeguarding resources

  (See https://thecpsu.org.uk/help-advice/deal-with-a-concern#contact-your-active-partnership)

Child Protection in Sport Unit (England, N Ireland and Wales)

- Contact details of most NGB and AP safeguarding lead officers
- Information about the safeguarding context for sport and physical activity, and for all funded NGBs
- Enquiry service to answer general safeguarding queries and to answer questions about arrangements within specific sports
- Website providing sport specific guidance, resources and advice that is freely available to all organisations and individuals

  (See www.thecpsu.org.uk or cpsu@nspcc.org.uk)

Ann Craft Trust

- Sport specific templates and resources relating to safeguarding adults in sport
- Access to advice about sports-linked adult safeguarding cases

  (See http://www.anncrafttrust.org/safeguarding-adults-sport-activity/)

Children 1st Safeguarding in Sport Team (Scotland)

- Contact details of most Scottish NGB safeguarding lead officers
- Information about the safeguarding context for sport and physical activity in Scotland, and for all Sports Scotland funded NGBs
- Enquiry service to answer general safeguarding queries and to answer questions about arrangements within specific Scottish sports
- Website providing sport specific guidance, resources and advice that is freely available to all Scottish organisations and individuals

REFERENCES

About the Whyte Review. https://www.sportengland.org/guidance-and-support/safeguarding/whyte-review.

BBC, 2018. Larry Nassar Abuse Report: USOC Apologises for Failing to Protect Athletes. https://www.bbc.co.uk/sport/gymnastics/46519353.

British Cycling, 2017. Independent Review into the Climate and Culture of the World Class Programme (WCP) at British Cycling. British Cycling, Manchester. https://www.britishcycling.org.uk/about/article/20170614-about-bc-news-British-Cycling-publishes-the-cycling-independent-review-0.

CPSU, 2020. Mental Health and Wellbeing in Sport. CPSU, London. https://thecpsu.org.uk/help-advice/topics/mental-health-and-wellbeing/.

CPSU, 2021. Resource Library for Safeguarding Children in Sport. CPSU, London. thecpsu.org.uk.

Department of Education (DfE), 2018. Working Together to Safeguard Children. Department of Education, London. https://www.gov.uk/government/publications/working-together-to-safeguard-children--2.

Football Association, 2018. Respect Programme. https://www.teamgrassroots.co.uk/the-fa-respect-programme-2018/.

Geoff Nichols, P., Taylor, M., James, R., Garrett, K., Holmes, L., King, C., et al., 2004. Voluntary activity in UK sport. Voluntary Action 6 (2).

Harthill, M., Lang, M., 2018. Official report of child protection and safeguarding concerns in sport and leisure settings: An analysis of English local authority data. Leisure Studies 37. https://doi.org/10.1080/02614367.2018.1497076.

Irish Sports Council & Sports Council of Northern Ireland, 2013. All Ireland Safeguarding Framework (N Ireland). http://www.sportni.net/wp-content/uploads/2013/03/2-2014ClubFrameworkForSafeguardingStandardsInSport.doc.

Jones, L., Bellis, M.A., Wood, S., Hughes, K., McCoy, E., Eckley, L., et al., 2012. Prevalence and risk of violence against children with disabilities: A systematic review and meta-analysis of observational studies. Lancet (London, England) 380 (9845), 899–907.

NPCC, 2018. https://www.npcc.police.uk/our-work/work-of-npcc-committees/Crime-Operations-coordination-committee/hydrant-programme/.

NSPCC, 2015. Standards for Safeguarding and Protecting Children in Sport (England). NSPCC Child Protection in Sport Unit, London. https://thecpsu.org.uk/resource-library/tools/standards-for-safeguarding-and-protecting-children-in-sport/.

NSPCC, 2021. Government to Close Loophole Allowing Sports Coaches and Faith Leaders to Have Sex with 16 and 17-Year-Olds in Their Care, NSPCC. London. https://www.nspcc.org.uk/about-us/news-opinion/2021/close-the-loophole-positions-of-trust-law/.

Sport Scotland, 2017. Standards for Child Wellbeing and Protection in Sport (Scotland). Children 1st, Edinburgh. https://sportscotland.org.uk/safeguarding-in-sport/child-wellbeing-and-protection/standards-for-child-wellbeing-and-protection-in-sport/.

Sport England, 2018. Safeguarding Code for Martial Arts. https://www.safeguardingcode.com/.

Sullivan, P.M., Knutson, J.F., 2000. Maltreatment and disabilities: A population-based epidemiological study. Child Abuse & Neglect 24 (10), 1257–1273.

Tackling Inactivity and Economic Disadvantage | Sport England. https://www.sportengland.org/research-and-data/research/lower-socio-economic-groups#:~:text=Tackling%20Inactivity%20and%20Economic%20Disadvantage,people%20in%20different%20community%20settings.

Vertommen, T., Schipper-van Veldhoven, N., Wouters, K., Kampen, J.K., Brackenridge, C.H., Rhind, et al., 2016. Interpersonal violence against children in sport in the Netherlands and Belgium. Child Abuse & Neglect 51, 223–236.

UK Sport & Sport England, 2017. A Code for Sports Governance. https://www.sportengland.org/funds-and-campaigns/code-sports-governance#:~:text=The%20Code%20for%20Sports%20Governance,us%20and%2For%20UK%20Sport.

Uniting the Movement. Sport England. https://www.sportengland.org/about-us/uniting-movement.

23

EDITORS' FINAL THOUGHTS: CHILD PROTECTION BEYOND THE PANDEMIC

RACHAEL CLAWSON ■ LISA WARWICK ■ RACHEL FYSON

This fourth edition of the *Child Protection Handbook* was planned, and writing began, before the COVID-19 pandemic took hold across the world in 2020 and 2021. None of us could have foreseen the far-reaching changes to child protection practice that lay ahead, nor predicted how long those changes would last. During the early months of the pandemic, when the consequences of illness and death from contracting coronavirus were very real, fear permeated society – including those people tasked with safeguarding children. Following the UK Government announcement of a national 'lockdown' on 23rd March 2020 – when schools and non-essential businesses were closed and people were forbidden from mixing with others outside of their own household – the ways in which social workers and others engaged with children and families and with each other changed overnight. Key practitioners working across the public sector were suddenly faced with adapting their practice to comply with lockdown legislation and guidance. Interpersonal communication and relationship-based practice were tested to the limit, and any initial beliefs that changes would be temporary are now long gone. It is clear that child protection practice is now in a transitional phase. Many of the new ways of organising and delivering practice which emerged as a response to the pandemic are here to stay: child protection services, along with many other aspects of society, now operate in a 'new normal'. It is crucial, therefore, to pause for a moment, to reflect on what we have learned from the pandemic and to consider how we want to shape the child protection practices of the future.

WHAT HAPPENED TO CHILD PROTECTION PRACTICE DURING THE PANDEMIC, AND WHAT CAN BE LEARNED FROM THIS?

As members of the 'helping professions' social workers and other safeguarding practitioners needed to swiftly adapt to the challenges presented by being in 'lockdown', a world of social distancing and, for many, both isolation and/or fear of social contact. The most immediate and arguably most significant change was the transition to online working across many areas of practice. Online activity permeated areas of practice where virtual working would previously have been considered impossible, unwelcome or both. Direct work with children, assessments and other activities mostly took place online, with only the highest risk cases being managed face to face. Practitioners had to improvise in creative ways to talk with children, families, carers colleagues and other professionals. However, these changes were also accompanied by a steep learning curve for many. Some practitioners and families were using virtual technology for the first time even as 'home' visits, court hearings and other sites of important decision-making took place using virtual platform; and even in situations where face-to-face visits were necessary and permitted, face masks impeded communication.

There was no universal experience of the impact of COVID-19. However, in the early months of lockdown, social workers talked about experiencing fear both for their own safety and for the safety of children they were seeking to protect. They also highlighted the emotional impact of the changes imposed upon them as support and therapeutic services provided to children and families either stopped or moved online (Ferguson et al., 2022). Many reported feelings of moral distress arising from bearing witness to the increasing stress and social need of families but being unable to undertake assessments or provide effective support. Practitioners also described how the pandemic had a significant impact their own mental health, largely as a result of the ways in which services were being managed (Barlow et al., 2020). Countless practitioners were working at home without a dedicated working space. Those living with their families or in shared accommodation reported often working from their bedrooms and feeling isolated and unsupported as opportunities for discussions with colleagues dwindled. Those living by themselves reported similar feelings of isolated from colleagues, but also had to manage the personal impacts of lack of human contact over an extended period of time. The erosion of the 'social' aspects of social work impacted upon staff retention. During the pandemic 5000 child and family social workers left their posts (a 16% increase from the previous year) and more than a third (39%) felt more negative about their work than the year before (House of Commons Library, 2021).

The practical challenges of online working had differential impacts on individuals and communities. Both some practitioners and many families were marginalised by the reliance on remote working practices which required a reliable broadband connection. Those without adequate hardware and software to run programmes such as Zoom or Microsoft Teams had to rely on less formal communication tools such as WhatsApp or FaceTime. Those without home Wi-Fi relied on mobile phones, which often entailed paying for expensive data packages. Even when the practicalities and financial costs of online working were overcome, they could still create difficulties for communication, including the inability of social workers to control (or even know) who else was in the room when an online meeting took place. Concerns were also raised about the possibility of re-traumatising vulnerable children and families through the impact of talking about traumatic experiences on a video call (Cook and Zschomler, 2020).

This edition of the *Child Protection Handbook* has repeatedly illustrated the complexities of protecting children from abuse and neglect. The British Association of Social Workers' Annual Survey (BASW, 2021) found that the COVID-19 pandemic had further increased the complexity of child protection work due to the interplay of numerous factors including not only social distancing, mask wearing and increased working from home, but also the wider impacts of the pandemic on the well-being of children and families. Research undertaken during the pandemic revealed practitioners' concerns with the negative impact of being unable to visit children at home – not being able to see, hear or smell the living environment and not being able to observe body language. These changes materially affected the way practitioners were able to assess a child's situation and any risk of abuse which the child may have been experiencing (Cook and Zschomler, 2020). At the same time, many practitioners reported increased caseloads and greater difficulties in getting to see children and families. Perhaps unsurprisingly, many also reported that their own mental health had been affected by new ways of practicing and the anxiety induced by being required to make decisions without full information (BASW, 2022). There were very real concerns about those children and families who either chose or were unable to engage with online ways of working. In August 2021, Anne Longfield (Children's Commissioner for England 2015–21) wrote about a children's care system that was 'broken', with children and families left to 'fend for themselves' and children at greatest risk being 'out of sight' during the pandemic (Longfield, 2021). As the UK gradually emerge from the repeated lockdowns, Longfield's fears were proven to be tragically well-founded: Arthur Labinjo-Hughes and Star Hobson were killed during lockdown by people who should have been caring for them. Media reports on both cases placed considerable emphasis on the perceived failings of child protection practitioners. Death is the most extreme outcome of child abuse and neglect, and many other children will have suffered during the pandemic without their stories coming to the attention of the public. At the time of writing there is limited data available to help us understand the prevalence of child abuse during the pandemic, but the indications are that some forms of abuse increased (NSPCC, 2022).

Despite the many adverse consequences of the pandemic in relation to child protection, there were also some constructive changes to working practice that need to be acknowledged. Not all of the pandemic-induced changes to child protection were viewed negatively by practitioners. Many positives emerged which may help inform more innovative ways of working in the future. For example, social workers reported that their work during periods of lockdown was supported by a rekindling of social work values and an easing of the bureaucratic burdens which had previously stifled creativity within practice (Ferguson et al., 2022). The pandemic also provided practitioners with time to reflect on their new ways of working. Holding inter-professional and multiagency meetings online often meant that more people, from a wider range of services, could attend, with the result that a more holistic perspective could be gained. As the use of virtual meetings increased, the time saved on travel freed up more time for direct work with children and families. Practitioners were more in control of managing their time and could do so more effectively. Professionals were able to build relationships by being in contact with families 'little and often'; they could be more responsive in a timely way with families using text, WhatsApp, and so on as a means of staying in touch. Children and young people responded well to more frequent, less formal styles of communication with child protection professionals, and also to 'walking visits' in open spaces which often enabled them to talk more freely than they would have in a more formal setting (Cook & Zschomler, 2020; Ferguson et al., 2022; Kingstone and Dikomitris, 2021).

LOOKING BEYOND THE PANDEMIC

The COVID-19 pandemic and national lockdown forced practitioners to work differently, often more creatively, and supercharged use of diverse communication technologies. It also, in some teams, afforded time for reflection. The challenge now, as the world returns to a greater semblance of 'normality', is to harness the positive aspects of pandemic practice and consider how best to embed these going forward. We do not yet know what the long-term impact of the pandemic will be on child protection, but we are in a transitional phase. Many child protection practitioners have yet to

return to working in their offices full time; most either continue to work from home or have adopted a hybrid model with some home working coupled with limited days in the office. The long-term implications – for both child outcomes and staff well-being – of social workers spending less time in team offices which enable the naturally-occurring micro-discussion, micro-reflection and micro-support are yet to be fully understood. However, as social work educators we are already aware of the significant impact on social work students of remote or hybrid working practices which have reduced opportunities for some important types of learning. The implications of changing practices need to consider not only outcomes for children and well-being of the existing workforce, but also how the next generation of practitioners can be supported to qualify and be nurtured through their early years in practice.

To conclude, we have identified a number of issues which we regard as key challenges for child protection:

1. How can services designed to work with individual children and families adjust their practices to better address needs arising from the impacts of poverty and social inequality, made ever more acute by the cost-of-living crisis?
2. How can the benefits of technological change be harnessed without leaving behind or losing sight of those members of society who are 'digitally excluded' through poverty, disability or lack of education? How can the workforce be upskilled to work more effectively with a generation of children who have grown up using digital technologies?
3. How can early help services, including playgroups, children's centres and youth clubs, be expanded so that preventative outreach reduces the prevalence of abuse and neglect, meaning fewer children are in need of higher-level child protection interventions?
4. How does the qualifying training and continuing professional development of child protection practitioners – including but not limited to social workers – need to change to better address the realities of post-pandemic working practices?
5. What can be done to attract more people to work in child protection and to retain experienced

staff? Improved pay may be part of the solution, but this needs to be coupled with serious consideration of how better to support the well-being of frontline staff who are making difficult, often life-changing, decisions on a daily basis.

This edition of *The Child Protection Handbook* is underpinned by a call for a more humane and compassionate approach to children and families, which respects their inherent worth as human beings. Notwithstanding the challenges outlined earlier, we have an opportunity now to re-set the foundations of child protection practice by creating services which respect human rights, uphold principles of social justice, and allow professionals to work with integrity and to practice ethically.

REFERENCES

Barlow, J., Bach-Mortenson, A., Homonchuk, O., Woodman, J., 2020. The Impact of the COVID-19 Pandemic on Services From Pregnancy Through Age 5 Years for Families Who Are High Risk Of Poor Outcomes or Who Have Complex Social Needs: Final Report. NIHR/UCL, London. https://www.ucl.ac.uk/children-policy-research/projects/impact-covid-19-pandemic-services-pregnancy-through-age-5-years.

BASW, 2021. The BASW Annual Survey of Social Workers and Social Work: 2021. BASW, London. https://www.basw.co.uk/resources/basw-annual-survey-social-workers-and-social-work-2021.

BASW. 2022. The BASW Annual Survey of Social Workers and Social Work: 2021 – A summary report. Birmingham: BASW.

Cook, L., Zschomler, D., 2020. Virtual home visits during the COVID-19 pandemic: Social workers' perspectives. Practice 32 (5), 401–408.

Ferguson, H., Kelly, L., Pink, S., 2022. Social work and child protection for a post-pandemic world: The re-making of practice during COVID-19 and its renewal beyond it. J. Soc. Work Pract. 36 (1), 5–24.

House of Commons Library, 2021. Research Briefing: Impact of the COVID-19 Pandemic on Social Work. https://commonslibrary.parliament.uk/research-briefings/cdp-2022-0059/.

Kingstone & Dikomitis, 2021. The pandemic transformed how social work was delivered – and these changes could be here to stay. The Conversation. https://theconversation.com/the-pandemic-transformed-how-social-work-was-delivered-and-these-changes-could-be-here-to-stay-165993.

Longfield, A., 2021. No government hoping to level up can ignore the social care crisis harming England's children. The Guardian. 11 August 2021. https://www.theguardian.com/commentisfree/2021/aug/11/government-level-up-ignore-crisis-england-children-social-care.

NSPCC, 2022. Statistics Briefing: The Impact of Coronavirus. NSPCC, London. https://learning.nspcc.org.uk/media/2747/statistics-briefing-impact-of-coronavirus.pdf.

INDEX